DOSAGE CALCULATIONS

Second Canadian Edition

DOSAGE CALCULATIONS

Second Canadian Edition

Gloria D. Pickar
President and Chief Academic Officer,
Compass Knowledge Group
Orlando, Florida
Former Academic Dean
Seminole Community College
Sanford, Florida

Beth Swart
Ryerson University

Hope Graham
St. Francis Xavier University

Margaret Swedish
Grant MacEwan College

NELSON EDUCATION

NELSON EDUCATION

Dosage Calculations, Second Canadian Edition
by Gloria D. Pickar, Beth Swart, Hope Graham, and Margaret Swedish

Vice President, Editorial Director:
Evelyn Veitch

Editor-in-Chief, Higher Education:
Anne Williams

Publisher:
Paul Fam

Executive Editor:
Jackie Wood

Senior Marketing Manager:
Alexis Hood

Senior Developmental Editor:
Mark Grzeskowiak

Permissions Coordinator:
Lynn McLeod

Content Production Manager:
Claire Horsnell

Production Service:
Integra Software Services

Copy Editor:
Wendy Yano

Technical Checker
Heather LeBlanc

Proofreader:
Integra Software Services

Indexer:
Integra Software Services

Senior Manufacturing Coordinator:
Joanne McNeil

Design Director:
Ken Phipps

Managing Designer:
Franca Amore

Interior Design:
Peter Papayanakis

Cover Design:
Peter Papayanakis

Cover Image:
PhotoAlto/Alamy Images

Compositor:
Integra Software Services

Printer:
RR Donnelley

Adapted from *Dosage Calculations*, Seventh Edition, by Gloria D. Pickar, published by Delmar, a part of Cengage Learning. Copyright ©2004 by Delmar.

Printed and bound in the United States of America
4 5 6 7 15 14 13 12

For more information contact Nelson Education Ltd., 1120 Birchmount Road, Toronto, Ontario, M1K 5G4. Or you can visit our Internet site at http://www.nelson.com

Notice to the Reader

Publisher does not warrant or guarantee any of the products described herein or perform any independent analysis in connection with any of the product information contained herein. Publisher does not assume, and expressly disclaims, any obligation to obtain and include information other than that provided to it by the manufacturer.

The reader is expressly warned to consider and adopt all safety precautions that might be indicated by the activities described herein and to avoid all potential hazards. By following the instructions contained herein, the reader willingly assumes all risks in connection with such instructions.

The publisher makes no representations or warranties of any kind, including but not limited to, the warranties of fitness for particular purpose or merchantability, nor are any such representations implied with respect to the material set forth herein, and the publisher takes no responsibility with respect to such material. The publisher shall not be liable for any special, consequential, or exemplary damages resulting, in whole or in part, from the reader's use of, or reliance upon, this material.

The drug labels that were included in this textbook were chosen for the purposes of instruction only, and thus may not necessarily represent the most current labels found in practice. Nurses and other healthcare professionals must always read labels to identify precise dosage amounts when calculating and administering medication.

Library and Archives Canada Cataloguing in Publication Data

Dosage calculations / Gloria D. Pickar... [et al.]—2nd Canadian ed.

Includes index.
ISBN 978-0-17-650259-1

1. Pharmaceutical arithmetic—Textbooks. I. Pickar, Gloria D., 1946–

RS57.D669 2011 615'.1401513
C2010-907882-9

ISBN-13: 978-0-17-650259-1
ISBN-10: 0-17-650259-9

Contents

PREFACE

Introduction

Dosage Calculations, Second Canadian Edition, offers a clear and concise method of calculating drug dosages. The text is directed to the student or professional who feels uncomfortable with mathematics. The previous Canadian and seven U.S. editions have been classroom tested and reviewed by well over 600 000 faculty and students, who report that it helped them allay math anxiety and promoted confidence in their ability to perform accurate calculations. As one reviewer noted, "I have looked at others [texts] and I don't feel they can compare."

The only math prerequisite is the ability to do basic arithmetic. For those who need a review, Chapters 1 and 2 offer an overview of basic arithmetic calculations with extensive exercises for practice. The student is encouraged to use a three-step method for calculating dosages:

1. convert measurements to the same system and same size units;
2. consider what dosage is reasonable; and
3. calculate

Based on feedback from Canadian reviewers, the authors of the Second Canadian Edition of *Dosage Calculations* have transcended provincial practices to come to consensus with regard to nationwide practices. This revision was designed with the beginning Canadian healthcare professional in mind. The International System (SI) of units is used almost exclusively. The medication dosages and drug labels have been vetted with the current Canadian drug database so that beginning professionals will be able to recognize names and dosages. (In the event copyright for a Canadian label was not available at time of printing, retention of the US label may occur in a few instances.) The importance of avoiding medication errors is highlighted by the incorporation of applied critical thinking skills based on patient care situations.

Organization of Content

The text is organized in a natural progression of basic to more complex information. Learners gain self-confidence as they master content in small increments with ample review and reinforcement. Many learners claim that while using this text, for the very first time they did not fear math.

The Table of Contents of the Second Canadian Edition has been revised by the authors to provide users with a more streamlined organization of the content. The fourteen chapters are divided into four sections.

Section 1 includes a mathematics diagnostic evaluation and a mathematics review in Chapters 1 and 2. The *mathematics diagnostic evaluation* allows learners to determine their computational strengths and weaknesses. *Chapters 1* to *3* provide a review of basic arithmetic procedures and systems of measurement. *Chapter 4* provides an overview of the three major calculation methods. This review is accompanied by numerous examples and practice problems to ensure that students can apply the procedures. This section introduces conversion from one unit of measurement to another. The SI system of measurement is stressed because of its use exclusively in Canada's health sector. However, to challenge students and prepare them for real life, a small number of questions require the student to convert Imperial values to metric. Even though metric is used in Canada, many individuals still give their weight in pounds and height in feet and inches, which require conversion to metric. Questions using Imperial values also emphasize attention to detail. The use of the apothecary and household system is de-emphasized with additional information in the Appendices. The ratio-proportion method of performing conversions is also included. International or 24-hour time and Fahrenheit and Celsius temperature conversions are presented in Section 1 also.

Section 2 includes Chapters 5 to 7. This section provides a foundation of information essential for measuring drug dosages and understanding drug orders and labels.

In *Chapter 5,* users learn to recognize and select appropriate equipment for the administration of medications based on the drug, dosage, and the method of administration. Emphasis is placed on interpreting syringe calibrations to ensure that the dosage to be administered is accurate. All photos and drawings have been enhanced for improved clarity.

Chapter 6 presents the common abbreviations used in healthcare so that learners can become proficient in interpreting medical orders. Generic medication administration records have been used, as appropriate, for examples. Additionally, the content on computerized medication administration records has been updated.

It is essential that learners are able to read medication labels to calculate dosages accurately. This ability is developed by having students interpret the medication labels provided beginning in *Chapter 7*. These labels represent current commonly prescribed medications and are presented in full colour and actual size (except in a few instances where the label is enlarged to improve readability).

In *Section 3*, the user learns and practices the skill of dosage calculations applied to patients across the life span. *Chapters 8* and *9* guide the learner to apply all the skills mastered to achieve accurate oral and injectable drug dosage calculations. Users learn to think through the problem logically for the right answer and then to apply a simple formula to double-check their thinking. When this logical but unique system is applied every time to every problem, experience has shown that decreased math anxiety and increased accuracy result.

Insulin content (types, species, and manufacturers) are expanded and updated to include the rapid-acting (lispro, aspart) and the extended long-acting insulins (glargine and detemer). An expanded discussion of premixed insulin combinations is included as well as the use of pens or pumps to deliver insulin.

Chapter 10 introduces the concepts of solutions. Users learn the calculations associated with diluting solutions and reconstitution of injectable drugs. This chapter provides a segue to intravenous calculations by fully describing the preparation of solutions. With the expanding role of the nurse and other healthcare workers in the home setting, clinical calculations for home care, such as nutritional feedings, are also emphasized.

Chapter 11 covers the calculation of pediatric and adult dosages and concentrates on the body weight method. Emphasis is placed on verifying safe dosages and applying concepts across the life span.

Advanced clinical calculations applicable to both adults and children are presented in *Section 4*. Intravenous administration calculations are presented in *Chapters 12* through *14*. Coverage reflects the greater application of IVs in drug therapy. Shortcut calculation methods are presented and explained fully. More electronic infusion devices are included. Saline locks, types of IV solutions, IV monitoring, IV administration records, and IV push drugs are presented in *Chapter 12*. Pediatric IV calculations are presented in *Chapter 13* while obstetric, heparin, and critical care IV calculations are covered in *Chapter 14*. Ample problems help students master the necessary calculations.

Each chapter begins with Learning Objectives that reflect clear expectations that help the student focus on what is expected to achieve the learning objectives. The learning can readily be transferred from the classroom environment to the workplace environment. Procedures in the text are introduced using several examples. Key concepts are summarized and highlighted in quick review boxes before each set of review problems to give learners an opportunity to review major concepts prior to working through the problems. Rationale for Practice boxes identify the "why" a specific strategy will help to solve a problem. Math tips provide memory joggers to assist learners in accurately solving problems. Learning is reinforced by practice problems that conclude each chapter. The importance of calculation accuracy and patient safety are emphasized by patient scenarios that apply critical thinking skills. Critical thinking skill scenarios have also been added to chapter practice problems and comprehensive exams to further emphasize accuracy and safety.

Information to be memorized is identified in Remember boxes, and Caution boxes alert learners to critical procedures.

Section Self-Evaluations found at the end of each section provide learners with an opportunity to test their mastery of chapter objectives prior to proceeding to the next section. Two *posttests* at the conclusion of the text serve to evaluate the learner's overall skill in dosage calculations. The first posttest covers essential skills commonly tested by employers, and the second serves as a comprehensive examination. Both are presented in a case study format to simulate actual clinical calculations.

An *answer key* at the back of the text provides all answers and selected solutions to problems in the Review Sets, Practice Problems, Section Self-Evaluations, and posttests.

Note about the Text

Throughout this book, the authors have chosen to refer to the recipient of nursing care as "patient" rather than "client." Since nurses function as members of interdisciplinary healthcare teams and the term *patient* is commonly used by other healthcare providers, using a common language fosters better communication, understanding, and collegiality. In addition, the American Nurses Association (1996) Nursing's Social Policy Statement notes that although the term *client* is preferred by some nurses, it implies that the recipient of care is able to choose one nurse from among many, a choice that typically does not occur. The authors recognize that the terms *client*, *person*, or *individual* may be the better choice in some circumstances and encourage the reader to make that distinction if needed.

The authors have used the Drug Product Database, Health Canada (http://www.hc-sc.gc.ca/dhp-mps/prodpharma/databasdon/index-eng.php) for the recommended dosages in this text. There may be some discrepancies between Health Canada and the

Compendium of Pharmaceuticals and Specialties (CPS) in dosage range requirements for drugs used as examples in the text. The purpose of this calculations text is for practising calculations. The authors have endeavoured to be as accurate as possible; however, it is the responsibility of the individual administering the drug to make sure that the dosage administered is safe.

Features of the Second Canadian Edition

- Canadian labels have been added throughout the book to reflect current drugs on the market.
- Generic drug names are included, although labels may reflect both generic and brand/trade names.
- Current safety recommendations of the Institute for Safe Medication Practices are reflected; for example, *units* instead of *U; daily* instead of *q.d.*
- Questions have been reviewed and updated throughout to reflect current drugs and protocols.
- Content is divided into four main sections to help learners better organize their studies.
- More than 2050 problems are included for learners to practice their skills and reinforce their learning; problems reflect current drugs and protocols.
- Critical thinking skills are applied to real-life patient care situations to emphasize the importance of accurate dosage calculations and the avoidance of medication errors.
- Full colour is used to make the text user friendly. Chapter elements such as Rules, Rationale for Practice, Math Tips, Cautions, Remember boxes, Quick Reviews, and Examples are colour-coded for easy recognition and use. Colour also highlights review sets and practice problems.
- All syringes and measuring devices are drawn to full size to provide accurate scale renderings to help learners master the measurement and reading of dosages.
- An amber colour has been added to selected syringe drawings throughout the text to *simulate a specific amount of medication,* as indicated in the example or problem. Because the colour used may not correspond to the actual colour of the medications named, *it must not be used as a reference for identifying medications.*
- Photos and drug labels are presented in full colour; colour is used to highlight and enhance the visual presentation of content to improve readability. Special attention is given to visual clarity with labels enlarged to ensure legibility.
- The math review has been expanded to bring learners up to the required level of basic math competence.
- Measurable objectives at the beginning of each chapter emphasize the content to be learned.
- SI units are used (household system of measurement is de-emphasized but are still included).
- RULE boxes draw the learner's attention to pertinent instructions. RATIONALE FOR PRACTICE boxes provide the reasoning for a specific action or decision when calculating drug dosages.
- REMEMBER boxes highlight information to be memorized.
- QUICK REVIEW boxes summarize critical information throughout the chapters before Review Sets are solved.
- CAUTION boxes alert learners to critical information.
- MATH TIPS serve to point out math shortcuts and reminders.
- Content is presented from simple to complex concepts in small increments followed by Review Sets and chapter Practice Problems for better understanding and to reinforce learning.
- Many problems involving the interpretation of syringe scales are included to ensure that the proper dosage is administered. Once the dosage is calculated, the learner is directed to draw an arrow on a syringe at the proper value. Syringe photos and illustrations have been updated.
- Labels of current and commonly prescribed medications are included to help users learn how to select the proper information required to determine correct dosage. There are over 375 labels included.
- Solved examples are included to demonstrate the $\frac{D}{H} \times Q = X$ formula method of calculating dosages.
- The dimensional analysis method is expanded by popular demand.
- The ratio-proportion method is included, giving instructors and students a choice of which method to use in calculating dosages.
- The IV equipment and calculations content has been expanded.
- Clear instructions are included for calculating IV medications administered in milligram per kilogram per minute.
- Clinical situations are simulated using actual medication labels, syringes, patient care order forms, and medication administration records.
- Case study format of posttests simulates actual clinical calculations and scenarios.
- Essential skills posttest simulates exams commonly administered by employers for new-hires.
- The index facilitates learner and instructor access to content and skills.

Instructor Resources

Instructor's Resource CD-ROM

ISBN # 0-17-661684-5

The *Instructor's Resource CD-ROM* to accompany *Dosage Calculations*, Second Canadian Edition, contains a variety of tools to successfully prepare lectures and teach within this subject area. The following components, available in CD-ROM format, are all free to adopters of *Dosage Calculations*:

Instructor's Solutions Manual—locate solutions for the review sets, practice problems, section evaluations, and posttests from the book.

Computerized Test Bank—additional questions not found in the book are available for further assessment. The software also allows for the creation of test items, tests, and coding for difficulty level.

PowerPoint Slides—depiction of administration tools and inclusion of calculation tips helpful to classroom lecture of dosage calculations.

Learner Resources

Tutorial Software

An electronic study aid is available FREE to each user of *Dosage Calculations*! The online Student Tutorial Software available with the book features:

- A bank of over 2000 questions from *Dosage Calculations*
- A clean menu structure to immediately access the program's items
- Enhanced short-answer functionality that will accept several variations of correct answers
- Interactive question navigator displays what questions you have answered correctly and incorrectly
- Review Sets and Practice Problems that operate within a tutorial mode, which allows two tries before the correct solution is provided. The Quick Review link offers tips for giving an accurate response
- Self-Evaluation Tests and posttests operate as a true testing environment that allow only one opportunity for correct answers
- Drop-down calculator available at a click of a button

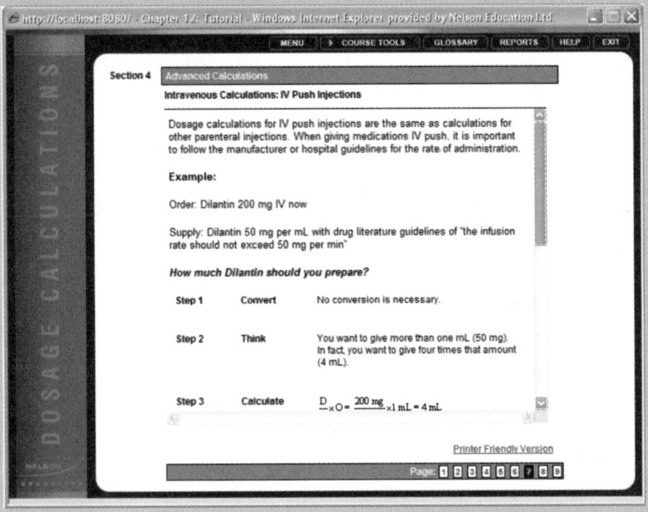

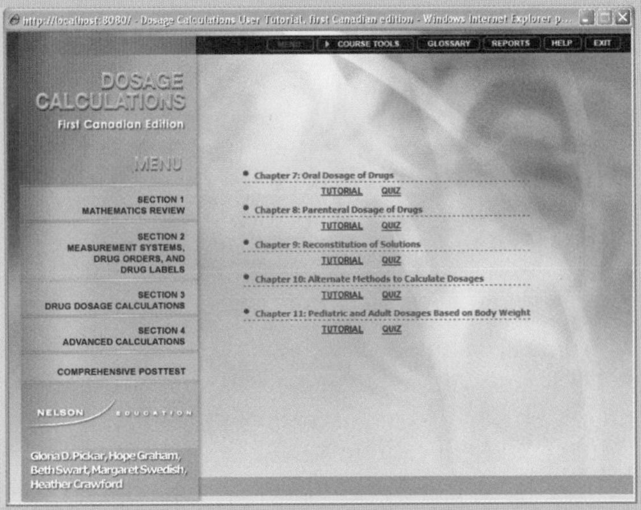

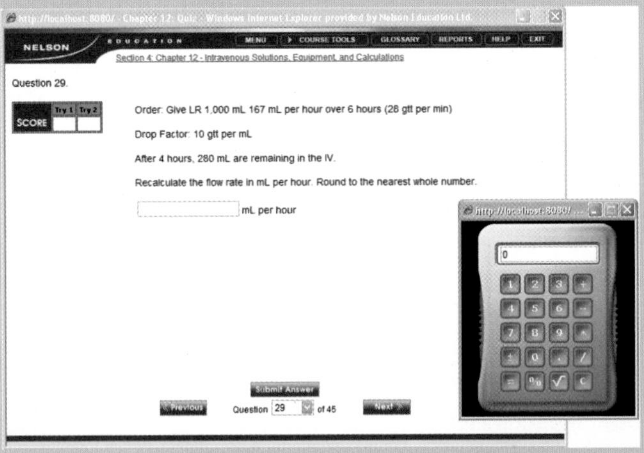

Reviewers

Nelson Education Ltd. would like to thank the following reviewers for their insightful comments during the development of this Canadian Edition:

Stephanie Langford
University of Ottawa

Lynne Harwood-Lunn
York University

Verona Francis-Barrett
Centennial College

Willy Kabotoff
University of Alberta

Carl Gray
Algonquin College

Technical Accuracy Check

We would like to thank Heather LeBlanc, BSc CCPE, Lead Instructor, Pharmacy Technician Program, Oulton College, who checked the accuracy of the dosage calculations, for her invaluable contribution to the development of this book. Invaluable feedback regarding the accuracy of the dosage calculations in preparing the new edition was also provided by Marcia Brown, Cindy Skolud, and Nadia Torresan-Doodnaught of Seneca College.

Credits

The following companies and individuals have provided technical data, photographs, syringes, drug labels, package inserts, or packaging to illustrate examples, problems, and posttests.

Abbott Laboratories, Abbott Park, IL

Biaxin, Synthroid, Lifecare Patient-Controlled Analgesia Plus II Infusion System, Primary I.V. set, vented 70 inchwith Y-Injection site MIRCRODRIP(R), Primary I.V. set, convertible pin, 80 inch with backcheck valve and 2 Injection sites piggback, Hema(R) II Y-Type Blood set, nonvented, 100 inch with 2 prepierced injection sites and secure lock, Continu-Flo(R) Solution Set, 60 drops/mL, Continu-Flo (R) Solution Set with DUO-VENT Spike, 10 drops/mL, ADD-Vantage System, Primary I.V. Set Nonvented, 100 inch, 60 drops/mL.

Alaris Medical Systems, San Diego, CA

Volumetric Infusion controller/pump, Infusion pump, Syringe Pump

Amgen Canada Inc., Mississauga, ON

Filgrastim

Apotex Inc., Weston, ON

Haloperidol, Procainamide HCl, Sucralfate, Amoxicillin, Allopurinol, Hydrochlorthiazide, Indomethacin, Erythromycin Ethylsuccinate

Astellas Pharma Canada, Inc., Markham, ON

Prograf

AstraZeneca Canada Inc., Mississauga, ON

Meropenem

Baxter Corporation, Mississauga, ON

5% Dextrose Injection, 5% Dextrose and 0.2% Sodium Chloride Injection, 5% Dextrose and 0.45% Sodium Chloride Injection, 0.45% Sodium Chloride Injection, 0.9% Sodium Chloride Injection, Continu-Flo Solution Set, Lactated Ringer's and 5% Dextrose Injection, Metronidazole, Potassium Chloride in 0.9% Sodium Chloride Injection, 5% Dextrose and 0.9% Sodium Chloride Injection, CC3 Volumetric Infusion Pump, Metronidazole

Bayer Inc., Toronto, ON

Avelox, Cipro

Becton, Dickinson and Company, Franklin Lake, NJ

(Courtesy and © Becton, Dickinson and Company) Safety Syringes, Intravenous Syringes

Bristol-Myers Squibb Canada, Montreal, QC

Amphotericin B, Erbitux, Percocet

Catherine Thomson

Parenteral Solutions

Cengage Learning

IV Systems, Insulin Syringes, Oral Medication Devices

Cytex Pharmaceuticals, Halifax, NS

Cyanocobalamin

Eli Lilly Canada Inc., Toronto, ON

(Humalog and Humulin are trademarks of Eli Lilly and Company and are used with permission.)

Humalog, Humulin N, Humulin R, Humulin 50/50, Humulin 30/70

Eli Lilly and Company, Indianapolis, IN

Atropine Sulfate, Cefaclor, Nebcin, Phenobarbital

Erfa Canada Inc., Westmount, QC

Procan SR

GlaxoSmithKline Inc., Mississauga, ON

Cortisporin, Clavulin Hycamtin, K10, Timentin, Zantac, Zofran

GlaxoSmithKline Inc, Research Triangle Park, NC

(Labels reproduced with permission of GlaxoSmithKline) Amoxicillin

Hoffman-LaRoche Limited (Roche Canada), Mississauga, ON

(© Copyright 2007, Hoffman-La Roche Limited)

Fuzeon, Rivotril, Rocephin, Toradol

Hoffman-La Roche, Inc., Nutley, NJ

Syringe, Labels submitted by manufacturer for general information and may change; please always refer to the latest product monograph/label. © Copyright 2007, Hoffman-LaRoche Limited.

Hospira Healthcare Corporation, Saint-Laurent, QC

Epinephrine, Heparin Sodium in 5% dextrose Lidocaine HCl Injection, Morphine, Potassium Chloride Injection, Sodium Bicarbonate Injection, Sterile Water, Vancomycin Hydrochloride

Janssen-Ortho Inc., Toronto, ON

Eprex, Levaquin

Johnson & Johnson Inc., Markham, ON

(Courtesy of Johnson & Johnson Inc. All Rights Reserved) Infant's TYLENOL® Concentrated Drops

Knoll Pharmaceutical Company, Mount Olive, NJ

Synthroid

LEO Pharma Inc., Thornhill, ON

Heparin

Mayne Pharma (Canada) Inc., Montreal, QC

Vincristine Sulfate Injection

McNeil Consumer Health, Raritan NJ

(Courtesy of McNeil Consumer and Specialty Pharmaceuticals) Tylenol

Merck Frosst Canada Ltd., Kirkland, QC

Prinivil

Novartis Pharmaceuticals Corporation, Summit NJ

Lopressor

Novo Nordisk Canada Inc., Mississauga, ON

NovoRapid ®, Levemir®, Novolin®

The Proctor and Gamble Company, Cincinnati, OH

Metamucil

Teva Canada formerly Novopharm Limited, Toronto, ON

Erythromycin, Hydrocortisone Sodium Succinate for Injection, Methotrexate, Methylprednisolone Sodium Succinate for Injection, Naproxen, Novo-Amoxin, Novo-Carbamaz, Novo-Doxylin, Novo-Lexin, Novo-Lorazepam, Novo-Pranol, Novo-Rythro Estolate, Novo-Tamoxifen, Novo-Trimel, Novo-Veramil, Pen VK Tablets

Organon Canada Ltd., Scarborough, ON

Hepalean

Pfizer Canada Inc., Kirkland QC

(©Pfizer Canada Inc.)

Aldactazide, Aldactone, Bacitracin, Depo-Provera, Dilantin, Lincomycin, Lopid, Nitrostat, Zithromax

Pharmaceutical Partners of Canada, Richmond Hill, ON

Ampicillin, Calcitriol, Cefazolin Injection, Ceftazidime Injection, Midazolam, Oxytocin, Penicillin G sodium, Piperacillin, Tobramycin, Vancomycin

Pharmascience Inc., Montreal, QC

Dexamethasone, Hydroxyzine HCl, Lorazepam, Potassium Chloride, Salbutamol, Valproic Acid

Ratiopharm Inc., Mississauga, ON

Amoxicillin and Clavulanate Potassium, Morphine

Sandoz Canada Inc., Bourcherville, QC

(© Copyright of Sandoz Canada Inc. All rights reserved)

Amikacin Sulfate Injection, Clindamycin Injection, Chlorpromazine, Diazepam, Digoxin, Droperidol, Furosemide, Gentamicin Injection, Glycopyrrolate, Haloperidol, Hydroxyzine HCl Injection, Meperidine, Methylprednisolone, Metoclopramide, Midazolam, Morphine Sulfate Injection, Morphine Sulfate Solution, Naloxone HCl Injection, Nubain, Promethazine, Ranitidine Injection, Tobramycin

sanofi-aventis, Laval, QC

Allegra 12, Cefotaxime, Diabeta, Lantus, Lasix, Lovenox, Suprax, Tussionex

Summit Pharmaceuticals

Slow K

TimeMed, Burr Ridge, IL

Flo-Meter infusion label

Triton Pharma Inc., Concord, ON

Eltroxin

UCB Pharma, Inc., Smyrna, GA

Lortab

Wyeth Consumer Healthcare Inc., Mississauga, ON

Robitussin Children's Cough and Cold

Text Credits

Inside front cover: Top 10 Drugs Reported as Causing Harm through Medication: Reprinted with permission from ISMP Canada

Page 182: Insulin Types Table 9-2, Reprinted with permission from Canadian Diabetes Association 2008 Clinical Practice Guidelines for the Prevention and Management of Diabetes in Canada. Can J Diabetes, 2008;32 (suppl 1): S1-201

Pages 337, 352 and 413: West Nomogram for Estimation of Body Surface Area. This chart was published in Nelson Textbook of Pediatrics, 16th ed., R. E. Behrman, R. M. Kliegman & H. B. Jenson, West Nomogram for Estimation of Body Surface Area, Copyright Elsevier, (2000).

Page 95: ISMP Canada's List of Dangerous Abbreviations, Symbols, and Dose Designations [February 2006, Volume 6 Issue 1]. Reprinted with permission from ISMP Canada.

USING THIS BOOK . . .

- Content is presented from simple to complex concepts in small increments followed by a quick review and solved examples. Review sets and practice problems provide opportunities to reinforce learning.
- All syringes are drawn to full size to provide accurate scale renderings to help learners master the reading of injectable dosages.

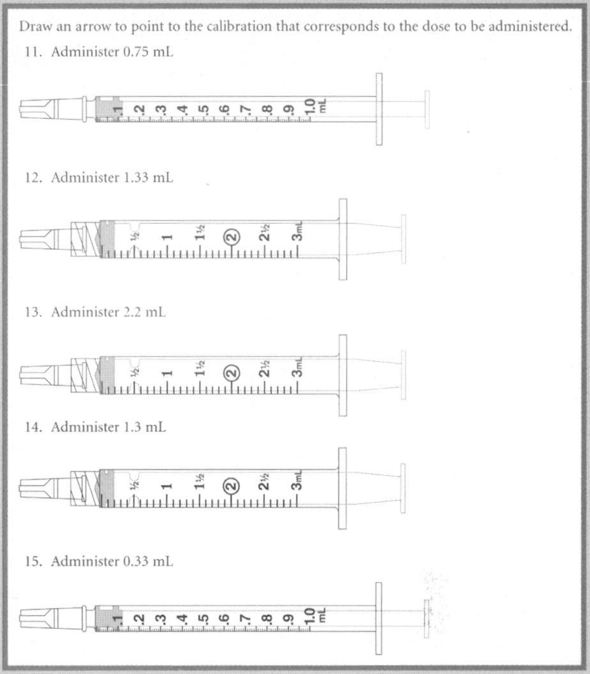

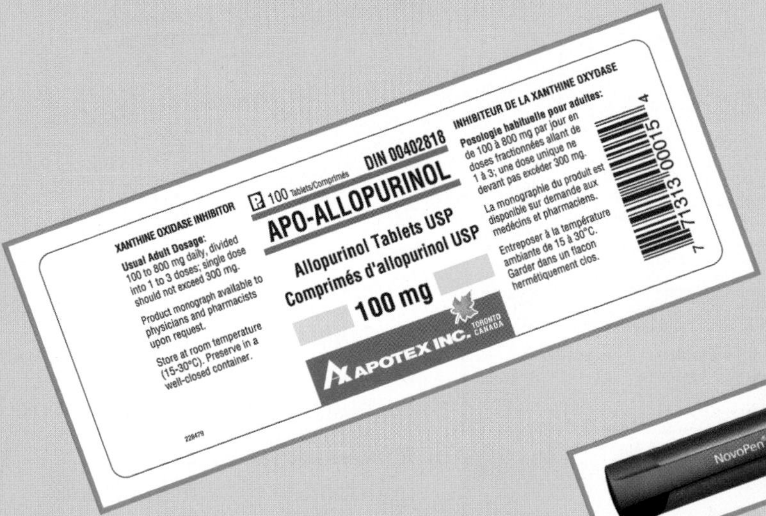

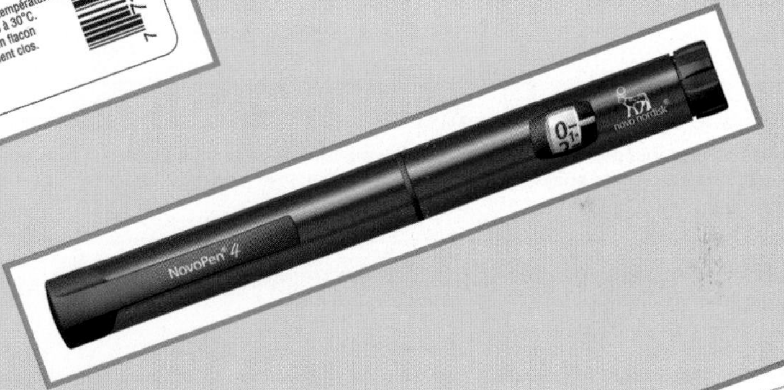

- Photos and drug labels are presented in full colour; colour is used to highlight and enhance the visual presentation of content and to improve readability. Special attention is given to visual clarity.

- ***Math tip*** boxes provide clues to essential computations.
- ***Caution*** boxes alert learners to critical information and safety concerns.

MATH TIP

When converting pounds to kilograms, round kilogram weight to one decimal place (tenths).

CAUTION

Those who administer drugs to patients are legally responsible for recognizing incorrect and unsafe dosages and for alerting the prescribing practitioner.

- ***Critical Thinking Skills*** are applied to real-life patient care situations to emphasize the importance of accurate dosage calculations and the avoidance of medication errors. As an added benefit, critical thinking scenarios that allow learners to present their own prevention strategy are included in end-of-chapter tests.

CRITICAL THINKING SKILLS

Many insulin errors occur when the nurse fails to clarify an incomplete order. Let us look at an example of an insulin error when the order did not include the type of insulin to be given.

Error

Failing to clarify an insulin order when the type of insulin is not specified.

Possible Scenario

Suppose the physician wrote an insulin order this way:

Humulin 100-unit insulin 50 units before breakfast

Because the physician did not specify the type of insulin, the nurse assumed it was short-acting insulin and noted that on the medication administration record. Suppose the patient was given the short-acting insulin for 3 days. On the morning of the third day, the patient developed signs of hypoglycemia (low blood glucose), including shakiness, tremors, confusion, and sweating.

Potential Outcome

A stat blood glucose would likely reveal a dangerously low glucose level. The patient would be given a glucose infusion to increase the blood sugar. The nurse may not realize the error until she and the doctor check the original order and find that the incomplete order was filled in by the nurse. When the doctor did not specify the type of insulin, the nurse assumed the physician meant regular, which is short-acting, when in fact intermediate-acting NPH insulin was desired.

Prevention

This error could have been avoided by remembering all the essential components of an insulin order: species, type of insulin (such as short-acting or NPH), supply dosage, the amount to give in units, and the frequency. When the nurse fills in an incomplete order, the nurse is essentially practising medicine outside the scope of practice. This would be a clear error of execution. It does not make sense to put you and your patient in such jeopardy. Communicating with the physician verbally or by phone would clarify the situation for everyone involved. Further, the nurse should have double-checked the dosage with another registered health care practitioner. Had the nurse done so, the error could have been discovered prior to administration.

RATIONALE FOR PRACTICE

When solving dosage problems for drugs supplied in tablets or capsules, Q (quantity) is always 1, because the supply dosage is per one tablet or capsule. Therefore, Q = 1 tablet or capsule.

- ***Rationale for Practice*** boxes highlight and draw the learners' attention to pertinent instructions.

REMEMBER

1 kg = 2.2 lb and 1 lb = 16 oz

Simply stated, weight in pounds is approximately twice the metric weight in kilograms; or weight in kilograms is approximately $\frac{1}{2}$ of weight in pounds. You can estimate kilograms by halving the weight in pounds.

- ***Remember*** boxes highlight information to be memorized.

QUICK REVIEW

To solve parenteral dosage problems, apply the three steps to dosage calculations:

Step 1 **Convert**
Step 2 **Think**
Step 3 **Calculate** $\frac{\textbf{D}\text{ (desired)}}{\textbf{H}\text{ (have)}} \times \textbf{Q}\text{ (quantity)} = \textbf{X}\text{ (amount)}$

Prepare a maximum of 5 mL per IM ventrogluteal injection site for an average-size adult, 2 mL per site for children age 2 through 12, 1 mL for children older than seven months to 2 years, and 0.5 mL for infants less than 7 months old. Refer to Table 9-1 for recommendations for the vastus lateralis and deltoid injecton sites.

Calculate dose volumes and prepare injectable fractional doses in a syringe using these guidelines:

Standard doses more than 1 mL: Round to *tenths* and measure in a 3-mL syringe. The 3-mL syringe is calibrated to 0.1-mL increments. Example: 1.53 mL is rounded to 1.5 mL and drawn up in a 3-mL syringe.

Small (less than 0.5 mL) doses: Round to *hundredths* and measure in a 1-mL syringe. Critical care and children's doses less than 1 mL calculated in hundredths should also be measured in a 1-mL syringe. The 1-mL syringe is calibrated in 0.01-mL increments. Example: 0.257 mL is rounded to 0.26 mL and drawn up in a 1-mL syringe.

Amounts of 0.5–1 mL, calculated in tenths, can be accurately measured in either a 1-mL or 3-mL syringe.

- ***Quick review*** boxes summarize critical information.

SECTION 1

Mathematics Review

Mathematics Diagnostic Evaluation

As a prerequisite objective, *Dosage Calculations* takes into account that you can add, subtract, multiply, and divide whole numbers. You should have a working knowledge of fractions, decimals, ratios, percents, and basic problem solving as well. This text reviews these important mathematical operations, which support all dosage calculations in health care.

Set aside $1\frac{1}{2}$ hours in a quiet place to complete the 50 items in the following diagnostic evaluation. You will need scratch paper and a pencil to work the problems.

Use your results to determine your current computational strengths and weaknesses to guide your review. A minimum score of 86 is recommended as an indicator of readiness for dosage calculations. If you achieve that score, you may proceed directly to Chapter 3. However, note any problems that you answered incorrectly, and use the related review materials in Chapters 1 and 2 to refresh your skills.

This mathematics diagnostic evaluation and the review that follows are provided to enhance your confidence and proficiency in arithmetic skills, thereby helping you to avoid careless mistakes later when you perform dosage calculations.

Good luck!

Directions:

1. Carry answers to three decimal places and round to two places.

   (Examples: 5.175 = 5.18; 5.174 = 5.17)

2. Express fractions in their lowest terms.

   (Example: $\frac{6}{10} = \frac{3}{5}$)

Mathematics Diagnostic Evaluation

1. $1517 + 0.63 =$ ________
2. Express the value of $0.7 + 0.035 + 20.006$ rounded to two decimal places. ________
3. $9.5 + 17.06 + 32 + 41.11 + 0.99 =$ ________
4. $\$19.69 + \$304.03 =$ ________
5. $93.2 - 47.09 =$ ________
6. $1005 - 250.5 =$ ________
7. Express the value of $17.156 - 0.25$ rounded to two decimal places. ________
8. $509 \times 38.3 =$ ________
9. $\$4.12 \times 42 =$ ________
10. $17.16 \times 23.5 =$ ________
11. $972 \div 27 =$ ________

12. $2.5 \div 0.001 =$ ________

13. Express the value of $\frac{1}{4} \div \frac{3}{8}$ as a fraction reduced to its lowest terms. ________

14. Express $\frac{1500}{240}$ as a decimal. ________

15. Express 0.8 as a fraction. ________

16. Express $\frac{2}{5}$ as a percent. ________

17. Express 0.004 as a percent. ________

18. Express 5% as a decimal. ________

19. Express $33\frac{1}{3}\%$ as a ratio in lowest terms. ________

20. Express 1:50 as a decimal. ________

21. $\frac{1}{2} + \frac{3}{4} =$ ________

22. $1\frac{2}{3} + 4\frac{7}{8} =$ ________

23. $1\frac{5}{6} - \frac{2}{9} =$ ________

24. Express the value of $\frac{1}{100} \times 60$ as a fraction. ________

25. Express the value of $4\frac{1}{4} \times 3\frac{1}{2}$ as a mixed number. ________

26. Identify the fraction with the greatest value: $\frac{1}{150}, \frac{1}{200}, \frac{1}{100}$ ________

27. Identify the decimal with the least value: 0.009, 0.19, 0.9 ________

28. $\frac{6.4}{0.02} =$ ________

29. $\frac{0.02 + 0.16}{0.4 - 0.34} =$ ________

30. Express the value of $\frac{3}{12 + 3} \times 0.25$ as a decimal. ________

31. 8% of 50 = ________

32. $\frac{1}{2}\%$ of 18 = ________

33. 0.9% of 24 = ________

Find the value of "X." Express your answer as a decimal.

34. $\frac{1:1000}{1:100} \times 250 = X$ ________

35. $\frac{300}{150} \times 2 = X$ ________

36. $\frac{2.5}{5} \times 1.5 = X$ ________

37. $\frac{1\,000\,000}{250\,000} \times X = 12$ ________

38. $\frac{0.51}{1.7} \times X = 150$ ________

39. $X = (82.4 - 52)\frac{3}{5}$ ________

40. $\frac{\frac{1}{150}}{\frac{1}{300}} \times 1.2 = X$ ________

41. Express 2:10 as a fraction in its lowest terms. ________

42. Express 2% as a ratio in its lowest terms. ________

43. If 5 equal medication containers contain 25 tablets total, how many tablets are in each container? ________

44. A person is receiving 0.5 milligrams of a medication four times a day. What is the total amount of medication in milligrams given each day? ________

45. If 1 kilogram equals 2.2 pounds, how many kilograms does a 66-pound child weigh? ________

46. If 1 kilogram equals 2.2 pounds, how many pounds are in 1.5 kilograms? (Express your answer as a decimal.) ________

47. If 1 centimetre equals $\frac{2}{5}$ inch, how many centimetres are in $2\frac{1}{2}$ inches? (Express your answer as a decimal.) ________

48. If 2.5 centimetres equal 1 inch, how long in centimetres is a 3-inch wound? ________

49. This diagnostic test has a total of 50 problems. If you incorrectly answer 5 problems, what percentage will you have answered correctly? ________

50. For every 5 female student nurses in a nursing class, there is 1 male student nurse. What is the ratio of female to male student nurses? ________

After completing these problems, see page 451 in the answer section to check your answers. Give yourself 2 points for each correct answer.

Perfect score = 100 My score = ________

Readiness score = 86 (43 correct)

CHAPTER 1

Fractions and Decimals

LEARNING OBJECTIVES

1. Compare the values of fractions and decimals.
2. Identify types of fractions.
3. Read and write fractions and decimals.
4. Reduce fractions to lowest terms.
5. Round decimals.
6. Add, subtract, multiply, and divide fractions and decimals.
7. Convert between fractions and decimals.
8. Compare values expressed in fractions and decimals.

FRACTIONS

Healthcare professionals need to understand fractions to be able to interpret and act on medical orders, read prescriptions, and understand patient records and information in healthcare literature. You will see fractions used in household measures. Proficiency with fractions is essential to success in medication calculations.

A *fraction* is a part of a whole number. (See example below.) Fractions are composed of two parts: a *numerator,* which is the top number and a *denominator,* which is the bottom number. The denominator refers to the total number of parts. The larger the number in the denominator, the smaller the value of the pieces (or fraction) of the whole. The numerator refers to a part of the whole that is being considered. The larger the number in the numerator, the more parts of the whole that are being considered. The fraction may also be read as the "numerator divided by the denominator."

Example:

$\frac{1}{4}$ $\frac{\text{numerator}}{\text{denominator}}$

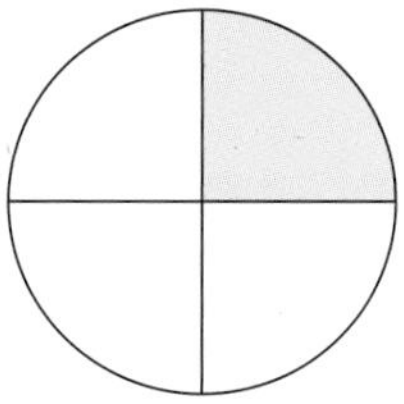

The whole is divided into four equal parts (denominator), and one part (numerator) is considered.

$\frac{1}{4}$ = 1 part of 4 parts, or $\frac{1}{4}$ of the whole.

The fraction $\frac{1}{4}$ may also be read as "1 divided by 4."

> **MATH TIP**
>
> The *d*enominator begins with *d* and is *d*own below the line in a fraction.

Types of Fractions

There are four types of common fractions: proper, improper, mixed, and complex. Whole numbers can also be expressed as fractions.

Proper Fractions

Proper fractions are fractions in which the value of the numerator is less than the value of the denominator. The value of the proper fraction is also less than 1.

RULE

Whenever the numerator is less than the denominator, the value of the fraction must be less than 1.

Example:

$\frac{5}{8} \ \frac{\text{numerator}}{\text{denominator}}$ is less than 1

Improper Fractions

Improper fractions are fractions in which the value of the numerator is greater than or equal to the value of the denominator. The value of the improper fraction is greater than or equal to 1.

RULE

If the numerator is greater than the denominator, the value of the fraction must be greater than 1.

Example:

$\frac{8}{5}$ is greater than 1

RULE

If the numerator and denominator are equal, the value of the improper fraction is always equal to 1.

Example:

$$\frac{5}{5} = 1$$

Mixed Numbers

When a whole number and a proper fraction are combined, the result is referred to as a *mixed number.* The value of the mixed number is always greater than 1.

RULE

If a fraction and a whole number are written together, the fraction value is always greater than 1.

Example:

$1\frac{5}{8} = 1 + \frac{5}{8}$; $1\frac{5}{8}$ is greater than 1

Complex Fractions

Complex fractions include fractions in which the numerator, the denominator, or both may be a proper fraction, improper fraction, or mixed number. The value may be less than, greater than, or equal to 1.

Examples:

$\frac{\frac{5}{8}}{\frac{1}{2}}$ is greater than 1 $\frac{\frac{5}{8}}{2}$ is less than 1 $\frac{1\frac{5}{8}}{\frac{1}{5}}$ is greater than 1 $\frac{\frac{1}{2}}{\frac{2}{4}} = 1$

Whole Numbers

Whole numbers have an unexpressed denominator of one (1).

Examples:

$1 = \frac{1}{1}$ $3 = \frac{3}{1}$ $6 = \frac{6}{1}$ $100 = \frac{100}{1}$

Fractions at Work

Being able to *convert* is a skill that must be mastered in order to become competent in medication calculation. In this chapter, you will learn to convert among the various types of fractions. Later in this chapter you will learn to convert fractions to decimals and decimals to fractions. In later chapters, you will learn to convert between units of measurement. Conversion among the different types of fractions simplifies calculations.

Besides conversion, other requisite skills of mastery in fractions for use in medication calculations include comparing fractions, finding *equivalent fractions,* reducing fractions to their *lowest terms,* and finding *lowest common denominators* (LCDs).

Equivalent Fractions

Fractions of equal value can be expressed in several ways. If the numerator and denominator of a fraction are either multiplied or divided by the same *nonzero* number, the fraction does not change in value. The resulting fraction has the same value as the original fraction and can be called an *equivalent fraction.*

MATH TIP

When changing a fraction, if you want to keep the same equivalent value, you must do the same thing (multiply or divide by the same number) to the numerator and to the denominator.

Examples:

$\frac{2}{4} = \frac{2 \div 2}{4 \div 2} = \frac{1}{2}$ $\frac{1}{3} = \frac{1 \times 3}{3 \times 3} = \frac{3}{9}$

Reducing Fractions to Lowest Terms

When calculating dosages, it is usually easier to work with fractions using the smallest numbers possible. Finding these equivalent fractions is called *reducing the fraction to the lowest terms* or *simplifying the fraction.*

RULE

To reduce a fraction to lowest terms, *divide* both the numerator and denominator by the *largest nonzero whole number* that will go evenly into both

Patience is required to reduce a fraction with large numbers. Sometimes the procedure for reducing fractions to their lowest terms seems like trial and error. You may have to reduce several times. Guidelines for reducing fractions include:

- Even numbers are divisible by 2 and sometimes by multiples of 2.
- Numbers ending in 5 or 0 are divisible by 5 and sometimes by multiples of 5.
- Certain numbers are called prime numbers because they cannot be reduced any further. Examples are 2, 3, 7, 11, 13, 17. See if a prime number will divide evenly into the numerator and denominator.

Example:

Reduce $\frac{7}{28}$ to lowest terms.

7 can evenly divide into both the numerator (7) and the denominator (28).

$$\frac{7 \text{ divided by } 7}{28 \text{ divided by } 7} = \frac{1}{4}$$

Example:

Reduce $\frac{6}{12}$ to lowest terms.

6 is the largest number that will divide evenly into both 6 (numerator) and 12 (denominator).

$$\frac{6}{12} = \frac{6 \div 6}{12 \div 6} = \frac{1}{2} \text{ in lowest terms}$$

MATH TIP

If *both* the numerator and denominator *cannot* be divided evenly by a nonzero number other than 1, then the fraction is already in lowest terms.

Finding Common Denominators for Two or More Fractions

To compare, add, or subtract fractions, the denominators must be the same. Such computations are made easier when the *lowest common denominator* (LCD) is used. The LCD is the smallest whole number that can be divided equally by all denominators within the problem.

To find the lowest common denominator, first check to see if the largest denominator in the problem is evenly divisible by each of the other denominators. If so, this largest denominator is the LCD.

Example 1:

$\frac{1}{8}$ and $\frac{1}{4}$

You find that 8 is evenly divisible by 4. Therefore, 8 is the LCD.

$\frac{2}{7}$ and $\frac{5}{14}$ and $\frac{1}{28}$

You find that 28 is evenly divided by 7 and 14. Therefore, 28 is the LCD.

If the largest denominator is not evenly divisible, you can find a common denominator by multiplying all the denominators together. This may not give you the LCD. You can then try to reduce the fraction by following the rule described above for *reducing fractions to lowest terms.*

Example 2:

$\frac{3}{8}$ and $\frac{1}{3}$

You find that 8 is *not* divisible evenly by 3. Therefore, you multiply 8 times 3, which equals 24. The number 24 is a common denominator for these two fractions. In this case the common denominator is the LCD.

$\frac{2}{3}$ and $\frac{1}{4}$ and $\frac{1}{6}$

You find that 6 is evenly divisible by 3 but is not evenly divisible by 4. You can multiply 3 by 4 by 6 (which equals 72) and reduce the fraction to its lowest terms, as described earlier. An alternative is to only multiply 4 by 6 (which equals 24) because you know that the largest denominator is evenly divisible by the remaining denominator (3) in the problem.

Example 3:

Enlarge $\frac{3}{5}$ to the equivalent fraction in tenths.

$$\frac{3}{5} = \frac{3 \times 2}{5 \times 2} = \frac{6}{10}$$

Converting Mixed Numbers to Improper Fractions

You need to know how to convert a variety of fraction to calculate medication dosages. Mixed numbers can be converted to improper fractions and improper fraction can be converted to mixed numbers.

RULE

To change or convert a mixed number to an improper fraction, multiply the whole number by the denominator and add the numerator.

Example:

$$1\frac{5}{8} = \frac{(1 \times 8) + 5}{8} = \frac{13}{8}$$

Converting Improper Fractions to Mixed Numbers

RULE

To change or convert an improper fraction to mixed number or whole number, divide the numerator by the denominator.

Examples:

$$\frac{8}{5} = 8 \div 5 = 1\frac{3}{5}$$

$$\frac{10}{4} = 10 \div 4 = 2\frac{2}{4} = 2\frac{1}{2}$$

Comparing Fractions

Now that you have learned to find equivalent fractions and LCDs, convert mixed numbers and improper fractions, and reduce fractions to their lowest terms, you can compare the relative sizes of fractions. You will know when the value of one fraction is greater or less than another. You can compare fractions when the denominators are the same or the numerators are the same.

RULE

If the numerators are the same, the fraction with the smaller denominator has the greater value.

Example:

Compare $\frac{1}{2}$ and $\frac{1}{4}$.

Numerators are both 1.

Denominators: 2 is greater than 4.

$\frac{1}{2}$ has a greater value.

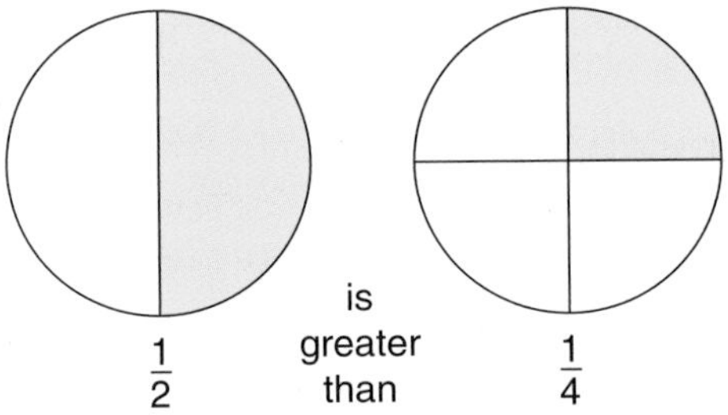
1/2
is greater than
1/4

RULE

If the denominators are both the same, the fraction with the smaller numerator has the lesser value.

Example:

Compare $\frac{2}{5}$ and $\frac{3}{5}$.

Denominators are both 5.

Numerators: 2 is less than 3.

$\frac{2}{5}$ has a lesser value.

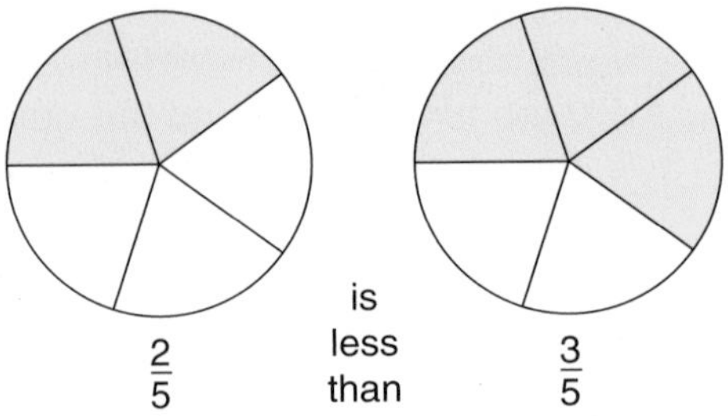
2/5
is less than
3/5

If neither the numerators nor denominators are the same, convert the fractions to equivalent fractions using the LCD. Then compare the numerators as noted in the previous example.

Example:

$\frac{2}{3}$ and $\frac{3}{8}$ and $\frac{7}{24}$

You find the LCD is 24. $\frac{2}{3}$ is the equivalent of $\frac{16}{24}$; $\frac{3}{8}$ is the equivalent of $\frac{9}{24}$. Therefore, the largest fraction is $\frac{2}{3}$ or $\frac{16}{24}$; the smallest fraction is $\frac{7}{24}$.

QUICK REVIEW

- Proper fraction: numerator is less than denominator; value is less than 1. Example: $\frac{1}{2}$
- Improper fraction: numerator is greater than denominator; value is greater than 1. Example: $\frac{4}{3}$. Or numerator = denominator; value = 1. Example: $\frac{5}{5}$
- Mixed number: whole number + a fraction; value is greater than 1. Example: $1\frac{1}{2}$
- Complex fraction: numerator and/or denominator composed of fractions; value is greater than, less than, or = 1. Example: $\frac{\frac{1}{2}}{\frac{1}{50}}$
- To change the form of a fraction without changing its value, multiply or divide both the numerator and the denominator by the same nonzero number. Example: $\frac{1}{12} = \frac{1 \times 2}{12 \times 2} = \frac{2}{24}$
- To reduce a fraction to its lowest terms, divide both terms by the largest nonzero whole number that will divide both the numerator and denominator evenly. Value remains the same. Example: $\frac{6}{10} = \frac{6 \div 2}{10 \div 2} = \frac{3}{5}$
- To convert a mixed number to an improper fraction, multiply the whole number by the denominator and add the numerator; use the original denominator in the fractional part. Example: $1\frac{1}{3} = \frac{4}{3}$
- To convert an improper fraction to a mixed number, divide the numerator by the denominator. Express any remainder as a proper fraction reduced to lowest terms. Example: $\frac{21}{9} = 2\frac{3}{9} = 2\frac{1}{3}$
- When numerators are equal, the fraction with the smaller denominator is greater. Example: $\frac{1}{2}$ is greater than $\frac{1}{3}$
- When denominators are equal, the fraction with the larger numerator is greater. Example: $\frac{2}{3}$ is greater than $\frac{1}{3}$

REVIEW SET 1

1. Circle the *improper* fraction(s).

   $\frac{2}{3}$ $\quad 1\frac{3}{4}$ $\quad \frac{6}{6}$ $\quad \frac{7}{5}$ $\quad \frac{16}{17}$ $\quad \frac{\frac{1}{9}}{\frac{2}{3}}$

2. Circle the *proper* fraction(s).

   $\frac{1}{4}$ $\quad \frac{1}{14}$ $\quad \frac{14}{1}$ $\quad \frac{14}{14}$ $\quad \frac{144}{14}$

3. Circle the *mixed* number(s) *reduced to the lowest terms.*

   $3\frac{4}{8}$ $\quad \frac{2}{3}$ $\quad 1\frac{2}{9}$ $\quad \frac{1}{3}$ $\quad 1\frac{1}{4}$ $\quad 5\frac{7}{8}$

4. Circle the pair(s) of *equivalent* fractions.

   $\frac{3}{4} = \frac{6}{8}$ $\quad \frac{1}{5} = \frac{2}{10}$ $\quad \frac{3}{9} = \frac{1}{3}$ $\quad \frac{3}{4} = \frac{4}{3}$ $\quad 1\frac{4}{9} = 1\frac{2}{3}$

Change the following mixed numbers to improper fractions.

5. $6\frac{1}{2}$ = ________

7. $10\frac{2}{3}$ = ________

6. $1\frac{1}{5}$ = ________

8. $7\frac{5}{6}$ = ________

Change the following improper fractions to whole numbers or mixed numbers; reduce to their lowest terms.

9. $\frac{24}{12}$ = ________

11. $\frac{30}{9}$ = ________

10. $\frac{8}{8}$ = ________

12. $\frac{100}{75}$ = ________

Convert the following fractions to equivalent fractions with the number of parts indicated.

13. $\frac{3}{4}$ to eighths ________

15. $\frac{2}{5}$ to tenths ________

14. $\frac{1}{4}$ to sixteenths ________

16. $\frac{2}{3}$ to ninths ________

Circle the correct answer.

17. Which is larger? $\frac{1}{150}, \frac{1}{100}$

18. Which is smaller? $\frac{1}{1000}, \frac{1}{10\,000}$

19. Which is larger? $\frac{2}{9}, \frac{5}{9}$

20. Which is smaller? $\frac{3}{10}, \frac{5}{10}$

21. A patient is supposed to drink a 300-mL bottle of magnesium citrate prior to his X-ray study. He has been able to drink 180 mL. What portion of the bottle remains? (Express your answer as a fraction reduced to lowest terms.) ________

22. Mrs. Gardiner is 3 days post-colon resection and has positive bowel sounds. She is tolerating ice chips well. Her fluid intake has been changed to 200 mL twice daily and is to be increased by $\frac{1}{2}$ daily for 3 days. What is the total for day 2, day 3, and day 4?
Day 2________ Day 3________ Day 4________

23. A respiratory therapy class consists of 3 men and 57 women. What fraction of the students in the class are men? (Express your answer as a fraction reduced to lowest terms.)
____

24. A nursing student answers 18 out of 20 questions correctly on a test. Write a proper fraction (reduced to lowest terms) to represent the portion of the test questions that were answered correctly. ________

25. Mr. Lee is informed that it is safe to reduce his caloric intake by $\frac{1}{8}, \frac{1}{6}$, or $\frac{1}{4}$. If Mr. Lee chooses to reduce his caloric intake by the maximum amount, he will choose to reduce his intake by which fraction? ________

After completing these problems, see page 452 in the answer section to check your answers.

Addition and Subtraction of Fractions

To add or subtract fractions, all the denominators must be the same. First, determine the LCD. Then convert the fractions to equivalent fractions with the LCD. These operations were examined in the last section. Finding the LCD is the first step in adding or subtracting fractions.

RULE

To add or subtract fractions:

1. **Convert all fractions to equivalent fractions with the LCDs; then**
2. **Add or subtract the numerators, place that value in the numerator, and use the LCD as the denominator; and**
3. **Convert to a mixed number or reduce the fraction to its lowest terms.**

MATH TIP

To *add or subtract fractions*, no calculations are performed on the denominators. Once they are all converted to LCDs, perform the mathematical operation (addition or subtraction) on the *numerators* only, and use the LCD as the denominator.

Adding Fractions

Example 1:

$$\frac{3}{4} + \frac{1}{4} + \frac{2}{4}$$

1. Find the LCD. This step is not necessary in this example, because the fractions already have the same denominator.
2. Add the numerators: $\dfrac{3 + 1 + 2}{4} = \dfrac{6}{4}$
3. Convert to a mixed number and reduce to its lowest terms: $\dfrac{6}{4} = 1\dfrac{2}{4} = 1\dfrac{1}{2}$

Example 2:

$$\frac{1}{3} + \frac{3}{4} + \frac{1}{6}$$

1. Find the LCD: 12. The number 12 is the LCD that 3, 4, and 6 will all equally divide into.

   Convert to equivalent fractions in twelfths.

   $$\frac{1}{3} = \frac{1 \times 4}{3 \times 4} = \frac{4}{12}$$

   $$\frac{3}{4} = \frac{3 \times 3}{4 \times 3} = \frac{9}{12}$$

   $$\frac{1}{6} = \frac{1 \times 2}{6 \times 2} = \frac{2}{12}$$

2. Add the numerators, and use the common denominator: $\frac{4+9+2}{12} = \frac{15}{12}$

3. Convert to a mixed number, and reduce to its lowest terms: $\frac{15}{12} = 1\frac{3}{12} = 1\frac{1}{4}$

Subtracting Fractions

Example 1:

$$\frac{15}{18} - \frac{8}{18}$$

1. Find the LCD. This is not necessary in this example, because the denominators are the same.
2. Subtract the numerators, and use the common denominator: $\frac{15-8}{18} = \frac{7}{18}$
3. Reduce to lowest terms: not necessary. No further reduction is possible.

Example 2:

$$1\frac{1}{10} - \frac{3}{5}$$

1. Find the LCD: 10. The number 10 is the lowest common denominator that both 10 and 5 will equally divide into.

   Convert to equivalent fractions in tenths:

   $$1\frac{1}{10} = \frac{11}{10}$$

   $$\frac{3}{5} = \frac{3 \times 2}{5 \times 2} = \frac{6}{10}$$

2. Subtract the numerators, and use the common denominator: $\frac{11-6}{10} = \frac{5}{10}$
3. Reduce to its lowest terms: $\frac{5}{10} = \frac{1}{2}$

   Let us review one more time how to add and subtract fractions.

QUICK REVIEW

To add or subtract fractions:

- Convert to equivalent fractions with LCD.
- Add or subtract the numerators; place that value in the numerator. Use the LCD as the denominator.
- Convert the answer to a mixed number or reduce to its lowest terms.

REVIEW SET 2

Add, and reduce the answers to their lowest terms.

1. $7\frac{4}{5} + \frac{2}{3} =$ ________
2. $\frac{3}{4} + \frac{2}{3} =$ ________
3. $4\frac{2}{3} + 5\frac{1}{24} + 7\frac{1}{2} =$ ________
4. $\frac{3}{4} + \frac{1}{8} + \frac{1}{6} =$ ________

5. $12\frac{1}{2} + 20\frac{1}{3} =$ ________

6. $\frac{1}{7} + \frac{2}{3} + \frac{11}{21} =$ ________

7. $\frac{4}{9} + \frac{5}{8} + 4\frac{2}{3} =$ ________

8. $34\frac{1}{2} + 8\frac{1}{2} =$ ________

9. $\frac{12}{17} + 5\frac{2}{7} =$ ________

10. $\frac{6}{5} + 1\frac{1}{3} =$ ________

Subtract, and reduce the answers to its lowest terms.

11. $\frac{3}{4} - \frac{1}{4} =$ ________

12. $8\frac{1}{12} - 3\frac{1}{4} =$ ________

13. $\frac{1}{8} - \frac{1}{12} =$ ________

14. $100 - 36\frac{1}{3} =$ ________

15. $\frac{1}{3} - \frac{1}{6} =$ ________

16. $2\frac{3}{5} - 1\frac{1}{5} =$ ________

17. $14\frac{3}{16} - 7\frac{1}{8} =$ ________

18. $25 - 17\frac{7}{9} =$ ________

19. $4\frac{7}{10} - 3\frac{9}{20} =$ ________

20. The central supply stock clerk finds there are $17\frac{1}{2}$ litres of hydrogen peroxide on the shelf. If the fully stocked shelf held 27 litres of hydrogen peroxide, how many litres were used?

____

21. Ms. Lewenski's medical regime includes fluid restriction. She is to receive $\frac{2}{3}$ of her total day's fluids in the morning and $\frac{1}{4}$ of the fluids in the afternoon. What fraction of the day's fluids does Ms. Lewenski have left to take in the evening? ________

22. Mr. Booth is receiving $\frac{1}{2}$ tablets three times daily. How many tablets is he receiving daily?

____

23. Ms. Coady is trying to make sure she drinks sufficient fluids daily. She drinks $1\frac{1}{2}$ glasses before breakfast, 1 glass at breakfast, $\frac{2}{3}$ glass in mid morning and $1\frac{3}{4}$ glasses at noon. What is the total number of glasses (including fraction of glasses) has Ms. Coady had to drink by afternoon? ________

24. Mr. Grady is recording his walking achievements in a rehabilitation program. His goal is to walk 8 kilometres this week. So far he has walked $1\frac{1}{4}$ km, $1\frac{1}{3}$, $1\frac{1}{2}$ km, and 1 km. How many kilometres are left for him to walk in order to meet his goal for this week?

____

25. As camp nurse, you are encouraging healthy eating. Apples are sectioned and available at meals and snack breaks. In the last two days, the number of apples consumed are $54\frac{1}{2}$ and $57\frac{3}{4}$. How many total apples have been consumed in the past two days? ________

After completing these problems, see page 452 in the answer section to check your answers.

Multiplication and Division of Fractions

Multiplying Fractions

To multiply fractions, multiply numerators (for the numerator of the answer), and multiply denominators (for the denominator of the answer).

Simplification of fractions is helpful in reducing math errors. Cancelling fractions is a method of simplifying fraction multiplication by reducing numerators and denominators by a common factor. Cancellation (like reducing to lowest terms) is based on the fact that the division of both the numerator and denominator by the same whole number does not change the value of the resulting number. In fact, it makes the calculation simpler, because you are working with smaller numbers.

Example:

$\frac{1}{3} \times \frac{250}{500}$ (numerator and denominator of $\frac{250}{500}$ are both divisible by 250)

$$= \frac{1}{3} \times \frac{\overset{1}{\cancel{250}}}{\underset{2}{\cancel{500}}} = \frac{1}{3} \times \frac{1}{2} = \frac{1}{6}$$

Also, a numerator and a denominator of any of the fractions involved in the multiplication may be cancelled when they can be divided by the same whole number. This is called *cross-cancellation.*

Example:

$$\frac{1}{8} \times \frac{8}{9} = \frac{1}{\underset{1}{\cancel{8}}} \times \frac{\overset{1}{\cancel{8}}}{9} = \frac{1}{1} \times \frac{1}{9} = \frac{1}{9}$$

Cultural Note: In some countries, the word *of* is used instead of *times* for multiplication of fractions. It might be simpler to understand multiplication of fractions by substituting *of* for times. For example, 1/2 of 4 is 2, 1/2 of 1/4 is 1/8, and 1/4 of 1/2 is 1/8.

RULE

To multiply fractions:

1. **Cancel terms, if possible;**
2. **Multiply numerators for the numerator of the answer, multiply denominators for the denominator of the answer; and**
3. **Reduce the result (*product*) to lowest terms.**

Example 1:

$$\frac{3}{4} \times \frac{2}{6}$$

1. Cancel terms: Divide 2 and 6 by 2

$$\frac{3}{4} \times \frac{\overset{1}{\cancel{2}}}{\underset{3}{\cancel{6}}} = \frac{3}{4} \times \frac{1}{3}$$

Divide 3 and 3 by 3

$$\frac{\overset{1}{\cancel{3}}}{4} \times \frac{1}{\underset{1}{\cancel{3}}} = \frac{1}{4} \times \frac{1}{1}$$

2. Multiply numerators and denominators:

$$\frac{1}{4} \times \frac{1}{1} = \frac{1}{4}$$

3. Reduce to lowest terms: not necessary. Product is in lowest terms.

Example 2:

$$\frac{15}{30} \times \frac{2}{5}$$

1. Cancel terms: Divide 15 and 30 by 15

$$\frac{\overset{1}{\cancel{15}}}{\underset{2}{\cancel{30}}} \times \frac{2}{5} = \frac{1}{2} \times \frac{2}{5}$$

Divide 2 and 2 by 2

$$\frac{1}{\underset{1}{\cancel{2}}} \times \frac{\overset{1}{\cancel{2}}}{5} = \frac{1}{1} \times \frac{1}{5}$$

2. Multiply numerators and denominators:

$$\frac{1}{1} \times \frac{1}{5} = \frac{1}{5}$$

3. Reduce to lowest terms: not necessary. Product is in lowest terms.

> **MATH TIP**
>
> When multiplying a fraction by a nonzero whole number, the same rule applies as for multiplying fractions. First convert the whole number to a fraction with a denominator of 1; the value of the number remains the same.

Example 3:

$$\frac{2}{3} \times 4$$

1. No terms to cancel. (You cannot cancel 2 and 4, because both are numerators. To do so would change the value.) Convert the whole number to a fraction.

$$\frac{2}{3} \times 4 = \frac{2}{3} \times \frac{4}{1}$$

2. Multiply numerators and denominators:

$$\frac{2}{3} \times \frac{4}{1} = \frac{8}{3}$$

3. Convert to a mixed number.

$$\frac{8}{3} = 8 \div 3 = 2\frac{2}{3}$$

MATH TIP

To multiply mixed numbers, first convert them to improper fractions, and then multiply.

Example 4:

$3\frac{1}{2} \times 4\frac{1}{3}$

1. Convert: $3\frac{1}{2} = \frac{7}{2}$

   $4\frac{1}{3} = \frac{13}{3}$

   Therefore, $3\frac{1}{2} \times 4\frac{1}{3} = \frac{7}{2} \times \frac{13}{3}$
2. Cancel: not necessary. No numbers can be cancelled.
3. Multiply: $\frac{7}{2} \times \frac{13}{3} = \frac{91}{6}$
4. Convert to a mixed number: $\frac{91}{6} = 15\frac{1}{6}$

Dividing Fractions

The division of fractions uses three terms: *dividend, divisor,* and *quotient.* The *dividend* is the fraction being divided or the first number. The *divisor,* the number to the right of the division sign, is the fraction the dividend is divided by. The *quotient* is the result of the division. To divide fractions, the divisor is inverted, and the operation is changed to multiplication. Once inverted, the calculation is the same as for multiplication of fractions.

Example:

$$\frac{1}{4} \div \frac{2}{7} = \frac{1}{4} \times \frac{7}{2} = \frac{7}{8}$$

$\frac{1}{4}$	$\div$	$\frac{2}{7}$	=	$\frac{1}{4}$	$\times$	$\frac{7}{2}$	=	$\frac{7}{8}$
↑ **Dividend**		↑ **Divisor**			↑ ÷ Changed to ×	↑ Inverted Divisor		↑ **Quotient**

RULE

To divide fractions,
1. Invert the terms of the divisor, change ÷ to ×;
2. Cancel terms, if possible;
3. Multiply the resulting fractions; and
4. Convert the result (quotient) to a mixed number, or reduce to lowest terms.

Example 1:

$$\frac{3}{4} \div \frac{1}{3}$$

1. Invert divisor, and change ÷ to ×: $\frac{3}{4} \div \frac{1}{3} = \frac{3}{4} \times \frac{3}{1}$
2. Cancel: not necessary. No numbers can be cancelled.
3. Multiply: $\frac{3}{4} \times \frac{3}{1} = \frac{9}{4}$
4. Convert to mixed number: $\frac{9}{4} = 2\frac{1}{4}$

Example 2:

$$\frac{2}{3} \div 4$$

1. Invert divisor, and change ÷ to ×: $\frac{2}{3} \div \frac{4}{1} = \frac{2}{3} \times \frac{1}{4}$
2. Cancel terms: $\frac{\overset{1}{\cancel{2}}}{3} \times \frac{1}{\underset{2}{\cancel{4}}} = \frac{1}{3} \times \frac{1}{2}$
3. Multiply: $\frac{1}{3} \times \frac{1}{2} = \frac{1}{6}$
4. Reduce: not necessary; already reduced to lowest terms.

> **MATH TIP**
>
> To divide mixed numbers, first convert them to improper fractions.

Example 3:

$$1\frac{1}{2} \div \frac{3}{4}$$

1. Convert: $1\frac{1}{2} = \frac{3}{2}$
2. Invert divisor, and change ÷ to ×: $\frac{3}{2} \times \frac{4}{3}$
3. Cancel: $\frac{\overset{1}{\cancel{3}}}{\underset{1}{\cancel{2}}} \times \frac{\overset{2}{\cancel{4}}}{\underset{1}{\cancel{3}}} = \frac{1}{1} \times \frac{2}{1}$
4. Multiply: $\frac{1}{1} \times \frac{2}{1} = \frac{2}{1}$
5. Reduce: $\frac{2}{1} = 2$

> **MATH TIP**
>
> Multiplying complex fractions also involves the division of fractions. Study this carefully.

Example 4:

$$\frac{\frac{1}{150}}{\frac{1}{100}} \times 2$$

1. Convert: Express 2 as a fraction. $\frac{\frac{1}{150}}{\frac{1}{100}} \times \frac{2}{1}$
2. Rewrite complex fraction as division: $\frac{1}{150} \div \frac{1}{100} \times \frac{2}{1}$
3. Invert divisor and change ÷ to ×: $\frac{1}{150} \times \frac{100}{1} \times \frac{2}{1}$
4. Cancel: $\frac{1}{\cancel{150}_{3}} \times \frac{\cancel{100}^{2}}{1} \times \frac{2}{1} = \frac{1}{3} \times \frac{2}{1} \times \frac{2}{1}$
5. Multiply: $\frac{1}{3} \times \frac{2}{1} \times \frac{2}{1} = \frac{4}{3}$
6. Convert to mixed number: $\frac{4}{3} = 1\frac{1}{3}$

This example appears difficult at first, but when solved logically, one step at a time, it is just like the others.

QUICK REVIEW

- To multiply fractions, cancel terms, multiply numerators, and multiply denominators.
- To divide fractions, invert the divisor, cancel terms, and multiply.
- Convert to a mixed number or reduce to lowest terms.

REVIEW SET 3

Multiply, and reduce the answers to their lowest terms.

1. $\frac{3}{10} \times \frac{1}{12} =$ ______
2. $\frac{12}{25} \times \frac{3}{5} =$ ______
3. $\frac{5}{8} \times 1\frac{1}{6} =$ ______
4. $\frac{1}{100} \times 3 =$ ______
5. $\frac{\frac{1}{6}}{\frac{1}{4}} \times \frac{3}{\frac{2}{3}} =$ ______
6. $\frac{\frac{1}{150}}{\frac{1}{100}} \times 2\frac{1}{2} =$ ______
7. $\frac{30}{75} \times 2 =$ ______
8. $9\frac{4}{5} \times \frac{2}{3} =$ ______
9. $\frac{3}{4} \times \frac{2}{3} =$ ______
10. $4\frac{2}{3} \times 5\frac{1}{24} =$ ______
11. $\frac{3}{4} \times \frac{1}{8} =$ ______

Divide, and reduce the answers to their lowest terms.

12. $\frac{3}{4} \div \frac{1}{4} =$ ______
13. $6\frac{1}{12} \div 3\frac{1}{4} =$ ______

14. $\frac{1}{8} \div \frac{7}{12} =$ ________

15. $\frac{1}{33} \div \frac{1}{3} =$ ________

16. $5\frac{1}{4} \div 10\frac{1}{2} =$ ________

17. $\frac{1}{60} \div \frac{1}{2} =$ ________

18. $2\frac{1}{2} \div \frac{3}{4} =$ ________

19. $\dfrac{\frac{1}{20}}{\frac{1}{3}} =$ ________

20. $\dfrac{\frac{3}{5}}{\frac{3}{4}} \div \dfrac{\frac{4}{5}}{1\frac{1}{9}} =$ ________

21. The nurse is maintaining calorie counts (or counting calories) for a patient who is not eating well. The patient ate $\frac{3}{4}$ of an apple. If one large apple contains 80 calories, how many calories did he consume? ________________

22. How many seconds are there in $9\frac{1}{3}$ minutes? ________________

23. A bottle of children's acetaminophen contains 30 tablets. If each dose for a 2-year-old child is $1\frac{1}{2}$ tablets, how many doses are available in this bottle? ________

24. Ms. Flynn needs to take $1\frac{1}{2}$ tablets of medication 3 times per day for 7 days. Over the 7 days, how many tablets will she take? ________________

25. The nurse aide observes that Mr. Suzuki's water pitcher is still $\frac{1}{3}$ full. If he drank 850 millilitres of water, how many millilitres does the pitcher hold? ($\frac{1}{3}$ of the pitcher.)

____

After completing these problems, see page 453 in the answer section to check your answers.

DECIMALS

The Arabic system of numeration (which we use) is positional. This means that the value of any numeral is affected by the position it occupies in a number. Starting at the right and moving to the left, the value assigned to the numerical places is 10 times greater than the value of the place that preceded it. The number 6 724 925 is assigned the places as you can see in the following example:

6	7	2	4	9	2	5
millions	hundred thousands	ten thousands	thousands	hundreds	tens	ones

Decimals numbers, commonly called *decimals,* are numeric values that include a whole number, a decimal point, and a decimal fraction. Numbers to the left of the decimal point have a value greater than 1. They are also known as *whole numbers.* Numbers to the right of the decimal point have a value less than 1.

Since many medications involve dosages that contain decimals, it is essential that healthcare professionals understand decimals, recognize the relative values of decimals, and understand the importance of correct decimal placement to be able to add, subtract, multiply, and divide decimals. Identifying the relative value enables you to think about your answer to the calculation before you do the math. Being able to think about the answer and evaluate the math is important in administering correct medication dosages. A common error associated with medication administration is improper decimal placement.

RULE

When dealing with decimals, think of the decimal point as the *centre* that separates whole and fractional amounts. The position of the numbers in relation to the decimal point indicates the place value of the numbers.

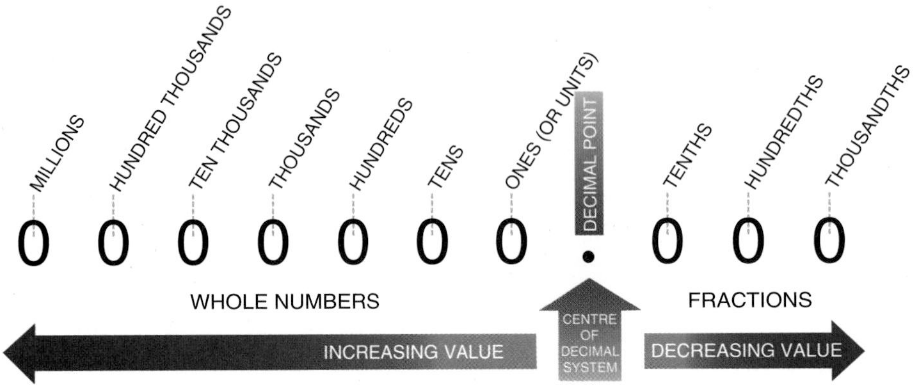

Example 1:

10.1 is higher than 9.15

Example 2:

3.2 is higher than 2.99

Example 3:

7.01 is higher than 6.99

MATH TIP

The decimal portion of the number ends in th(s).

Examples:

0.001 = one thousand*th*

0.02 = two hundred*ths*

0.7 = seven ten*ths*

Decimal fractions are numbers that are less than 1. They are fractions with a denominator of 10, 100, 1000, or any power of 10.

Examples:

Decimal	Fraction
0.1	$= \frac{1}{10}$
0.01	$= \frac{1}{100}$
0.001	$= \frac{1}{1000}$

Decimal numbers are numeric values that include a whole number, a decimal point, and a decimal fraction.

Examples:

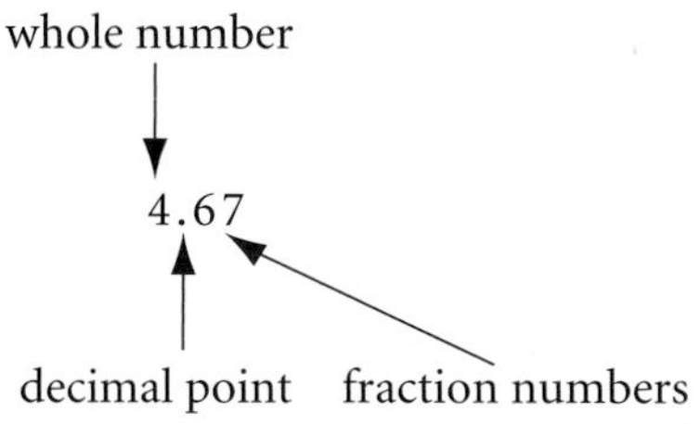
whole number
4.67
decimal point
fraction numbers

> **RULE**
>
> **The decimal number is read by stating the whole number first, the decimal point as *and*, and then the decimal fraction by naming the value of the last decimal place.**

Example:

Look carefully at the decimal number 4.125. The last decimal place is thousandths. Therefore, the number is read as "four and one hundred twenty-five thousandths."

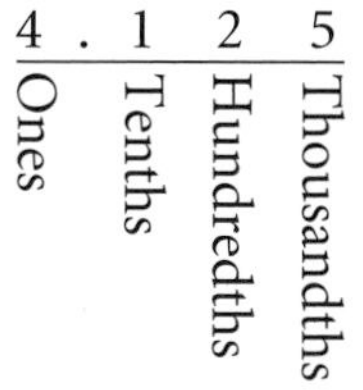
4 . 1 2 5
Ones
Tenths
Hundredths
Thousandths

Examples:

The number 6.2 is read as "six and two tenths."

The number 10.03 is read as "ten and three hundredths."

Writing Decimals

The fraction portion of the number indicates an understood denominator of 10 or some power of 10. To eliminate possible confusion and avoid errors when the number is less than 1, you must always place a zero to the left of the decimal point.

Example:

Decimal Number	Fraction
0.3	3/10
0.18	18/100
0.175	175/1000

> **CAUTION**
>
> Whenever a decimal fraction (whose value is less than 1) is written in medical notations, the zero MUST precede the decimal point. This practice highlights the decimal point and the fact that the value of the number is less than 1.

CAUTION

There should not be a zero at the end of a decimal.

RULE

Zeros added *after* the last digit of a decimal fraction *do not* change its value.

Reading Decimals

When there is a zero (0) to the left of the decimal, the zero is not read aloud *except* when the nurse is taking a verbal order over the phone from a prescriber. When repeating back an order for a medication involving a decimal, the zero should be read aloud to prevent a medication error.

For example, "zero point three" would be the verbal interpretation of the first example in the above series.

Comparing Decimals

Being able to understand the relative value of decimals and recognizing the high and low values of each decimal number is key to calculating and administering accurate medication dosages. The relative value of a number is determined by the spaces to the left of the decimal point—the more spaces, the higher the value. If the spaces are the same, then compare the actual numbers. The first place from the left where they differ determines the relative value of each number.

For example, if you compare 23.5 and 25.3, the first place from the left where the two numbers differ is in the ones value; that is, the number three is less than the number five. Therefore, the number 23.5 is less than 25.3. If the numbers to the right of the decimal point do not differ, begin comparing numbers to the right of the decimal point until you find a difference in the numbers. For example, compare 31.53 and 31.64. Since the numbers to the left of the decimal point are the same (both are 31), then you notice that in the first space to the right of the decimal point, they differ. Since 5 is less than 6, then the number with the lesser value is 31.53.

CAUTION

A common error in comparing decimals is to overlook the decimal place values and misinterpret higher numbers for greater amounts and lower numbers for lesser amounts.

MATH TIP

You can accurately compare decimal amounts by aligning the decimal points and adding zeros, so that the numbers to be compared have the same number of decimal places. Remember that adding zeros at the end of a decimal fraction does not change the original value.

Example 1:

Compare 0.125, 0.05, and 0.2 to find which decimal fraction is largest.

Align decimal points and add zeros.

$0.125 = \frac{125}{1000}$ or one hundred twenty-five thousandths

$0.05\mathbf{0} = \frac{50}{1000}$ or fifty thousandths

$0.2\mathbf{00} = \frac{200}{1000}$ or two hundred thousandths

Now it is easy to see that 0.2 is the greater amount and 0.05 is the least. But at first glance, you might have been tricked into thinking that 0.2 was the least amount and 0.125 was the greater amount. This kind of error can have dire consequences in dosage calculations and healthcare.

Example 2:

Suppose 0.5 microgram of a drug has been ordered. The recommended maximum dosage of the drug is 0.25 microgram, and the minimum recommended dosage is 0.125 microgram. Comparing decimals, you can see that the ordered dosage is not within the allowable range.

0.125 microgram (recommended minimum dosage)

0.25**0** microgram (recommended maximum dosage)

0.5**00** microgram (ordered dosage)

Now you can see that 0.5 microgram is outside the allowable limits of the safe dosage range of 0.125 to 0.25 microgram for this medication. In fact, it is twice the allowable maximum dosage.

Example 3:

0.25 = 0.25**0**

Twenty-five hundredths equals two hundred fifty thousandths.

The last zero does not change the value of the decimal, therefore it is not necessary. The preferred notation is 0.25 rather than 0.250.

Conversion between Fractions and Decimals

To expedite medication calculations, it is frequently necessary to be able to know equivalency between fractions and decimal numbers and/or to use both fractions and decimal numbers in the required medication calculation.

RULE

To convert a fraction to a decimal, divide the numerator by the denominator.

Example 1:

Convert $\frac{1}{4}$ to a decimal.

$$\frac{1}{4} = 4\overline{)1.00} = 0.25$$

(quotient .25; 8, 20, 20)

Example 2:

Convert $\frac{2}{5}$ to a decimal.

$$\frac{2}{5} = 5\overline{)2.0} = 0.4$$

(quotient .4; 20)

RULE

To convert a decimal to a fraction:

1. **Express the decimal number as a whole number in the numerator of the fraction,**
2. **Express the denominator of the fraction as the number 1 followed by as many zeros as there are places to the right of the decimal point, and**
3. **Reduce the resulting fraction to its lowest terms.**

Example 1:

Convert 0.125 to a fraction.

1. Numerator: 125
2. Denominator: 1 followed by 3 zeros = 1000
3. Reduce: $\frac{125}{1000} = \frac{1}{8}$

Example 2:

Convert 0.65 to a fraction.

1. Numerator: 65
2. Denominator: 1 followed by 2 zeros = 100
3. Reduce: $\frac{65}{100} = \frac{13}{20}$

QUICK REVIEW

- In decimal fractions, zeros added before the decimal point or at the end of the decimal fraction *do not* change the value. Example: .5 = **0**.5 = 0.5**0**. However, using the leading zero is the only acceptable notation (such as 0.5).
- In a decimal number, zeros added before and/or after the decimal point may change the value. Example: 1.5 ≠ 1.**0**5 and 1.5 ≠ 1**0**.5
- To avoid a medication error, *always* place a zero to the left of the decimal point in a decimal fraction. *Always* read aloud the zero in a medication order involving a decimal fraction. Example: 0.5
- The number of places in a decimal fraction indicates the power of 10.

  Examples:
  0.5 = five tenths
  0.05 = five hundredths
  0.005 = five thousandths

- Compare decimals by aligning decimal points and adding zeros.

  Example:
  Compare 0.5, 0.05, and 0.005
  0.500 = five hundred thousandths (greatest)
  0.050 = fifty thousandths
  0.005 = five thousandths (least)

- To convert a fraction to a decimal, divide the numerator by the denominator.
- To convert a decimal to a fraction, express the decimal number as a whole number in the numerator and the denominator as the correct power of 10. Reduce the fraction to its lowest terms.

  Example:

$$0.04 = \frac{4\,(\text{numerator is a whole number})}{100\,(\text{denominator is 1 followed by two zeros})} = \frac{\overset{1}{\cancel{4}}}{\underset{25}{\cancel{100}}} = \frac{1}{25}$$

REVIEW SET 4

Complete the following table of equivalent fractions and decimals. Reduce fractions to their lowest terms.

Fraction	Decimal	The decimal number is read as:
1. $\frac{1}{5}$	________	____________________
2. ________	________	eighty-five hundredths
3. ________	1.05	____________________
4. ________	0.006	____________________
5. $10\frac{3}{200}$	________	____________________
6. ________	1.9	____________________
7. ________	________	five and one tenth
8. $\frac{4}{5}$	________	____________________
9. ________	250.5	____________________
10. $33\frac{3}{100}$	________	____________________
11. ________	0.95	____________________
12. $2\frac{3}{4}$	________	____________________

Fraction	Decimal	The decimal number is read as:
13. ________	________	seven and five thousandths
14. $1000\frac{1}{200}$	________	____________________
15. ________	________	four thousand eighty-five and seventy-five thousandths

16. Change 0.017 to a four-place decimal. ____________________

17. Change 0.2500 to a two-place decimal. ____________________

18. Convert $\frac{75}{100}$ to a decimal. ____________________

19. Convert 0.045 to a fraction reduced to lowest terms. ____________________

Circle the correct answer.

20. Which is largest?	0.012	0.120	0.021
21. Which is smallest?	0.635	0.6	0.063

22. True or false? $0.375 = 0.0375$

23. True or false? 2.2 grams = 2.02 grams

24. True or false? 6.5 ounces = 6.500 ounces

25. For a certain medication, the safe dosage should be greater than or equal to 0.5 gram but less than or equal to 2 grams. Circle each dosage that falls within this range.

    0.8 gram 0.25 gram 2.5 grams 1.25 grams

After completing these problems, see page 453 in the answer section to check your answers.

Addition and Subtraction of Decimals

Addition and subtraction is used in the clinical setting when adding dosages, intake of fluids, hourly outputs, and in restricted diets (fluid, electrolyte, carbohydrate). The addition and subtraction of decimals is very similar to addition and subtraction of whole numbers. There are only two simple but essential rules that are different. Healthcare professionals must use these two rules to perform accurate dosage calculations for some medications.

You have learned to compare decimals by aligning the decimal points vertically. Similarly, you need to align the decimals to add and subtract decimals. Whenever there is an unequal number of spaces to the right and left of the decimal point, add a zero wherever there is a blank space. (These added zeros do not change the value of the number.) Then add and subtract the numbers the same as you add and subtract whole numbers.

RULE

To add and subtract decimals, line up the decimal points.

CAUTION

In final answers, eliminate unnecessary zeros at the end of a decimal to avoid confusion.

Example 1:

$$1.25 + 1.75 = \begin{array}{r} 1.25 \\ +1.7 \\ \hline 3.00 \end{array} = 3$$

Example 2:

$$1.25 - 0.13 = \begin{array}{r} 1.25 \\ -0.13 \\ \hline 1.12 \end{array}$$

Example 3:

$$3.54 + 1.26 = \begin{array}{r} 3.54 \\ +1.26 \\ \hline 4.80 \end{array} = 4.8$$

Example 4:

$$2.54 - 1.04 = \begin{array}{r} 2.54 \\ -1.04 \\ \hline 1.50 \end{array} = 1.5$$

RULE

To add and subtract decimals, add zeros at the end of decimal fractions if necessary to make all decimal numbers of equal length.

Example 1:

$$\begin{array}{r} 3.75 - 2.1 = 3.75 \\ -2.10 \\ \hline 1.65 \end{array}$$

Example 2:

Add 0.9, 0.65, 0.27, 4.712

$$\begin{array}{r} 0.900 \\ 0.650 \\ 0.270 \\ +4.712 \\ \hline 6.532 \end{array}$$

Example 3:

$$\begin{array}{r} 5.25 - 3.6 = 5.25 \\ -3.60 \\ \hline 1.65 \end{array}$$

Example 4:

$$\begin{array}{r} 66.96 + 32 = 66.96 \\ +32.00 \\ \hline 98.96 \end{array}$$

QUICK REVIEW

- To add or subtract decimals, align the decimal points and add zeros, making all decimals of equal length. Eliminate unnecessary zeros in the final answer.

Examples:

$$\begin{array}{r} 1.5 + 0.05 = 1.50 \\ +0.05 \\ \hline 1.55 \end{array}$$

$$\begin{array}{r} 7.8 + 1.12 = 7.80 \\ +1.12 \\ \hline 8.92 \end{array}$$

$$\begin{array}{r} 0.725 - 0.5 = 0.725 \\ -0.500 \\ \hline 0.225 \end{array}$$

$$\begin{array}{r} 12.5 - 1.5 = 12.5 \\ -1.5 \\ \hline 11.0 = 11 \end{array}$$

REVIEW SET 5

Find the result of the following problems.

1. 0.16 + 5.375 + 1.05 + 16 = ________
2. 7.517 + 3.2 + 0.16 + 33.3 = ________
3. 13.009 − 0.7 = ________
4. 5.125 + 6.025 + 0.15 = ________
5. 175.1 + 0.099 = ________
6. 25.2 − 0.193 = ________
7. 0.58 − 0.062 = ________
8. \$10.10 − \$0.62 = ________
9. \$19 − \$0.09 = ________
10. \$5.05 + \$0.17 + \$17.49 = ________
11. 4 + 1.98 + 0.42 + 0.003 = ________

12. 0.3 − 0.03 = ________

13. 16.3 − 12.15 = ________

14. 2.5 − 0.99 = ________

15. 5 + 2.5 + 0.05 + 0.15 + 2.55 = ________

16. 0.03 + 0.16 + 2.327 = ________

17. 700 − 325.65 = ________

18. 645.32 − 40.9 = ________

19. 18 + 2.35 + 7.006 + 0.093 = ________

20. 13.529 + 10.09 = ________

21. A dietitian calculates the sodium in a patient's breakfast: raisin bran cereal = 0.1 gram, 250 mL 2% milk = 0.125 gram, 180 mL orange juice = 0.001 gram, 1 corn muffin = 0.35 gram, and butter = 0.121 gram. How many grams of sodium did the patient consume?

____

22. The prescription is for 30 mg. The stock supply has one tablet of 7.5 mg and one tablet of 15 mg. How many more milligrams of the medication must the nurse get from the pharmacy? ____

23. Ms. Brisson has a hospital bill for $16 709.43. Her insurance company pays $14 651.37. What is her balance due? ____

24. A pharmacist weighs a tube of antibiotic ointment and discovers it weighs 0.15 kg. How much would 20 tubes weigh? ____

25. A home health nurse accounts for her day of work. If she spent 3 hours and 20 minutes at the office, 40 minutes travelling, $3\frac{1}{2}$ hours caring for patients, 24 minutes for lunch, and took a 12-minute break, what is her total number of hours including the break? Express your answer as a decimal. (HINT: First convert each time to hours and minutes.)

____

After completing these problems, see pages 453–454 in the answer section to check your answers.

Multiplication and Division of Decimals

Multiplying Decimals

The procedure for multiplication of decimals is very similar to that used for whole numbers. The only difference is the decimal point, which must be properly placed in the product or answer. Use the following simple rule.

RULE

To multiply decimals:

1. **Multiply the decimals without concern for decimal point placement,**
2. **Count off the total number of decimal places in the numbers multiplied, and**
3. **Place the decimal point in the product to the left of the total number of places counted. If the product has insufficient numbers for correct placement of the decimal point, add as many zeros as necessary to the left of the product to correct this.**

Example 1:

$1.5 \times 0.5 = 1.5$ (1 decimal place)

$\times\ 0.5$ (1 decimal place)

0.75 (The decimal point is located 2 places to the left, because a total of 2 decimal places are counted.)

Example 2:

$1.72 \times 0.9 = 1.72$ (2 decimal places)

$\times\ 0.9$ (1 decimal place)

1.548 (The decimal point is located 3 places to the left, because a total of 3 decimal places are counted.)

Example 3:

$5.06 \times 1.3 = 5.06$ (2 decimal places)

$\times\ 1.3$ (1 decimal place)

1518

506

6.578 (The decimal point is located 3 places to the left, because a total of 3 decimal places are counted.)

Example 4:

$1.8 \times 0.05 = 1.8$ (1 decimal place)

$\times\ 0.05$ (2 decimal places)

0.090 (The decimal point is located 3 places to the left. Notice that a zero has to be inserted between the decimal point and the 9 to allow for enough decimal places.)

$0.090 = 0.09$ (Eliminate unnecessary zero.)

RULE

When multiplying a decimal by a power of 10, move the decimal point as many places to the right as there are zeros in the multiplier.

Example 1:

1.25×10

The multiplier 10 has 1 zero; move the decimal point 1 place to the right.

$1.25 \times 10 = 1.2.5 = 12.5$

Example 2:

2.3×100

The multiplier 100 has 2 zeros; move the decimal point 2 places to the right. (Note: Add zeros as necessary to complete the operation.)

$2.3 \times 100 = 2.30. = 230$

Example 3:

0.001×1000

The multiplier 1000 has 3 zeros; move the decimal point 3 places to the right.

$0.001 \times 1000 = 0.001. = 1$

Dividing Decimals

Decimal fractions occur frequently in calculations as common fractions, which require division. Remember two things we have learned about fractions and decimals:

1. The value of the fraction is not changed when the numerator and denominator are multiplied by the same number.
2. When multiplying a decimal by a power of 10, move the decimal point as many places to the right as there are zeros in the multiplier.

Now follow the steps in the Rule box below to divide fractions.

RULE

To divide decimals:

1. **Eliminate the decimal point in the divisor (number divided by or denominator) by moving the decimal point as many places as necessary to make the divisor a whole number.**
2. **Move the decimal point the same number of places to the right in the numerator (dividend) as you did in the denominator.**
3. **Reduce the fraction to its lowest terms and then divide if necessary.**
4. **Place the decimal point in the *quotient* (answer) above the *new* decimal point place in the *dividend*.**

Example 1:

$0.25 \div 0.125$

$= \frac{0.25}{0.125}$

Multiply the numerator and denominator by 1000, and move decimal point 3 places to the right.

$= \frac{250}{125}$

Divide both the numerator and denominator by 25 to reduce the fraction to its lowest terms.

$= \frac{10}{5}$ can be reduced further by dividing both the numerator and denominator by 5

$= 2$

Therefore, $0.25 \div 0.125 = 2$

Example 2:

$$100.75 \div 2.5 = 2.5.\overline{)100.7.5} = 40.3$$

(dividend) (divisor)

40.3 (quotient)

100
07
00
75
75

Example 3:

$$56.5 \div 0.02 = 0.02.\overline{)56.50.} = 2825$$

2825.

4
16
16
5
4
10
10

MATH TIP

Recall that adding a zero at the end of a decimal number does not change its value (56.5 = 56.50). Adding a zero was necessary in the last example to complete the operation.

RULE

When dividing a decimal by a power of 10, move the decimal point to the left as many places as there are zeros in the divisor.

Example 1:

$0.65 \div 10$

The divisor 10 has 1 zero; move the decimal point 1 place to the left.

$0.65 \div 10 = .0.65 = 0.065$

(Note: Place the zero to the left of the decimal point to avoid confusion and to emphasize that this is a decimal.)

Example 2:

$7.3 \div 100$

The divisor 100 has 2 zeros; move the decimal point 2 places to the left.

$7.3 \div 100 = .07.3 = 0.073$

(Note: Add zeros as necessary to complete the operation.)

Example 3:

0.5 ÷ 1,000

The divisor 1,000 has 3 zeros; move the decimal point 3 places to the left.

0.5 ÷ 1000 = .000.5 = 0.0005

CAUTION:

A decimal point placed incorrectly is a major cause of medication error. It is important to always place the decimal point clearly and correctly.

Rounding Decimals

When dividing, the answer may not "come out even." In some cases you could keep dividing and end up with an answer that is very long! Sometimes it is convenient and safe to round an answer—that is, to use an approximate answer instead of an exact one.

Rounding Off

Rounding off numbers produces results, which can be either larger or smaller the given number. For many calculations, it is necessary to compute calculations to thousandths (three decimal places) and round off to hundredths (two places). In this text, instructions will usually be given as to how many places to carry out your division.

How many places is it necessary to carry out the division? The answer depends on the way the medication is dispensed and the equipment needed to administer it. Some tablets can be broken in half. Some liquids are prepared in units of measurement: tenths, hundredths, or thousandths. Some syringes are marked to the nearest tenth, hundredth, or thousandth place. Intravenous rates are usually rounded to the nearest whole number.

RULE

To round off a number:
If the first number to the right of the number to be rounded is greater than 5, then you round up to the next number. If the first number beyond the number to be rounded is less than 5, then you round down.

When rounding for dosage calculations, unnecessary zeros can be dropped. For example, 5.20 rounded to hundredths place should be written as 5.2 because the 0 is not needed to clarify the number.

Examples:

Tenths Hundredths Thousandths — All rounded to hundredths (two places)

0 . 1 2 3 = 0.12

1 . 7 4 4 = 1.74

5 . 3 2 5 = 5.33

0 . 6 6 6 = 0.67

0 . 3 0 = 0.3 (When this is rounded to hundredths, the final zero should be dropped. It is not needed to clarify the number.)

RULE

To obtain an answer that is rounded off to the nearest tenth, look at the number in the hundredth place and follow the above rule for rounding off.

Examples:

Tenths Hundredths — All rounded to tenths (one place)

0 . 1 3 = 0.1

5 . 6 4 = 5.6

0 . 7 5 = 0.8

1 . 6 6 = 1.7

0 . 9 5 = 1.0 = 1 (Zero at the end of a decimal is unnecessary.)

Rounding Down

The danger of a medication overdose must always be guarded against. Therefore, the amount of medication is often rounded down instead of rounding up. Rounding down is routinely done in pediatrics and when administering high-alert medications to adults.

To round down a number to a particular place, merely drop all the digits after that place. In particular, to round down to the tenths place, merely drop all the digits after the tenths place.

Example:

Round 5.6685 to the nearest hundredth, tenth and whole number.

5.6685 rounded down to the nearest hundredth = 5.66

5.6685 rounded down to the nearest tenth = 5.6

5.6685 rounded down to the nearest whole number = 5

NOTE: This is done to avoid medication overdose only. Routinely, in other applications, you will follow the above rules for rounding off: if the first number beyond the number to be rounded is greater than 5, then you round up to the next number; if the first number beyond the number to be rounded is less than 5, then you round down.

QUICK REVIEW

- To multiply decimals, place the decimal point in the product to the *left* as many decimal places as there are in the total of the number of places counted in the two decimals multiplied.

  Example:
  0.25 × 0.2 = 0.050 = 0.05 (Zeros at the end of the decimal are unnecessary.)

- To divide decimals, move the decimal point in the divisor and dividend the number of decimal places that will make the divisor a whole number and align it in the quotient.

  Example: 24 ÷ 1.2

  ```
       20.
  1.2.)24.0.
  ```

- To multiply or divide decimals by a power of 10, move the decimal point to the *right* (to *multiply*) or to the *left* (to *divide*) the number of decimal places as there are zeros in the power of 10.

  Examples:
  5.06 × 10 = 5.0.6 = 50.6

  2.1 ÷ 100 = .02.1 = 0.021

- When rounding decimals, add 1 to the place value considered if the next decimal place is 5 or greater.

  Examples:

  Rounded to hundredths: 3.054 = 3.05; 0.566 = 0.57. Rounded to tenths: 3.05 = 3.1; 0.54 = 0.5

REVIEW SET 6

Multiply, and round your answers to two decimal places.

1. 1.16 × 5.03 = ________
2. 0.314 × 7 = ________
3. 1.71 × 25 = ________
4. 3.002 × 0.05 = ________
5. 75.1 × 1000.01 = ________
6. 16.03 × 2.05 = ________
7. 55.50 × 0.05 = ________
8. 23.2 × 15.025 = ________

Divide, and round your answers to two decimal places.

9. 16 ÷ 0.04 = ________
10. 25.3 ÷ 6.76 = ________
11. 0.02 ÷ 0.004 = ________
12. 45.5 ÷ 15.25 = ________
13. 73 ÷ 13.40 = ________
14. 16.36 ÷ 0.06 = ________
15. 0.375 ÷ 0.25 = ________
16. 100.04 ÷ 0.002 = ________

Multiply or divide by the power of 10 indicated. Draw an arrow to demonstrate movement of the decimal point.

17. $562.5 \times 100 =$ ________

18. $16 \times 10 =$ ________

19. $25 \div 1000 =$ ________

20. $32.005 \div 1000 =$ ________

21. $23.25 \times 10 =$ ________

22. $717.717 \div 10 =$ ________

23. $83.16 \times 10 =$ ________

24. $0.33 \times 100 =$ ________

25. $14.106 \times 1000 =$ ________

After completing these problems, see page 454 in the answer section to check your answers.

PRACTICE PROBLEMS—CHAPTER 1

1. Convert 0.35 to a fraction to its lowest terms. ________

2. Convert $\frac{3}{8}$ to a decimal. ________

Find the least common denominator for the following pairs of fractions.

3. $\frac{5}{7}; \frac{2}{3}$ ________

4. $\frac{1}{5}, \frac{4}{11} =$ ________

5. $\frac{4}{9}; \frac{5}{6}$ ________

6. $\frac{1}{3}, \frac{3}{5} =$ ________

Perform the indicated operation, and reduce fractions to lowest terms.

7. $1\frac{2}{3} + \frac{9}{5} =$ ________

8. $4\frac{5}{12} + 3\frac{1}{15} =$ ________

9. $\frac{7}{9} - \frac{5}{18} =$ ________

10. $5\frac{1}{6} - 2\frac{7}{8} =$ ________

11. $\frac{4}{9} \times \frac{7}{12} =$ ________

12. $1\frac{1}{2} \times 6\frac{3}{4} =$ ________

13. $7\frac{1}{5} \div 1\frac{7}{10} =$ ________

14. $\frac{3}{16} + \frac{3}{10} =$ ________

15. $8\frac{4}{11}$ divided by $1\frac{2}{3}$ = ________

16. $\frac{9\frac{1}{2}}{1\frac{4}{5}} =$ ________

17. $\frac{13\frac{1}{3}}{4\frac{6}{13}} =$ ________

18. $\frac{\frac{1}{10}}{\frac{2}{3}} =$ ________

19. $\frac{1}{125} \times \frac{1}{25} =$ ________

20. $\frac{\frac{7}{8}}{\frac{1}{3}} \div \frac{3\frac{1}{2}}{\frac{1}{3}} =$ ________

21. $\frac{20}{35} \times 3 =$ ________

22. $2\frac{1}{4} \times 7\frac{1}{8} =$ ________

Perform the indicated operation, and round the answer to two decimal places.

23. $11.33 + 29.16 + 19.78 =$ ________

24. $93.712 - 26.97 =$ ________

25. $43.69 - 0.7083 =$ ________

26. $66.4 \times 72.8 =$ ________

27. $360 \times 0.53 =$ ________

28. $268.4 \div 14 =$ ________

29. $10.10 - 0.62 =$ ________

30. $5 + 2.5 + 0.05 + 0.15 =$ ________

31. $1.71 \times 25 =$ ________

32. $45 \div 0.15 =$ ________

33. $2974 \div 0.23 =$ ________

34. $51.21 \div 0.016 =$ ________

35. $0.74 \div 0.37 =$ ________

36. $1.5 + 146.73 + 1.9 + 0.832 =$ ________

Multiply or divide by the power of 10 indicated. Draw an arrow to demonstrate movement of the decimal point.

37. $9.716 \times 1000 =$ ________

38. $50.25 \div 100 =$ ________

39. $0.25 \times 100 =$ ________

40. $5.75 \times 1000 =$ ________

41. $0.25 \div 10 =$ ________

42. $11.525 \times 10 =$ ________

43. You are to administer 4 tablets with a dosage strength of 0.04 mg each. What total dosage will you give? ________

44. After your five-student team completes 1/2 of an assignment together, one member becomes ill and cannot complete his share. Write a fraction, reduced to the lowest terms, of the remaining portion of the assignment that each student must now do in order to complete the assignment.

____

45. Tablets are labelled 0.1 mg and you are to give $3\frac{1}{2}$ (3.5) tablets. What total dosage is this?

____

46. Last week a nurse earning $17.43 per hour gross pay worked 40 hours plus 6.25 hours of overtime, which is paid at twice the hourly rate. What is the total gross pay for last week for this nurse, including regular and overtime pay? ________

47. The instructional assistant is ordering supplies for the nursing skills laboratory. A single box of 12 urinary catheters costs $98.76. A case of 12 boxes of these catheters costs $975. Calculate the savings per catheter when a case is purchased. ________

48. You are to administer 1.25 mg of a medication. Each tablet of that medication has a strength of 0.5 mg. How many tablets do you need to administer? ________

49. Mr. Makela is to receive 1200 millilitres of fluid in a 24-hour period. How many millilitres should he drink between the hours of 7:00 AM and 7:00 PM if he is to receive $\frac{2}{3}$ of the total amount during that time? ________

50. A baby weighed 3.7 kilograms at birth. The baby now weighs 6.65 kilograms. How many kilograms did the baby gain? ________

After completing these problems, see page 454 in the answer section to check your answers.

CHAPTER

2

Ratios and Percents

LEARNING OBJECTIVES

1. Interpret values expressed in ratios and percentages.
2. Read and write ratios and percents.
3. Calculate the percent of a quantity.
4. Interpret values expressed in ratios and percentages.
5. Compare values expressed in fractions, decimals, ratios, and percents.
6. Convert among fractions, decimals, ratios, and percentages.

Healthcare professionals may use fractions, decimals, percents, and ratios to calculate a variety of medications and treatments. It is important to be able to quickly and accurately convert among them.

RATIOS

A *ratio* is another way of indicating the relationship between two numbers. In other words, it is another way to express a fraction. Ratios can be written as a fraction (1/10) or as two numbers separated by a colon (1:10). The latter can be read "one is to ten". The colon is a traditional way to write the division sign within a ratio.

Example 1:

3:4 is read "three *is to* four"

Example 2:

On an evening shift, if there are 5 nurses and 35 patients, what is the ratio of nurses to patients?
5 nurses to 35 patients = 5 nurses per 35 patients = $\frac{5}{35} = \frac{1}{7}$. This is the same as a ratio of 5:35 or 1:7.

> **MATH TIP**
>
> The terms of a ratio are the *numerator* (always to the left of the colon) and the *denominator* (always to the right of the colon) of a fraction. Like fractions, ratios should be stated in lowest terms.

Example 3:

Epinephrine 1:1000 for injection = 1 part epinephrine to 1000 total parts of solution. It is a fact that 1:1000 is the same as $\frac{1}{1000}$ and 0.001.

In some drug solutions such as epinephrine 1:1000, the ratio is used to indicate the drug's concentration. This will be covered in more detail later in this chapter.

The strength of a drug that is diluted can be expressed as a ratio—that is, a numerical relationship between two quantities.

Example 1:

The ratio 1:2 (one to two) indicates that there is 1 part drug to 2 parts of solution. This solution can also be expressed as $\frac{1}{2}$ strength solution.

Example 2:

The ratio 1:10 (one to ten) indicates that there is 1 part drug to 10 parts of solution. This solution can also be expressed as $\frac{1}{10}$ strength solution.

Ratio and Proportion

Proportion is an equation that contains two ratios of equal value. You may recognize this as calculations done in elementary and/or secondary classrooms. Proportions can be used to calculate medication dosages. Although the method is not difficult to learn and use, healthcare professionals and researchers who have studied calculations methods used by beginning and seasoned healthcare professionals have repeatedly found that using this method seems to result in more medication errors than using dimensional analysis or what is called the "formula method." These latter two methods will be discussed in more detail in Chapter 4.

CAUTION

Although ratios and a medication calculation method called "ratio and proportion" is one way of calculating drug dosages and is still used successfully by some healthcare practitioners, evidence is emerging that this methodology holds extra difficulties for the beginning nurse professional who is learning medication calculations (Kohtz & Gowda, 2010; Koohestani & Baghcheghi, 2010; Rice & Bell, 2005).[1] Therefore, in this text, although the writers acknowledge information about ratios, describe them, and show how to read, write, and convert them in this chapter, for the remainder of this text, students will not be encouraged to use ratios in their calculation of medication dosages.

PERCENTS

A percent is a fourth way to show a fractional relationship. Fractions, decimals, ratios, and percents can all be converted from one form to the others. *Percent* comes from the Latin phrase *per centum*, which means *per hundred.* Conversions of fractions and decimals were discussed in Chapter 1. A percent indicates a value equal to the number of hundredths. That is, when a percent is written as a fraction, the denominator is always 100.

---

[1] Kohtz, C., & Gowda, C. (2010). Teaching drug calculation in nursing education. *Nurse Educator*, *35*(2), 83–86. doi:10.1097/NNE.0b013e3181ced8a8

Koohestani, H., & Baghcheghi, N. (2010). Comparing the effects of two educational methods of intravenous drug rate calculations on rapid and sustained learning of nursing students: Formula method and dimensional analysis method. *Nurse Education in Practice*, *10*(4), 233–237. doi:10.1016/j.nepr.2009.11.011

Rice, J. N., & Bell, M. L. (2005). Using dimensional analysis to improve drug dosage calculation ability. *Journal of Nursing Education*, *44*(7), 315–318.

MATH TIP

To remember the value of a given percent, replace the % symbol with "/" for *per* and "100" for *cent*. THINK: *Percent* (%) means "/100."

Example:

$$3\% = 3 \text{ percent} = 3/100 = \frac{3}{100} = 0.03$$

Converting between Ratios, Percents, Fractions, and Decimals

When you understand the relationship of ratios, percents, fractions, and decimals, you can readily convert from one to the other. Let's begin by converting a percent to a fraction.

RULE

To convert a percent to a fraction:
1. **Delete the % sign,**
2. **Write the remaining number as the numerator,**
3. **Write 100 as the denominator, and**
4. **Reduce the result to lowest terms.**

Example:

$$5\% = \frac{5}{100} = \frac{1}{20}$$

It is also easy to express a percent as a ratio.

RULE

To convert a percent to a ratio:
1. **Delete the % sign,**
2. **Write the remaining number as the numerator,**
3. **Write "100" as the denominator,**
4. **Reduce the result to lowest terms, and**
5. **Express the fraction as a ratio.**

Example:

$$25\% = \frac{25}{100} = \frac{1}{4} = 1{:}4$$

In reading a ratio, the colon is read *is to.*

Because the denominator of a percent is always 100, it is easy to find the equivalent decimal. Recall that to divide by 100, you move the decimal point two places to the left, the number of places equal to the number of zeros in the denominator. This is the hundredths place.

RULE

To convert a percent to a decimal:
1. **Delete the % sign, and**
2. **Divide the remaining number by 100, which is the same as moving the decimal point 2 places to the left.**

Example:

$$25\% = \frac{25}{100} = 25 \div 100 = .25. = 0.25$$

Conversely, it is easy to change a decimal to a percent.

RULE

To convert a decimal to a percent:
1. **Multiply the decimal number by 100 (move the decimal point 2 places to the right), and**
2. **Add the % sign.**

Example:

$$0.25 \times 100 = 0.25. = 25\%$$

Now you know all the steps to change a ratio to the equivalent percent.

RULE

To convert a ratio to a percent:
1. **Convert the ratio to a fraction,**
2. **Convert the fraction to a decimal, and**
3. **Convert the decimal to a percent.**

Example:

Convert 1:1000 epinephrine solution to the equivalent concentration expressed as a percent.

1. $1{:}1000 = \frac{1}{1000}$ (ratio converted to fraction)
2. $\frac{1}{1000} = .001. = 0.001$ (fraction converted to decimal)
3. $0.001 = 0.00.1 = 0.1\%$ (decimal converted to percent)

Thus, 1:1000 epinephrine solution = 0.1% epinephrine solution.

Review the preceding example again slowly until it is clear. Ask your instructor for assistance, as needed. If you go over this one step at a time, you can master these important calculations. You need never fear fractions, decimals, ratios, and percents again.

Comparing Percents and Ratios

Nurses and other healthcare professionals frequently administer solutions with the concentration expressed as a percent or ratio. Consider two intravenous solutions given directly into a person's vein: one that is 0.9%; the other 5%. It is important to be clear that 0.9% is *smaller* than 5%. A 0.9% solution means that there are 0.9 parts of the solid per 100 total parts (0.9 parts is less than one whole part, so it is less than 1%). Compare this to the 5% solution, with 5 parts of the solid (or more than 5 times 0.9 parts) per 100 total parts. Therefore, the 5% solution is much more concentrated, or stronger, than the 0.9% solution. A misunderstanding of these numbers and the quantities they represent can have dire consequences.

Likewise, you may see a solution concentration expressed as $\frac{1}{3}$ % and another expressed as 0.45%. Convert these amounts to equivalent decimals to clarify values and compare concentrations.

$$\frac{1}{3}\% = \frac{\frac{1}{3}}{100} = \frac{1}{3} \div \frac{100}{1} = \frac{1}{3} \times \frac{1}{100} = \frac{1}{300} = 0.0033$$

$$0.45\% = \frac{0.45}{100} = 0.0045 \text{ (greater value, stronger concentration)}$$

Compare solution concentrations expressed as a ratio, such as 1:1000 and 1:100.

$$1{:}1000 = \frac{1}{1000} = 0.001$$

$1{:}100 = \frac{1}{100} = 0.01$ or 0.010 (add zero for comparison) 1:100 is a stronger concentration.

QUICK REVIEW

- Fractions, decimals, ratios, and percents are related equivalents.

  Example: $1{:}2 = \frac{1}{2} = 0.5 = 50\%$
- Like fractions, ratios should be reduced to their lowest terms.

  Example: $2{:}4 = 1{:}2$
- To express a ratio as a fraction, the number to the left of the colon becomes the numerator, and the number to the right of the colon becomes the denominator. The colon in a ratio is equivalent to the division sign in a fraction.

  Example: $2{:}3 = \frac{2}{3}$
- To change a ratio to a decimal, convert the ratio to a fraction, and divide the numerator by the denominator.

  Example: $1{:}4 = \frac{1}{4} = 1 \div 4 = 0.25$
- To change a percent to a fraction, drop the % sign and place the remaining number as the numerator over the denominator 100. Reduce the fraction to its lowest terms. THINK: per (/) cent (100).

  Example: $75\% = \frac{75}{100} = \frac{3}{4}$
- To change a percent to a ratio, first convert the percent to a fraction in its lowest terms. Then, place the numerator to the left of a colon and the denominator to the right of that colon.

  Example: $35\% = \frac{35}{100} = \frac{7}{20} = 7{:}20$
- To change a percent to a decimal, drop the % sign, and divide by 100.

  Example: 4% = .04. = 0.04
- To change a decimal to a percent, multiply by 100, and add the % sign.

  Example: 0.5 = 0.50. = 50%
- To change a ratio to a percent, first convert the ratio to a fraction. Convert the fraction to a decimal and then the decimal to a percent.

  Example: $1{:}2 = \frac{1}{2} = 1 \div 2 = 0.5 =$ 0.50. = 50%

REVIEW SET 7

Change the following ratios to fractions that are reduced to their lowest terms.

1. $3:150 =$ ________
2. $6:10 =$ ________
3. $0.05:0.15 =$ ________

Change the following ratios to decimals; round to two decimal places, if needed.

4. $20:40 =$ ________
5. $\frac{1}{1000}:\frac{1}{150} =$ ________
6. $0.3:4.5 =$ ________
7. $1\frac{1}{2}:6\frac{2}{9} =$ ________

Change the following ratios to percents; round to two decimal places, if needed.

8. $12:48 =$ ________
9. $0.08:0.64 =$ ________
10. $7:10 =$ ________
11. $50:100 =$ ________

Change the following percents to fractions that are reduced to their lowest terms.

12. $45\% =$ ________
13. $0.5\% =$ ________
14. $1\% =$ ________
15. $66\frac{2}{3}\% =$ ________

Change the following percents to decimals; round to two decimal places, if needed.

16. $2.94\% =$ ________
17. $33\% =$ ________
18. $0.9\% =$ ________

Change the following percents to ratios that are reduced to their lowest terms.

19. $16\% =$ ________
20. $25\% =$ ________
21. $50\% =$ ________

Which of the following is largest? Circle your answer.

22. 0.9% 0.9 1:9 $\frac{1}{90}$
23. 0.05 $\frac{200}{400}$ 0.025 1:25
24. 0.0125% 0.25% 0.1% 0.02%
25. $\frac{1}{150}$ $\frac{1}{300}$ 0.5 $\frac{2}{3}\%$

After completing these problems, see page 455 in the answer section to check your answers.

PERCENTAGE MEASURES

Percentage strengths are used extensively in intravenous solutions, and for a variety of other medications, such as eye drops and ointments and other topical (for external use) ointments. Since percentage (%) means "parts per hundred," the higher the percentage strength, the stronger the solution or ointment. Note: Percentage notations are made with no space between the quantity and the symbol, for example 15%.

Another way the healthcare professional uses percentages is in calculating an amount. For example, a patient reports that he drank 75% of his 200-mL cup of coffee for breakfast. To record the amount he actually drank in his chart, you must determine what amount is 75% of 200 mL.

RULE

To find a percentage (part) of a whole = *Percent × Whole Quantity*

1. **Change the percent to a fraction multiplied by (×) the whole quantity.**
2. **Reduce the fraction to its lowest terms; and**
3. **Multiply the fraction by the whole quantity, using the skill you learned in Chapter 1, i.e.,**
    a. **Cancel terms;**
    b. **Multiply numerators for the numerator of the answer, multiply denominators for the denominator of the answer; and**
    c. **Reduce the result (product) to its lowest terms.**

To continue with the example:

Percentage (Part) = Percent × Whole Quantity

1. Change 75% to a fraction and multiply by the whole quantity:

    $$\frac{75}{100} \times 200\,\text{mL}$$

2. Reduce the fraction to its lowest terms:

    reduces down by dividing each number by 25 i.e. 75 divided by 25 → 3; 100 divided by 25 → 4

    $$\frac{\overset{3}{\cancel{75}}}{\underset{4}{\cancel{100}}} \times 200\text{ mL}$$

3. Multiply $\frac{3}{4} \times 200$:

    a. 4 reduces to 1 and 200 reduces to 50 when each is divided by 4

    $$\frac{3}{\underset{1}{\cancel{4}}} \times \overset{50}{\cancel{200}}$$

    b. Multiply 3 × 50 = 150 mL

    c. Note that denominator is 1.

4. Therefore, 75% of 200 mL is 150 mL.

Percentage (Part) = Percent × Whole Quantity

To find a percentage or part of a whole quantity:

MATH TIP

In a mathematical expression, the word *of* means *times* and indicates that you should multiply.

QUICK REVIEW

Percentage (Part) = Percent × Whole Quantity

Example: What is 15% of 48? $X = 15\% \times 48 = \frac{15}{100} \times 48$

$$= \frac{\overset{}{15}}{\underset{25}{\cancel{100}}} \times \overset{12}{\cancel{48}} = \frac{\overset{3}{\cancel{15}}}{\underset{5}{\cancel{25}}} \times 12 = \frac{3}{5} \times 12 = \frac{36}{5} = 7.2$$

REVIEW SET 8

Perform the indicated operation; round decimals to hundredths place.

1. What is 0.25% of 520? ________
2. What is 5% of 95? ________
3. What is 40% of 140? ________
4. What is 0.7% of 62? ________
5. What is 3% of 889? ________
6. What is 20% of 75? ________
7. What is 4% of 20? ________
8. What is 7% of 34? ________
9. What is 15% of 250? ________
10. What is 75% of 150? ________
11. Mr. Ping has an order for an anti-infective in the amount of 500 milligrams by mouth twice a day for 10 days to treat pneumonia. He received a bottle of 20 pills. How many pills has Mr. Ping taken if he has used 40% of the 20 pills? ________
12. Ms. Cho is on oral fluid restrictions of 1200 millilitres for a 24-hour period. For breakfast and lunch she has consumed 60% of the total fluid allowance. How many millilitres has she had? ________
13. Ms. Little's hospital bill for surgery is $17 651.07. Her insurance company pays 80%. How much will she owe? ________
14. Table salt (sodium chloride) is 40% sodium by weight. If a box of salt weighs 750 grams, how much sodium is in the box of salt? ________
15. Mr. Yoder has an average daily intake of 3500 calories. At breakfast he eats 20% of the total daily caloric allowance. How many calories did he ingest? ________

After completing these problems, see page 455 in the answer section to check your answers.

PRACTICE PROBLEMS—CHAPTER 2

Find the equivalent decimal, fraction, percent, and ratio forms. Reduce fractions and ratios to their lowest terms; round decimals to two places.

	Decimal	Fraction	Percent	Ratio
1.	________	$\frac{2}{5}$	________	________
2.	0.05	________	________	________
3.	________	________	17%	________
4.	________	________	________	1:4

5. ________	________	6%	________
6. ________	$\frac{1}{6}$	________	________
7. ________	________	50%	________
8. ________	________	________	1:100
9. 0.09	________	________	________
10. ________	$\frac{3}{8}$	________	________
11. ________	________	________	2:3
12. ________	$\frac{1}{3}$	________	________
13. 0.52	________	________	________
14. ________	________	________	9:20
15. ________	$\frac{6}{7}$	________	________
16. ________	________	________	3:10
17. ________	$\frac{1}{50}$	________	________
18. 0.06	________	________	________
19. 0.04	________	________	________
20. ________	________	10%	________

Convert as indicated.

21. 1:25 to a decimal ________
22. $\frac{10}{400}$ to a ratio ________
23. 0.075 to a percent ________
24. 17:34 to a fraction ________
25. 75% to a ratio ________

Perform the indicated operation. Round decimals to hundredths.

26. What is 35% of 750? ________
27. What is 7% of 52? ________
28. What is 8.3% of 24? ________

Identify the strongest solution in each of the following:

29. 1:40 1:400 1:4 ________
30. 1:10 1:200 1:50 ________

To calculate the following, use your skills of reducing terms, multiplying and dividing fractions, and converting fractions to decimals. Express your answers as decimals rounded to the nearest hundredth.

31. $1680 \times \frac{20}{400} =$ ________
32. $\frac{4}{75} \div \frac{1}{300} =$ ________
33. $\frac{3}{15} \times 5 =$ ________
34. $2.2 \times 250 \div 500 =$ ________

35. $0.6 \times \frac{200}{1.2} =$ ______

36. $11\frac{7}{9} \times 3 =$ ______

37. $\frac{1}{8} \div \frac{1}{3} \times 2 =$ ______

38. $\frac{7}{4} \times 12 =$ ______

39. $\frac{9}{0.6} \times 8 =$ ______

40. $\frac{0.4}{0.1} \times 22.5 =$ ______

41. There are 368 people employed at Riverview Clinic. If $\frac{3}{8}$ of the employees are nurses, $\frac{1}{8}$ are maintenance/cleaners, $\frac{1}{4}$ are technicians, and $\frac{1}{4}$ are all other employees, calculate the number of employees that each fraction represents. ______

42. A portion of meat totalling 125 grams contains 20% protein and 5% fat. How many grams each of protein and fat does the meat contain? ______ protein ______ fat

43. The total points for a course in a nursing program is 308. A nursing student needs to achieve 75% of the total points to pass the semester. How many points are required to pass? ______

44. To work off 90 calories, Angie must walk for 27 minutes. How many minutes would she need to walk to work off 200 calories? ______

45. The doctor orders a record of the patient's fluid intake and output. The patient drinks 25% of a bowl of broth. How many millilitres of intake will be recorded if the bowl holds 200 millilitres?

______

46. The recommended daily allowance (RDA) of a particular vitamin is 60 milligrams. If a multivitamin tablet claims to provide 45% of the RDA, how many milligrams of the particular vitamin would a patient receive from the multivitamin tablet? ______

47. A patient received an intravenous medication at a rate of 6.75 milligrams per minute. After 42 minutes, how much medication had she received? ______

48. A person weighed 60 kilograms at his last doctor's office visit. At today's visit the patient has lost 5% of his weight. How many kilograms has the patient lost? ______

49. The cost of a certain medication is expected to decrease by 17% next year. If the cost is $12.56 now, how much would you expect it to cost at this time next year? ______

50. A patient is to be started on 150 milligrams of a medication and then decreased by 10% of the original dose for each dose until he is receiving 75 milligrams. When he takes his 75-milligram dose, how many total doses will he have taken? HINT: Be sure to count his first (150 milligrams) and last (75 milligrams) doses. ______

After completing these problems, see pages 455–456 in the answer section to check your answers.

CHAPTER

3

Systems of Measurement

LEARNING OBJECTIVES

1. Identify the International System of Units (SI).
2. Accurately express the SI units commonly used in the health sector.
3. Accurately interpret the relationship between selected SI prefixes.
4. Recognize common equivalents among the SI and household system.
5. Identify and accurately express non-SI units used in the health sector.
6. Convert between traditional and international time.

Measurement systems have been developed and modified by custom and local adaptations throughout history. Three measurement systems for calculating drug dosages have been used in Canada in the past century. They include the household system, the apothecary system, and the current, International System of Units (SI).

Converting among the systems is less common now in the health sector but there are a few instances in which this may still be necessary. One instance is if the healthcare professional is working in the community and/or giving instructions to a patient or family. In everyday life, Canadians use a variety of measurement systems. It is not uncommon to measure sugar by the teaspoon, a picture frame in inches, or buy grocery produce by the pound. Similarly, a Canadian-educated healthcare professional may choose to work in a country whose health sector uses a variety of measurement systems. So it is still important for Canadian healthcare professionals to understand some approximate conversions among the various systems.

THE INTERNATIONAL SYSTEM OF UNITS

The decimal metric system, based on the metre and kilogram, can be historically traced to the French Revolution (1789–1799). In 1875, the Bureau International des Poids et Mesures (BIPM) was established in France. Its mandate was to provide "the basis for a single, coherent system of measurement to be used throughout the world."[1] Over time, the system evolved and, even today, continues to be refined. In 1960, after a long series of international discussions, the Système International d'Unités was established. In English, the system was known as the *International System of Units.*

It is believed that 98% of the world population uses metric units. The SI is considered the most up-to-date version of the metric system.[2] The advantages of the SI include the following: It is coherent, logical, and simpler to use than other systems. Its globally uniform descriptions, terms, and symbols enhance international communication. It has only seven base units instead of the countless units of the various other systems. These factors, plus the elimination of the need to convert between various systems, can help ensure safety in healthcare.

---

[1] BIPM. (2006). *A concise summary of the International System of Units, the SI.* Retrieved from the BIPM website: http://www.bipm.org.

[2] U.S. Metric Association (USMA), Inc. (2009). Metric usage and metrication in other countries. Retrieved from http://lamar.colostate.edu/~hillger/internat.htm

Although use of the metric system was legalized in Canada in 1871, it was 100 years before Canada proclaimed a Weights and Measures Act to start the process of ensuring "all units of measurement used in Canada shall be determined on the basis of [SI]."[1] Ten years after this proclamation, after much discussion and planning, the health sector implemented its plan for conversion to SI. Due to government flip-flopping, customer apathy, and administrative stubbornness, Canadian metrication stumbled and stalled. Finally, in 1983, a moratorium on metrication was declared. Today, even though a hodgepodge of SI and imperial systems is used in everyday life in Canada, the health sector has maintained the conversion to SI.

One of the features of the SI is its use of only seven *base units.* Five of these units are commonly used in the health sector: length, mass, amount of substance, time, and thermodynamic temperature.

Base Quantity	Base Unit	Symbol
length	metre[2]	m
mass	gram	g
time, duration	second	s
thermodynamic temperature	Kelvin[3]	K
amount of substance	mole[4]	mol

FIGURE 3-1 SI Units Used in the Health Sector[5]

One of the advantages of SI noted previously is that it is logical. Since the SI is based on the decimal system, prefixes are used to express numbers that are much larger or much smaller than the base unit. The only exception is the gram, which, for historical reasons, is considered a base unit. To express multiples and submultiples of the gram, attach the desired prefix to the unit name *gram.* Multiples and submultiples commonly used in the health sector and their respective symbols and values are in the table that follows.

Prefix	Symbol	Numerical Value	Alternative Way of Expressing
kilo	k	1000	10^{3}
centi	c	0.01	10^{-2}
milli	m	0.001	10^{-3}
micro	μ[6] or mcg	0.000 001	10^{-6}

FIGURE 3-2 SI Prefixes[7]

Even where the SI system is officially recognized as the only system of units, some non-SI units, defined in terms of SI units, are still widely used because of historical reasons or because they are deeply embedded in our culture. Two that are commonly used in the health sector are units of time and volume.

---

[1] Weights and Measures Act, R.S.C. 1970-71-72, c. 36, s. 4(1).

[2] *Metre* and *meter* are both correct spellings. Most nations use the former while the latter is commonly used in the United States.

[3] Note: The temperature commonly used in SI is Celsius, a derivative of the base unit, Kelvin. Celsius, Kelvin, and Fahrenheit temperature units are discussed in more detail in Appendix D.

[4] Mole is defined as the number of atoms in exactly 12 g of carbon-12 isotope. Many chemistry reports of blood tests are expressed in molar units. Drug plasma levels are reported in molar units in SI, for example, minimoles per litre (mmol/L).

[5] See Appendix B for the complete list of base units and a reference for additional information to explore the other units.

[6] The official symbol is μ (Greek small letter *mu*) but, to avoid confusion in expressing medication dosages, *mc* (without the italics) is recommended.

[7] See Appendix A for a complete list of SI multiple and submultiple prefixes.

Quantity	Unit	Symbol	Relation to SI
time	minute	min	1 min = 60 s
	hour	h	1 h = 3600 s
	day	d	1 d = 86 400 s
volume	litre[1]	L or l[2]	1 L = 1 dm^3

FIGURE 3-3 Commonly used non-SI units

RULE

To express SI units:

- **Symbols of units are written in lower case except when they are named for a person or at the beginning of a sentence.**
- **Prefixes are in lower case except at the beginning of a sentence.**
- **Symbols of units and prefixes are printed in non-italics.**
- **Prefix symbols are attached to the unit symbols without a space.**
- **Neither symbols of units nor prefixes are pluralized.**
- **Prefix names and symbols can be used with many non-SI units except for units of time.**
- **A space must separate the digits from the symbols.**
- **In the English language, the decimal marker is a period (.). (In a number of European languages and in some other countries a comma is used as the decimal marker.)**
- **In writing numbers with many digits, group the digits in threes around the decimal point and separate the groups with a space. In Canada, instead of a space, you will often see commas used to separate groups of three digits.**
- **In four-digit numbers, leaving a space is optional (e.g., both 1 000 and 1000 are correct).**

REMEMBER

To avoid confusion:

- Always use the capitalized *L* to indicate litre. The lower case *l* is easily confused with the number one (1).
- Always use *mcg* to indicate microgram. The μ symbol is easily misunderstood.

CAUTION

You may see *gram* abbreviated as *Gm* or *gm*, litre as lowercase *l*, or millilitre as *ml*. These abbreviations are considered unsafe because they are too easily misinterpreted. You should only use the standardized SI abbreviations. Use *g* for gram, *L* for litre, and *mL* for millilitre.[3]

CAUTION

The SI abbreviations for milligram (*mg*) and millilitre (*mL*) appear to be somewhat similar, but in fact mg is a weight unit and mL is a volume unit. Confusing these two units can have dire consequences in dosage calculations. Learn to clearly differentiate them now.

The metric system is the most common and the only standardized system of measurement in health-care. Take a few minutes to review these essential points.

---

[1] *Litre* and *liter* are both correct spellings. Most nations use the former while the latter is used in the United States.

[2] To avoid confusion with the number one, the symbol for the litre should be capital L.

[3] Institute for Safe Medication Practices. (2010). ISMP's list of error-prone abbreviations, symbols, and dose designations. Retrieved from ISMP_Canada Website: www.ismp-canada.org/.

QUICK REVIEW

In SI:

- The common units are gram, litre, metre, and mole.
- Subunits are designated by the appropriate prefix and the base unit (such as *milli*gram) and standardized abbreviations (such as *mg*).
- The unit or abbreviation always follows the amount.
- Decimals are used to designate fractional amounts.
- Use a zero to emphasize the decimal point for fractional amounts of less than 1.
- Omit unnecessary zeros.
- Multiply or divide by 1000 to derive most equivalents needed for dosage calculations.
- When in doubt about the exact amount or the abbreviation used, do not guess. Ask the writer to clarify.

REVIEW SET 9

1. The system of measurement most commonly used for prescribing and administering medications is the ________ system.
2. Litre and millilitre are SI units that measure ________.
3. Gram and milligram are SI units that measure ________.
4. Metre and millimetre are SI units that measure ________.
5. 1 mg is ________ of a g.
6. There are ________ mL in a litre.
7. 10 mL = ________ cc
8. Which is largest—kilogram, gram, or milligram? ________
9. Which is smallest—kilogram, gram, or milligram? ________
10. 1 litre = ________ mL
11. 1000 mcg = ________ mg
12. 1 kg = ________ g
13. 1 cm = ________ mm

Select the *correct* metric notation.

14. .3 g, 0.3 Gm, 0.3 g, .3 Gm, 0.30 g ________
15. $1\frac{1}{3}$ ml, 1.33 mL, 1.33 ML, $1\frac{1}{3}$ ML, 1.330 mL ________
16. 5 Kg, 5.0 kg, kg 05, 5 kg, 5 kG ________
17. 1.5 mm, $1\frac{1}{2}$ mm, 1.5 Mm, 1.50 MM, $1\frac{1}{2}$ MM ________
18. mg 10, 10 mG, 10.0 mg, 10 mg, 10 MG ________

Interpret these SI abbreviations.

19. mcg ________
20. mL ________
21. mmol ________
22. g ________
23. mm ________
24. kg ________
25. cm ________

After completing these problems, see page 456 in the answer section to check your answers.

HOUSEHOLD AND APOTHECARY SYSTEMS OF MEASUREMENT

As noted in the opening of this chapter, Canadians use a variety of measurement units in everyday life even though SI units are the only units used in the healthcare system. Sometimes Canadian healthcare professionals work in the community, so it is appropriate to know equivalent measurement units for common measurements that could be more familiar to the individual patient and/or family. For this purpose, the following table notes four units of volume, two units of mass, and one unit of length with which Canadian healthcare professionals working in a community context should be aware. The values shown are approximate equivalents. A more complete explanation and an alternative approximate equivalency (some would argue "more accurate equivalents") can be found in Appendixes B and C (pages 527–529), respectively.

REMEMBER

Approximate equivalent	*SI measurement*
1 teaspoon (t)	5 mL
1 tablespoon (Tbs)	15 mL
1 cup	240 mL
1 quart (qt)	1 litre
1 fluid ounce (oz)	30 mL
2.2 pounds (lb or #)	1 kg
1 inch (in or ")	2.54 cm

SPECIAL CLASSES OF UNITS OF MEASUREMENT

Units and milliequivalents are measurements used to indicate the strength or potency of a drug. Neither can be directly converted into any other system of measurement.

Units describe biological effects that cannot yet be known or defined precisely in SI units. Since medications measured this way are important for human health and safety, the World Health Organization takes responsibility to define International Units (IU) for these substances. Technically, the *unit* is a measurement of standardized potency versus a weight per volume, as in the majority of medications. Insulin, hormones, vitamins, anticoagulants, and penicillin are common examples of medications measured in units. Some drugs that were once standardized by units may later be synthesized to their chemical composition but still retain units as the indicator of their potency.

Milliequivalents compose a measurement of combining or reacting value or power versus weight per volume. Technically, the milliequivalent measures the strength of an ion concentration. It is the expression of the number of grams of a drug contained in 1 mL of a normal solution. Milliequivalents are used to measure a variety of mineral and electrolyte replacements and supplements. Also, the milliequivalent is the unit used when referring to the concentration of serum electrolytes. Potassium chloride is a common electrolyte replacement that is ordered in milliequivalents.

The official abbreviation for units is *u,* but it is now recommended, in order to avoid confusion, that the word *units* be written out.[1] The prefix *milli* is sometimes used with the term *unit,* to indicate 0.001 units. The abbreviation for *international units* is *IU.* The abbreviations for milliequivalents is *mEq.*

It is not necessary to learn conversions for the international unit, unit, or milliequivalent because medications prescribed in these measurements are also prepared and administered in the same system.

---

[1] ISMP Canada, 2010.

Example 1:

Heparin sodium *800 units* subcutaneously are prescribed, and *heparin* sodium *1000 units/mL* is the stock drug.

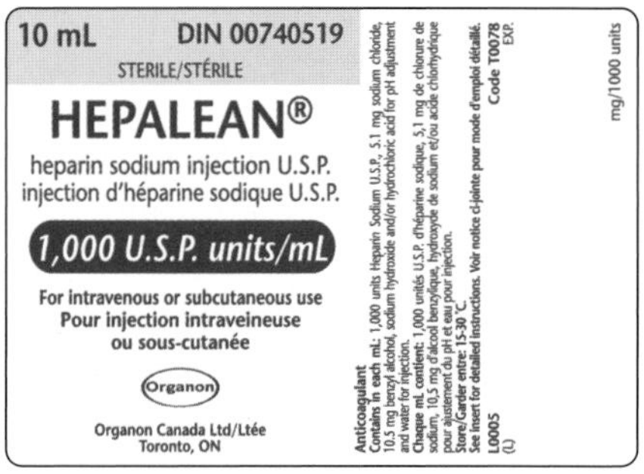

Example 2:

Potassium chloride 10 mEq orally is prescribed, and *potassium chloride 20 mEq/15 mL* is the stock drug.

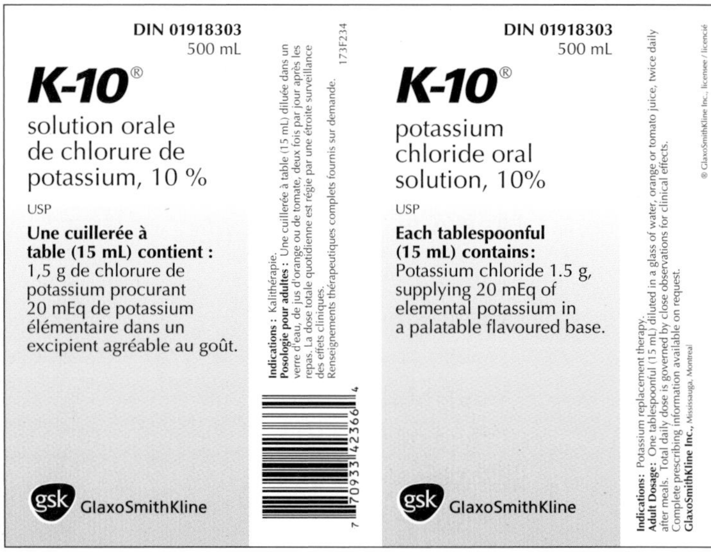

Example 3:

Oxytocin 2 milliunits (0.002 units) intravenous per minute is prescribed and *oxytocin 10 units/mL* to be added to 1000-mL intravenous solution is available.

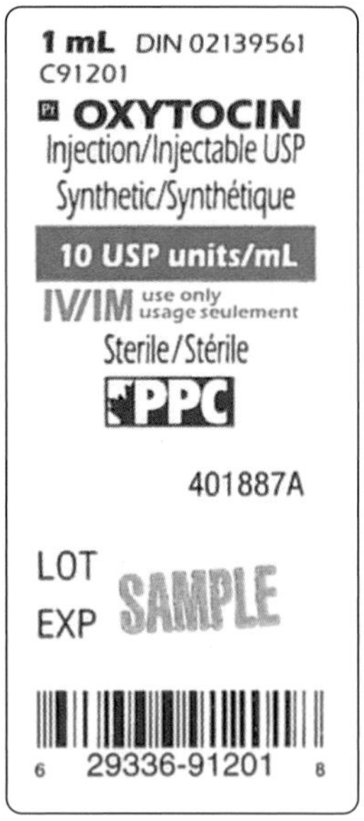

QUICK REVIEW

- The international unit (IU), unit, milliunit (mU), and milliequivalent (mEq) are specially measured quantities expressed in Arabic numbers followed by the unit or symbol.
- No conversion is necessary for units, IU, and mEq, because the ordered dosage and supply dosage are in the same system.
- 1 unit = 1000 mU.

REVIEW SET 10

Interpret the following notations.

1. 1000 units ________
2. 10 mEq ________

Express the following using correct notation.

3. 30 milliequivalents ________
4. 1500 units ________

5. The household system of measurement is commonly used in hospital dosage calculations. (True) (False)
6. Drugs such as heparin and insulin are commonly measured in ________, which is abbreviated ________.
7. The unit of potency used to measure vitamins and chemicals is the ________, and is abbreviated ________.
8. The unit frequently used to express the concentration of replacement electrolytes is ________.
9. 100 milliunits = ________ units.

After completing these problems, see page 456 in the answer section to check your answers.

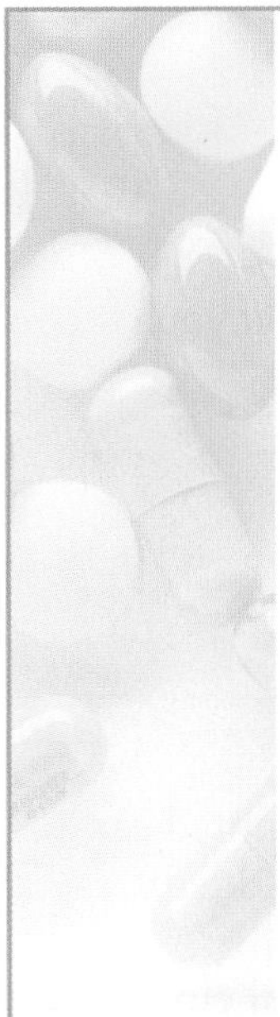

CRITICAL THINKING SKILLS

The importance of the placement of the decimal point cannot be overemphasized. Let's look at some examples of potential medication errors related to placement of the decimal point.

error 1

Not placing a zero before a decimal point on medication orders.

possible scenario

An emergency room physician wrote an order for the bronchodilator epinephrine for a patient with severe asthma. The order was written as follows:

epinephrine .5 mg subcutaneously now, repeat dose in 20 minutes if no improvement

Suppose the nurse, not noticing the faint decimal point, administered 5 mg of epinephrine subcutaneously instead of 0.5 mg. The patient would receive 10 times the dose intended by the physician.

potential outcome

Within minutes of receiving the injection, the patient would likely complain of headache and develop tachycardia, hypertension, nausea, and vomiting. The patient's hospital stay would be lengthened due to the need to recover from the overdose.

prevention

This type of medication error is avoided by remembering the rule to place a 0 in front of a decimal to avoid confusion regarding the dosage: 0.5 mg. Further, remember to question orders that are unclear or seem unreasonable.

CRITICAL THINKING SKILLS

Many medication errors occur by confusing mg and mL. Remember that mg is the weight of the medication, and mL is the volume of the medication preparation.

error 2

Confusing mg and mL.

possible scenario

Suppose a physician ordered morphine hydrochloride syrup (an opioid analgesic) 20 mg by mouth every 3–4 h for a patient with cancer. Morphine hydrochloride syrup is supplied in a concentration of 20 mg in 2 mL. The pharmacist supplied a bottle of morphine hydrochloride syrup containing a total volume of 250 mL with 20 mg of morphine hydrochloride in every 2 mL. The nurse, in a rush to give her medications on time, misread the order as 20 mL and gave the patient 20 mL of morphine hydrochloride syrup instead of 2 mL. Therefore, the patient received 200 mg of morphine hydrochloride syrup or 10 times the correct dosage.

potential outcome

The patient could develop a number of complications related to a high dosage of opiates: respiratory depression, hypotension, hallucinations, nausea, and vomiting, to name a few.

prevention

The mg is the weight of a medication, and mL is the volume you prepare. Do not allow yourself to get rushed or distracted so that you would confuse milligrams with millilitres. When you know you are distracted or stressed, have another nurse double-check the calculation of the dose.

TIME AND TEMPERATURE CONVERSIONS

Converting between Traditional and International Time

Any discussion on measurement units and medications must include the unit of *time.* As noted earlier in this chapter, the SI base unit of time is the second (s). However, due to deeply embedded tradition, the use of non-SI units such as minute, hour, and day are used with the SI.

Time is an important part of a medication regimen. Canada uses the 12-hour traditional clock in everyday life, the same as the United States and the United Kingdom. Two exceptions in Canada are French speakers in Quebec and around our national capital, Ottawa, where 24-hour time is commonly used. A third exception in Canada is the healthcare system. Several decades ago, Canada's healthcare system adopted the 24-hour clock as the standard for its system of time. This 24-hour clock system is also known as *international time.*

Look at a variation of the 24-hour clock (Figure 3-4). The figure uses an inner and outer circle of numbers. The numbers of the inner circle correlate with traditional AM time (12:00 midnight to 11:59 AM), time periods that are *ante meridian* or *before noon.* The numbers on the outer circle correlate with traditional PM time (12:00 noon to 11:59 PM), time periods that are *post meridian* or *after noon.*

Use of the 24-hour clock decreases the possibility for error in administering medications and documenting time of medication administration because no two times are expressed by the same number. Using the 24-hour clock decreases the risk for misinterpreting time. Two other advantages of the 24-hour clock include its computer compatibility and the greater ease of calculating the duration of time intervals.

In Canadian health institutions that display time, the time is either digitally displayed in the 24-hour clock format or as a traditional 12-hour clock with a second ring of numbers representing the hours between 1 PM (1300 hours) and midnight (2400 hours).

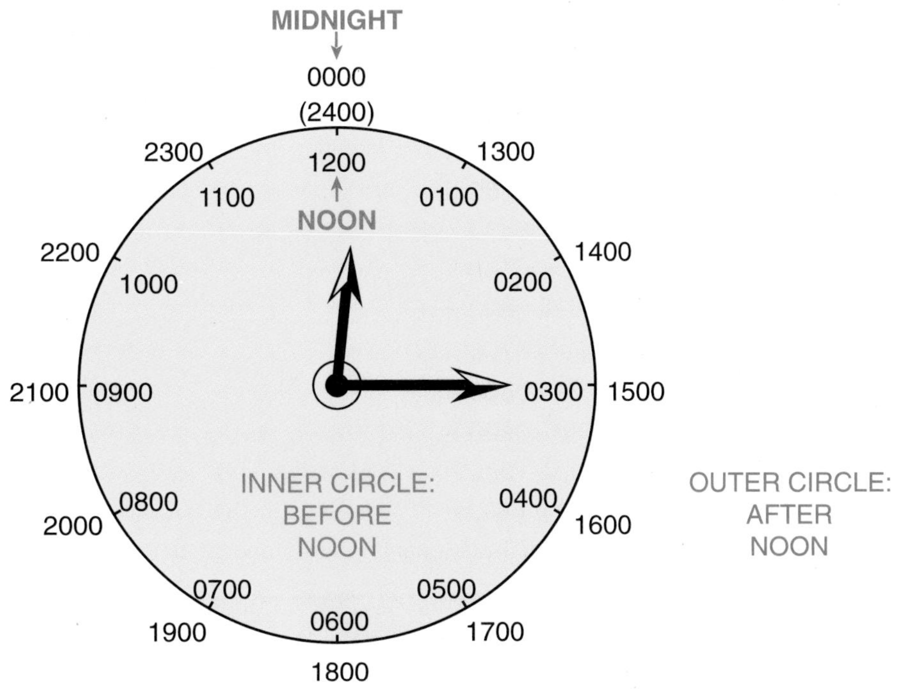

FIGURE 3-4 24-hour Clock Depicting 0015 h (12:15 AM) and 1215 h (12:15 PM)

All 24-hour clock times are expressed sequentially with 4 digits without colons and without AM and PM labels. The system starts at midnight. The first two digits express the number of hours since midnight. Midnight can be expressed as 2400 hours or as 0000 hours. It is most frequently written as 2400 hours but each minute after midnight is written as if midnight were 0000 hours. The term *hours* (or its abbreviation *h*) should always be written following the digits indicating the time.

RULE

- **For the minutes between 2400 h (midnight) and 0100 h (1 AM), state each zero before the number of minutes but label it hours.**
- **For hours after 0059 h, state the number in *hundreds* if the minutes are zero.**
- **For single digit hours, state the word *zero* before the hours.**
- **To indicate minutes and hours, state the hour (preceded by the *zero* if the hours is single digit), number of minutes, and follow this with the word *hours*.**

Examples:

0001 h (1 minute after midnight) is read *zero zero zero one hour*

0014 h (14 minutes after midnight) is read *zero zero fourteen hours*

0100 h (1 AM) is read *zero one hundred hours*

0630 h (6:30 AM) is read *zero six thirty hours*

1400 h (2 PM) is read *fourteen hundred hours*

1840 h (6:40 PM) is read *eighteen forty hours*

AM	Int'l. Time	PM	Int'l. Time
12:00 midnight	2400 h	12:00 noon	1200 h
1:00	0100 h	1:00	1300 h
2:00	0200 h	2:00	1400 h
3:00	0300 h	3:00	1500 h
4:00	0400 h	4:00	1600 h
5:00	0500 h	5:00	1700 h
6:00	0600 h	6:00	1800 h
7:00	0700 h	7:00	1900 h
8:00	0800 h	8:00	2000 h
9:00	0900 h	9:00	2100 h
10:00	1000 h	10:00	2200 h
11:00	1100 h	11:00	2300 h

FIGURE 3-5 Comparison of Traditional and International Time

RULE

1. **International time is designated by a unique four-digit number.**
2. **No punctuation is used between the numbers in international time.**
3. **Minutes after 12:00 AM (midnight) and before 1:00 AM are 0001 h through 0059 h in international time.**
4. **Traditional time and international time are the same hours starting with 1:00 AM (0100) through 12:59 PM (1259 h).**
5. **Hours starting with 1:00 PM through 12:00 AM (midnight) are 12:00 hours greater in international time (1300 h through 2400 h).**

MATH TIP

For the hours between 1:00 PM (1300 h) and 12:00 AM (2400 h), add 1200 h to the traditional time to find the equivalent international time; subtract 1200 h from the international time to convert to the equivalent traditional time.

Let us apply these rules to convert between the two time systems.

Example 1:

3:00 PM = 3:00 + 12:00 = 1500 h

Example 2:

2212 h = 2212 h – 1200 h = 10:12 PM

Example 3:

12:45 AM = 0045 h

Example 4:

0004 h = 12:04 AM

Example 5:

0130 h = 1:30 AM

Example 6:

11:00 AM = 1100 h

QUICK REVIEW

- The hours from 1:00 PM through 12:00 midnight are 12:00 hours greater in international time (1300 h through 2400 h).

CRITICAL THINKING SKILLS

error

Incorrect interpretation of order due to misunderstanding of traditional time.

possible scenario

A physician prescribed a mild sedative for an anxious patient who is scheduled for a sigmoidoscopy in the morning. The order read "*diazepam 5 mg orally at 6:00 × 1 dose.*" The evening nurse might have assumed that the physician intended this medication to reduce the client's anxiety and aid them in sleeping the night before the procedure. However, the nurse knew that sleeping aids are usually administered at bedtime, not at the time of evening preparations. The nurse practised critical thinking and contacted the physician to clarify the order. The physician said she meant for the diazepam to be given at 6 o'clock AM to help the patient relax prior to the actual test.

potential outcome

Diazepam would help the patient relax during the enema and make the patient sleepy. But it is not desirable for the patient to be drowsy or sedated during the evening preparations. Because of the omission of the AM designation, the patient would not benefit from this mild sedative at the intended time if the medication had been administered the evening before the test. The patient would have likely experienced unnecessary anxiety both before and during the test.

prevention

This scenario emphasizes the benefit of the 24-hour clock. If international time had been in use at this facility, the order would have been written as "*diazepam 5 mg orally at 0600 h × 1 dose,*" clearly indicating the exact time of administration, reducing the risk of error.

REVIEW SET 11

Give the following time equivalents as indicated.

AM/PM Clock	24-Hour Clock	AM/PM Clock	24-Hour Clock
1. ________	0257 h	11. 7:31 PM	________
2. 3:10 AM	________	12. 12:00 midnight	________
3. 4:22 PM	________	13. 6:45 AM	________
4. ________	2001 h	14. ________	0915 h
5. ________	1102 h	15. ________	2107 h
6. 12:33 AM	________	16. ________	1823 h
7. 2:16 AM	________	17. ________	0540 h
8. ________	1642 h	18. 11:55 AM	________
9. ________	2356 h	19. 10:12 PM	________
10. 4:20 AM	________	20. 9:06 PM	________

Fill in the blanks by writing out the words as indicated.

21. 24-hour time 0623 h is stated "________________________."
22. 24-hour time 0041 h is stated "________________________."
23. 24-hour time 1903 h is stated "________________________."
24. 24-hour time 2311 h is stated "________________________."

Find the length of each time interval for questions 25 through 33.

25. 0200 h to 0600 h ________
26. 1100 h to 1800 h ________
27. 1500 h to 2330 h ________
28. 0935 h to 2150 h ________
29. 0003 h to 1453 h ________
30. 2316 h to 0328 h ________
31. 8:22 AM to 1:10 PM ________
32. 4:35 PM to 8:16 PM ________
33. 10:05 AM Friday to 2:43 AM Saturday ________

34. The 24-hour clock is imprecise and not suited to healthcare. (True) (False)
35. Indicate whether these international times would be AM or PM when converted to traditional time.

a. 1030 h ________
b. 1920 h ________
c. 0158 h ________
d. 1230 h ________

After completing these problems, see page 456 in the answer section to check your answers.

Measurement of Temperature: Converting between the Fahrenheit and Celsius scales

In Canada, most people today are familiar with Celsius scale in everyday life, as well as in the health-care setting. Therefore, converting between the Fahrenheit and Celsius scales is mostly an academic exercise that does not have to be learned as an additional competency.

For information about these scales and formulas for conversion please refer to Appendix D, pages 530–532.

PRACTICE PROBLEMS—CHAPTER 3

Give the SI prefix for the following parts of the base units.

1. 0.001 ________
2. 0.000001 ________
3. 0.01 ________
4. 1000 ________

Identify the equivalent unit with a value of 1 that is indicated by the following amounts (such as 1000 mU = 1 unit).

5. 0.001 gram ________
6. 1000 grams ________
7. 0.001 milligram ________
8. 0.01 metre ________

Identify the SI base unit for the following.

9. length ________
10. weight ________
11. volume ________

Interpret the following notations.

12. mg ________
13. mcg ________
14. unit ________
15. mEq ________
16. mL ________
17. km ________
18. mm ________
19. g ________
20. cm ________
21. L ________
22. m ________
23. kg ________
24. IU ________

Express the following amounts in proper notation.

25. five hundred milligrams ________
26. one-half litre ________
27. five hundredths of a milligram ________

Express the following numeric amounts in words.

28. 375 units ________
29. 2.6 mL ________
30. 20 mEq ________
31. 0.4 L ________
32. 0.17 mg ________
33. If you drank 0.25 L, how many mL would you have consumed? ________
34. How many mg are in a medication that contains 150 mcg? ________
35. A baby weights 1.5 kg. How many grams would be the equivalent? ________
36. The physician has prescribed 0.1 g of a medication. How many mg would be the equivalent? ________
37. If a scar measured 15 mm, how many centimetres would be the equivalent? ________
38. The physician ordered 0.2 mg of a medication. How many mcg would be the equivalent? ________
39. How many mL are in a half litre? ________
40. How many g are in 256 000 mcg? ________
41. The physician prescribed 0.15 g of a medication. How many mg would be the equivalent? ________

Convert the following traditional times to international times.

42. 1:30 PM
43. 12:04 AM
44. 12:00 midnight
45. 6:20 AM

Write out the words to express the following times.

46. 0041 h ________
47. 1115 h ________
48. 0623 h ________

49. Critical Thinking Skill: Describe the strategy that would prevent a medication error in the following scenario.

possible scenario

Suppose a physician prescribed oral warfarin (an anticoagulant) for a patient with a history of phlebitis. The physician wrote an order for 1 mg, but while writing the order placed a decimal point after the 1 and added a 0:

warfarin 1.0 mg orally once per day

Warfarin 1.0 mg was transcribed on the medication record as warfarin 10 mg. The patient received 10 times the correct dosage.

potential outcome

The patient would likely begin hemorrhaging. An antidote, such as vitamin K, would be necessary to reverse the effects of the overdose. However, it is important to remember that not all drugs have antidotes.

prevention

____

____

50. Critical Thinking Skill: Describe the strategy that would prevent a medication error or the need to notify the prescribing practitioner.

possible scenario

Suppose a physician prescribed oral codeine (a potent narcotic analgesic) for an adult patient recovering from extensive nasal surgery. The physician wrote the following order for 60 mg of oral solution.

Codeine solution 60 mg orally every four to six hours as needed for pain

The surgical unit stocks codeine solution in two strengths: 10 mg/5 mL and 15 mg/5 mL. The nurse chose the 10 mg/5 mL, confused the mg and mL in calculating, and calculated that he needed 12 mL. Even though the nurse was in a rush to help ease the patient's pain, the nurse regularly practised critical thinking and felt uneasy about the total volume of medication in his original calculation. It seemed that 12 mL of an oral solution usually used for pediatric patients was a smaller amount than seemed normal. Following the unit's policy of double-checking medication calculations when a stock supply of high-alert medication was being used, a colleague calculated the dosage as 30 mL. They compared their calculation differences, looked back at the original order, and re-read the stock medicine label.

potential outcome

Because the nurse chose the 10 mg/5 mL strength, the nurse needs six times the 5 mL to give the 60 mg ordered (10 mg $\times$ 6 = 60 mg). That means the nurse needs to administer 30 mL(5 mL $\times$ 6 = 30 mL) of this medication. Otherwise, the patient will receive only 20% ($\frac{1}{5}$) of the intended amount. The nurse correctly felt uneasy about the amount and followed the surgical unit's protocol, thus avoiding under-medicating his patient for post-operative pain.

prevention

____

____

After completing these problems, see page 457 in the answer section to check your answers

CHAPTER

4

Calculation Methods Used in Determining Drug Dosages

LEARNING OBJECTIVES

1. Solve simple calculation problems using the formula method.
2. Solve simple calculation problems using the dimensional analysis method.
3. Solve simple calculation problems using the ratio and proportion method.
4. Select a method for solving drug dosage problems.

Healthcare professionals use different methods to safely calculate medication dosages. This chapter is focused on teaching this text's first method *dimensional analysis.* In Chapter 8, you will learn a second method, the *formula method.* Then you can choose the method that you find easiest to use.

It is important to mention a third method of medication calculation here, the *ratio and proportion,* as noted in Chapter 2.[1] You may find healthcare professionals who still use this method. This method is admittedly useful in the most simple medication calculations. However, an increasing body of research is now demonstrating what the writers of this text have been noticing among the students they have been teaching for a number of years, that students who use the ratio and proportion method for calculating medication dosages are more prone to calculation errors than those who use dimensional analysis. For one thing, in more complicated calculation problems, it becomes necessary to do a series of ratio and proportion calculations to calculate the required medication dosage. In response to this mounting evidence, the writers of this text decided to reduce the emphasis placed on the ratio and proportion method in this edition of the text.

In addition to doing your own research and literature review on the topic, you can start by reading the journal articles noted in Chapter 2 on this topic. In summary, beginning research among nursing students shows a significantly better sustained learning rate among students taught dimensional analysis when compared with those taught the formula method of medication calculation (Koohestani & Baghcheghi, 2010). In earlier research, Rice and Bell (2005) found evidence of the value of teaching dimensional analysis to increase the confidence and accuracy of medication calculation ability among nursing students. Although Kohtz and Gowda (2010) did not find a "significant" difference, they did find that students who used dimensional analysis made fewer mistakes than students who used other methods, even though both groups used calculators.

METHOD 1: DIMENSIONAL ANALYSIS

Dimensional analysis is a centuries' old calculation method known as *units conversion.* It is the method most commonly used in the physical sciences. This method is also known by a variety of other names such as *factor labelling, factor analysis,* the *unit factor method,* the *label-factor method, scientific method,* and the *conversion factor method. Dimension* refers to a unit of mass (or weight), volume, length, time, and so on. Examples include milligram (mg), litre (L), metre (m), and minute (min).

[1] See references listed in Chapter 2, page 44.

Dimensional analysis is a commonsense approach to drug calculations. It is a fast, simple, and organized system for setting up problems. It can be used for all medication problems. Finally, dimensional analysis also assists with preventing medication errors by allowing you to visualize all parts of the medication problem and to critically think your way through the problem. It also eliminates the need to memorize formulas. Only one easy-to-solve equation is needed to determine each answer. At first, you might notice a similarity with the formula method.Dimensional analysis is particularly useful when a medication is ordered in one unit and available in a different unit.

Being able to correctly convert from one unit of measurement to another is a strength of dimensional analysis. This skill is frequently needed in calculating medication dosages when a medication is ordered in one unit but only available in a different unit. In the next two examples you can see the calculation problem of such conversions being built step by step using dimensional analysis. It is important to master the steps so you can apply them in a variety of medication calculation situations.

Example 1:

You have 700 mL of liquid and need to know how many litres equals 700 mL.

Step 1 Identify the desired answer unit and write it to the left of an equal sign.

$$L =$$

Step 2 Identify the given quantity in the problem and the desired quantity and write them to the right of the equal sign. (In this example, we have the *desired quantity* only.)

$$L = 700 \text{ mL}$$

Step 3 Establish the "unit path" from the given quantity to the wanted quantity using equivalents as "conversion factors." Make sure that the unit of the desired quantity is in the numerator of either the given quantity or in the unit path.

$$L = 700 \text{ mL} \times \frac{1 \text{ L}}{1000 \text{ mL}}$$

Remember, what you learned in Chapter 2 about the metric system and SI units: 1 L = 1000 mL. Therefore, when you include this information in your problem above, you are really only multiplying the numerator and the denominator by the same value, and thus not changing the value of the equation.

Step 4 Carefully check each conversion factor and ensure that it is correctly placed in the numerator or denominator portion of the problem to allow the unwanted units to be cancelled from the problem.

Yes, there is millilitre (mL) in the numerator and denominator that can be cancelled and leave only the litre (L), which is the desired unit for the answer. This equation is set up correctly to calculate the answer in litres (L).

Step 5 Cancel terms.

$$L = 700 \cancel{\text{mL}} \times \frac{1 \text{ L}}{1000 \cancel{\text{mL}}}$$

Step 6 Reduce the fraction to its lowest terms. (Divide both the numerator and denominator by 100.) Multiply the numerators and the denominators (7 × 1L, & 10, respectively). Divide the numerator by the denominator. (Remember how to divide by the power of 10—move the decimal point one place to the left for every power of 10.) Insert zero before the decimal point to emphasize that the quantity is less than 1.

$$L = \overset{7}{\cancel{700}} \times \frac{1 \text{ L}}{\underset{10}{\cancel{1000}}} = \frac{7 \text{ L}}{\cancel{10}} = .7 \text{ mL} = 0.7 \text{ mL}$$

Therefore, 700 mL = 0.7 L

MATH TIP

When setting up the problem, be sure to always include the units. Carry out the calculations and add the appropriate units to the answer as well. The units that are in the numerator stay above the line and those in the denominator stay below the line.

Example 2:

Suppose you want to know how many milligrams (mg) are in 6 grams (g). You may use the following format to set up the problem, using the steps discussed above:

Step 1 Identify the desired answer units and write it to the left of an equal sign.

$$\text{mg} =$$

Step 2 Identify the given quantity in the problem and the desired quantity and write them to the right of the equal sign. (In this example, we have the *desired quantity* only.)

$$\text{mg} = 6\text{ g}$$

Step 3 Establish the "unit path" from the given quantity to the wanted quantity using equivalents as "conversion factors." Make sure that the unit of the desired quantity is in the numerator of either the given quantity or in the unit path.

$$\text{mg} = 6\text{ g} \times \frac{1000\text{ mg}}{1\text{ g}}$$

Step 4 Carefully check each conversion factor and ensure that it is correctly placed in the numerator or denominator portion of the problem to allow the unwanted units to be cancelled from the problem.

Yes, there are grams in the numerator and denominator that can be cancelled and leave only the milligrams, which is the desired unit for the answer. This equation is set up correctly to calculate the answer in milligrams (mg).

Step 5 Cancel terms.

$$\text{mg} = 6\,\cancel{\text{g}} \times \frac{1000\text{ mg}}{1\,\cancel{\text{g}}}$$

The grams (g) are cancelled in the numerator and denominator. In this case, what remains is already reduced to its lowest terms. Note: you are left with milligrams (mg) in the answer, which is the desired unit for the answer, as it is the same as the unit to the right of the equation.

Step 6 Multiply the numerators and denominators and divide the product of the numerator by the product of the denominator.

$$\text{mg} = 6 \times \frac{1000\text{ mg}}{1} = \frac{6000\text{ mg}}{1} = 6000\text{ mg}$$

In this case the denominator is 1, so the final division result is 6000 mg.

Therefore, in 6 g, there are 6000 mg.

RULE

1. Identify the *desired answer* unit and write it to the left of the equal sign.
2. Identify the *given quantity* in the problem and the *desired quantity* and write them to the right of the equal sign so that the desired quantity is a numerator and the given quantity is written to allow cancellation of units.
3. Establish the *unit path* from the given quantity to the wanted quantity using equivalents as "conversion factors." Make sure that the unit of the desired quantity is in the numerator of either the given quantity or in the unit path.
4. Carefully check each conversion factor and ensure that it is correctly placed in the numerator or denominator portion of the problem to allow the unwanted units to be cancelled from the problem.
5. Cancel the terms as per fraction multiplication in Chapter 1. The remaining unit(s) should match the unit(s) on the left of the equation and be the unit(s) desired. If all the units except the answer unit(s) are not eliminated, recheck the equation.
6. Reduce the fractions to their lowest terms; multiply the numerators and denominators; and divide the denominator into the numerator to provide the numerical value of the wanted quantity.

MATH TIP

Units may be cancelled the same as numbers and letters in arithmetic and algebra.

MATH TIP

Incorrect placement of units of measurement can result in an incorrect answer. Even when calculating with dimensional analysis, thinking and reasoning are essential.

REVIEW SET 12

Use the dimensional analysis method to convert each of the following to the equivalent indicated.

1. 500 mL = ________ L
2. 0.015 g = ________ mg
3. 8 mg = ________ g
4. 10 mg = ________ g
5. 60 mg = ________ g
6. 300 mg = ________ g
7. 0.2 mg = ________ g
8. 1.2 g = ________ mg
9. 0.0025 kg = ________ g
10. 0.065 g = ________ mg
11. 0.005 L = ________ mL
12. 1.5 L = ________ mL
13. 250 mL = ________ L
14. 2 kg = ________ g
15. 5000 mL = ________ L
16. 1 L = ________ mL
17. 1 g = ________ mg
18. 1 mL = ________ L
19. 23 mcg = ________ mg
20. 1.05 g = ________ kg
21. 18 mcg = ________ mg
22. 0.4 mg = ________ mcg
23. 25 g = ________ kg
24. 50 cm = ________ m
25. 10 L = ________ mL

After completing these problems, see page 457 in the answer section to check your answers.

The dimensional analysis method requires three elements: given quantity, desired quantity, and unit path, using equivalent "conversion factors" when necessary to convert units from one unit to another. When setting up the calculation problem, set up the conversion factors to permit cancellation of unwanted units. Carefully choose each conversion factor and ensure that it is correctly placed in the numerator and denominator portion of the problem to allow the unwanted units to be cancelled from the problem. Finally, cancel the units and reduce the numbers to their lowest terms as you learned in Chapter 1, then multiply the numerators, multiply the denominators, and divide the product of the numerators by the product of the denominators to provide the numerical value of the wanted quantity.

CAUTION

Starting the calculation incorrectly will not allow you to eliminate the undesired units. Knowing when the equation is set up correctly is an essential part of the dimensional analysis method.

METHOD 2: FORMULA

The formula method is commonly used method for calculating drug dosages.

$$\frac{D}{H} \times Q = \text{Amount to give}$$

D or *desired* dose: drug dose prescribed
H or *have* dose: drug dose available
Q or *quantity:* form and amount in which the drug comes

Example 1:

Prescribed: 500 mg of Drug A

Dosage available: 250 mg of Drug A in 1 tablet

Using the formula method calculate the amount of Drug A to administer

$$\frac{\overset{2}{\cancel{500}}\ \text{mg}}{\underset{1}{\cancel{250}}\ \text{mg}} \times 1\ \text{tab} = 2\ \text{tablets of Drug A}$$

Example 2:

Prescribed: 80 mg of Drug B

Dosage available: 100 mg of Drug B in 2 mL

Using the formula method, calculate the amount of Drug B to administer

$$\frac{8\cancel{0}\ \text{mg}}{\underset{5}{\cancel{100}}\ \text{mg}} \times \cancel{2}\ \text{mL} = \frac{8}{5}\ \text{mL} = 1.6\ \text{mL}$$

MATH TIP

When putting numbers into a formula, it is important to also include the units. Carry out the calculations and add the appropriate units to the answer as well. The units that are in the numerator stay above the line and those in the denominator stay below the line.

RULE

To calculate a drug dosage using the formula method:

1. **Memorize the formula, or verify the formula from a resource.**
2. **Place the information from the problem into the formula in the correct position, with all terms in the formula labelled correctly.**
3. **Make sure all measurements are in the same units and systems of measurement, or a conversion must be done *before* calculating the formula.**
4. **Think logically and consider what a reasonable amount to administer would be.**
5. **Calculate the answer.**
6. **Label all answers with the correct units.**
7. **Double-check the math of the calculation.**

REVIEW SET 13

Use the formula method to calculate the quantity of drug to administer in the following:

1. A dosage of 0.8 g has been prescribed. The strength available is 1 g in 2.5 mL. ________
2. You have available a dosage strength of 250 mg in 1.5 mL. The prescription is for 200 mg. ________
3. The strength available is 1 g in 5 mL. The prescription is for 0.2 g. ________
4. A dosage of 300 mcg is prescribed. The strength available is 500 mcg in 1.2 mL. ________
5. A dosage strength of 1000 units per 1.5 mL is available. Prepare a 1250-unit dose. ________
6. The intravenous solution available has a strength of 200 mEq per 20 mL. You are to prepare a 50-mEq dosage. ________
7. A dosage of 0.2 mg per 2 mL is available. Prepare a 0.25-mg dosage. ________

After completing these problems, see page 458 to check your answers.

If you feel you do not understand the concept of conversions within the SI, review the decimal section in Chapter 1 and the SI section in Chapter 2 again. Get help from your instructor before proceeding further.

METHOD 3: RATIO AND PROPORTION

Ratio and proportion is another method of calculating dosage problems used by healthcare professionals. This method is useful in simple medication calculations. In more complicated calculation problems, a series of ratio and proportion calculations become necessary to calculate the required medication dosage.

As noted in Chapter 2, a *ratio* is the numerical relationship between two quantities. When two equal ratios are expressed as an equation, they are said to be a *proportion.*

RULE

In a proportion, the product of the *means* (the two inside numbers) equals the product of the *extremes* (the two outside numbers). Finding the product of the means and the extremes is called *cross-multiplying*.

Example:

Extremes

5:10 = 10:20

Means

$5 \times 20 = 10 \times 10$

$100 = 100$

Because ratios are the same as fractions, the same proportion can be expressed like this: $\frac{5}{10} = \frac{10}{20}$. The fractions are *equivalent,* or equal. The numerator of the first fraction and the denominator of the second fraction are the extremes, and the denominator of the first fraction and the numerator of the second fraction are the means.

Example:

Extreme	5	10	Mean
Mean	10	20	Extreme

Cross-multiply to find the equal products of the means and extremes.

RULE

If two fractions are *equivalent*, or equal, their cross-products are also equal.

Example:

$\frac{5}{10} \times \frac{10}{20}$

$5 \times 20 = 10 \times 10$

$100 = 100$

When one of the quantities in a proportion is unknown, a letter, such as "X," may be substituted for this unknown quantity. You would solve the equation to find the value of "X." In addition to cross-multiplying, there is one more rule you need to know to solve for "X" in a proportion.

RULE

Dividing or multiplying each side (*member*) of an equation by the same nonzero number produces an equivalent equation.

MATH TIP

Dividing each side of an equation by the same nonzero number is the same as reducing or simplifying the equation. Multiplying each side by the same nonzero number enlarges the equation.

Let us examine how to simplify an equation.

Example:

25X = 100 (25X means 25 × X)

Simplify the equation to find "X." Divide both sides by 25, the number before "X." Reduce to lowest terms.

$$\frac{\overset{1}{\cancel{25}}X}{\underset{1}{\cancel{25}}} = \frac{\overset{4}{\cancel{100}}}{\underset{1}{\cancel{25}}}$$

$\frac{1X}{1} = \frac{4}{1}$ (Dividing or multiplying a number by 1 does not change its value. "1X" is understood to be simply "X.")

X = 4

Replace "X" with 4 in the same equation, and you can prove that the calculations are correct.

25 × **4** = 100

Now you are ready to apply the concepts of cross-multiplying and simplifying an equation to solve for "X" in a proportion.

Example 1:

$$\frac{90}{2} = \frac{45}{X}$$

You have a proportion with an unknown quantity "X" in the denominator of the second fraction. Find the value of "X."

1. Cross-multiply: $\frac{90}{2} \times \frac{45}{X}$
2. Multiply terms: 90 × X = 2 × 45

   90X = 90 (90X means 90 × X)

3. Simplify the equation: Divide both sides of the equation by the number before the unknown "X." You are equally reducing the terms on both sides of the equation.

$$\frac{\overset{1}{\cancel{90}}X}{\underset{1}{\cancel{90}}} = \frac{\overset{1}{\cancel{90}}}{\underset{1}{\cancel{90}}}$$

X = 1

Try another one. The unknown "X" is a different term.

Example 2:

$$\frac{80}{X} \times 60 = 20$$

1. Convert: Express 60 as a fraction.

$$\frac{80}{X} \times \frac{60}{1} = 20$$

2. Multiply fractions: $\frac{80}{X} \times \frac{60}{1} = 20$

$$\frac{4800}{X} = 20$$

3. Convert: Express 20 as a fraction.

$$\frac{4800}{X} = \frac{20}{1}$$

You now have a proportion.

4. Cross-multiply: $\frac{4800}{X} \times \frac{20}{1}$

$$20X = 4800$$

5. Simplify: Divide both sides of the equation by the number before the unknown "X."

$$\frac{\overset{1}{\cancel{20}}X}{\underset{1}{\cancel{20}}} = \frac{\overset{240}{\cancel{4800}}}{\underset{1}{\cancel{20}}}$$

$$X = 240$$

Example 3:

$$\frac{X}{160} = \frac{2.5}{80}$$

1. Cross-multiply: $\frac{X}{160} \times \frac{2.5}{80}$

$$80 \times X = 2.5 \times 160$$

$$80X = 400$$

2. Simplify: $\frac{\overset{1}{\cancel{80}}X}{\underset{1}{\cancel{80}}} = \frac{\overset{5}{\cancel{400}}}{\underset{1}{\cancel{80}}}$

$$X = 5$$

Example 4:

$$\frac{40}{100} = \frac{X}{2}$$

1. Cross-multiply: $\frac{40}{100} \times \frac{X}{2}$

2. Multiply terms: $100 \times X = 40 \times 2$

   $100X = 80$

3. Simplify the equation: $\frac{\cancel{100}^{1}X}{\cancel{100}_{1}} = \frac{8\cancel{0}}{10\cancel{0}}$

   $X = 0.8$

Calculations that result in an amount less than 1 should be expressed as a decimal. Most medications are ordered and supplied in SI units. SI is a decimal-based system.

QUICK REVIEW

- A *proportion* is an equation of two equal ratios. The ratios may be expressed as fractions.

  Example: 1:4 = X:8 or $\frac{1}{4} = \frac{X}{8}$

- In a proportion, the product of the means equals the product of the extremes.

  Example: 1:4 = X:8 (Extremes: 1 and 8; Means: 4 and X) Therefore, $4 \times X = 1 \times 8$

- If two fractions are equal, their cross-products are equal. This operation is referred to as *cross-multiplying*.

  Example: $\frac{1}{4} \times \frac{X}{8}$ Therefore, $4 \times X = 1 \times 8$ or $4X = 8$

- Dividing each side of an equation by the same number produces an equivalent equation. This operation is referred to as *simplifying the equation*.

  Example: If $4X = 8$, then $\frac{4X}{4} = \frac{8}{4}$, and $X = 2$

REVIEW SET 14

Find the value of "X." Express answers as decimals rounded to two places.

1. $\frac{1000}{2} = \frac{125}{X}$ ________
2. $\frac{0.5}{2} = \frac{250}{X}$ ________
3. $\frac{75}{1.5} = \frac{35}{X}$ ________
4. $\frac{1200}{X} \times 12 = 28$ ________
5. $\frac{250}{1} = \frac{750}{X}$ ________
6. $\frac{80}{5} = \frac{10}{X}$ ________

7. $\dfrac{5}{20} = \dfrac{X}{40}$ ________

8. $\dfrac{\frac{1}{100}}{1} = \dfrac{\frac{1}{150}}{X}$ ________

9. $\dfrac{2.2}{X} = \dfrac{8.8}{5}$ ________

10. $\dfrac{60}{10} = \dfrac{100}{X}$ ________

11. $\dfrac{X}{0.5} = \dfrac{6}{4}$ ________

12. $\dfrac{25\%}{30\%} = \dfrac{5}{X}$ ________

13. In any group of 100 nurses, you would expect to find 45 nurses who will specialize in a particular field of nursing. In a class of 240 graduating nurses, how many would you expect to specialize? ________________

14. If a patient receives 450 mg of a medication given evenly over 5.5 hours, how many milligrams did the patient receive per hour? ________________

15. How much salt should you add to 500 mL of water to make a solution that contains 5g of salt for every 250 mL? ________________

After completing these problems, see page 458 to check your answers.

Each ratio in a proportion must have the same relationship and follow the same sequence. A proportion compares like things to like things. Be sure the units in the numerators match and the units in the denominators match. Label the units in each ratio.

Example:

How many grams are equivalent to 3.5 kg?

The first ratio of the proportion contains the *known equivalent,* for example 1 kg : 1000 g. The second ratio contains the *desired unit of measure* and the *unknown equivalent* expressed as "X," for example 3.5 kg : X g. This proportion in fractional form looks like this:

$$\frac{1\text{ kg}}{1000\text{ g}} = \frac{3.5\text{ kg}}{X\text{ g}}$$

CAUTION

Notice that the ratios follow the same sequence. *THIS IS ESSENTIAL*. The proportion is set up so that like units are across from each other. The units in the numerators match (kg) and the units in the denominators match (g).

Cross-multiply to solve the proportion for "X."

$$\frac{1\text{ kg}}{1000\text{ g}} \times \frac{3.5\text{ kg}}{X\text{ g}}$$

$X = 3.5 \times 1000 = 3500$ g

You know the answer is in grams because grams is the unknown equivalent.

3.5 kg = 3500 g

QUICK REVIEW

To use the ratio-proportion method to convert from one unit to another or between systems of measurement:

- Recall the equivalent.
- Set up a proportion: Ratio for known equivalent equals ratio for unknown equivalent.
- Label the units and match the units in the numerators and denominators.
- Cross-multiply to find the value of the unknown "X" equivalent.

REVIEW SET 15

Use the ratio-proportion method to calculate the amount you will prepare for each of the following questions.

1. Prescription: 0.2 g of a drug

   Stock dosage: 100 mg per tablet

   How many tablets should be given in one dose? __2__

2. Prescription: 600 000 units

   Stock dosage: 400 000 units per mL

   How many mL should be given in one dose? ________

3. Prescription: 160 mg

   Stock dosage: 80 mg per 5 mL

   How many mL should be given in one dose? ________

4. Prescription: 7.5 mg

   Stock dosage: 2.5 mg per tablet

   How many tablets should be given in one dose? __3__

5. Prescription: 0.125 mg

   Stock dosage: 250 mcg per tablet

   How many tablets should be given in one dose? __0.5__

6. Order: *conjugated estrogens 1.25 mg PO daily*

   Supply: conjugated estrogens 0.625 mg tablets

   Give: __2__ tablet(s)

7. Order: *cimetidine HCl 150 mg PO QID with meals & bedtime*

   Supply: cimetidine HCl liquid 300 mg per 5 mL

   Give: ________ mL

8. Order: *thiamine hydrochloride 80 mg IM stat*

   Supply: thiamine hydrochloride 100 mg per 1 mL

   Give: ________ mL

9. Order: *meperidine hydrochloride 35 mg IM q4h prn for pain*

   Supply: meperidine hydrochloride 50 mg per 1 mL

   Give: ________ mL

10. Order: *lithium carbonate 12 mEq PO TID*

    Supply: lithium carbonate 8 mEq per 5 mL

    Give: ________ mL

11. Order: *lorazepam 2.4 mg IM bedtime prn for anxiety*

    Supply: lorazepam 4 mg per 1 mL

    Give: ________ mL

12. Order: *prednisone 7.5 mg PO daily*

    Supply: prednisone 5 mg (scored) tablets

    Give: ________ tablet(s)

13. Order: *hydrochlorothiazide 30 mg PO BID*

    Supply: hydrochlorothiazide 50 mg/5 mL

    Give: ________ mL

14. Order: *theophylline 160 mg PO q6h*

    Supply: theophylline 80 mg per 15 mL

    Give: ________ mL

15. Order: *imipramine hydrochloride 20 mg IM bedtime*

    Supply: imipramine hydrochloride 25 mg per 2 mL

    Give: ________ mL

16. Order: *indomethacin 15 mg PO TID*

    Supply: indomethacin suspension 25 mg/5 mL

    Give: ________ mL

17. Order: *lorazepam 2 mg IM 2 h pre-op*

    Supply: lorazepam 4 mg per mL

    Give: ________ mL

18. Order: *phenobarbital 30 mg PO TID*

    Supply: phenobarbital 15 mg tablets

    Give: ________ tablet(s)

19. Order: *glyburide 2.5 mg PO daily*

    Supply: glyburide 1.25 mg

    Give: ________ tablet(s)

20. Order: *chlorpromazine 60 mg IM stat*

    Supply: chlorpromazine 25 mg per mL

    Give: ________ mL

21. Order: *levothyroxine 0.15 mg PO daily*

    Supply: levothyroxine 75 mcg tablets

    Give: ________ tablet(s)

22. Order: *oxtriphylline 160 mg PO q6h*

    Supply: oxtriphylline 100 mg per 5 mL

    Give: ________ mL

23. Order: *methylprednisolone sodium succinate 100 mg IV q6h*

    Supply: methylprednisolone sodium succinate 125 mg per 2 mL

    Give: ________ mL

24. Order: *fluphenazine hydrochloride elixir 8 mg PO q8h*

    Supply: fluphenazine hydrochloride elixir 2.5 mg per 5 mL

    Give: ________ mL

25. Order: *amoxicillin 350 mg PO q8h*

    Supply: amoxicillin 250 mg per 5 mL

    Give: ________ mL

After completing these problems, see pages 458–459 in the answer section to check your answers.

MATH TIP

A proportion is written as two ratios separated by an equal sign, such as 5:10 = 10:20. The two ratios in a proportion may also be separated by a double colon sign, such as 5:10 :: 10:20.

SUMMARY

At this point, you should be quite familiar with a variety of methods to use in calculating medication dosages. From memory, you should be able to recall quickly and accurately the equivalents for conversions. If you are having difficulty understanding the concept of converting from one unit of measurement to another, review the previous chapters and seek additional help from your instructor.

Choose one method that you find consistently works accurately and most easily for you. Work the practice problems for Chapter 4. Concentrate on accuracy. One error can be a serious mistake when calculating the dosages of medicines or performing critical measurements of health status.

PRACTICE PROBLEMS—CHAPTER 4

Use dimension analysis to calculate the amount you prepare for each dose.

1. Order: *lactulose 30 g in 100 mL fluid pr TID*

   Supply: lactulose 3.33 g per 5 mL

   Give: ________ mL in 100 mL

2. Order: *penicillin G potassium 500 000 units IM QID*

   Supply: penicillin G potassium 5 000 000 units per 20 mL

   Give: ________ mL

3. Order: *cephalexin 100 mg PO QID*

   Supply: cephalexin oral suspension 250 mg per 5 mL

   Give: ________ mL

4. Order: *amoxicillin 125 mg PO QID*

   Supply: amoxicillin 250 mg per 5 mL

   Give: ________ mL

5. Order: *diphenhydramine 25 mg IM stat*

   Supply: diphenhydramine 10 mg per 1 mL

   Give: ________ mL

6. Order: *diphenhydramine 40 mg PO stat*

   Supply: diphenhydramine 12.5 mg per 5 mL

   Give: ________ mL

7. Order: *penicillin G potassium 350 000 units IM BID*

   Supply: penicillin G potassium 500 000 units per 2 mL

   Give: ________ mL

8. Order: *diazepam 3.5 mg IM q6h prn for anxiety*

   Supply: diazepam 5 mg per 1 mL

   Give: ________ mL

9. Order: *tobramycin sulfate 90 mg IM q8h*

   Supply: tobramycin sulfate 80 mg per 2 mL

   Give: ________ mL

10. Order: *heparin 2500 units subcutaneously BID*

    Supply: heparin 20 000 units per mL

    Give: ________ mL

11. Order: *prochlorperazine 8 mg IM q6h prn for nausea*

    Supply: prochlorperazine 5 mg per 1 mL

    Give: ________ mL

12. Order: *gentamycin 60 mg IM q6h*

    Supply: gentamycin 80 mg per 2 mL

    Give: ________ mL

13. Order: *piperacillin sodium 500 mg IM BID*

    Supply: piperacillin sodium (reconstituted) 2 g per 10 mL

    Give: ________ mL

14. Order: *nystatin oral suspension 250 000 units PO QID*

    Supply: nystatin oral suspension 100 000 units per mL

    Give: ________ mL

15. Order: *erythromycin 80 mg PO q4h*

    Supply: erythromycin 250 mg per 5 mL

    Give: ________ mL

16. Order: *potassium chloride 10 mEq PO stat*

    Supply: potassium chloride 20 mEq per 15 mL

    Give: ________ mL

17. Order: *vancomycin 400 mg IV q6h*

    Supply: vancomycin 1 g per 20 mL

    Give: ________ mL

18. Order: *levothyroxine sodium 150 mcg PO daily*

    Supply: levothyroxine sodium 0.075 mg tablets

    Give: ________ tablet(s)

19. Order: *amoxicillin 400 mg PO q8h*

    Supply: amoxicillin 250 mg per 5 mL

    Give: ________ mL

20. Order: *fosphenytoin 225 mg IV stat*

    Supply: fosphenytoin 150 mg per 2 mL

    Give: ________ mL

21. Order: *chlorpromazine 35 mg IM stat*

    Supply: chlorpromazine 25 mg per mL

    Give: ________ mL

22. Order: *Add potassium chloride 30 mEq to 1000 mL D^5W IV*

    Supply: KCl (potassium chloride) 40 mEq per 20 mL

    Add: ________ mL

23. Order: *cefaclor 300 mg PO TID*

    Supply: cefaclor 125 mg per 5 mL

    Give: ________ mL

24. Critical Thinking Skill: Describe the strategy you would implement to prevent this medication error.

possible scenario

The physician prescribed *amoxicillin 50 mg PO QID* for a child with an upper respiratory infection. Amoxicillin is supplied in an oral suspension with 125 mg/5 mL. The nurse initially calculated the dose this way:

$$\frac{125\ \cancel{mg}}{50\ \cancel{mg}} \times 5\ mL = \frac{625\ mL}{50} = 12.5\ mL$$

potential outcome

The nurse asked a colleague to double-check the dosage, as per institution policy. The scenario became a "near miss" –an "almost error" was averted. The correct amount is 2 mL. If the patient received this large overdose, the child would likely develop complications from overdosage of amoxicillin. When the physician was notified of the error, she would likely have ordered the medication discontinued and had extra blood lab work done. An incident report would be filed and the family notified of the error. If you were the colleague asked to double-check the calculation of this medication, what method would you use to set up the calculation problem? Why? Show your calculation of the correct amount of Amoxicillin using dimensional analysis.

prevention

____

____

25. Critical Thinking Skill: Describe the strategy you would implement to prevent this medication error.

possible scenario

An attending physician prescribed *cefotaxime 2 g intravenously immediately* for a patient with a leg abscess. The supply dosage available is 1000 mg per 10 mL. The nurse was in a rush to give the medication and calculated the dose this way:

If: 1 g = 1000 mg

then: 2 g = 1000 ÷ 2 = 500 mg (per 5 mL)

As the nurse did a subsequent review of the patient care order, compared it with the dosage available, and considered what was reasonable, the nurse realized that 2 grams is equal to 2000 milligrams, which was twice the amount available in one vial (10 mL). That is, the dosage required would be 2 vials, or 2 × 10 ml = 20 mL of cefotaxime.

potential outcome

If the nurse had administered the 5 mL, as originally calculated, the patient would have received only $\frac{1}{4}$ or 25% of the dosage ordered. If this error had occurred, the leg abscess could progress to osteomyelitis (a severe bone infection) because of the underdosage.

prevention

____

____

After completing the problems, see pages 459–460 in the answer section to check your answers.

SECTION 1 SELF-EVALUATION

Directions:

1. Round decimals to two places, as needed.
2. Express fractions in their lowest terms.

Chapters 1 and 2: Mathematics Review

Multiply or divide by the power of 10 indicated. Draw an arrow to demonstrate movement of the decimal point.

1. $30.5 \div 10 =$ ________
2. $40.025 \times 100 =$ ________

Identify the lowest common denominator for the following sets of numbers.

3. $\frac{1}{6}, \frac{2}{3}, \frac{3}{4}$ ________
4. $\frac{2}{5}, \frac{3}{10}, \frac{3}{11}$ ________

Complete the operations indicated.

5. $\frac{1}{4} + \frac{2}{3} =$ ________
6. $\frac{6}{7} - \frac{1}{9} =$ ________
7. $1\frac{3}{5} \times \frac{5}{8} =$ ________
8. $\frac{3}{8} \div \frac{3}{4} =$ ________
9. $13.2 + 32.55 + 0.029 =$ ________
10. 20% of 0.09 = ________
11. $80.3 - 21.06 =$ ________
12. $0.3 \times 0.3 =$ ________
13. $\frac{1}{150} \div \frac{1}{100} =$ ________
14. $\dfrac{\frac{1}{120}}{\frac{1}{60}} =$ ________
15. $\dfrac{16\%}{\frac{1}{4}} =$ ________

Arrange in order from smallest to largest.

16. $\frac{1}{3}, \frac{1}{2}, \frac{1}{6}, \frac{1}{10}, \frac{1}{5}$ ________
17. 0.25, 0.125, 0.3, 0.009, 0.1909 ________
18. Identify the strongest solution of the following: 1:3, 1:60, 1:6 ________

Convert as indicated.

19. 1:100 to a decimal ________
20. $\frac{6}{150}$ to a decimal ________
21. 0.009 to a percent ________
22. $33\frac{1}{3}$ % to a fraction ________
23. 0.05 to a fraction ________
24. $\frac{1}{2}$ % to a ratio ________
25. 2:3 to a fraction ________
26. 3:4 to a percent ________
27. $\frac{2}{5}$ to a percent ________

Chapters 3 and 4: Systems of Measurement & Calculation Methods

Find the value of "X" in the following equations. Express your answers as decimals; round to the nearest hundredth.

28. $\frac{0.35}{1.3} \times 4.5 = X$ ________

29. $\frac{0.3}{2.6} = \frac{0.15}{X}$ ________

30. $\frac{0.25}{0.125} \times 2 = X$ ________

31. $\frac{10\%}{\frac{1}{2}\%} \times 1000 = X$ ________

32. $\frac{\frac{1}{100}}{\frac{1}{150}} \times 2.2 = X$ ________

Express the following amounts in proper medical notation.

33. one-half millilitre ________

Interpret the following notations.

34. 450 mg ________

35. 0.25 L ________

Choose one of the methods of medication calculation (dimensional analysis, formula method, or ratio-proportion) for solving the following calculation problems. The solutions for the calculation problems will focus on the dimensional analysis method. Fill in the missing decimal numbers next to each metric unit as indicated.

36. 7.13 kg = ________ g = ________ mg = ________ mcg

37. ________ kg = ________ g = ________ mg = 925 mcg

38. ________ kg = ________ g = 125 mg = ________ mcg

39. ________ kg = 16.4 g = ________ mg = ________ mcg

Convert each of the following to the equivalent units indicated.

40. 20 mg = ________ g

41. 56.2 mm = ________ cm

42. 11.59 kg = ________ g

43. Most adults have about 6000 mL of circulating blood volume. This is equivalent to ________ L of blood volume.

Convert the following times as indicated. Designate AM or PM where needed.

Traditional Time	*International Time*
44. 11:35 pm	________
45. ________	1844 h

46. Tetracycline 250 mg is ordered four times daily. The medication label indicates that one capsule contains 0.25 g. How many capsules should be given for one dose? ________

47. Meperidine 60 mg is needed postoperatively for pain. The vial contains 75 mg/mL. How many mL should be given? ________

48. Amoxicillin 500 mg is needed for pneumonia. The suspension is available in 125 mg/5 mL. How many mL need to be prepared? ________

49. Digoxin 125 mcg is needed. The vial label indicates a concentration of 0.5 mg in 2 mL. How many mL are needed? ________

50. A patient needs to receive methotrexate 175 mg intravenously. The vial label indicates a concentration of 50 mg/2 mL. How many mL of methotrexate need to be prepared?

____

After completing these problems, see page 460 to check your answers. Give yourself 2 points for each correct answer.

Perfect score = 100 My score = ________

Mastery score = 86 or higher (43 correct)

For more practice, go back to the beginning of this section and repeat the Mathematics Diagnostic Evaluation.

SECTION 2

Measurement Systems, Drug Orders, and Drug Labels

CHAPTER 5

Equipment Used in Dosage Measurement

LEARNING OBJECTIVES

1. Recognize and select the appropriate equipment for the medication, dosage, and method of administration ordered.
2. Read and interpret the calibrations of each utensil presented.

Now that you are familiar with the systems of measurement used in the calculation of dosages, let us take a look at the common measuring utensils. In this chapter, you will learn to recognize and read the calibrations of devices used in both oral and parenteral administration. The oral utensils include the medicine cup, pediatric oral devices, and calibrated droppers. The parenteral devices include the 3-mL syringe, prefilled syringe, 1-mL syringe, a variety of insulin syringes, and special safety and intravenous syringes.

ORAL ADMINISTRATION

Medicine Cup

Figure 5-1 shows the 30-mL medicine cup that is used to measure most liquids for oral administration. Notice that systems of measurement other than metric—the apothecary and household systems—are indicated on the cup. Individuals unfamiliar with the metric system may find comparison to the household system helpful in visualizing the amount to be measured. Use of the metric system is consistent with standards of practice in healthcare and is most accurate for measuring medication doses. For volumes less than 10 mL, a smaller, more accurate device should be used (see Figures 5-2, 5-3, and 5-4).

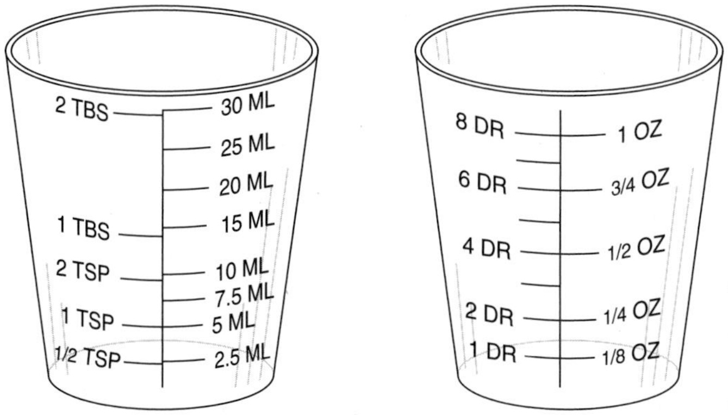

Cengage Learning

FIGURE 5-1 Medicine Cup with Approximate Equivalent Measures

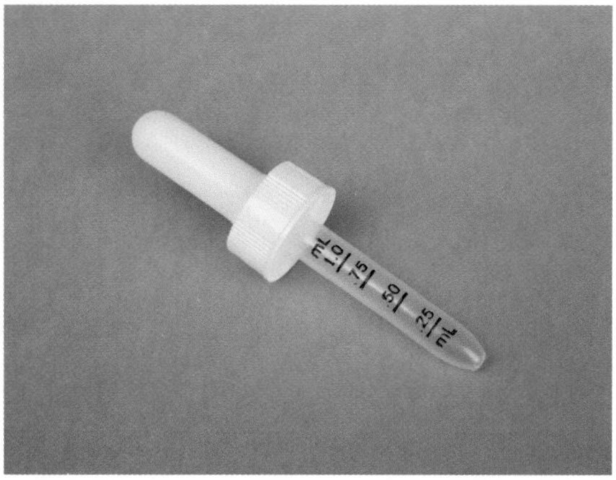

FIGURE 5-2 Calibrated Dropper

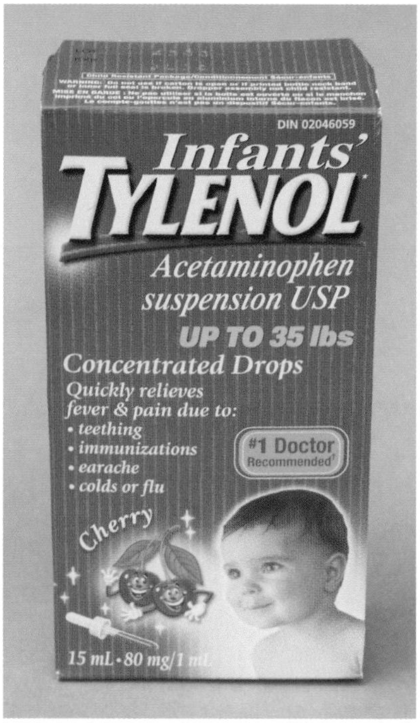

FIGURE 5-3 Infants' Tylenol Drops Label

Calibrated Dropper

Figure 5-2 shows the calibrated dropper, which is used to administer some small quantities. A dropper is used when giving medicine to children and older adults, and when adding small amounts of liquid to water or juice. Eye and ear medications are also dispensed from a medicine dropper or squeeze drop bottle.

The amount of the drop varies according to the diameter of the hole at the tip of the dropper. For this reason, a properly calibrated dropper usually accompanies the medicine. It is calibrated according to the way that drug is prescribed. The calibrations are usually given in millilitres, cubic centimetres, or drops.

> **CAUTION**
>
> To be safe, never interchange packaged droppers between medications, because drop size varies from one dropper to another.

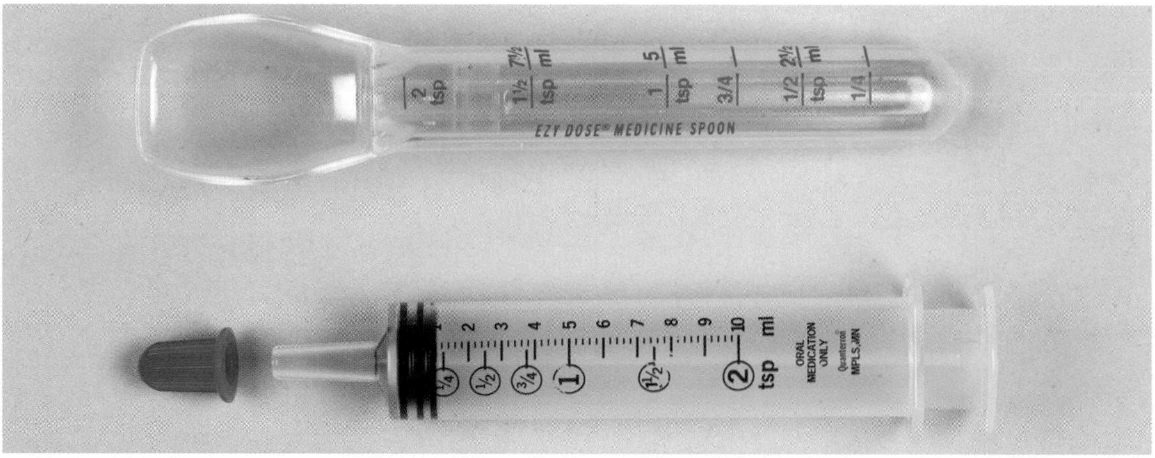

FIGURE 5-4 Devices for Administering Oral Medications to Children

Pediatric Oral Devices

Various types of calibrated equipment are available to administer oral medications to children. Several devices intended only for oral use are shown in Figure 5-4. Parents and child care givers should be taught always to use calibrated devices when administering medications to children.

CAUTION

Household spoons vary in size and are not reliable for accurate dosing.

CAUTION

To be safe, do not use syringes intended for injections in the administration of oral medications. Confusion about the route of administration may occur.

You can distinguish oral from parenteral syringes in two ways. Syringes intended for oral use typically do not have a luer lock hub and the tip is too large to ever accommodate a needle. They also usually have a cap on the tip that must be removed before administering the medication. Syringes intended for parenteral use have a luer lock hub that allows a needle to be secured tightly (see Figure 5-6).

PARENTERAL ADMINISTRATION

The term *parenteral* is used to designate routes of administration other than gastrointestinal, including intradermal, subcutaneous, intramuscular, and intravenous routes.

Three-millilitre or 3-cc Syringe

Figure 5-5 shows a 3-mL syringe assembled with needle unit. The parts of the syringe are identified in Figure 5-6. Notice that the black rubber tip of the suction plunger is visible. The nurse pulls back on the plunger to withdraw the medicine from the storage container. The calibrations are read from the top black ring, *not* the raised middle section and *not* the bottom ring. Look closely at the metric scale in Figure 5-5, which is calibrated in millilitres (mL) for each tenth (0.1) of a millilitre. Each 1/2 (or 0.5) millilitre is marked up to the maximum volume of 3 mL.

Standardized to the syringe calibrations, standard drug dosages of 1 mL or greater can be rounded to the nearest tenth (0.1) of a mL and measured on the mL scale. Refer to Chapter 1 to review the rules of decimal rounding. For example, 1.45 mL is rounded to 1.5 mL. Notice that the coloured liquid in Figure 5-5 identifies 1.5 mL.

Courtesy of Roche Laboratories, Inc.

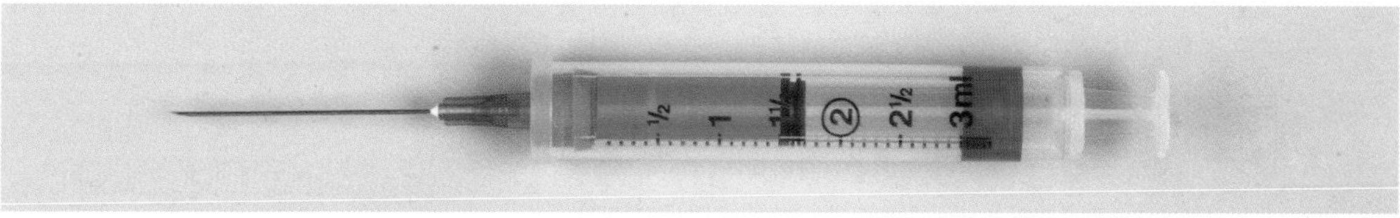

FIGURE 5-5 Three-mL Syringe with Needle Unit Measuring 1.5 mL

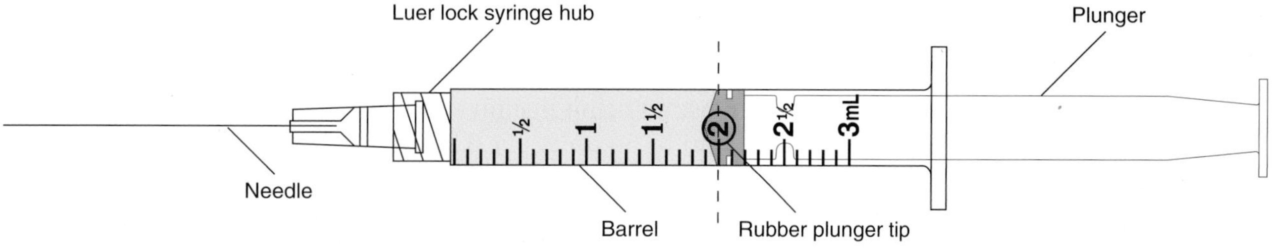

FIGURE 5-6 Three-mL Syringe with Needle Unit Measuring 2 mL

Prefilled, Single-Dose Syringe

Figure 5-7 is an example of a *prefilled, single-dose syringe.* Such syringes contain the usual single dose of a medication and are to be used only once. The syringe is discarded after the single use.

If you are to give *less than the full single dose* of a drug provided in a prefilled, single-dose syringe, you should discard the extra amount *before* injecting the patient.

Example:

The drug order prescribes 7.5 mg of diazepam to be administered to a patient. You have a prefilled, single-dose syringe of diazepam containing 10 mg per 2 mL of solution (as in Figure 5-7). You would discard 2.5 mg (0.5 mL) of the drug solution; then 7.5 mg would remain in the syringe. You will learn more about calculating drug dosages beginning in Chapter 8.

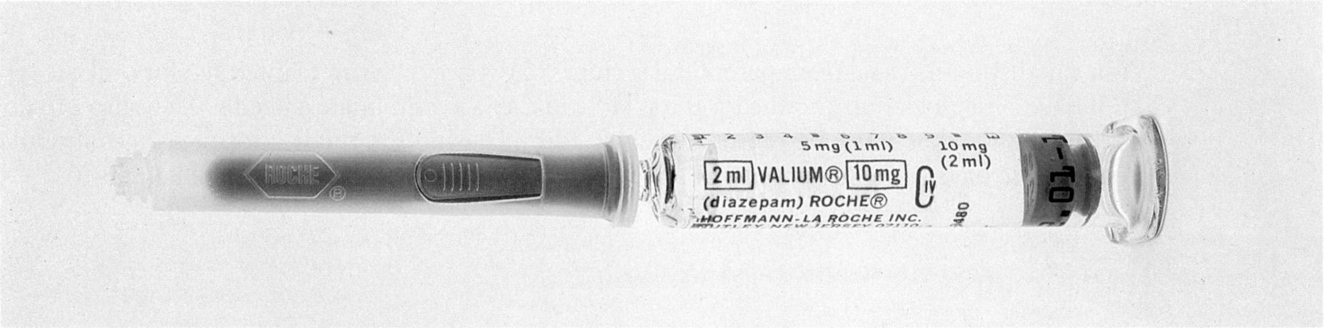

Courtesy of Roche Laboratories, Inc.

FIGURE 5-7 Prefilled, Single-Dose Syringe

RATIONALE FOR PRACTICE

Some syringes are marked in cubic centimetres (cc), whereas most drugs are prepared and labelled with the strength given per millilitre (mL). Remember that the cubic centimetre and millilitre are equivalent measurements in dosage calculations (1 cc = 1 mL).

Insulin Syringe

Figure 5-8(a) shows *both sides* of a standard 100-unit insulin syringe. This syringe is to be used for the measurement and administration of 100-unit insulin *only.* It must not be used to measure other medications that are measured in units.

CAUTION

One hundred–unit insulin should be measured only in a 100-unit insulin syringe.

Notice that Figure 5-8(a) pictures one side of the insulin syringe calibrated in odd-number 2-unit increments and the other side calibrated in even-number 2-unit increments. The plunger in Figure 5-9(a) simulates the measurement of 70 units of 100-unit insulin. It is important to note that for 100-unit insulin, 100 units equal 1 mL.

Figure 5-8(b) shows two Lo-Dose 100-unit insulin syringes. The enlarged scale is easier to read and is calibrated for each 1 unit (U) up to 50 units per 0.5 mL or 30 units per 0.3 mL. Every 5 units are labelled. The 30-unit syringe is commonly used for pediatric administration of insulin. The plunger in Figure 5-9(b) simulates the measurement of 19 units of 100-unit insulin.

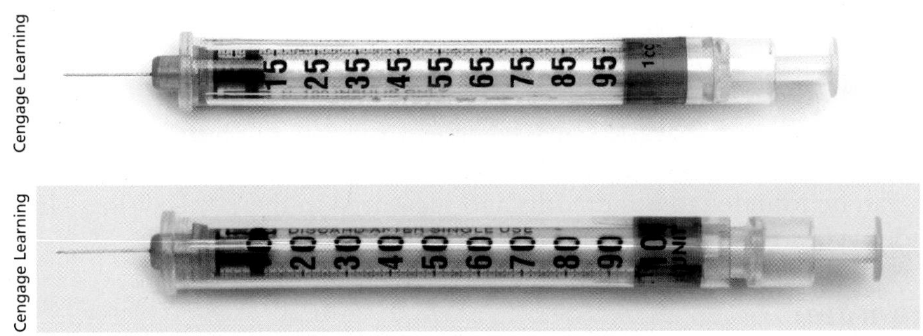
Cengage Learning
Cengage Learning

(a)

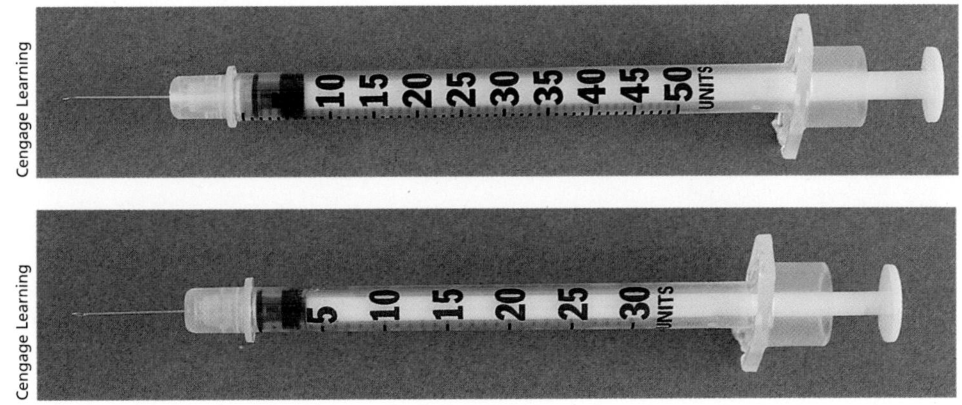
Cengage Learning
Cengage Learning

(b)

FIGURE 5-8 Insulin Syringes (a) Front and Reverse of a Standard 100-unit Insulin Syringe; (b) Lo-Dose 100-unit Insulin Syringes, 50 and 30 Units

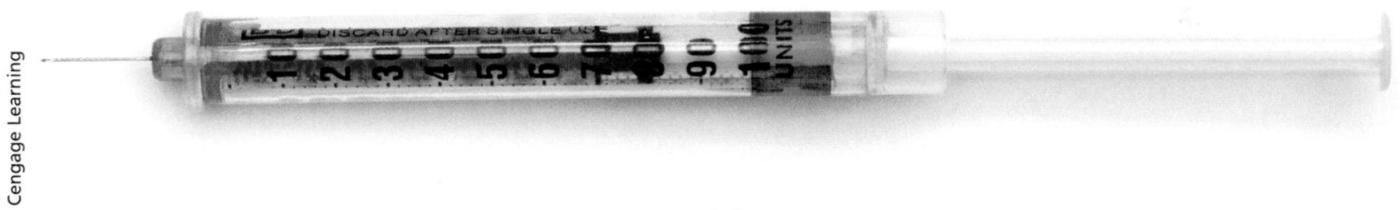
Cengage Learning

(a)

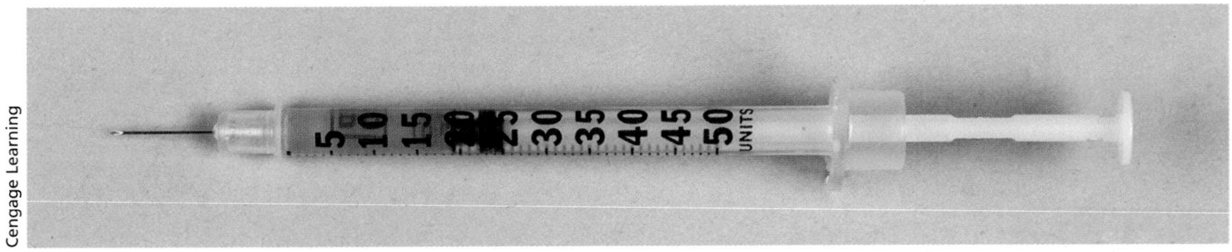
Cengage Learning

(b)

FIGURE 5-9 (a) Standard 100-unit Insulin Syringe Measuring 70 Units of 100-unit Insulin; (b) Lo-Dose 100-unit Insulin Syringe Measuring 19 Units of 100-unit Insulin

One-millilitre Syringe

Figure 5-10 shows the 1-mL syringe. This syringe is also referred to as the *tuberculin* or *TB syringe.* It is used when a small dose of a drug must be measured, such as an allergen extract, vaccine, or child's medication. Notice that the 1-mL syringe is calibrated in hundredths (0.01) of a millilitre, with each one-tenth (0.1) millilitre labelled on the metric scale. Pediatric and critical care doses of less than 1 mL can be rounded to hundredths and measured in the 1-mL syringe. It is preferable to measure all amounts less than 0.5 mL in a 1-mL syringe.

Example:

The amount 0.366 mL is rounded to 0.37 and measured in the 1-mL syringe.

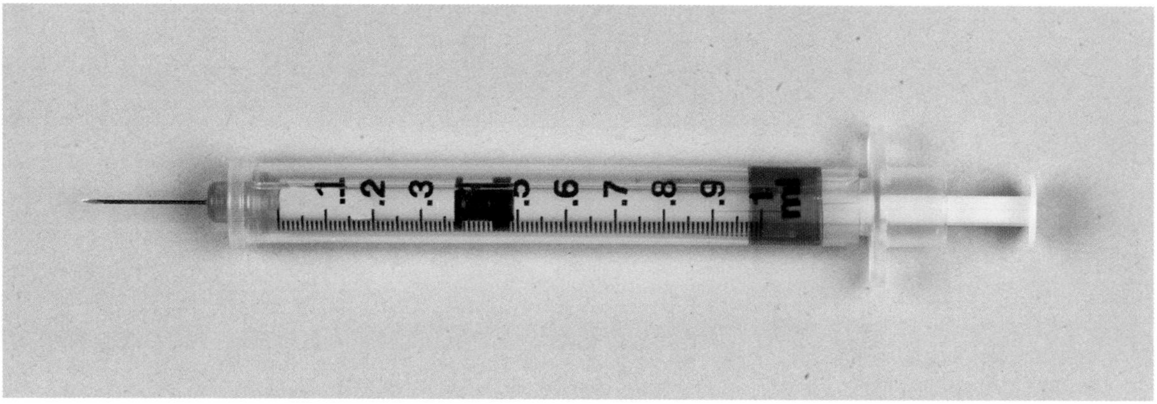

FIGURE 5-10 One-millilitre Syringe

Safety Syringe

Figure 5-11 shows 3-mL, 1-mL, and insulin safety syringes. Notice that the needle is protected by a shield to prevent accidental needlestick injury to the nurse after administering an injectable medication.

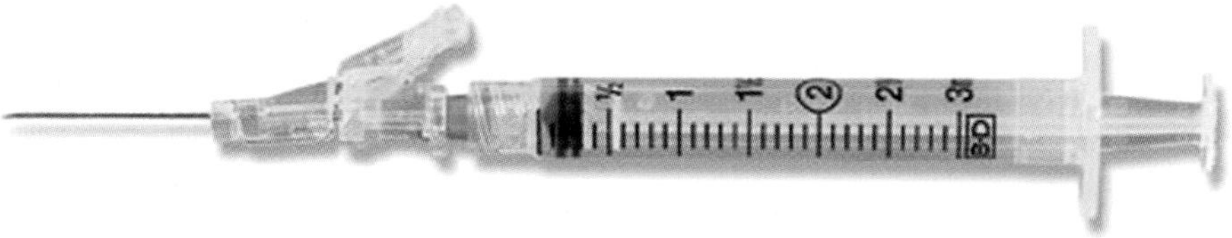

(a)

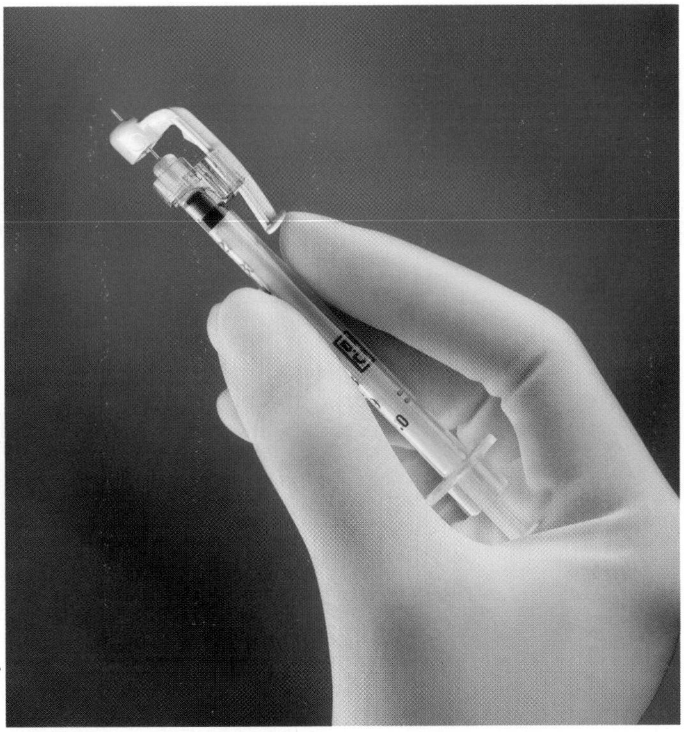

Courtesy ©Becton-Dickinson and Company

(b)

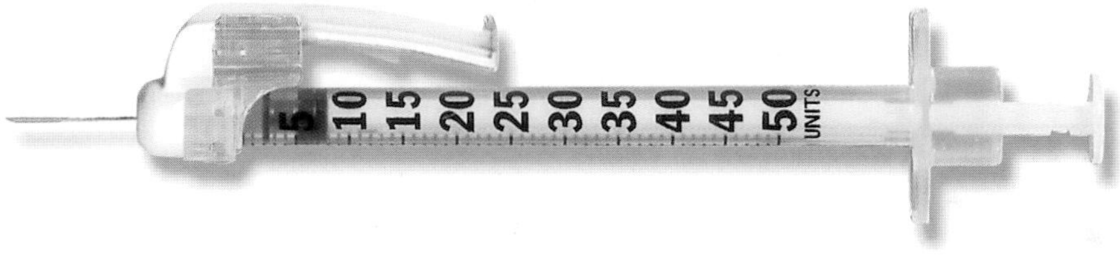

Courtesy ©Becton-Dickinson and Company

(c)

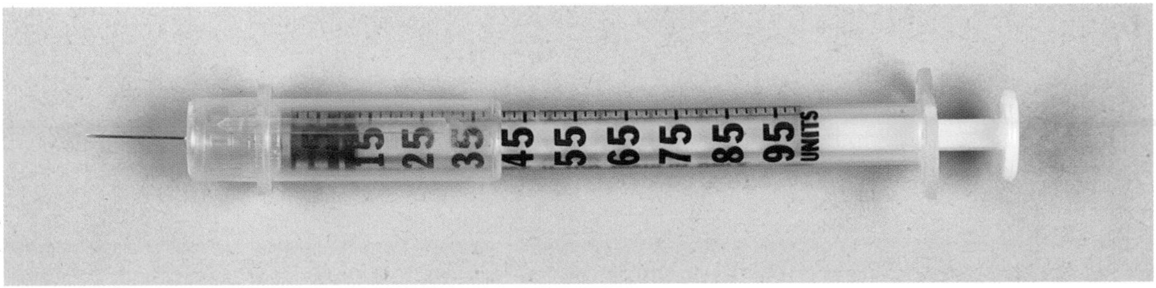

Courtesy ©Becton-Dickinson and Company

(d)

FIGURE 5-11 Safety Syringes (a) 3 mL; (b) 1 mL; (c) Lo-Dose 100-unit Insulin; (d) Standard 100-unit Insulin

Intravenous Syringe

Figures 5-12 and 5-13 show large syringes commonly used to prepare medications for intravenous administration. The volume and calibration of these syringes vary. To be safe, examine the calibrations of the syringes, and select the one best suited for the volume to be administered.

Courtesy ©Becton-Dickinson and Company

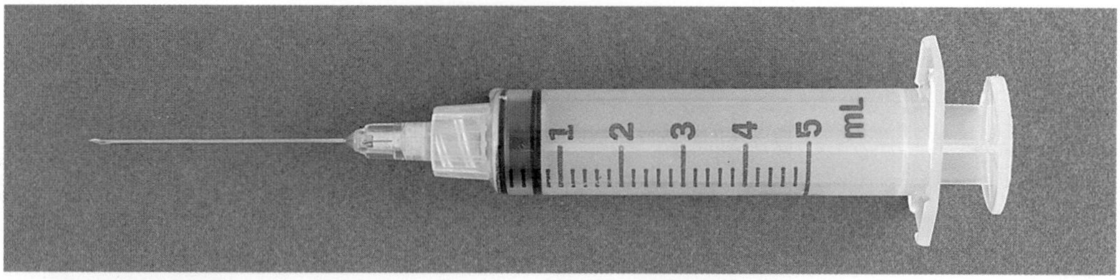

(a)

Courtesy ©Becton-Dickinson and Company

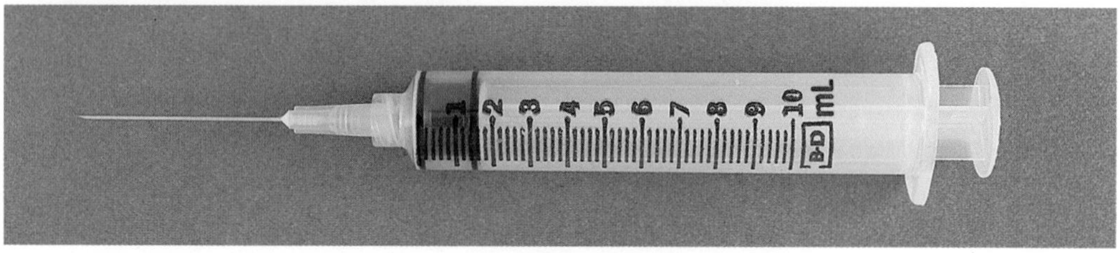

(b)

FIGURE 5-12 Intravenous Syringes (a) 5 mL; (b) 10 mL

Courtesy ©Becton-Dickinson and Company

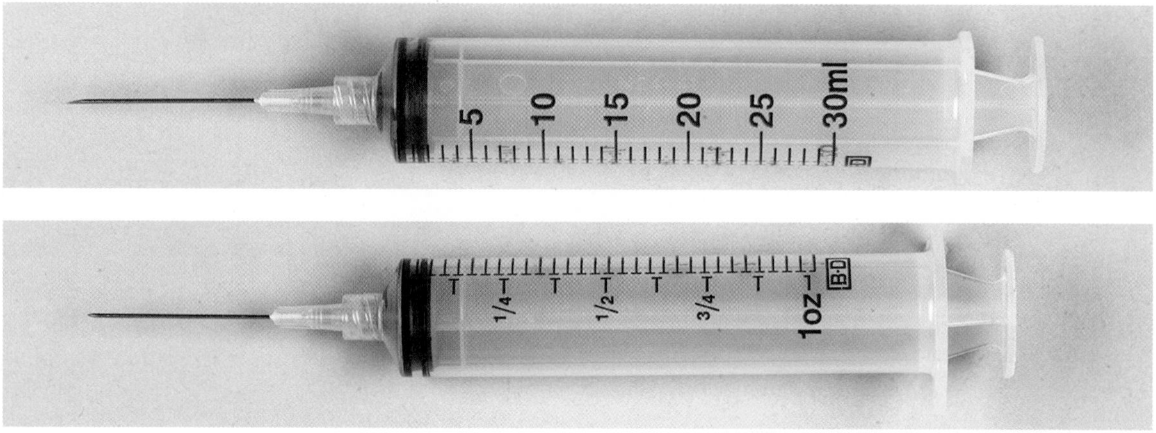

(a)

Courtesy ©Becton-Dickinson and Company

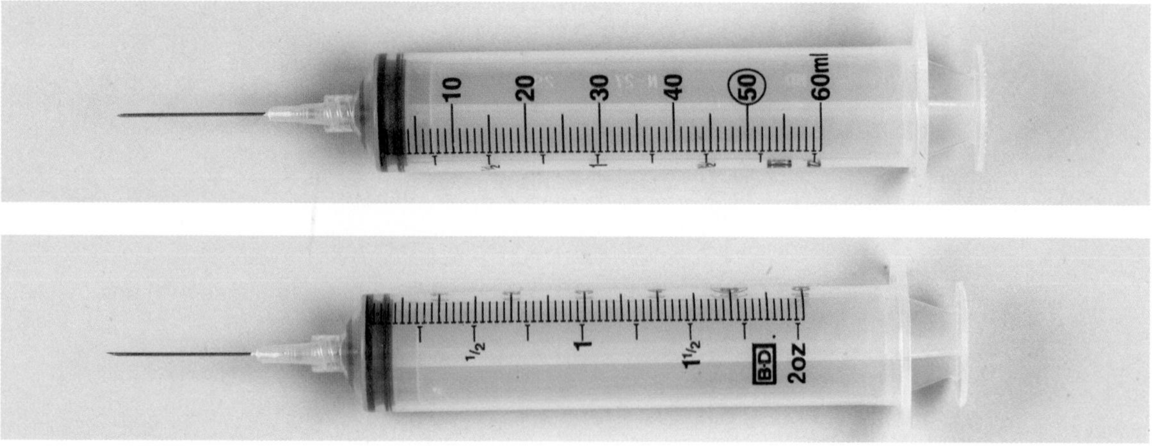

(b)

FIGURE 5-13 Intravenous Syringes (a) Front and Reverse of a 30 mL/1 oz Syringe; (b) Front and Reverse of a 60 mL/2 oz Syringe

Needleless Syringe

Figure 5-14 pictures a needleless syringe system designed to prevent accidental needlesticks during intravenous administration.

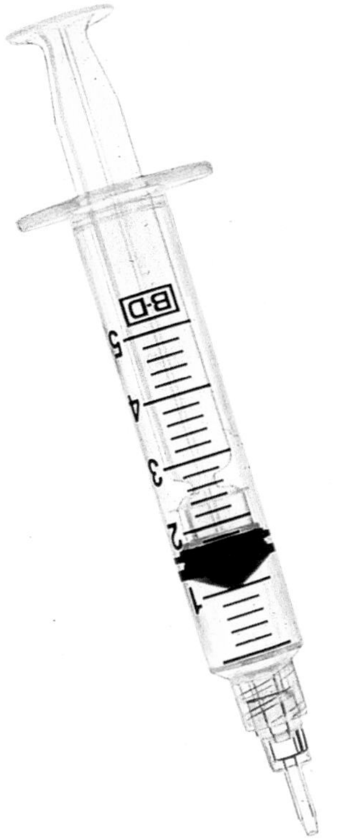

FIGURE 5-14 Example of a Needleless Syringe System

QUICK REVIEW

- The medicine cup has a 30-mL capacity for oral liquids. Amounts less than 10 mL should be measured in a smaller device, such as an oral syringe.
- The calibrated dropper measures small amounts of oral liquids. The size of the drop varies according to the diameter of the tip of the dropper.
- The standard 3-mL syringe is used to measure most injectable drugs. It is calibrated in tenths of a mL.
- The prefilled, single-dose syringe cartridge is to be used once and then discarded.
- The Standard 100-unit insulin syringe is used to measure 100-unit insulin only. It is calibrated for a total of 100 units per 1 mL.
- The Lo-Dose 100-unit insulin syringe is used for measuring small amounts of 100-unit insulin. It is calibrated for a total of 50 units per 0.5 mL or 30 units per 0.3 mL. The smaller syringe is commonly used for administering small amounts of insulin.
- The 1-mL syringe is used to measure small or critical amounts of injectable drugs. It is calibrated in hundredths of a mL.
- Syringes intended for injections should never be used to measure or administer oral medications.

REVIEW SET 16

1. In which syringe should 0.25 mL of a drug solution be measured? ____________
2. a. Can 1.25 mL be measured in the regular 3-mL syringe? ____________

   b. How? ____________
3. Should insulin be measured in a 1-mL syringe? ____________
4. Fifty (50) units of 100-unit insulin equals how many millilitres (mL)? ____________
5. a. The gtt is considered a consistent quantity for comparisons between different droppers. (True) (False)

   b. Why? ____________
6. Can you measure 3 mL in a medicine cup? ____________
7. How would you measure 3 mL of oral liquid to be administered to a child? ____________
8. The medicine cup indicates that each teaspoon is the equivalent of ________ mL.
9. Describe your action if you are to administer less than the full amount of a drug supplied in a prefilled, single-dose syringe. ____________
10. What is the primary purpose of the safety and needleless syringes? ____________

Note to Learner

The drawings of the syringes on subsequent pages represent actual sizes.

Draw an arrow to point to the calibration that corresponds to the dose to be administered.

11. Administer 0.75 mL

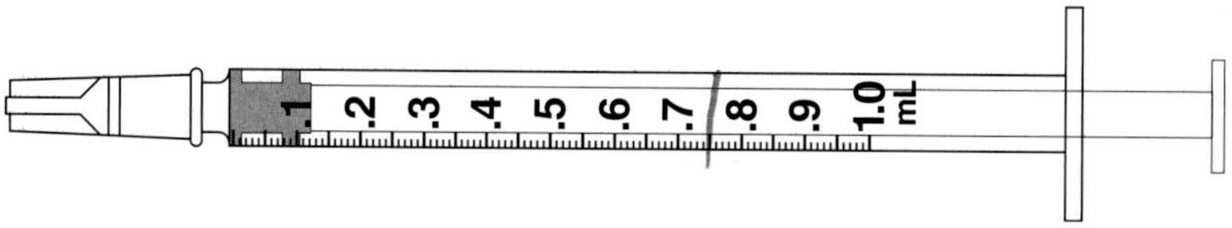

12. Administer 1.33 mL

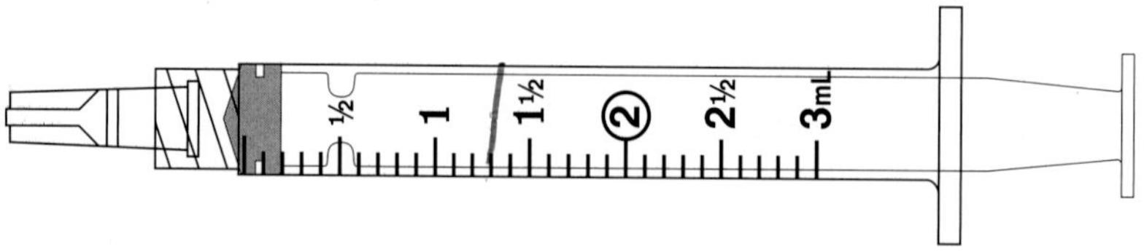

13. Administer 2.2 mL

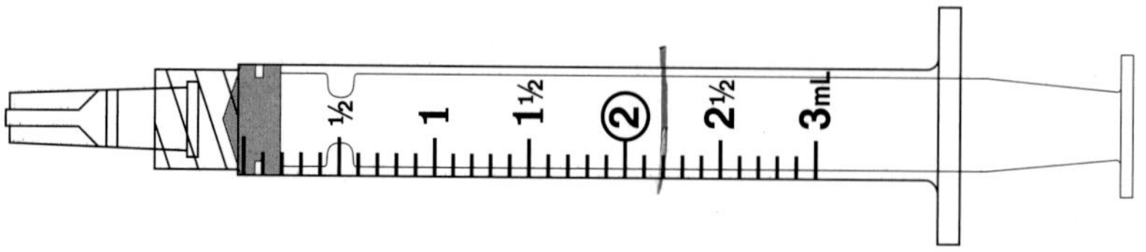

14. Administer 1.3 mL

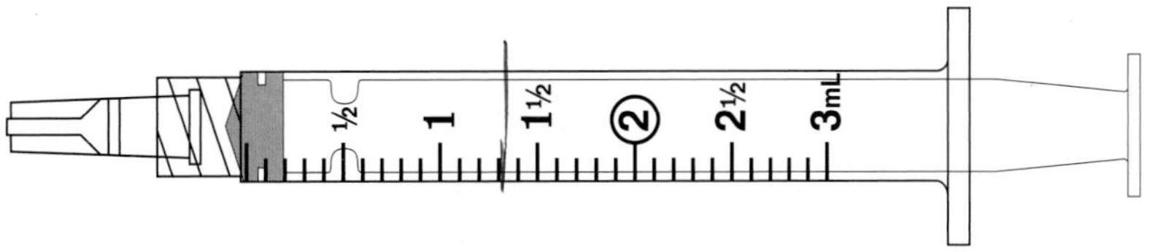

15. Administer 0.33 mL

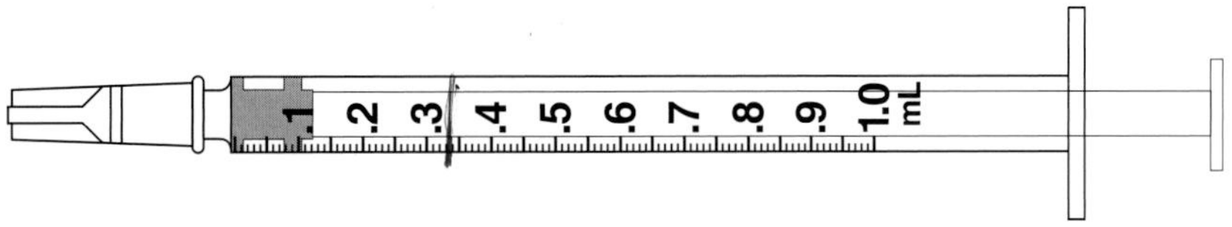

16. Administer 65 units of 100-unit insulin

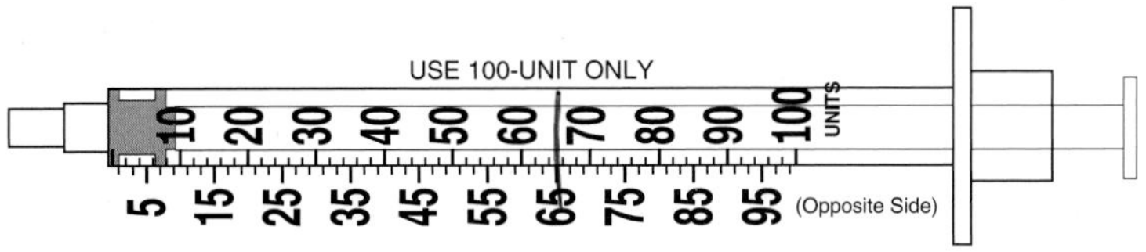

17. Administer 27 units of 100-unit insulin

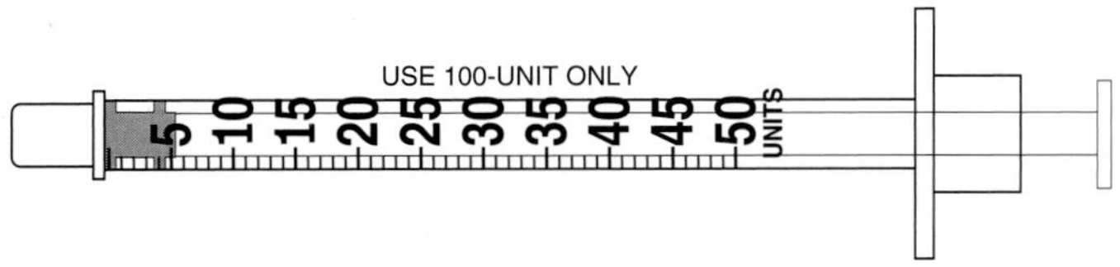

18. Administer 75 units of 100-unit insulin

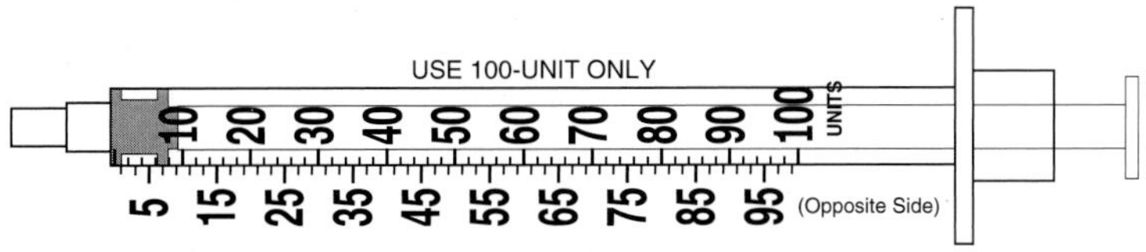

19. Administer 4.4 mL

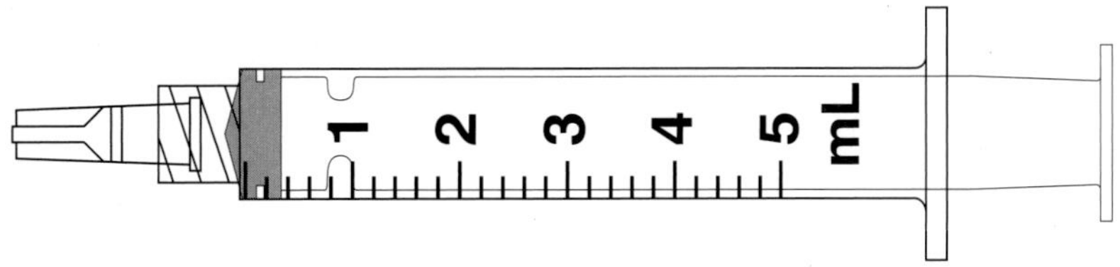

20. Administer 16 mL

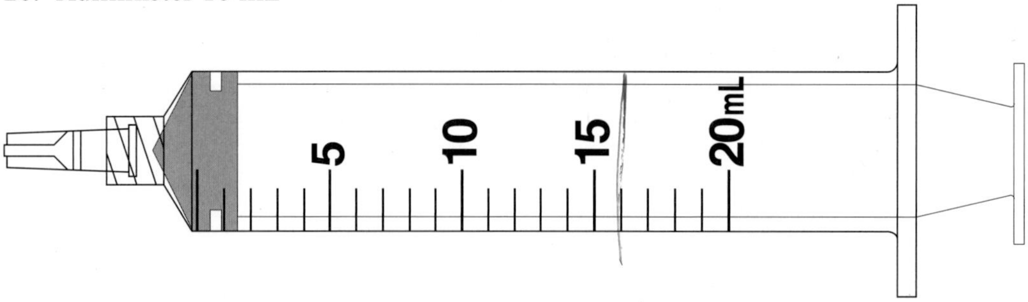

21. On the 5-mL syringe, each calibration is equal to ________. (Express the answer as a decimal.)

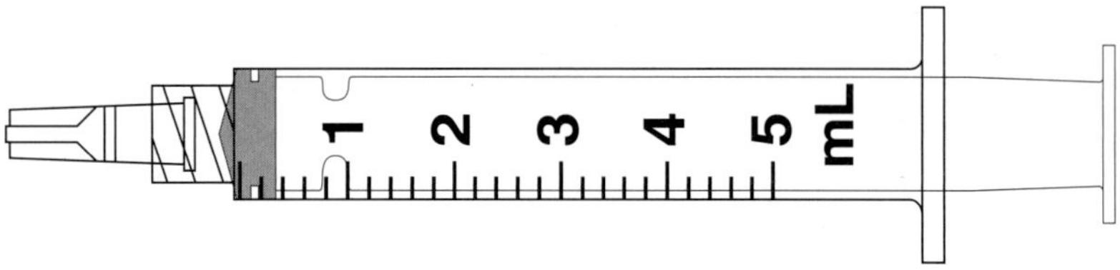

22. On the 20-mL syringe, each calibration is equal to ________.

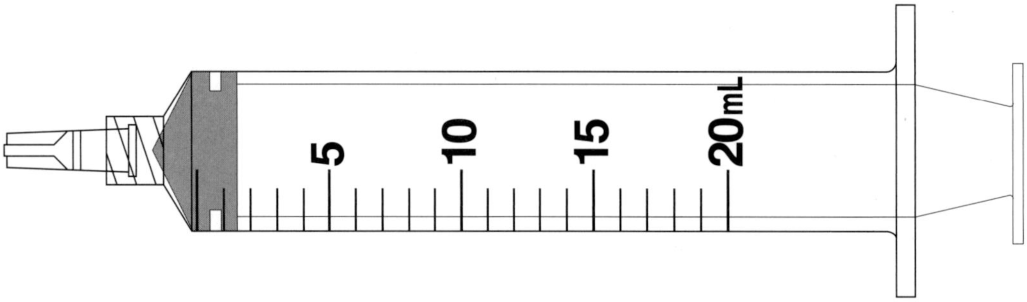

23. On the 10-mL syringe, each calibration is equal to ________. (Express the answer as a decimal.)

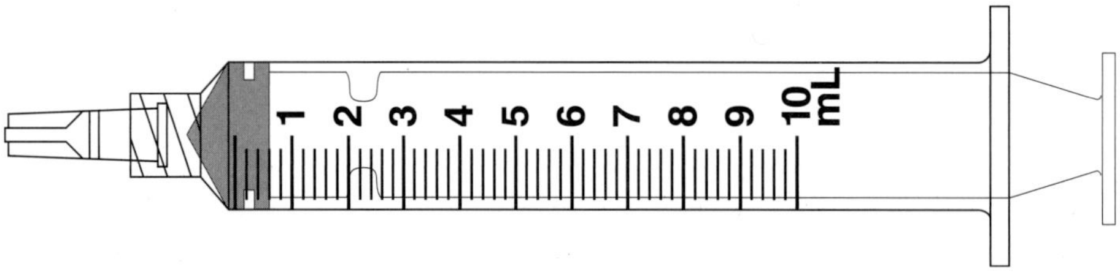

After completing these problems, see pages 461–462 of the answer section to check your answers.

CRITICAL THINKING SKILLS

Select correct equipment to prepare medications. In the following situation, the correct dosage was not given because an incorrect measuring device was used.

error

Using an inaccurate measuring device for oral medications.

possible scenario

Suppose a pediatrician ordered amoxicillin suspension 250 mg (5 mL or 1 teaspoon), every 8 hours, to be given to a child. The child should receive the medication for 10 days for otitis media, an ear infection. The pharmacy dispensed the medication in a bottle containing 150 mL, or a 10-day supply. The nurse did not clarify for the mother how to measure and administer the medication. The child returned to the clinic in 10 days for routine follow-up. The nurse asked whether the child had taken all the prescribed amoxicillin. The child's mother stated, "No, we have almost half of the bottle left." When the nurse asked how the medication had been given, the mother showed the bright pink plastic teaspoon she had obtained from the local ice cream parlor. The nurse measured the spoon's capacity and found it to be less than 3 mL. (Remember, 1 tsp = 5 mL.) The child would have received only 3/5, or 60%, of the correct dose.

potential outcome

The child did not receive a therapeutic dosage of the medication and was actually underdosed. The child could develop a super infection, which could lead to a more severe illness such as meningitis. Risk of bacterial resistance to the antibiotic is increased. Inadequate shaking of the suspension prior to measuring could also result in inaccurate dose of the drug.

prevention

Teach family members (and patients, as appropriate) to use calibrated measuring spoons or specially designed oral syringes to measure the correct dosage of medication. The volumes of serving spoons may vary considerably, as this situation illustrates. Also teach to adequately shake the medication before measuring and to take all of the medication as ordered to limit to risk of antibiotic resistance.

PRACTICE PROBLEMS—CHAPTER 5

1. In the 100-unit insulin syringe, 100 units = ________ mL.
2. The 1-mL syringe is calibrated in ________ of a mL.
3. Can you measure 1.25 mL in a single tuberculin syringe? ________ Explain. ________________

   ____

   ____
4. How would you measure 1.33 mL in a 3-mL syringe? ________________________
5. The medicine cup has a ________ mL capacity.
6. To administer exactly 0.52 mL to a child, select a ________ syringe.
7. Seventy-five units of 100-unit insulin equals ________ mL.
8. All droppers are calibrated to deliver standardized drops of equal amounts regardless of the dropper used. (True) (False)
9. The prefilled syringe is a multiple-dose system. (True) (False)
10. Insulin should be measured in an insulin syringe *only*. (True) (False)

11. The purpose of needleless syringes is ____.

12. Medications are measured in syringes by aligning the calibrations with the ________ of the black rubber tip of the plunger. (top ring, raised middle, or bottom ring)

13. The medicine cup calibrations indicate that 2 tsp are approximately ________ mL.

14. Some syringes are marked in cubic centimetres (cc) rather than millilitres (mL). (True) (False)

15. The ________ syringe(s) is(are) intended to measure parenteral doses of medications. (standard 3-mL, 1-mL, or insulin)

Draw an arrow to indicate the calibration that corresponds to the dose to be administered.

16. Administer 0.45 mL

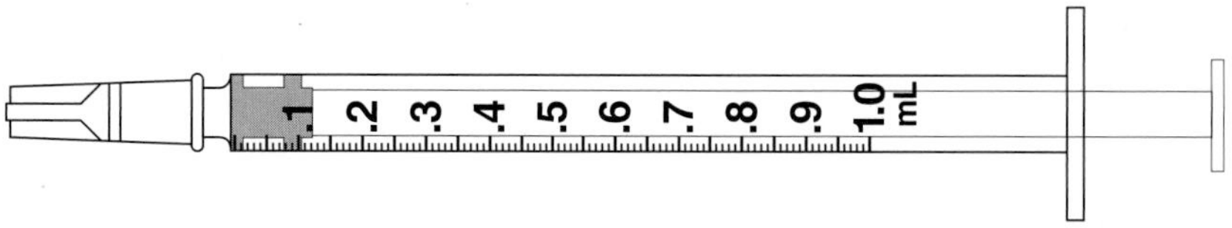

17. Administer 80 units of 100-unit insulin

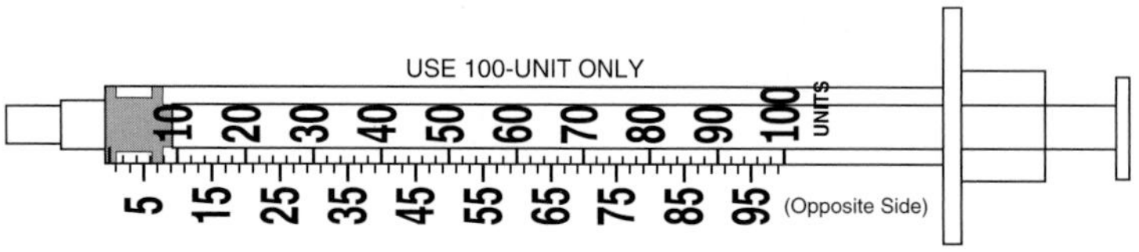

18. Administer 15 mL

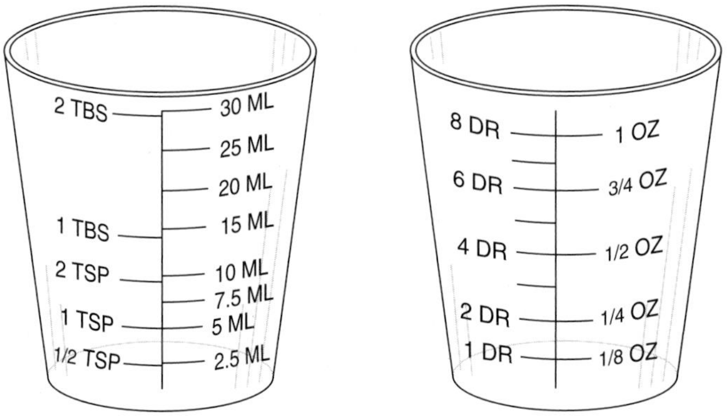

19. Administer 2.4 mL

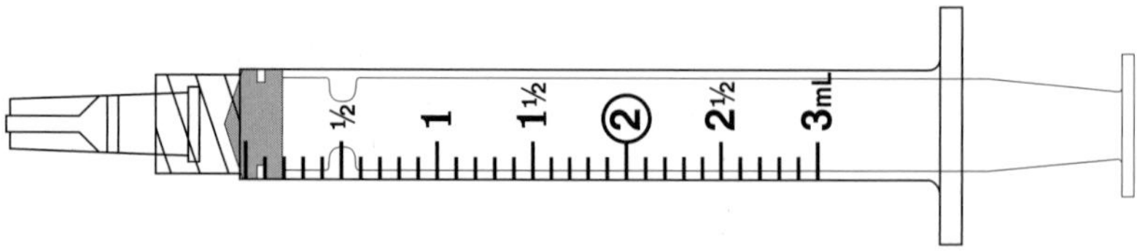

20. Administer 1.1 mL

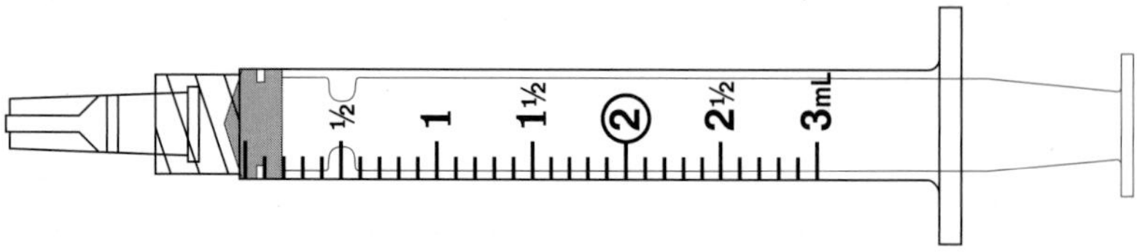

21. Administer 6.2 mL

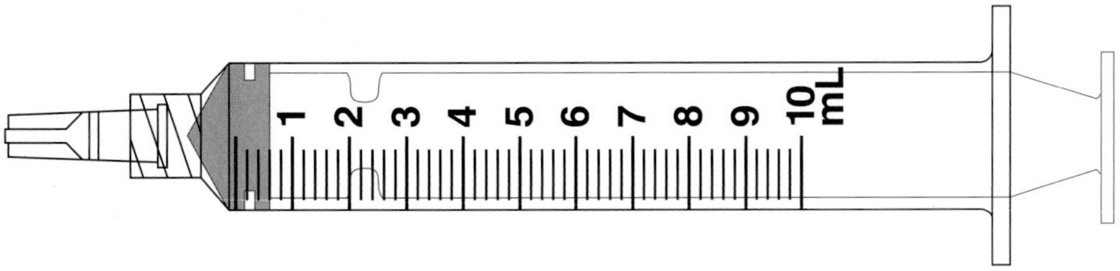

22. Administer 3.6 mL

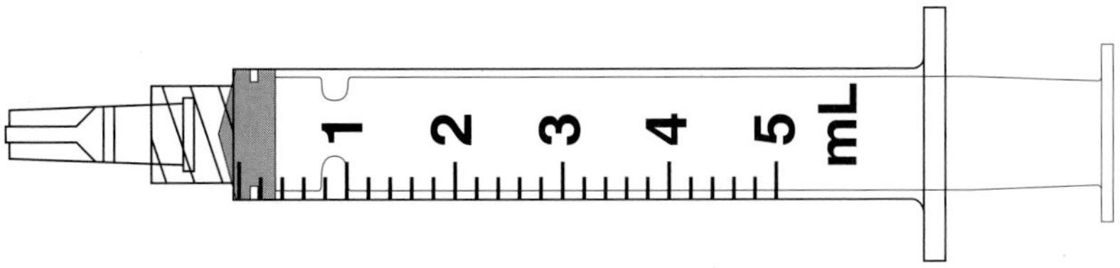

23. Administer 4.8 mL

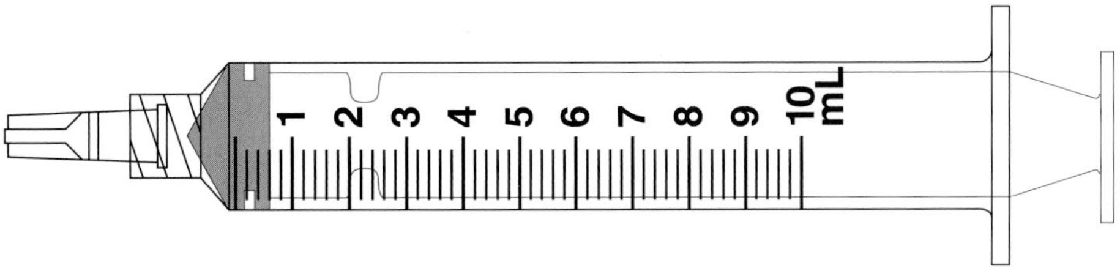

24. Administer 12 mL

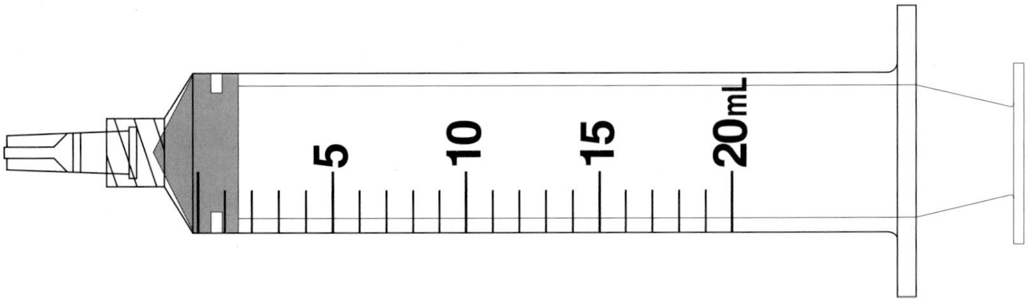

25. Critical Thinking Skill: Describe the strategy that would prevent this medication error.

possible scenario

Suppose a patient with cancer has oral prochlorperazine liquid ordered for nausea. Because the patient has had difficulty taking the medication, the nurse decided to draw up the medication in a syringe without a needle to facilitate giving the medication. An unexpected crisis situation disrupted the medication process. Once the crisis was resolved, the nurse attached a needle and injected the oral medication.

potential outcome

The medication would be absorbed systemically, and the patient could develop an abscess at the site of injection.

prevention

____

____

26. Critical Thinking Skill: Describe the strategy that would prevent this medication administration error.

possible scenario

A child with ear infections is to receive cefaclor oral liquid as an anti-infective. The medication is received in oral syringes for administration. The nurse fails to remove the cap on the tip of the syringe and attempts to administer the medication.

potential outcome

The nurse would exert enough pressure on the syringe plunger that the protective cap could pop off in the child's mouth and possibly cause the child to choke.

prevention

____

____

After completing these problems, see pages 462–464 of the answer section to check your answers.

CHAPTER

6

Interpreting Drug Orders

LEARNING OBJECTIVES

1. Read and write correct medical notation.
2. Interpret the standard medical abbreviation from a list of common terminology.
3. Classify the notation that specifies the dosage, route, and frequency of the medication to be administered.
4. Interpret physician and other prescribing practitioner patient care orders and medication administration records.

The focus in this chapter is on accurate interpretation of a prescription or medication patient care order. However, the goal of ensuring patient safety extends beyond interpretation to adherence to standards and best practices by healthcare professionals. In Canada, the responsibility for this for nursing is with the provincial/territorial nursing jurisdictions. Medication management and administration is continually reviewed and updated to support patient safety. Informed practice means being current. Use of sources such as one's specific jurisdictional documents on practice standards, information from the Institute for Safe Medication Practices (ISMP) (http://www.ismp.canada.org), and current Canadian nursing practice textbooks promotes accurate and effective medication administration practice.

The prescription or medication order conveys the therapeutic drug plan for the patient. It is the responsibility of the nurse to:

- Interpret the order
- Prepare the exact dosage of the prescribed drug
- Identify the patient
- Administer the proper dosage by the prescribed route, at the prescribed time intervals
- Record the administration of the prescribed drug
- Monitor and document the patient's response for desired (therapeutic) and adverse effects

Before you can prepare the correct dosage of the prescribed drug, you must learn to interpret or read the written patient care order. For brevity and speed, the healthcare professions have adopted certain standards and common abbreviations for use in notation. Recognition and interpretation of abbreviations is a skill that develops with practice. Abbreviations, symbols, and dose designations are potential sources for medication errors. Be sure that the interpretation is always correct; question and check if unsure.

An example of a typical written patient care order is:

9/4/XX amoxicillin 500 mg PO QID (pc & bedtime)
J. Physician, M.D.

This order means the patient should receive 500 milligrams of an antibiotic named amoxicillin orally four times a day (after meals and at bedtime). You can see that the medical notation considerably shortens the written-out order.

MEDICAL ABBREVIATIONS

Nurses, as well as other healthcare professionals, must practise to ensure safety in the administration of medications. Misinterpretation of abbreviations contributes to medication errors. In Canada, the Institute for Safe Medication Practices has identified abbreviations and dose designations that are problematic with recommendations to correct the potential for error. For specific information, see http://www.ismp-canada.org/download/ISMPCanadaListofDangerousAbbreviations.pdf

Medication policies developed by each healthcare facility inform the nurse which abbreviations are acceptable for use in that facility. When an abbreviation is not clearly written, it is the responsibility of the nurse to contact the writer of the order containing the abbreviation to obtain clarification and avoid the potential error.

CAUTION

It is essential to know and use only *current* abbreviations accepted in your practice setting.

REMEMBER

Common Medical Abbreviations

Abbreviation	Interpretation	Abbreviation	Interpretation
Route:		**Frequency:**	
IM	intramuscular	TID	three times a day[1]
IV	intravenous	QID	four times a day[1]
		min	minute
SL	sublingual, under the tongue	h/hr	hour
ID	intradermal	qh/qhr	every hour
SUBCUT	subcutaneously		
GT	gastrostomy tube	q2h	every two hours
NG	nasogastric tube	q3h	every three hours
NJ	nasojejunal tube	q4h	every four hours
PO	by mouth, orally	q6h	every six hours
pr	per rectum, rectally	q8h	every eight hours
pr subcut	rectally subcutaneous		
Frequency:		q12h	every twelve hours
ac	before meals	**General:**	
pc	after meals	q	every
ad lib	as desired, freely		
prn	when necessary	NPO	nothing by mouth
stat	immediately, at once	gtt	drop
BID	twice a day[1]	tab	tablet

[1] Some healthcare agencies continue to use bid, tid, qid; some references support avoiding these abbreviations, instead writing out information in full. BID, TIQ, QID appear in ISMP documents and are common in computerized medication administration sheets (MAR).

The above table lists some common medical abbreviations used in writing drug orders. The abbreviations are grouped according to those that refer to the route (or method) of administration, the frequency (time interval), and other general terms.

Do Not Use

Dangerous Abbreviations, Symbols and Dose Designations

The abbreviations, symbols, and dose designations found in this table have been reported as being frequently misinterpreted and involved in harmful medication errors. They should NEVER be used when communicating medication information.

Abbreviation	Intended Meaning	Problem	Correction
U	unit	Mistaken for "0" (zero), "4" (four), or cc.	Use "unit".
IU	international unit	Mistaken for "IV" (intravenous) or "10" (ten).	Use "unit".
Abbreviations for drug names		Misinterpreted because of similar abbreviations for multiple drugs; e.g., MS, MSO_4 (morphine sulfate), $MgSO_4$ (magnesium sulfate) may be confused for one another.	Do not abbreviate drug names.
QD QOD	Every day Everyother day	QD and QOD have been mistaken for each other, or as 'qid'. The Q has also been misinterpreted as "2" (two).	Use "daily" and "every other day".
OD	Every day	Mistaken for "right eye" (OD = oculus dexter).	Use "daily".
OS, OD, OU	Left eye, right eye, both eyes	May be confused with one another.	Use "left eye", "right eye" or "both eyes".
D/C	Discharge	Interpreted as "discontinue whatever medications follow" (typically discharge medications).	Use "discharge".
cc	cubic centimetre	Mistaken for "u" (units).	Use "mL" or "millilitre".
µg	microgram	Mistaken for "mg" (milligram) resulting in one thousand-fold overdose.	Use "mcg".
Symbol	**Intended Meaning**	**Potential Problem**	**Correction**
@	at	Mistaken for "2" (two) or "5" (five).	Use "at".
> <	Greater than Less than	Mistaken for "7"(seven) or the letter "L". Confused with each other.	Use "greater than"/"more than" or "less than"/"lower than".
Dose Designation	**Intended Meaning**	**Potential Problem**	**Correction**
Trailing zero	$\mathcal{X}$.0 mg	Decimal point is overlooked resulting in 10-fold dose error.	Never use a zero by itself after a decimal point. Use "**$\mathcal{X}$ mg**".
Lack of leading zero	.$\mathcal{X}$ mg	Decimal point is overlooked resulting in 10-fold dose error.	Always use a zero before a decimal point. Use "**0.**$\mathcal{X}$ mg".

Report actual and potential medication errors to ISMP Canada via the web at https://www.ismp-canada.org/err_report.htm or by calling 1-866-54-ISMPC. ISMP Canada guarantees confidentiality of information received and respects the reporter's wishes as to the level of detail included in publications.

ismp CANADA
Institute for Safe Medication Practices Canada
Institut pour l'utilisation sécuritaire des médicaments du Canada

THE DRUG ORDER

The drug order consists of seven parts:

1. Name of the *patient*
2. Name of the *drug* to be administered
3. *Dosage* of the drug
4. *Route* by which the drug is to be administered
5. *Frequency*, time, and special instructions related to administration
6. *Date and time* when the order was written
7. *Signature* of the person writing the order

CAUTION

If any of the seven parts is missing or unclear, the order is considered incomplete and is, therefore, not a legal patient care order. The nurse *must obtain* clarification of the order from the writer.

Parts 1 through 5 of the drug order comprise what is considered the original Five Rights of safe medication administration. They are essential and each one must be faithfully checked every time a medication is prepared and administered. Safe administration of medication requires the nurse or healthcare practitioner to accurately document the drug administration. Accurate documentation along with right reason, right frequency, and right site have been added to the Rights of safe medication administration with variance as to how this is expressed across provincial/territorial nursing jurisdictions.

REMEMBER

The Rights of safe and accurate medication administration:

The *right patient* must receive the *right drug* for the *right reason* in the *right amount* by the *right route* in the *right site* at the *right time* and *right frequency*, followed by the *right documentation*.

Each patient care order should follow a specific sequence. The name of the drug is written first, followed by the dosage, route, and frequency. Drugs are identified with generic (non-proprietary) and brand (trade or proprietary) names. The order may state generic or brand names, or both. Combination and over-the-counter drugs are often identified by brand name. When correctly written, the trade name of the drug begins with a capital or uppercase letter. The generic name begins with a lowercase letter.

CAUTION

Nurses must know current correct information about drugs, whether identified by generic or brand names. Authoritative resources include Compendium of Pharmaceuticals and Specialties, Health Canada's Drug Product Database website, drug package enclosures with the manufacturer's information, and licensed pharmacists.

Example:

Pen VK 300 mg PO QID for 7–10 days.

NOTE: This order could have been written using the generic name (recommended in some jurisdictions). It would look like *penicillin V potassium 300 mg PO QID for 7–10 days.*

1. *Pen VK* is the brand name of the drug
2. *300 mg* is the dosage
3. *PO* is the route
4. *QID* is the frequency
5. *For 7–10 days* indicates that there is a time limit on the use of this medication

This order means: Give 300 milligrams of *Penicillin V potassium* orally four times a day for 7 to 10 days.

CAUTION

If the nurse has difficulty understanding and interpreting the patient care order, the nurse *must* clarify the order with the writer. Usually this person is the physician or another authorized practitioner.

Let's practise reading and interpreting patient care orders.

Example 1:

Dilantin 100 mg PO TID

Reads: "Give 100 milligrams of Dilantin orally 3 times a day."

Example 2:

procaine penicillin G 400 000 units IM q6h

Reads: "Give 400 000 units of procaine penicillin G intramuscularly every 6 hours."

Example 3:

meperidine hydrochloride 75 mg IM q4h prn for pain

Reads: "Give 75 milligrams of meperidine hydrochloride intramuscularly every 4 hours when necessary for pain."

CAUTION

The *prn* frequency designates the minimum time allowed between doses. There is no maximum time other than automatic stops as defined by institution policy.

Example 4:

Humulin-R 100-unit insulin 5 units SUBCUT stat

Reads: "Give 5 units of Humulin R 100-unit insulin subcutaneously immediately."

Example 5:

Cephalexin 1 g IV q6h

Reads: "Give 1 gram of cephalexin by intravenous every 6 hours."

The administration times are designated by institution policy. For example, TID administration times may be 0900, 1300, and 1700.

QUICK REVIEW

- The *right patient* must receive the *right drug* for the *right reason* in the *right amount* by the *right route* in the *right site* at the *right time* and the *right frequency*, followed by the *right documentation*.
- Understanding patient care orders requires interpreting common medical abbreviations.
- The patient care order must contain (in this sequence): drug name, dosage, route, frequency.
- All parts of the patient care order must be stated clearly for accurate, exact interpretation.
- If you are ever in doubt as to the meaning of any part of a patient care order, ask the writer to clarify before proceeding.

REVIEW SET 17

Interpret the following medication (drug) orders:

1. *naproxen 250 mg PO BID* ____________________
2. *Humulin insulin 30 units SUBCUT daily 30 min before breakfast* ____________________
3. *cefaclor 500 mg PO stat, then 250 mg q8h* ____________________
4. *levothyroxine 25 mcg PO daily* ____________________
5. *lorazepam 10 mg IM q4h prn for agitation* ____________________
6. *cefazolin 500 mg intravenously per piggyback as per protocol* ____________________
7. *aluminum hydroxide 10 mL PO bedtime* ____________________
8. *atropine sulfate ophthalmic 1% 2 gtt right eye q15 min × 4* ____________________
9. *morphine sulfate 15 mg IM q3–4h prn for pain* ____________________
10. *Lanoxin 0.25 mg PO daily* ____________________
11. *tetracycline 250 mg PO QID* ____________________
12. *nitroglycerin 0.6 mg SL stat* ____________________
13. *Cortisporin otic suspension 2 gtt both ears TID and bedtime* ____________________

14. Compare and contrast *TID* and *q8h* administration times. Include sample administration times for each in your explanation. ______________________________

____

15. Describe your action if no method of administration is written. ______________________________

____

16. Do *QID* and *q4h* have the same meaning? __________ Explain. ______________________________

____

17. Who determines the medication administration times? ______________________________

____

18. Name the seven parts of a written medication prescription. ______________________________

____

19. In Canada, what are three sources of information on current medication practices? ______

____

20. State the Rights of safe and accurate medication administration as noted in this chapter. ______________________________

____

After completing these problems, see page 464 in the answer section to check your answers.

Medication Order and Administration Forms

Hospitals have a special form for recording drug orders. This form may be different in different healthcare settings. All settings require dating on these forms but the date format may vary. Figure 6-1 shows a sample physician's order form. In some jurisdictions and practice areas, orders may be written by other healthcare professionals and forms may be labelled Patient Care Orders. Find and name each of the seven parts of the patient care orders listed. Notice that the nurse or other healthcare professional must verify and initial each order, ensuring that each of the seven parts is accurate. In some places, the pharmacist may be responsible for verifying the order as part of the computerized record.

ENTERED	FILLED	CHECKED	VERIFIED

NOTE: A NON-PROPRIETARY DRUG OF EQUAL QUALITY MAY BE DISPENSED - IF THIS COLUMN IS NOT CHECKED!

DATE	TIME WRITTEN	PLEASE USE BALL POINT - PRESS FIRMLY	✓	TIME NOTED	NURSES SIGNATURE
11/3/xx	0815	cephalexin 250 mg PO q6h	✓	0830	G. Pickar, RN
		Humulin N Insulin 40 units SUBCUT ac breakfast	✓		
		meperidine hydrochloride 75 mg IV q3–4 h prn for severe pain	✓		
		Codeine 30 mg PO q4h prn for mild–mod pain	✓		
		acetaminophen 650 mg PO q4h prn for fever greater than 38.3°C	✓		
		furosemide 80 mg IV stat	✓		
		potassium chloride 300 mg PO BID	✓		
		J. Physician, MD			
11/3/xx	2200	Lasix 80 mg IV stat	✓		
		J. Physician, MD		2210	M. Smith, RN

AUTO STOP ORDERS: UNLESS REORDERED, FOLLOWING WILL BE D/C'D AT 0800 ON:

DATE	ORDER		
		☐ CONT ☐ D/C	PHYSICIAN SIGNATURE
		☐ CONT ☐ D/C	PHYSICIAN SIGNATURE
		☐ CONT ☐ D/C	PHYSICIAN SIGNATURE

CHECK WHEN ANTIBIOTICS ORDERED ☐ Prophylactic ☐ Empiric ☐ Therapeutic

Allergies: None Known

CLIENT DIAGNOSIS: Diabetes

HEIGHT 166 cm WEIGHT 59 kg

Patient, Mary Q.
#3-11316-7

1

FORM 959-708 (8-XX) PHYSICIANS ORDER Reynolds + Reynolds LITHO IN U.S.A. K41814 (7-XX) D339360

FIGURE 6-1 Physician's Order

The drug orders from the physician's order form are transcribed to a medication administration record (MAR), depicted in Figure 6-2. This form may be different in different healthcare settings. The nurse or other healthcare professional uses this record as a guide to:

- Check the patient care order,
- Prepare the correct dosage, and
- Record the drug administered.

These three check points help to ensure accurate medication administration.

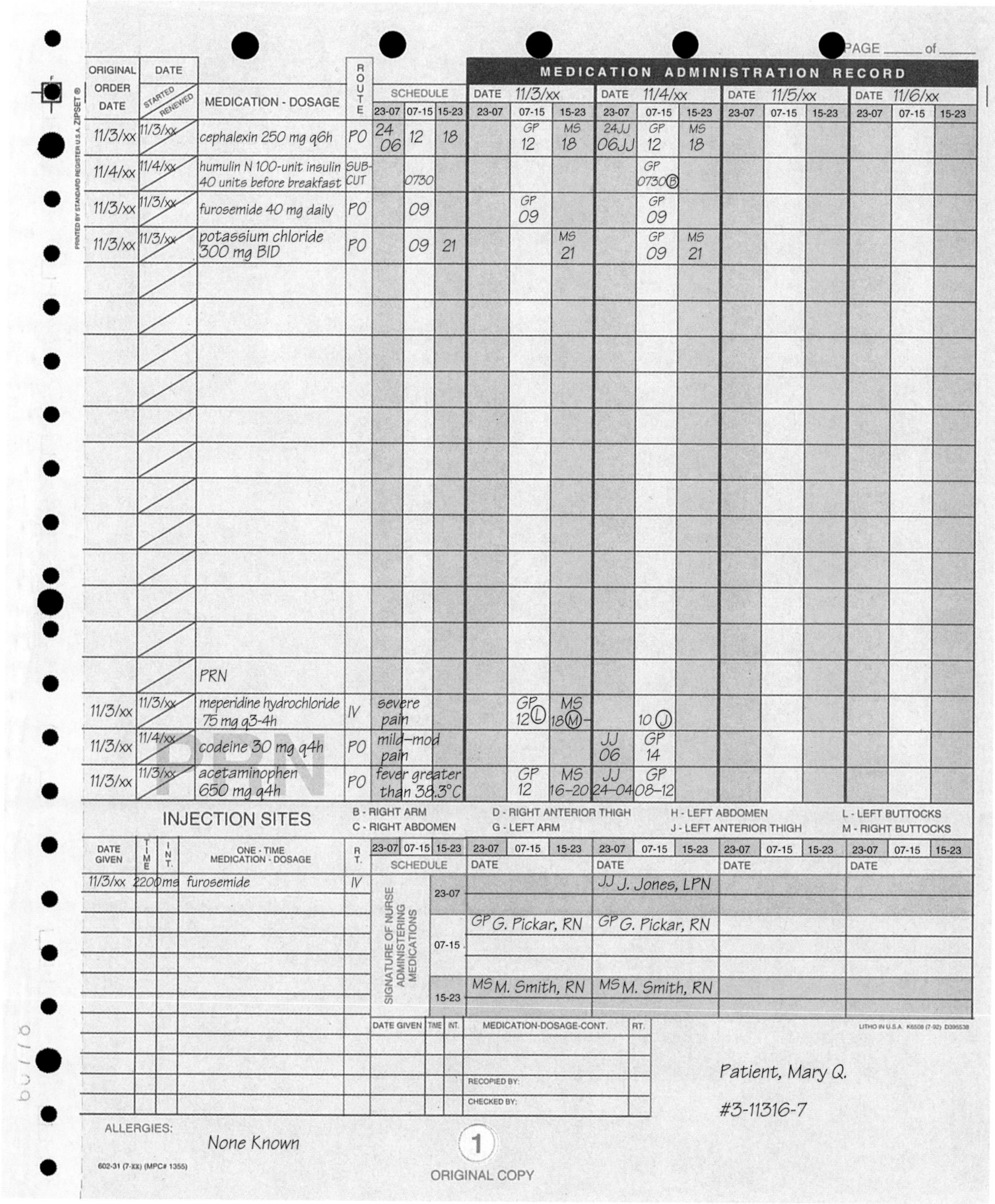

PAGE ____ of ____

MEDICATION ADMINISTRATION RECORD

ORIGINAL ORDER DATE	DATE STARTED / RENEWED	MEDICATION - DOSAGE	ROUTE	SCHEDULE 23-07	SCHEDULE 07-15	SCHEDULE 15-23	DATE 11/3/xx 23-07	11/3/xx 07-15	11/3/xx 15-23	DATE 11/4/xx 23-07	11/4/xx 07-15	11/4/xx 15-23	DATE 11/5/xx 23-07	11/5/xx 07-15	11/5/xx 15-23	DATE 11/6/xx 23-07	11/6/xx 07-15	11/6/xx 15-23
11/3/xx	11/3/xx	cephalexin 250 mg q6h	PO	24 06	12	18		GP 12	MS 18	24JJ 06JJ	GP 12	MS 18						
11/4/xx	11/4/xx	humulin N 100-unit insulin 40 units before breakfast	SUB-CUT		0730						GP 0730(B)							
11/3/xx	11/3/xx	furosemide 40 mg daily	PO		09			GP 09			GP 09							
11/3/xx	11/3/xx	potassium chloride 300 mg BID	PO		09	21			MS 21		GP 09	MS 21						
		PRN																
11/3/xx	11/3/xx	meperidine hydrochloride 75 mg q3-4h	IV	severe pain				GP 12(L)	MS 18(M)-		10(J)							
11/3/xx	11/4/xx	codeine 30 mg q4h	PO	mild–mod pain						JJ 06	GP 14							
11/3/xx	11/3/xx	acetaminophen 650 mg q4h	PO	fever greater than 38.3°C				GP 12	MS 16-20	JJ 24-04	GP 08-12							

INJECTION SITES: B - RIGHT ARM; C - RIGHT ABDOMEN; D - RIGHT ANTERIOR THIGH; G - LEFT ARM; H - LEFT ABDOMEN; J - LEFT ANTERIOR THIGH; L - LEFT BUTTOCKS; M - RIGHT BUTTOCKS

DATE GIVEN	TIME	INT.	ONE - TIME MEDICATION - DOSAGE	RT.
11/3/xx	2200	ms	furosemide	IV

SIGNATURE OF NURSE ADMINISTERING MEDICATIONS

	DATE 11/3/xx	DATE 11/4/xx
23-07		JJ J. Jones, LPN
07-15	GP G. Pickar, RN	GP G. Pickar, RN
15-23	MS M. Smith, RN	MS M. Smith, RN

DATE GIVEN | TIME | INT. | MEDICATION-DOSAGE-CONT. | RT.

RECOPIED BY:

CHECKED BY:

Patient, Mary Q.

#3-11316-7

ALLERGIES: None Known

602-31 (7-XX) (MPC# 1355)

ORIGINAL COPY

FIGURE 6-2 Medication Administration Record

COMPUTERIZED MEDICATION ADMINISTRATION SYSTEMS

Many healthcare facilities now use computers for processing patient care orders. Patient care orders are either electronically transmitted or manually entered into the computer from an order form, such as the one depicted in Figure 6-3. Through the computer, the nurse or other healthcare professional can transmit the order within seconds to the pharmacy for filling. The computer can keep track of drug stock and usage patterns. Most importantly, it can scan for information previously entered, such as drug

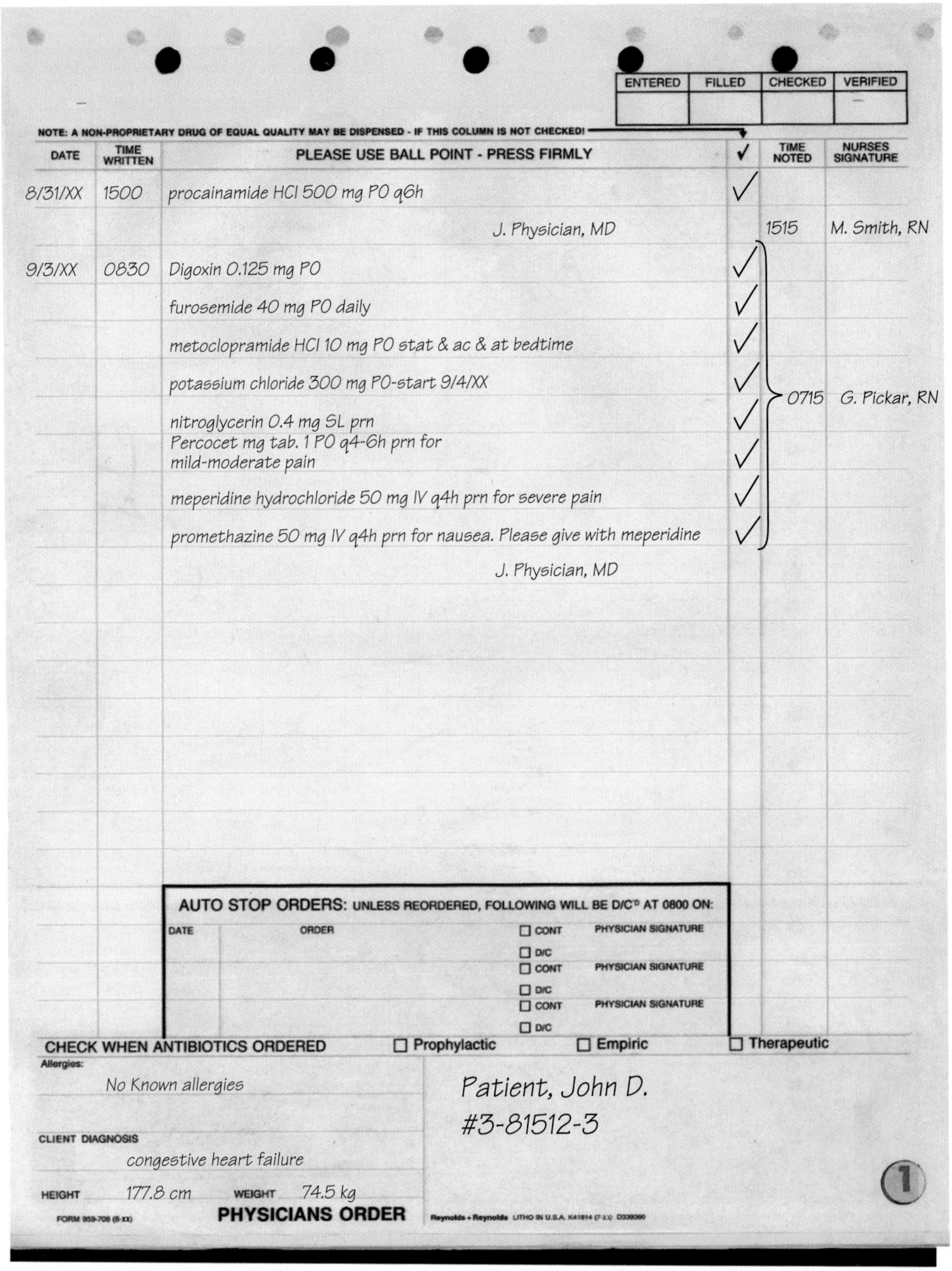

ENTERED	FILLED	CHECKED	VERIFIED

NOTE: A NON-PROPRIETARY DRUG OF EQUAL QUALITY MAY BE DISPENSED - IF THIS COLUMN IS NOT CHECKED!

DATE	TIME WRITTEN	PLEASE USE BALL POINT - PRESS FIRMLY	✓	TIME NOTED	NURSES SIGNATURE
8/31/XX	1500	procainamide HCl 500 mg PO q6h	✓		
		J. Physician, MD		1515	M. Smith, RN
9/3/XX	0830	Digoxin 0.125 mg PO	✓	0715	G. Pickar, RN
		furosemide 40 mg PO daily	✓		
		metoclopramide HCl 10 mg PO stat & ac & at bedtime	✓		
		potassium chloride 300 mg PO-start 9/4/XX	✓		
		nitroglycerin 0.4 mg SL prn	✓		
		Percocet mg tab. 1 PO q4-6h prn for mild-moderate pain	✓		
		meperidine hydrochloride 50 mg IV q4h prn for severe pain	✓		
		promethazine 50 mg IV q4h prn for nausea. Please give with meperidine	✓		
		J. Physician, MD			

AUTO STOP ORDERS: UNLESS REORDERED, FOLLOWING WILL BE D/C'D AT 0800 ON:

DATE	ORDER		PHYSICIAN SIGNATURE
		☐ CONT ☐ D/C	PHYSICIAN SIGNATURE
		☐ CONT ☐ D/C	PHYSICIAN SIGNATURE
		☐ CONT ☐ D/C	

CHECK WHEN ANTIBIOTICS ORDERED ☐ Prophylactic ☐ Empiric ☐ Therapeutic

Allergies: No Known allergies

Patient, John D.
#3-81512-3

CLIENT DIAGNOSIS congestive heart failure

HEIGHT 177.8 cm WEIGHT 74.5 kg

FORM 959-708 (8-XX) PHYSICIANS ORDER Reynolds + Reynolds LITHO IN U.S.A. K41814 (7-XX) D33080

1

FIGURE 6-3 Physician's Order

incompatibilities, drug allergies, safe dosage ranges, doses already given, or recommended administration times. The healthcare staff can be readily alerted to potential problems or inconsistencies. The corresponding medication administration record may also be printed directly from the computer (Figure 6-4).

The computerized MAR may be viewed at the computer or from a printed copy (Figure 6-4). The nurse may be able to look back at the patient's cumulative MAR, document administration times and comments at the computer terminal, and then keep a printed copy of the information obtained and entered. The data analysis, storage, and retrieval abilities of computers are making them essential tools for safe and accurate medication administration.

Note that in Figures 6-1, 6-2, 6-3, and 6-4, there is a patient care order that includes a range for interval to repeat medication. While this is still occurring in practice, there is a shift to indicate only the minimal interval for repeat, leaving the healthcare professional and patient to decide on a longer interval. Also, although the generic name is the preferred use for writing an order, brand or trade names still do appear especially with combination medications, e.g., Percocet.

REMEMBER

It is important to be aware and comply with practice in one's specific area of practice.

PHARMACY MAR

START	STOP	MEDICATION	SCHEDULED TIMES	OK'D BY	0001 HRS. TO 1200 HRS.	1201 HRS. TO 2400 HRS.
08/31/xx 1800 SCH		PROCAINAMIDE HCL (PROCAN SR) 500 MG TAB-SR 500 MG Q6H PO	0600 1200 1800 2400	JD	0600GP 1200 GP	1800 MS 2400 JD
09/03/xx 0900 SCH		DIGOXIN (LANOXIN) 0.125 MG TAB 1 TAB QOD PO ODD DAYS-SEPT	0900	JD	0900 GP	
09/03/xx 0900 SCH		FUROSEMIDE (LASIX) 40 MG TAB 1 TAB QD PO	0900	JD	0900 GP	
09/03/xx 0845 SCH		METOCLOPRAMIDE (MAXERAN) 10 MG TAB 10 MG AC&HS PO GIVE ONE NOW!!	0730 1130 1630 2100	JD	0730 GP 1130 GP	1630 MS 2100 MS
09/04/xx 0900 SCH		POTASSIUM CHLORIDE (K-LYTE) 25 MEQ EFFERVESCENT TAB 1 EFF. TAB BID PO DISSOLVE AS DIR START 9-4	0900 1700	JD	0900 GP	1700 GP
09/03/xx 1507 PRN		NITROGLYCERIN 0.4 mg TAB-SL 1 TABLET PRN* SL PRN CHEST PAIN		JD		
09/03/xx 1700 PRN		OXYCODONE 5 mg and ACETAMINOPHEN 325 mg Percocet 1 TAB Q4-6H PO PRN MILD–MODERATE PAIN		JD		
09/03/xx 2100 PRN		MEPERIDINE HYDROCHLORIDE INJ 50 MG Q4H IM PRN SEVERE PAIN W PHENERGAN		JD		2200 (H) MS
09/03/xx 2100 PRN		PROMETHAZINE (PHENERGAN) INJ 50 MG Q4H IM PRN NAUSEA W DEMEROL		JD		2200 (H) MS

Gluteus	Thigh
A. Right	H. Right
B. Left	I. Left
Ventro Gluteal	
C. Right	J. Right
D. Left	K. Left
E. Abdomen 1 | 2 / 3 | 4	

730-13 (12/xx)

	NURSE'S SIGNATURE	INITIAL
7–3	G. Pickar, RN	GP
3–11	M. Smith, RN	MS
11–7	J. Doe, RN	JD

ALLERGIES: NKA

DIAGNOSIS: CHF

Patient: Patient, John D.
Patient# 3-81512-3
Admitted: 08/31/xx
Physician: J. Physician, MD
Room: PCU-14 PCU

FIGURE 6-4 Computerized Medication Administration Record

QUICK REVIEW

- Drug orders are prescribed on the Physician's Orders form or similar forms, such as a Patient Care Orders form.
- The person who administers a drug records it on the MAR. This record may be handwritten or computerized.
- All parts of the patient care order must be stated clearly for accurate, exact interpretation. If you are ever in doubt as to the meaning of any part of a patient care order, ask the writer to clarify.

REVIEW SET 18

Refer to the **MAR (Figure 6-2)** on page 113 to answer questions 1 through 9.

1. What is the route of administration for the insulin? ______
2. How many times in a 24-hour period will furosemide be administered? ______
3. What is the only medication ordered to be given routinely at noon? ______
4. What time of day is the insulin to be administered? ______
5. A dosage of 300 mg of potassium is ordered. This is equivalent to 4 mEq of potassium chloride. What does *mEq* mean? ______
6. You work 1500–2300 on November 5. Which routine medications will you administer to Mary Q. Patient during your shift? ______
7. Mary Q. Patient has a temperature of 38.9°C. What medication should you administer? ______
8. How many times in a 24-hour period will potassium chloride be administered? ______
9. Identify the place on the MAR where the stat IV furosemide was charted. ______

Refer to the computerized **MAR (Figure 6-4)** on page 115 to answer questions 10 through 19. Convert the scheduled international time to traditional AM/PM time.

10. Scheduled times for administering procainamide HCl ______
11. Scheduled times for administering digoxin and furosemide ______
12. Scheduled times for administering metoclopramide ______
13. Scheduled times for administering potassium chloride ______
14. How often can the meperidine HCl be given? ______
15. If the digoxin was last given on 09/07/xx at 0900 h, when is the next time and date it will be given? ______
16. What is the ordered route of administration for the nitroglycerin? ______
17. How many times a day is furosemide ordered? ______
18. The equivalent dosage of digoxin is ______ mcg.
19. Which drugs are ordered to be administered "as necessary"? ______

After completing these problems, see page 465 to check your answers.

CRITICAL THINKING SKILLS

It is the responsibility of the nurse to clarify any patient care order that is incomplete; that is, an order that does not contain the essential seven parts discussed in this chapter. Let's look at an example in which this error occurred.

error

Failing to clarify incomplete orders.

possible scenario

Suppose a physician ordered *famotidine tablet PO at bedtime* for a patient with an active duodenal ulcer. You will note there is no dosage listed. The nurse thought the medication came in only one dosage strength, added 20 mg to the order, and sent it to the pharmacy. The pharmacist prepared the dosage written on the physician's order sheet. Two days later, during rounds, the physician noted that the patient had not responded well to the famotidine. When asked about the famotidine, the nurse explained that the patient had received 20 mg at bedtime. The physician informed the nurse that the patient should have received the 40-mg tablet.

potential outcome

Potentially, the delay in correct dosage could result in gastrointestinal bleeding or delayed healing of the ulcer.

prevention

This medication error could have been avoided simply by the physician writing the strength of the medication. When this was omitted, the nurse should have checked the dosage before sending the order to the pharmacy. When the nurse fills in an incomplete order, the nurse is essentially practising medicine without a licence, which is illegal and potentially dangerous.

PRACTICE PROBLEMS—CHAPTER 6

Interpret the following abbreviations and symbols without consulting another source.

1. NG ________
2. pr ________
3. ac ________
4. SL ________
5. TID ________
6. q4h ________
7. prn ________
8. PO ________
9. tab ________
10. stat ________
11. ad lib ________
12. IM ________
13. pc ________

Give the abbreviation or symbol for the following terms without consulting another source.

14. nothing by mouth ________
15. drop ________
16. millilitre ________
17. at bedtime ________
18. gram ________
19 four times a day ________
20. every hour ________
21. subcutaneous ________
22. intravenous ________
23. twice daily ________
24. every 3 hours ________
25. every 12 hours ________
26. capsule ________
27. kilogram ________

Interpret the following physician's drug orders without consulting another source.

28. *keterolac 60 mg IM stat and q6h* ______
29. *procaine penicillin G 300 000 units IM QID* ______
30. *Mylanta tab 1 PO 1 h ac, 1 h pc, at bedtime and q2h during the night prn for gastric upset* ______
31. *chlordiazepoxide 25 mg PO q6h prn for agitation* ______
32. *heparin 5000 units SUBCUT stat* ______
33. *meperidine hydrochloride 50 mg IM q3–4h prn for pain* ______
34. *digoxin 0.25 mg PO daily* ______
35. *Neo-Synephrine ophthalmic 10% 2 gtt left eye q30 min × 2* ______
36. *furosemide 40 mg IM stat* ______
37. *betamethasone 4 mg IV BID* ______

Refer to the **MAR in Figure 6-5** on page 119 to answer questions 38 through 41.

38. How many units of heparin will the patient receive at 2200 h? ______
39. What route is ordered for the Humulin R insulin? ______
40. Interpret the order for ciprofloxacin HCl. ______
41. If the administration times for the sliding scale insulin are accurate (30 minutes before meals), what times will meals be served? ______

Refer to the **Computerized Pharmacy MAR in Figure 6-6** on page 120 to answer questions 42 through 45.

42. The physician visited about 1700 h on 08/08/xx. What order did the physician write? ______
43. Interpret the order for ranitidine. ______
44. Which of the routine medications is(are) ordered for 1800 h? ______

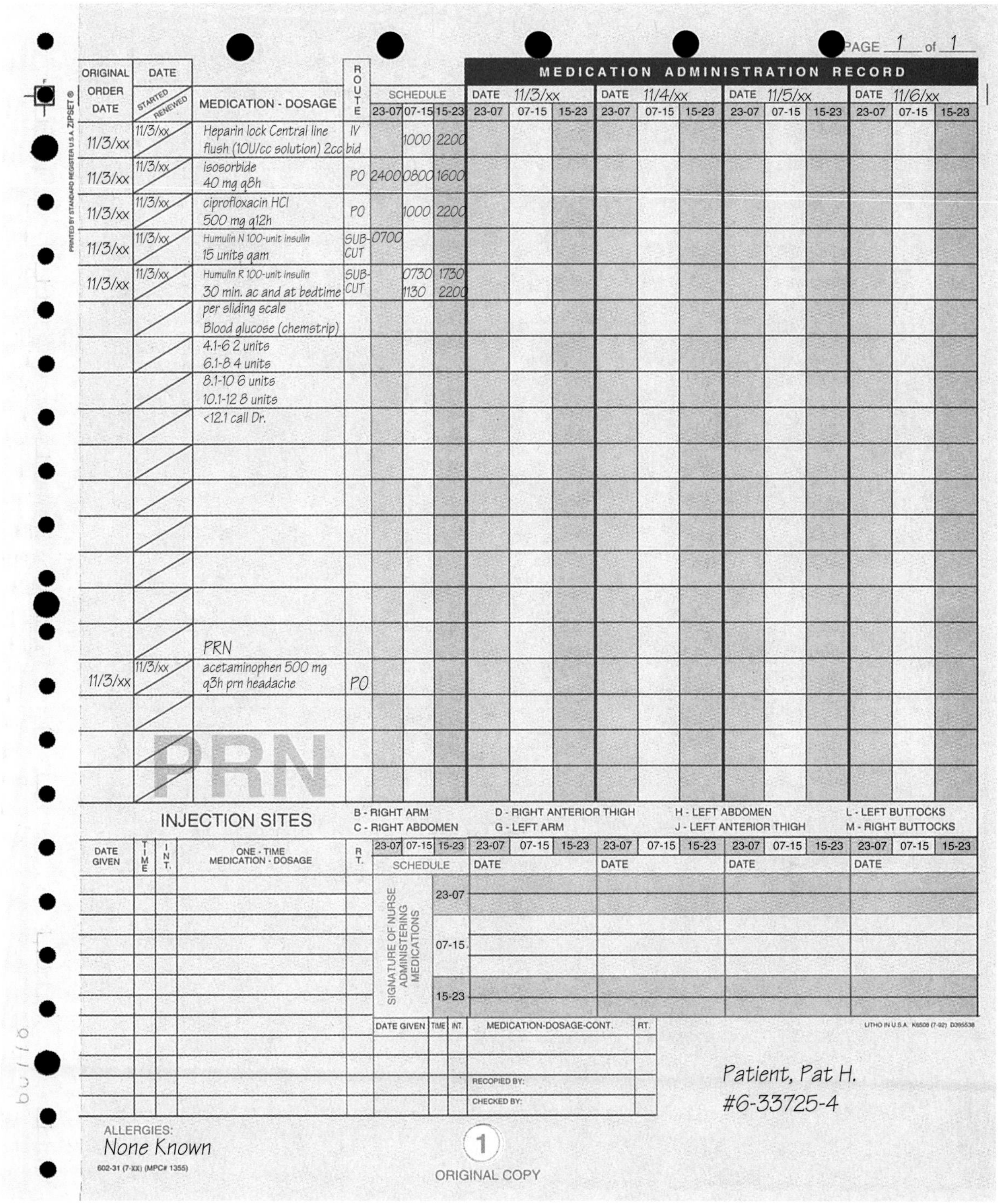
PAGE 1 of 1

MEDICATION ADMINISTRATION RECORD

ORIGINAL ORDER DATE	DATE STARTED / RENEWED	MEDICATION - DOSAGE	ROUTE	SCHEDULE 23-07	SCHEDULE 07-15	SCHEDULE 15-23	DATE 11/3/xx	DATE 11/4/xx	DATE 11/5/xx	DATE 11/6/xx
11/3/xx	11/3/xx	Heparin lock Central line flush (10U/cc solution) 2cc bid	IV		1000	2200				
11/3/xx	11/3/xx	isosorbide 40 mg q8h	PO	2400	0800	1600				
11/3/xx	11/3/xx	ciprofloxacin HCl 500 mg q12h	PO		1000	2200				
11/3/xx	11/3/xx	Humulin N 100-unit insulin 15 units qam	SUB-CUT	0700						
11/3/xx	11/3/xx	Humulin R 100-unit insulin 30 min. ac and at bedtime per sliding scale Blood glucose (chemstrip) 4.1-6 2 units 6.1-8 4 units 8.1-10 6 units 10.1-12 8 units <12.1 call Dr.	SUB-CUT		0730 1130	1730 2200				
		PRN								
11/3/xx	11/3/xx	acetaminophen 500 mg q3h prn headache	PO							

PRN

INJECTION SITES: B - RIGHT ARM; C - RIGHT ABDOMEN; D - RIGHT ANTERIOR THIGH; G - LEFT ARM; H - LEFT ABDOMEN; J - LEFT ANTERIOR THIGH; L - LEFT BUTTOCKS; M - RIGHT BUTTOCKS

DATE GIVEN | TIME | INT. | ONE - TIME MEDICATION - DOSAGE | RT.

SIGNATURE OF NURSE ADMINISTERING MEDICATIONS: 23-07, 07-15, 15-23

DATE GIVEN | TIME | INT. | MEDICATION-DOSAGE-CONT. | RT.

RECOPIED BY:
CHECKED BY:

Patient, Pat H.
#6-33725-4

ALLERGIES: None Known

602-31 (7-XX) (MPC# 1355)

ORIGINAL COPY

LITHO IN U.S.A. K6508 (7-92) D395538

PRINTED BY STANDARD REGISTER U.S.A. ZIPSET ®

FIGURE 6-5 Medication Administration Record for Chapter 6 Practice Problems (Questions 38–41)

PHARMACY MAR

START	STOP	MEDICATION	SCHEDULED TIMES	OK'D BY	0701 TO 1500	1501 TO 2300	2301 TO 0700
21:00 8/17/xx SCH		MEGESTROL ACETATE (APO-MEGESTROL) 40 MG TAB 2 TABS PO BID	0900 2100				
12:00 8/17/xx SCH		VANCOMYCIN 250 MG CAP 1 CAPSULE PO QID	0800 1200 1800 2200				
9:00 8/13/xx SCH		FLUCONAZOLE (DIFLUCAN) 100 MG TAB 100 MG PO QD	0900				
21:00 8/11/xx SCH		PERIDEX ORAL RINSE 480 ML 30 ML ORAL RINSE BID SWISH & SPIT	0900 2100				
17:00 8/10/xx SCH		RANITIDINE (ZANTAC-C) 150 MG TAB 1 TABLET PO BID WITH BREAK.&SUPPER	0800 1700				
17:00 8/08/xx SCH		DIGOXIN (LANOXIN) 0.125 MG TAB 1 TAB PO daily 1700	1700				
0:01 8/27/xx PRN		LIDOCAINE 5% UNG 35 G TUBE APPLY TOPICAL PRN* TO RECTAL AREA					
14:00 8/22/xx PRN		SODIUM CHLORIDE INJ 10 ML AS DIR IV TID DILUENT FOR ATIVAN IV					
14:00 8/22/xx PRN		LORAZEPAM (ATIVAN)*2 MG INJ 1 MG IV TID PRN ANXIETY					
9:30 8/21/xx PRN		TUCKS 40 PADS APPLY APPLY TOPICAL Q4-6H TO RECTUM PRN					
9:30 8/21/xx PRN		ANUSOL SUPP 1 SUPP 1 SUPP PR Q4-6H					
16:00 8/18/xx PRN		MEPERIDINE* (DEMEROL) INJ 25 MG 10 MG IV Q1H PRN PAIN IN ADDITION TO PCA					

Gluteus	Thigh
A. Right	H. Right
B. Left	I. Left
Ventro Gluteal	Deltoid
C. Right	J. Right
D. Left	K. Left
E. Abdomen	1 | 2 / 3 | 4 QD

Page 1 of 2

STANDARD TIMES
daily = 0900
BID = Q12H = 0900 & 2100
TID = 0800, 1400, 2200
Q8H = 0800, 1600, 2400
QID = 0800, 1200, 1800, 2200
Q6H = 0600, 1200, 1800, 2400
Q4H = 0400, 0800, 1200. . .
QD DIGOXIN = 1700
QD WARFARIN = 1600

NURSE'S SIGNATURE	INITIAL
0701-1500	
1501-2300	
2301-0700	
Ok'd by	

ALLERGIES: NAFCILLIN
Sulfamethoxazole/Trimethoprim DS
SULFA
TRIMETHOPRIM
CIPROFLOXACIN HCL

Patient: Smith, John
Patient #: 3-90301-4
Physician: J. Physician, M.D.
Room: 407-4 South

FROM: 08/30/xx 0701 TO: 08/31/xx 0700

FIGURE 6-6 Computerized Pharmacy MAR for Chapter 6 Practice Problems (Questions 42–45)

45. How many hours are between the scheduled administration times for megesterol acetate?

____

46. Critical Thinking Skill: Describe the strategy that would prevent this medication error.

possible scenario

Suppose a physician wrote an order for gentamicin 100 mg to be given IV q8h to a patient hospitalized with meningitis. The unit secretary transcribed the order as:

gentamicin 100 mg IV q8h

(0600, 1200, 1800, 2400)

The medication nurse checked the order without noticing the discrepancy in the administration times. Suppose the patient received the medication every 6 hours for 3 days before the error was noticed.

potential outcome

The patient would have received one extra dose each day, which is equivalent to one-third more medication daily. Most likely, the physician would be notified of the error, and the medication would be discontinued with serum gentamicin levels drawn. The levels would likely be in the toxic range, and the patient's gentamicin levels would be monitored until the levels returned to normal. This patient would be at risk of developing ototoxicity or nephrotoxicity from the overdose of gentamicin.

prevention

____

____

After completing these problems, see page 465 to check your answers.

CHAPTER

7

Understanding Drug Labels

LEARNING OBJECTIVES

1. Read and interpret medication labels.
2. Find and differentiate the trade and generic names of drugs.
3. Determine the dosage strength.
4. Determine the form in which the drug is supplied.
5. Determine the supply dosage or concentration.
6. Identify the total volume of the drug container.
7. Differentiate the total volume of the container from the supply dosage.
8. Find the directions for mixing or preparing the supply dosage of drugs, as needed.
9. Recognize and follow drug alerts.
10. Identify the administration route.
11. Check the expiration date.
12. Identify the lot or control number, Drug Identification Number, and bar code symbols.
13. Recognize the manufacturer's name.
14. Differentiate labels for multidose and unit-dose containers.
15. Identify combination drugs.
16. Describe supply dosage expressed as a ratio or percent.

The patient care order prescribes how much of a drug the patient is to receive. The nurse must prepare the order from the drugs on hand. The drug label tells how the available drug is supplied. Examine the various preparations, labels, and dosage strengths of tobramycin sulfate (Nebcin) injection (Figure 7-1).

Look at the following common drug labels to learn to recognize pertinent information about the drugs supplied.

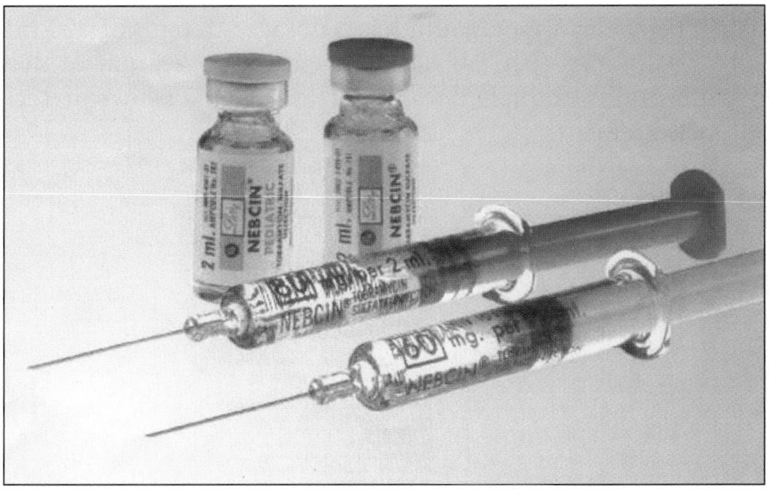

Courtesy Eli Lilly and Company

FIGURE 7-1 Various tobramycin sulfate samples

TRADE AND GENERIC NAMES

The trade, brand, or proprietary name is the manufacturer's name for a drug. Notice that the trade name is usually the most prominent word on the drug label—in large type and boldly visible to promote the product. It is often followed by the sign ® meaning that both the name and formulation are registered. The generic or established, nonproprietary name appears directly under the trade name. Sometimes the generic name is also placed inside parentheses. By law, the generic name must be identified on all drug labels.

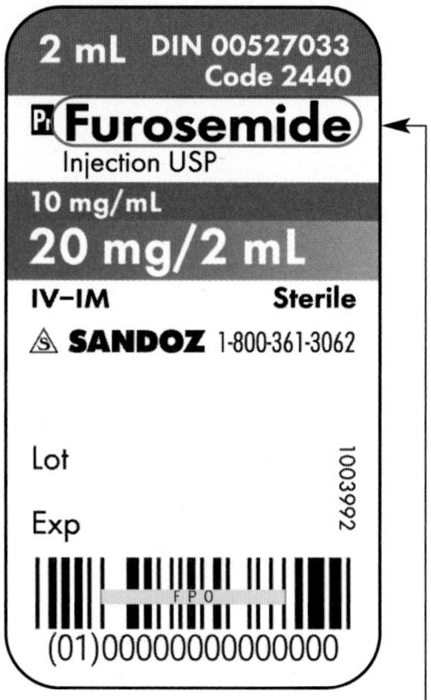

Generic Drug (furosemide)

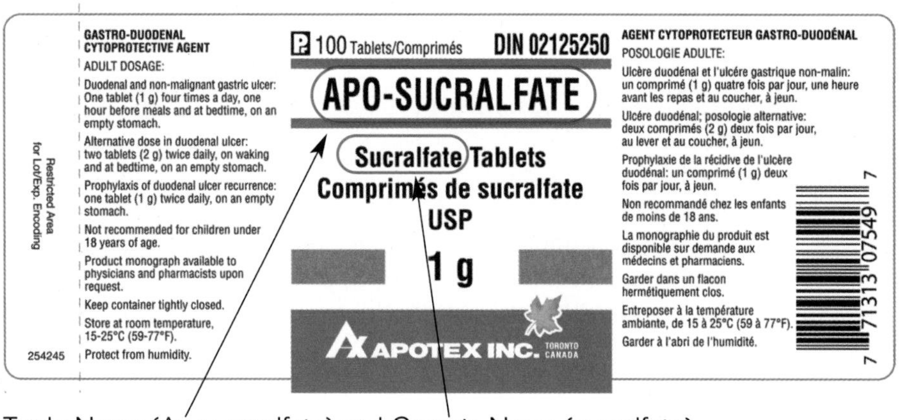

Trade Name (Apo-sucralfate) and Generic Name (sucralfate)

Generic equivalents of many trade-name drugs are ordered as substitutes by the prescribing practitioner's preference or pharmacy policy. Because only the generic name appears on these labels, nurses need to carefully cross-check all medications. Failure to do so could cause inaccurate drug identification.

DOSAGE STRENGTH

The dosage strength refers to the dosage *weight* or amount of drug provided in a specific unit of measurement. The dosage strength of gemfibrozil tablets is 600 milligrams (the weight and specific unit of measurement) per tablet. Some drugs often will have two different but equivalent dosage strengths. In the example label, Penicillin V potassium has a dosage strength of 300 milligrams (per tablet). This is equivalent to 500 000 units (per tablet). The label, however, may or may not include both units of measurements and in this example does not. This variable allows prescribers to order the drug using either unit of measurement.

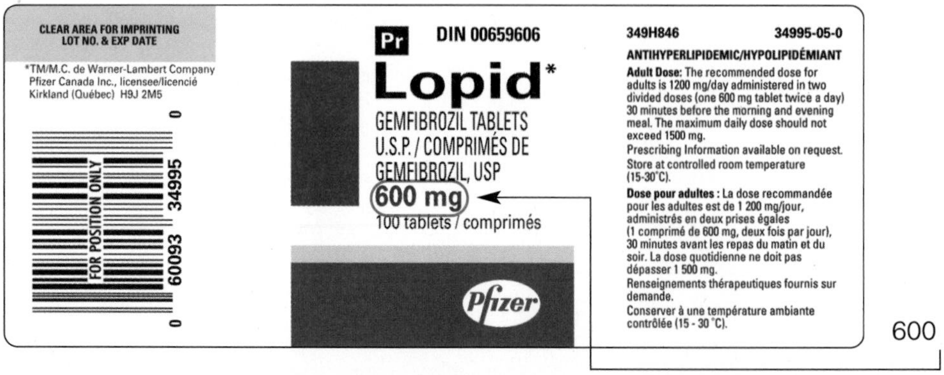

600 milligrams

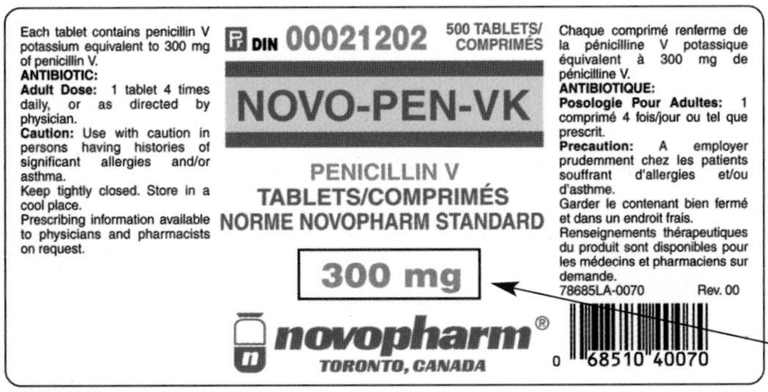

300 milligrams (500 000 units)

FORM

The form identifies the *structure* and *composition* of the drug. Solid dosage forms for oral use include tablets and capsules. Some powdered or granular medications that are not manufactured in tablet or capsule form can be directly combined with food or beverages and administered. Others must be reconstituted (liquefied) and measured in a precise liquid volume, such as millilitres, drops, or fluid ounces. They may be a crystalloid (clear solution) or a suspension (solid particles in liquid that separate when held in a container).

Injectable medications may be supplied in solution or dry powdered form to be reconstituted. Once reconstituted, they are measured in millilitres.

Medications are also supplied in a variety of other forms, such as suppositories, creams, and patches.

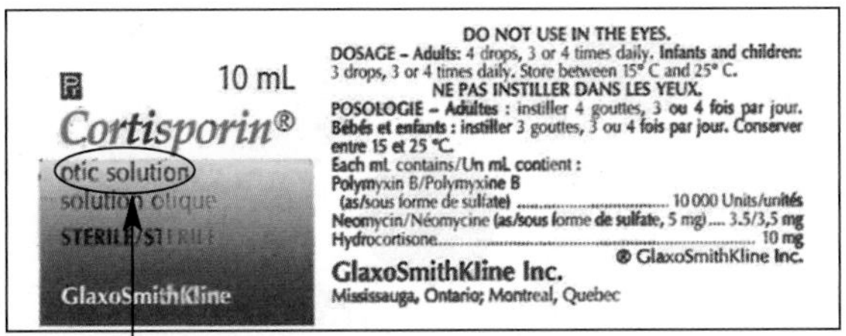

Otic Suspension Sterile Drops

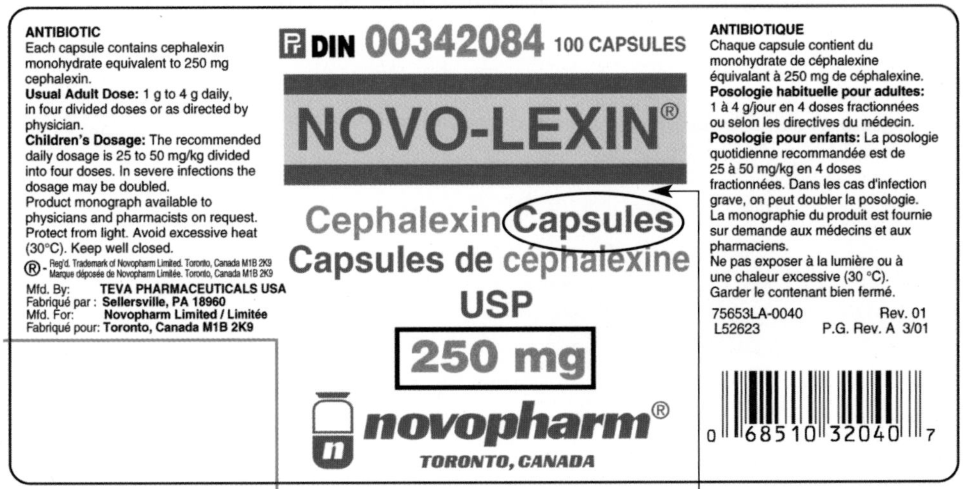

Capsules

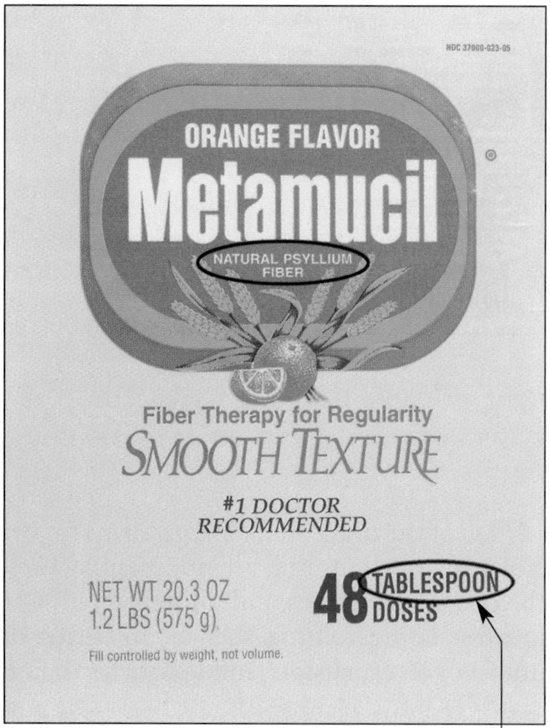

Metamucil, Proctor and Gamble Inc., 48 Tablespoon Doses

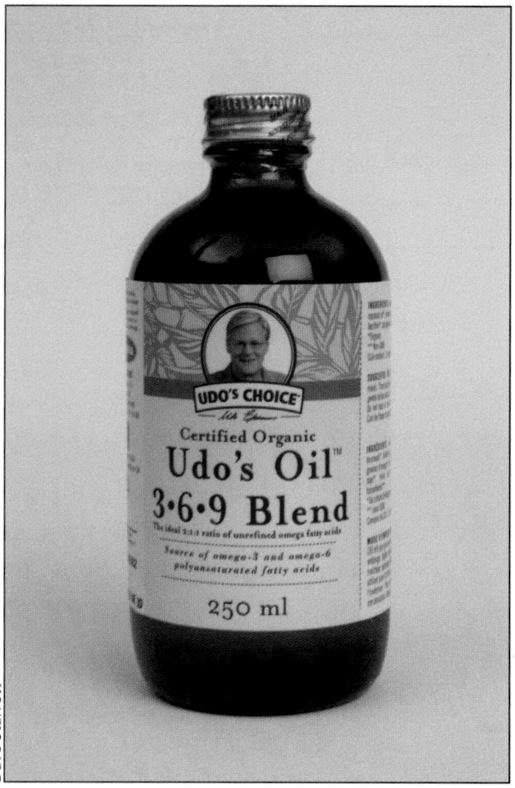

New Organic Certified Udo's 3-6-9 Liquid

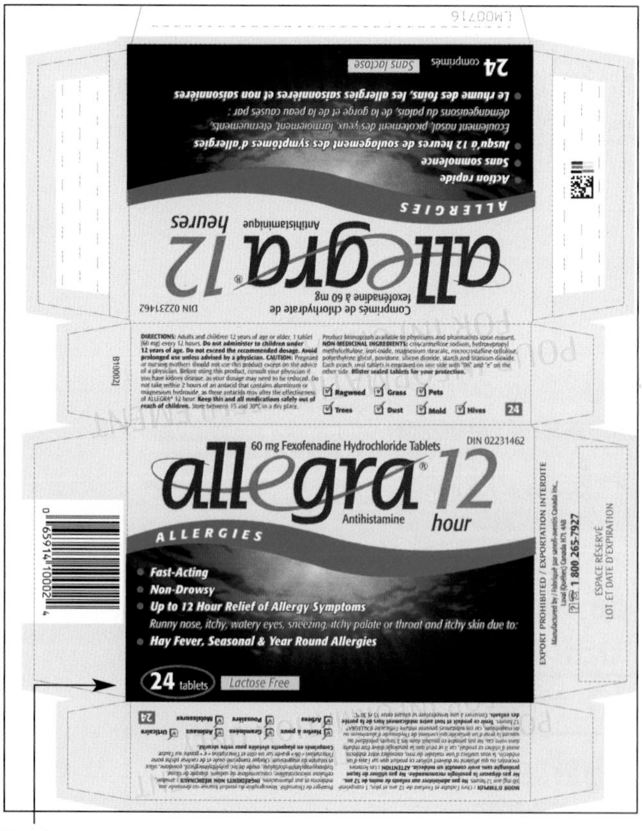

Tablets

Millilitres

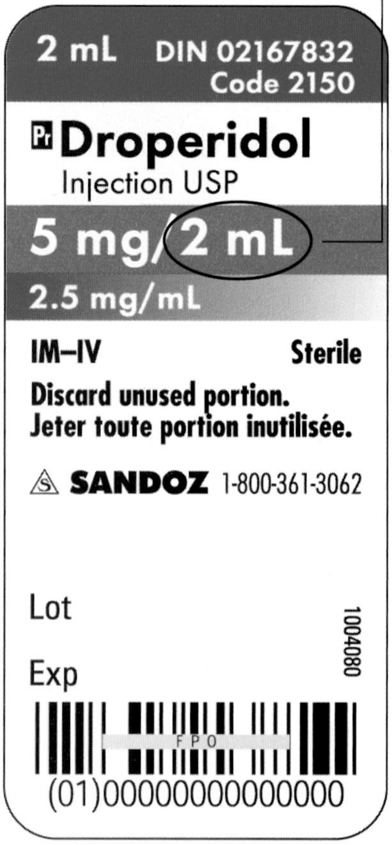

SUPPLY DOSAGE

The supply dosage refers to both *dosage strength* and *form.* It is read "X measured units per some quantity." For solid-form medications, such as tablets, the supply dosage is X measured units per tablet. For liquid medications, the supply dosage is the same as the medication's concentration, such as X measured units per millilitre. Take a minute to read the supply dosage printed on the following labels.

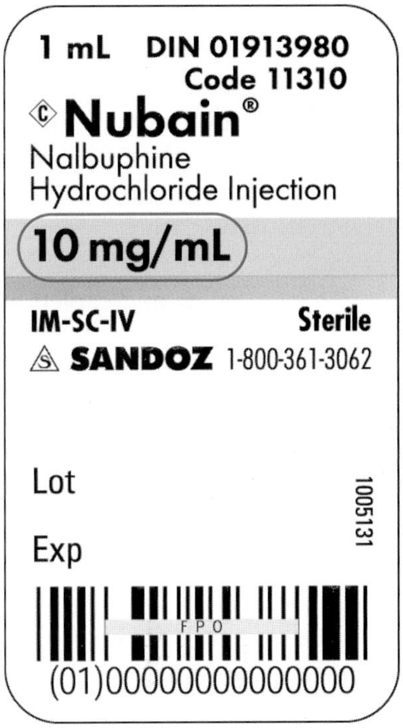

10 milligrams per millilitre

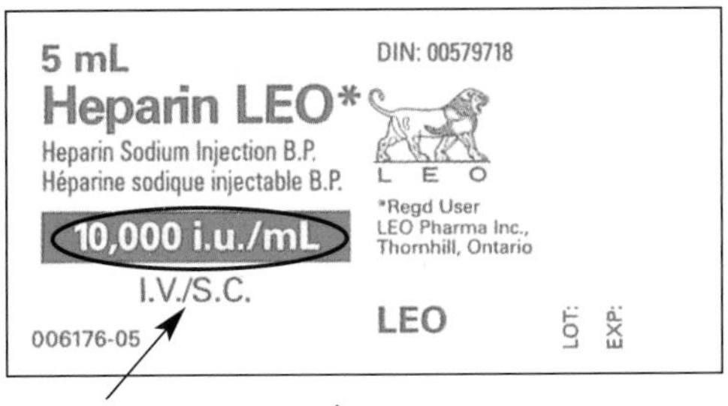

10 000 international units per millilitre

TOTAL VOLUME

The total volume refers to the *full quantity* contained in a package, bottle, or vial. For tablets and other solid medications, it is the total number of individual items. For liquids, it is the total fluid volume.

10 millilitres

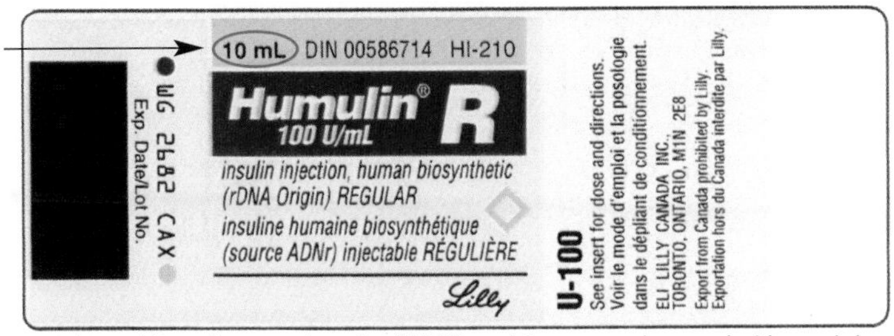

400 millilitres

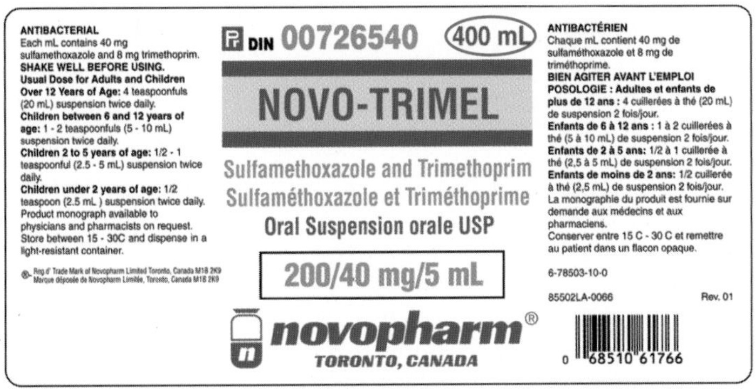

ADMINISTRATION ROUTE

The administration route refers to the *site* of the body or *method of drug delivery* into the patient. Examples of routes of administration include oral, enteral (into the gastrointestinal tract through a tube), sublingual, injection (IV, IM, SUBCUT), otic, optic, topical, rectal, vaginal, and others. Unless specified otherwise, tablets, capsules, and caplets are intended for oral use.

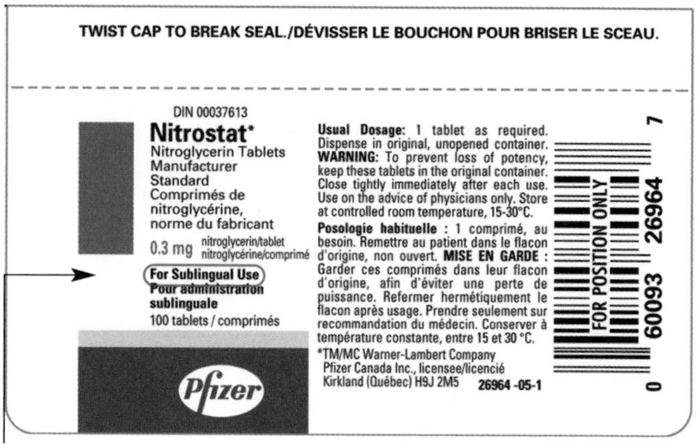

Sublingual

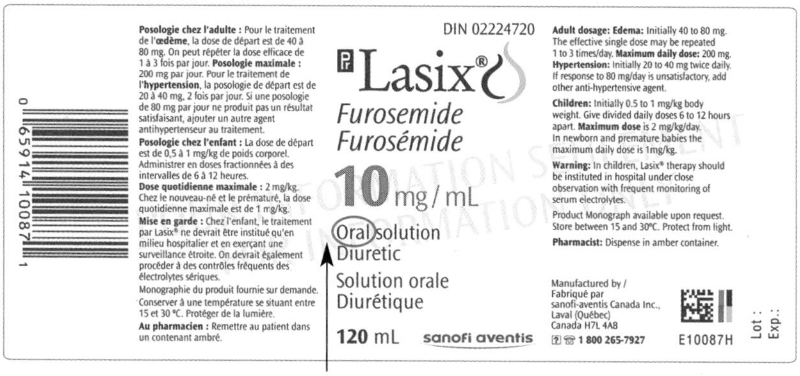

Oral

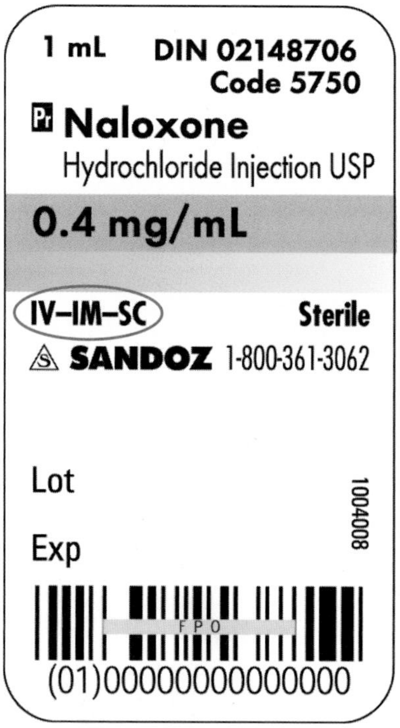

Intravenous (IV)
Intramuscular (IM)
Subcutaneous (SUBCUT or SC)

DIRECTIONS FOR MIXING OR RECONSTITUTING

Some drugs are dispensed in *powder form* and must be *reconstituted for use.* (Reconstitution is discussed further in Chapter 10.)

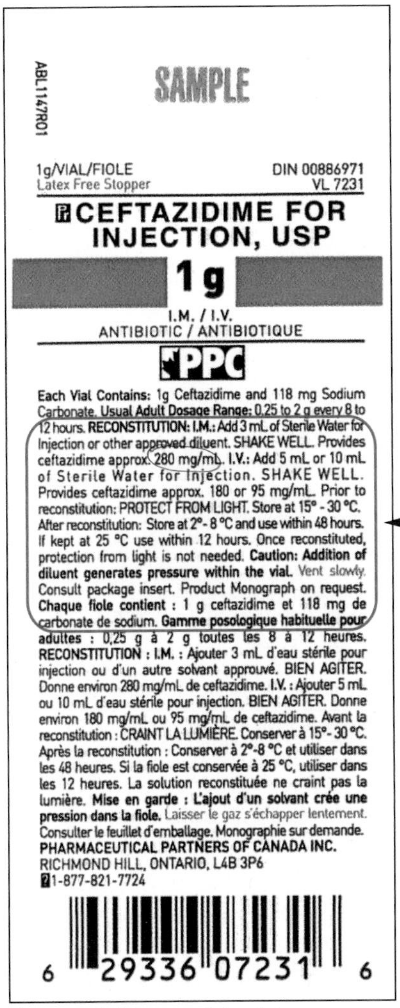

Pharmaceutical Partners of Canada Inc., Richmond Hill, ON

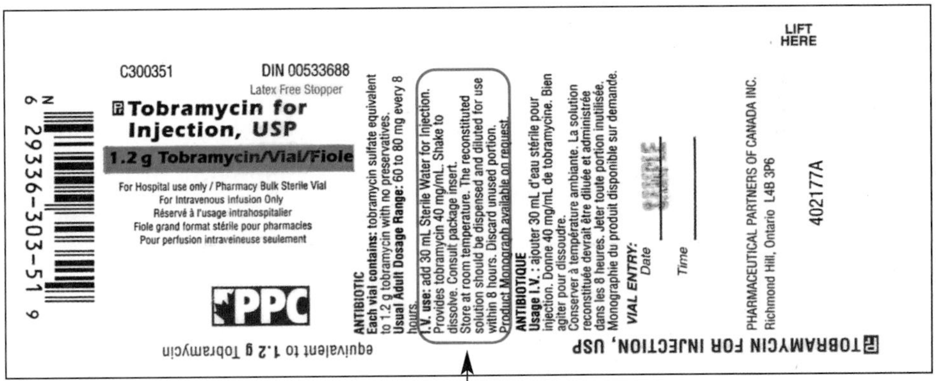

Pharmaceutical Partners of Canada Inc., Richmond Hill, ON

LABEL ALERTS

Manufacturers may print warnings on the packaging or special alerts may be added by the pharmacy before dispensing. Look for special storage alerts such as "refrigerate at all times," "keep in a dry place," "replace cap and close tightly before storing," or "protect from light." Reconstituted suspensions may be dispensed already prepared for use, and directions may instruct the healthcare professional to "shake well before using" as a reminder to remix the components. Read and follow all label instructions carefully.

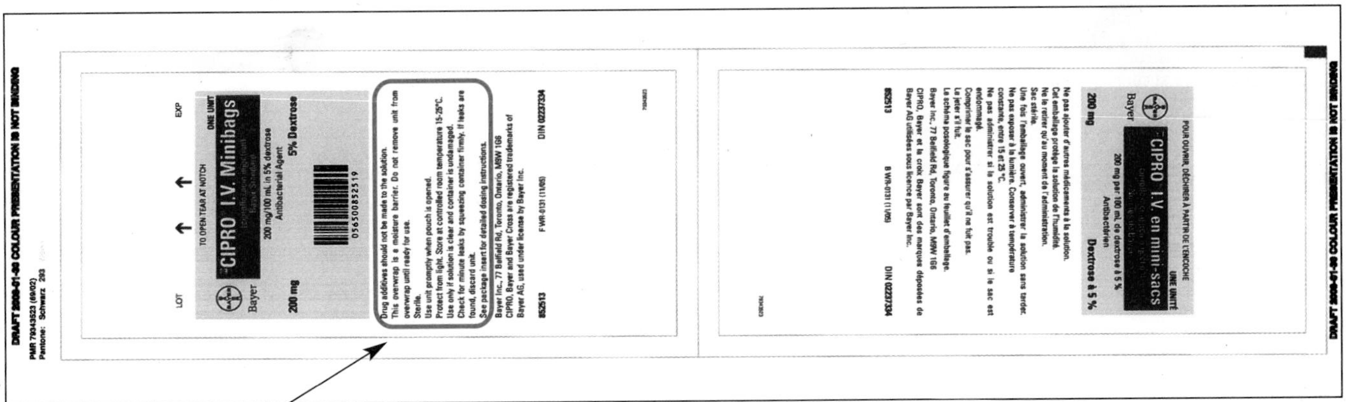

Bayer Inc., Toronto, ON

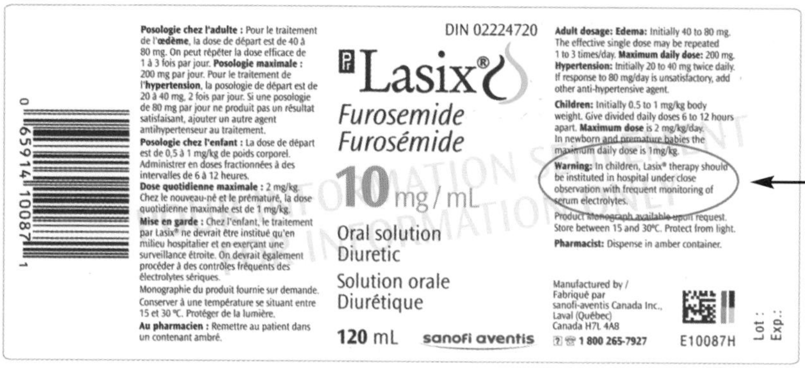

See Alert

Sanofi-aventis Canada, Laval , QUE

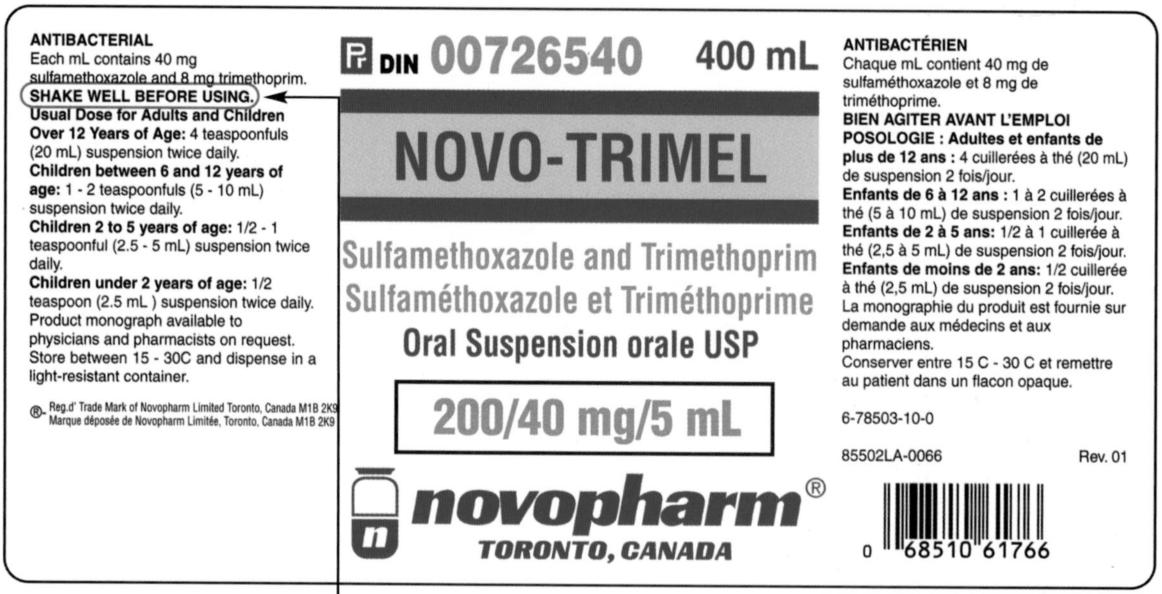

Novopharm Limited, Toronto, ON.

See Alert

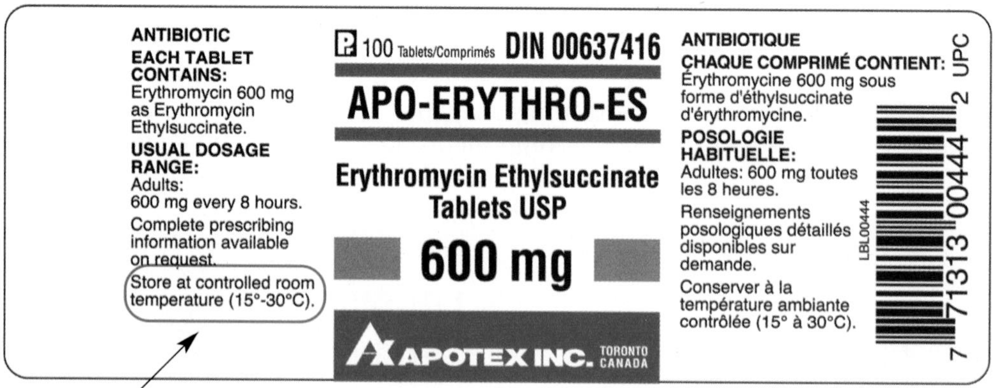

Apotex Inc., Weston, ON

See Alert

NAME OF THE MANUFACTURER

The name of the manufacturer is circled on the following labels.

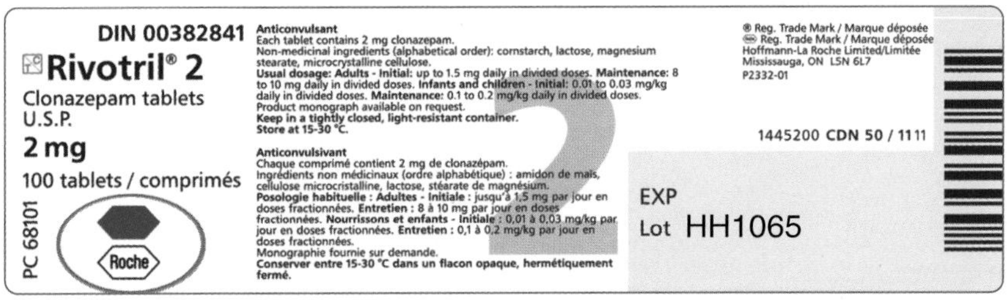

Hoffmann-LaRoche Limited

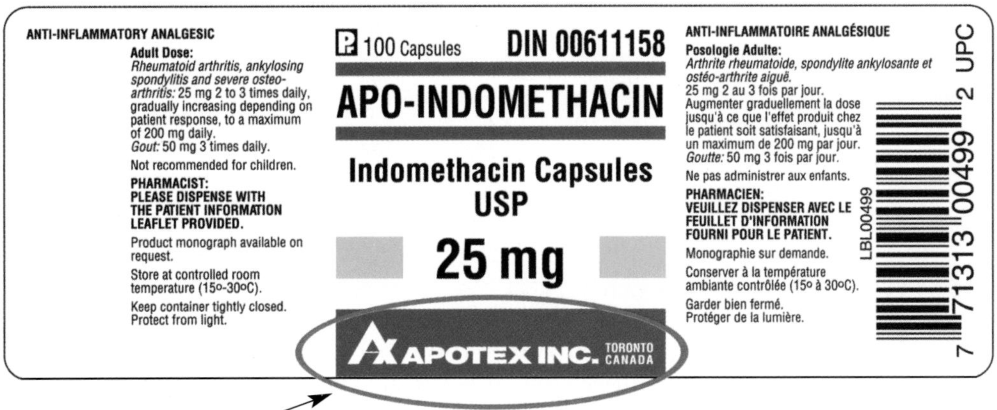

Apotex Incorporated

EXPIRATION DATE

The medication should be used, discarded, or returned to the pharmacy by the expiration date. Further, note the special expiration instructions given on labels for reconstituted medications. Note: If the day is not indicated on the expiry date, the product expires on the last day of the month indicated. For example, an expiry of 7/08 would mean July 31, 2008. Refer to the haloperidol label on the right.

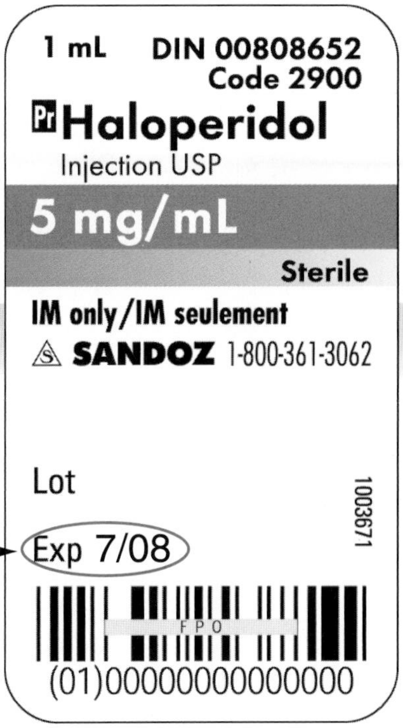

7/08

LOT OR CONTROL NUMBERS

Federal law requires all medication packages to be identified with a lot or control number. If a drug is recalled, for reasons such as damage or tampering, the lot number quickly identifies the particular group of medication packages to be removed from shelves. This number has been invaluable for vaccine and over-the-counter medication recalls.

Humalog and Humulin are trademarks of Eli Lilly and Company and are used with permission. Eli Lilly Canada Inc., Toronto, ON

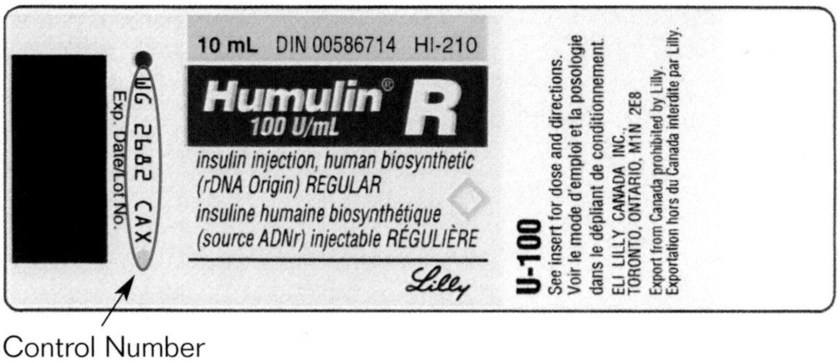

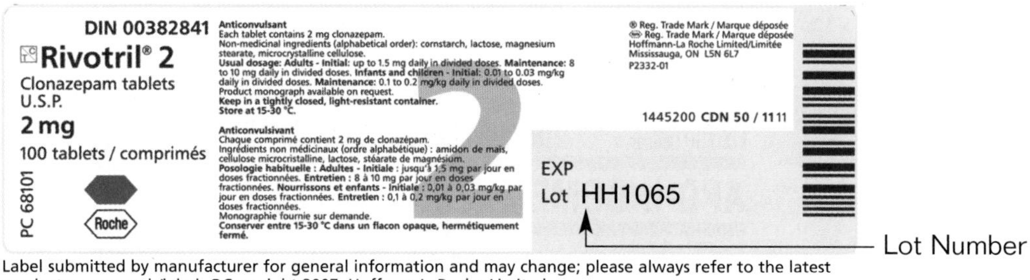

Label submitted by manufacturer for general information and may change; please always refer to the latest product monograph/label. ©Copyright 2007, Hoffman-LaRoche Limited.

DRUG IDENTIFICATION NUMBER

This number, assigned by the Therapeutic Products Directorate of Health Canada, indicates to healthcare professionals and consumers that this product has been evaluated as meeting safety and health benefit expectations. Prescription and over-the-counter drug products assigned this Drug Identification Number (DIN) number are approved for sale in Canada. In the label for Apo-Procainamide 500, this number is DIN 00713341. Related information may be accessed at http://www.hc-sc.gc.ca/hpb/drugs-dpd/.

Apotex Inc., Weston, ON

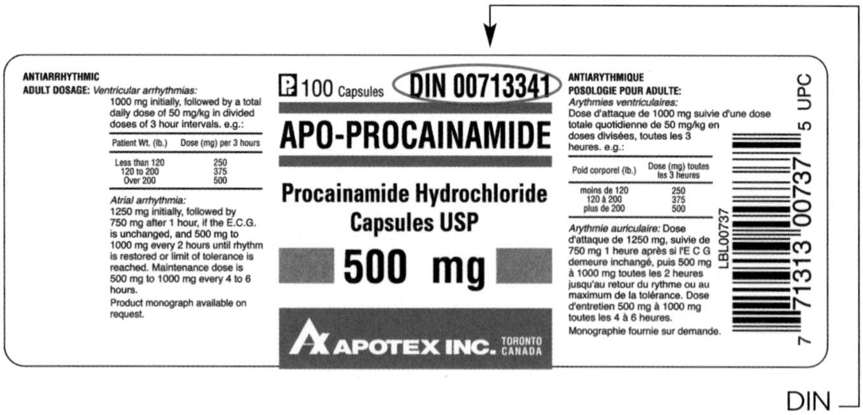

NATURAL PRODUCT NUMBER

Similarly, manufacturers of products considered to be alternative medicines must obtain approval and be licensed to market their products in Canada. Review and assignment of Natural Product Numbers (NPNs) is done by the Natural Health Products Directorate of Health Canada, which promotes consumer safety and awareness. In the label for Jamieson Calcium this number is NPN 80000248. Related information may be accessed at http://www.hc-sc.gc.ca/dhp-mps/prodnatur/applications/licen-prod/lnhpd-bdpsnh-eng.php.

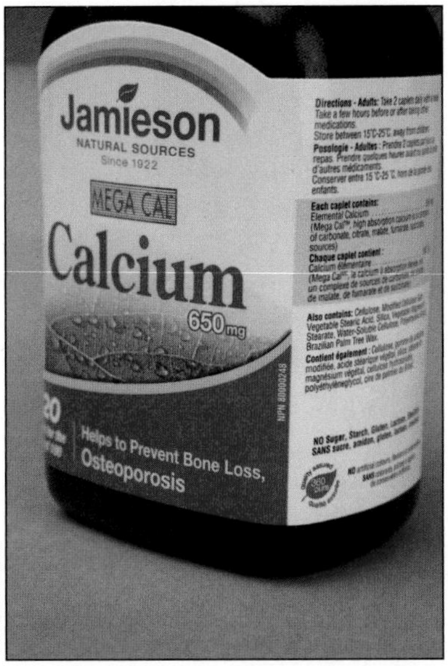

Dave Starrett

Products considered to be alternative medicines carry a Natural Product Number (NPN).

BAR CODE SYMBOLS

Bar code symbols are commonly used in retail sales. Bar code symbols also document drug dosing for recordkeeping and stock reorder, and may soon automate medication documentation right at the patient's bedside. The horizontal ones look like picket fences and the vertical ones look like ladders.

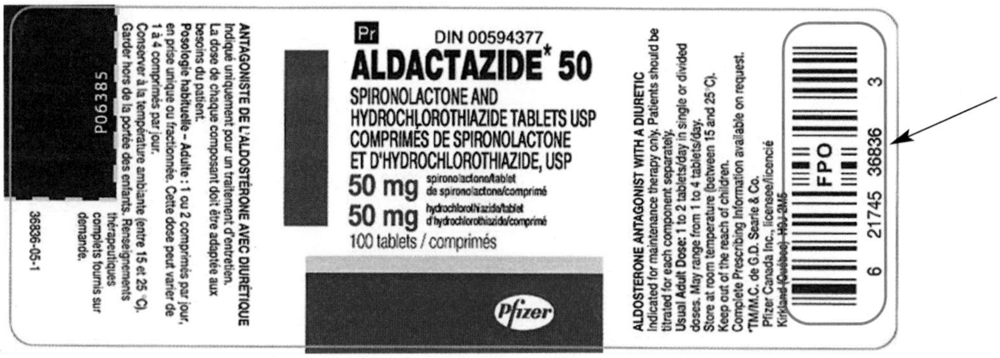

©Pfizer Canada Inc., Kirkland, Que

UNIT- OR SINGLE-DOSE LABELS

Most oral medications administered in the hospital setting are available in unit dosage, such as a single capsule or tablet packaged separately in a typical blister pack. The pharmacy provides a 24-hour supply of each drug for the patient. The only major difference in this form of labelling is that the total volume of the container is usually omitted, because the volume is *one* tablet or capsule. Likewise, the dosage strength is understood as *per one.* Further, injectable medicines are packaged in single-dose preparations.

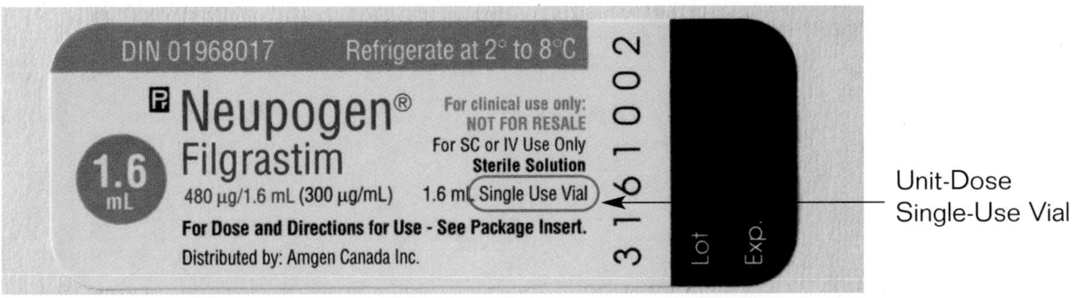

Amgen Canada Inc., Mississauga, ON

COMBINATION DRUGS

Some medications are a combination of two or more drugs in one form. Read the labels for acetaminophen/oxycodone HCl and sulfamethoxazole/trimethoprim and notice the different substances that are combined in each tablet. Combination drugs are usually prescribed by the number of tablets, capsules, or millilitres to be given rather than by the dosage strength. The combination medication represents the strength of each component. For example, Percocet contains 5 mg of oxycodone hydrochloride and 325 mg of acetaminophen; Novo-Trimel contains 200 mg of sulfamethoxazole and 40 mg of trimethoprim in every 5 mL of the suspension.

Bristol-Myers Squibb, Montreal, QUE

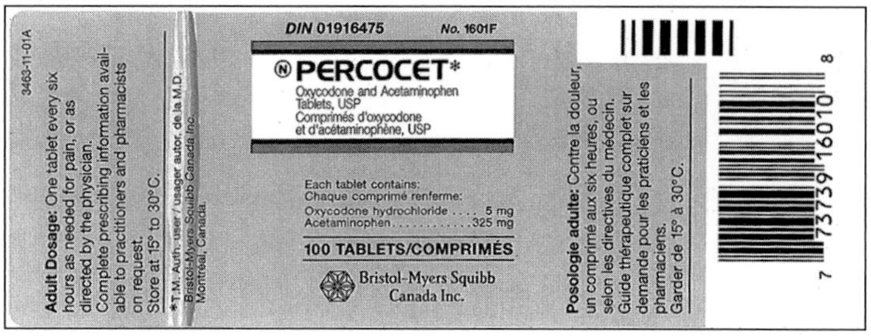

Combination Drugs

Novopharm Limited, Toronto, ON

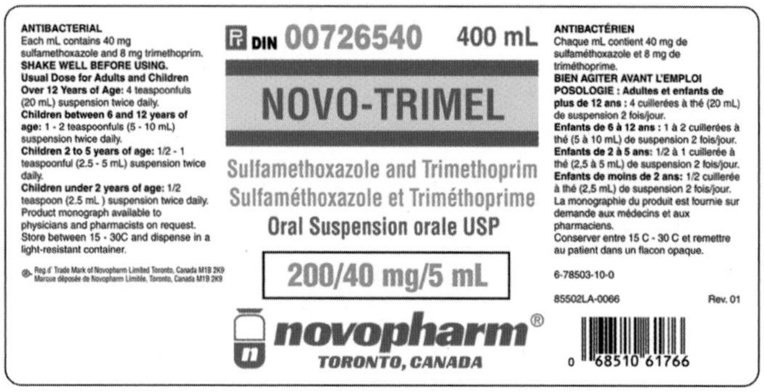

SUPPLY DOSAGE EXPRESSED AS A RATIO OR PERCENT

Occasionally, solutions will be ordered and/or manufactured in a supply dosage expressed as a ratio or percentage.

RULE

Ratio solutions express the *number of grams* of the drug *per total millilitres of solution*.

Example:

Epinephrine 1:1000 contains 1 g pure drug per 1000 mL solution,
1 g:1000 mL = 1000 mg:1000 mL = 1 mg:1 mL.

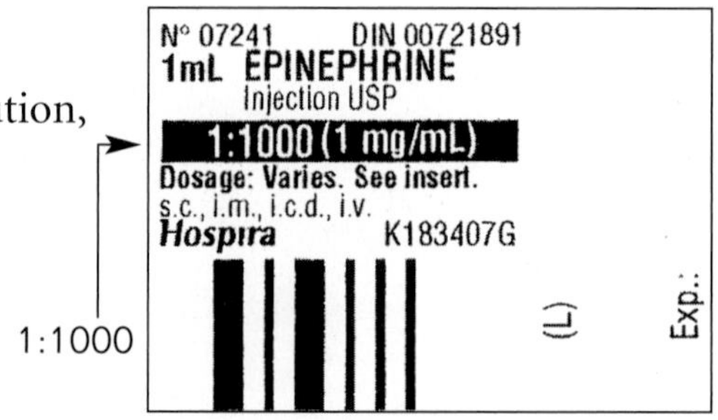

Hospira Healthcare Corporation, Saint-Laurent, QUE

RULE

Percentage (%) solutions express the *number of grams* of the drug *per 100 millilitres of solution*.

Example:

Lidocaine 2% contains 2 g pure drug per 100 mL solution,
2 g/100 mL = 2000 mg/100 mL = 100 mg/5 mL = 20 mg/mL.

2%

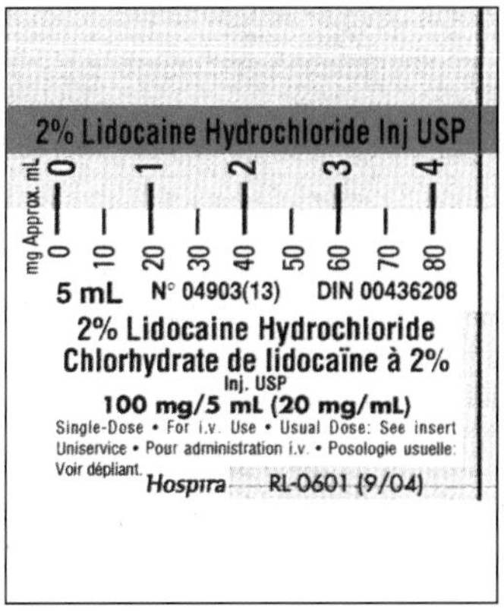

Hospira Healthcare Corporation, Saint-Laurent, QUE

Although these labels look different from many of the other labels, it is important to recognize that the supply dosage can still be determined. Many times the label will have a more commonly identified supply dosage and not just the ratio or percentage. Look at the epinephrine (on previous page) and lidocaine labels. On the epinephrine label, the ratio is 1:1000; the supply dosage also can be identified as 1 mg/mL. On the lidocaine label, the percentage is 2%; the supply dosage also can be identified as 20 mg/mL.

CHECKING LABELS

Recall the Rights of Medication Administration: The *right patient* must receive the *right drug* for the *right reason* in the *right amount* by the *right route* in the *right site* at the *right time* and *right frequency*, followed by the *right documentation*. To be absolutely sure the patient receives the right drug, check the label three times.

CAUTION

Before administering a medication to a patient, check the drug label three times:

1. Against the patient care order (or medication order, MAR).
2. Before preparing the medication.
3. After preparing the medication and before administering it.

QUICK REVIEW

Read labels carefully to:

- Identify the drug and the manufacturer.
- Differentiate between dosage strength, form, supply dosage, total container volume, and administration route.
- Recognize that the drug's supply dosage similarly refers to a drug's weight per unit of measure or *concentration*.
- Find the directions for reconstitution, as needed.
- Note expiration date.
- Describe lot or control number.
- Identify supply dosage on labels with ratios and percents.
- Be sure you administer the right drug.

REVIEW SET 19

Use the following labels A through G to find the information requested in questions 1 through 12. Indicate your answer by letter (A through G).

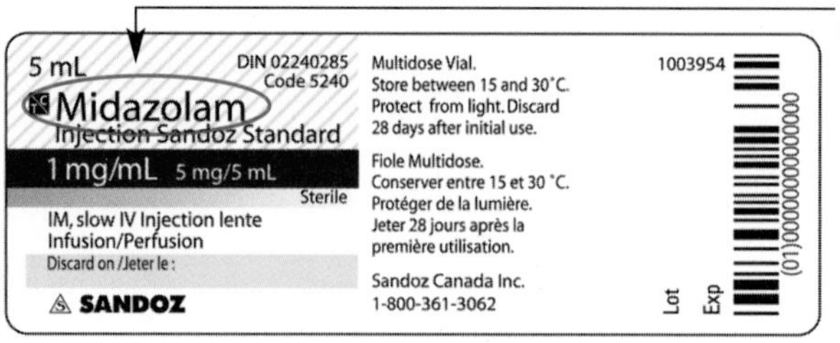

A

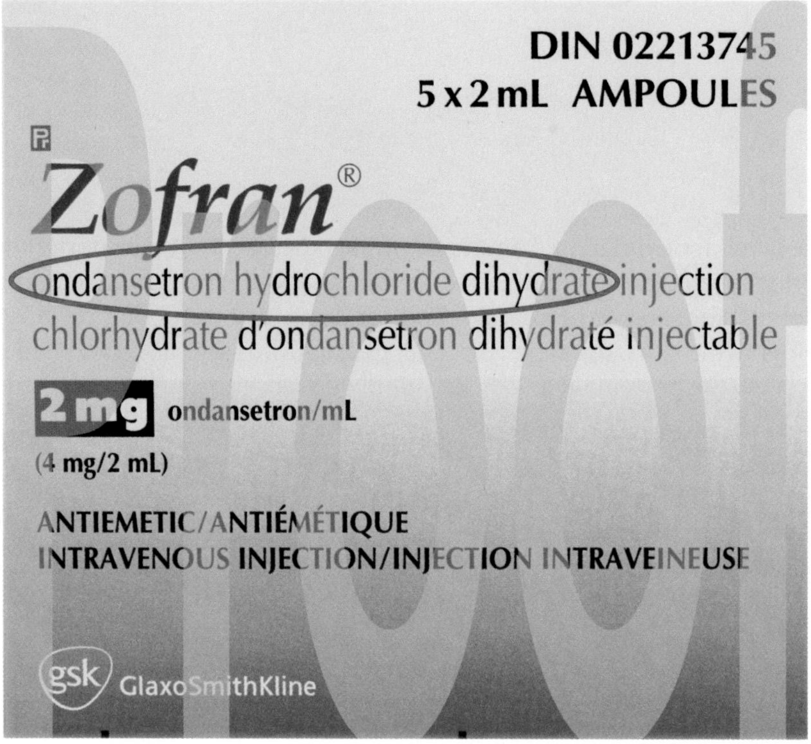

B

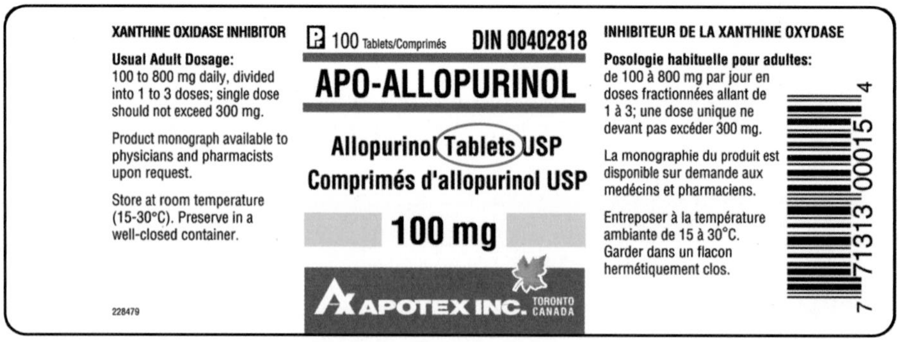

C

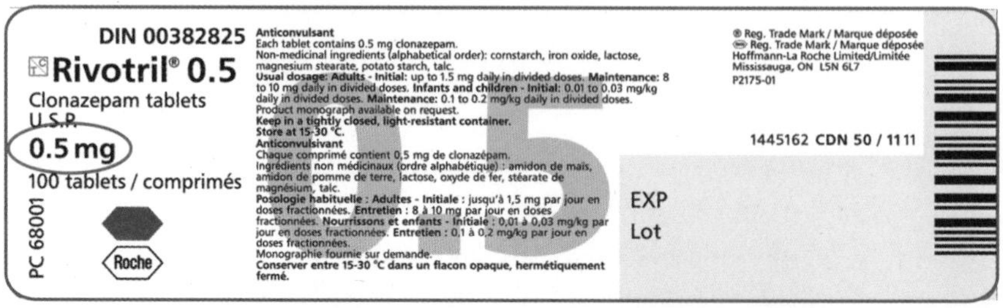

D

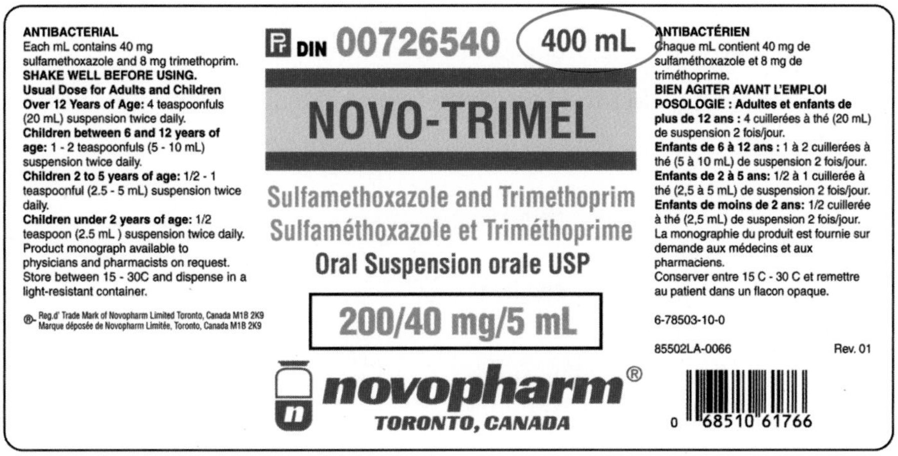
ANTIBACTERIAL
Each mL contains 40 mg sulfamethoxazole and 8 mg trimethoprim.
SHAKE WELL BEFORE USING.
Usual Dose for Adults and Children Over 12 Years of Age: 4 teaspoonfuls (20 mL) suspension twice daily.
Children between 6 and 12 years of age: 1 - 2 teaspoonfuls (5 - 10 mL) suspension twice daily.
Children 2 to 5 years of age: 1/2 - 1 teaspoonful (2.5 - 5 mL) suspension twice daily.
Children under 2 years of age: 1/2 teaspoon (2.5 mL) suspension twice daily.
Product monograph available to physicians and pharmacists on request.
Store between 15 - 30C and dispense in a light-resistant container.
®-Reg.d' Trade Mark of Novopharm Limited Toronto, Canada M1B 2K9 Marque déposée de Novopharm Limitée, Toronto, Canada M1B 2K9
DIN 00726540
400 mL
NOVO-TRIMEL
Sulfamethoxazole and Trimethoprim
Sulfaméthoxazole et Triméthoprime
Oral Suspension orale USP
200/40 mg/5 mL
novopharm®
TORONTO, CANADA
ANTIBACTÉRIEN
Chaque mL contient 40 mg de sulfaméthoxazole et 8 mg de triméthoprime.
BIEN AGITER AVANT L'EMPLOI
POSOLOGIE : Adultes et enfants de plus de 12 ans : 4 cuillerées à thé (20 mL) de suspension 2 fois/jour.
Enfants de 6 à 12 ans : 1 à 2 cuillerées à thé (5 à 10 mL) de suspension 2 fois/jour.
Enfants de 2 à 5 ans: 1/2 à 1 cuillerée à thé (2,5 à 5 mL) de suspension 2 fois/jour.
Enfants de moins de 2 ans: 1/2 cuillerée à thé (2,5 mL) de suspension 2 fois/jour.
La monographie du produit est fournie sur demande aux médecins et aux pharmaciens.
Conserver entre 15 C - 30 C et remettre au patient dans un flacon opaque.
6-78503-10-0
85502LA-0066
Rev. 01
0 68510 61766

Novopharm Limited, Toronto, ON

E

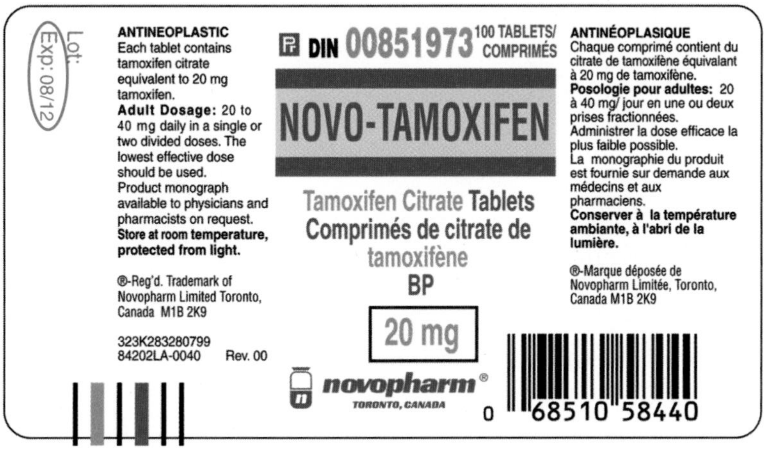
Lot:
Exp: 08/12
ANTINEOPLASTIC
Each tablet contains tamoxifen citrate equivalent to 20 mg tamoxifen.
Adult Dosage: 20 to 40 mg daily in a single or two divided doses. The lowest effective dose should be used.
Product monograph available to physicians and pharmacists on request.
Store at room temperature, protected from light.
®-Reg'd. Trademark of Novopharm Limited Toronto, Canada M1B 2K9
323K283280799
84202LA-0040
Rev. 00
DIN 00851973
100 TABLETS/ COMPRIMÉS
NOVO-TAMOXIFEN
Tamoxifen Citrate Tablets
Comprimés de citrate de tamoxifène
BP
20 mg
novopharm®
TORONTO, CANADA
ANTINÉOPLASIQUE
Chaque comprimé contient du citrate de tamoxifène équivalant à 20 mg de tamoxifène.
Posologie pour adultes: 20 à 40 mg/ jour en une ou deux prises fractionnées.
Administrer la dose efficace la plus faible possible.
La monographie du produit est fournie sur demande aux médecins et aux pharmaciens.
Conserver à la température ambiante, à l'abri de la lumière.
®-Marque déposée de Novopharm Limitée, Toronto, Canada M1B 2K9
0 68510 58440

Novopharm Limited, Toronto, ON

F

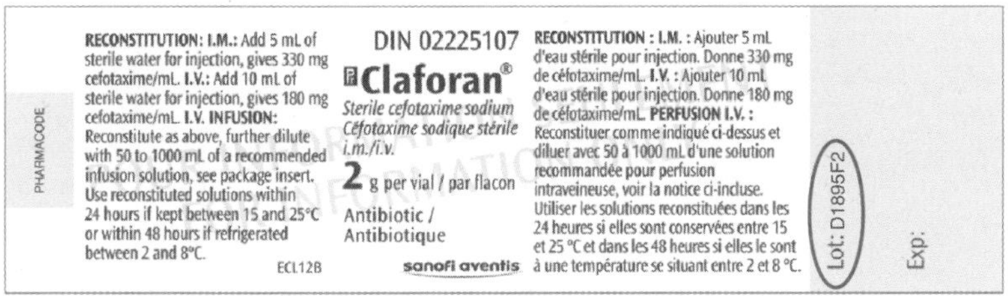
PHARMACODE
RECONSTITUTION: I.M.: Add 5 mL of sterile water for injection, gives 330 mg cefotaxime/mL. I.V.: Add 10 mL of sterile water for injection, gives 180 mg cefotaxime/mL. I.V. INFUSION: Reconstitute as above, further dilute with 50 to 1000 mL of a recommended infusion solution, see package insert. Use reconstituted solutions within 24 hours if kept between 15 and 25°C or within 48 hours if refrigerated between 2 and 8°C.
ECL12B
DIN 02225107
Claforan®
Sterile cefotaxime sodium
Céfotaxime sodique stérile
i.m./i.v.
2 g per vial / par flacon
Antibiotic / Antibiotique
sanofi aventis
RECONSTITUTION : I.M. : Ajouter 5 mL d'eau stérile pour injection. Donne 330 mg de céfotaxime/mL. I.V. : Ajouter 10 mL d'eau stérile pour injection. Donne 180 mg de céfotaxime/mL. PERFUSION I.V. : Reconstituer comme indiqué ci-dessus et diluer avec 50 à 1000 mL d'une solution recommandée pour perfusion intraveineuse, voir la notice ci-incluse. Utiliser les solutions reconstituées dans les 24 heures si elles sont conservées entre 15 et 25 °C et dans les 48 heures si elles le sont à une température se situant entre 2 et 8 °C.
Lot: D1895F2
Exp:

Sanofi-aventis Canada, Laval, QUE

G

1. The total volume of the liquid container is circled. E
2. The dosage strength is circled. D
3. The form of the drug is circled. C
4. The trade name of the drug is circled. A
5. The generic name of the drug is circled. B
6. The expiration date is circled. F
7. The lot number is circled. G
8. Look at label E and determine how much of the supply drug you will administer to the patient per dose for the order *sulfamethoxazole 100/20 mg*. 2.5 mL
9. Look at label A and determine the route of administration. IM
10. Indicate which labels have an imprinted bar code symbol. A,C,d,E,F
11. Look at label B, and determine the supply dosage. 4mg/2mL

12. Look at label F, and determine how much of the drug supplied you will administer to the patient per dose for the order *Tamoxifen 40 mg PO q12h.* ________

Refer to the following label to identify the specific drug information described in questions 13 through 17.

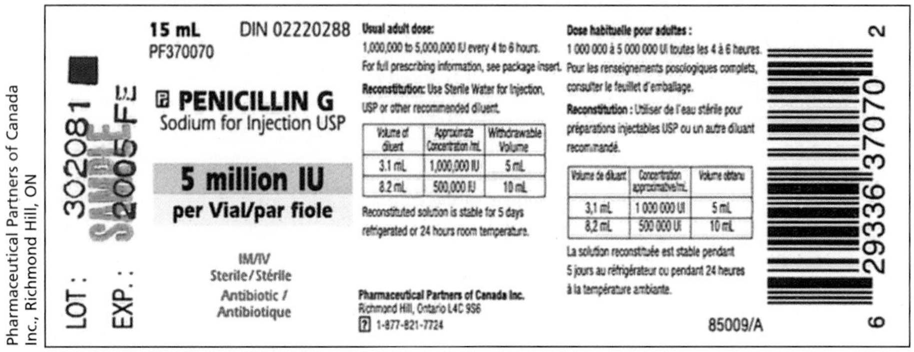

13. Generic name ________
14. Dosage strength ________
15. Route of administration ________
16. Drug Identification Number ________
17. Manufacturer ________

Refer to the following label to answer questions 18 through 20.

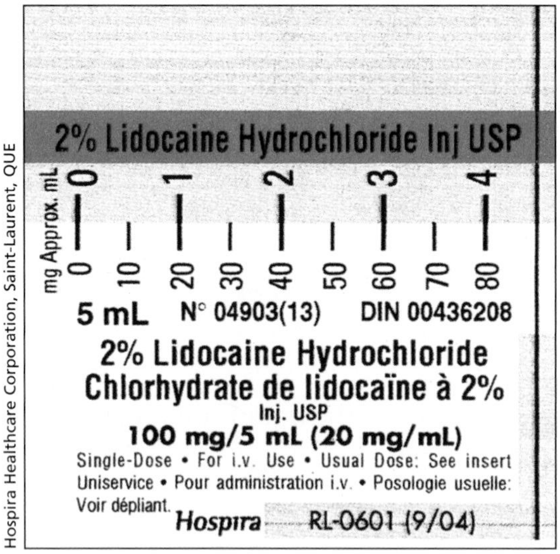

18. The supply dosage of the drug is __2__ %.
19. The supply dosage of the drug is ________ g per 100 mL.
20. The supply dosage of the drug is __20__ mg per mL.

After completing these problems, see page 466 in the answer section to check your answers.

CRITICAL THINKING SKILLS

Reading the labels of medications is critical. Make sure that the drug you want is what you have on hand before you prepare it. Let's look at an example of a medication error related to reading the label incorrectly.

error

Not checking the label for correct dosage.

possible scenario

A nurse flushed a triple central venous catheter (an IV with three ports). According to hospital policy, the nurse was to flush each port with 10 mL of normal saline followed by 2 mL of heparin flush solution in the concentration of 100 units/mL. The nurse mistakenly picked up a vial of heparin containing heparin 10000 units/mL. Without checking the label, she prepared the solution for all three ports. The patient received 60000 units of heparin instead of 600 units.

potential outcome

The patient in this case would be at great risk for hemorrhage, leading to shock and death. Protamine sulfate would be ordered to counteract the action of the heparin.

prevention

There is no substitute for checking the label before administering a medication. The nurse in this case had three opportunities to catch the error, having drawn three different syringes of medication for the three ports.

PRACTICE PROBLEMS—CHAPTER 7

Look at labels A through G, and identify the information requested.

Label A:

1. The supply dosage of the drug in percentage is 8.4 %.
2. The Drug Identification Number is 00261998.
3. The supply dosage of the drug in milligrams is 84 mg/mL.

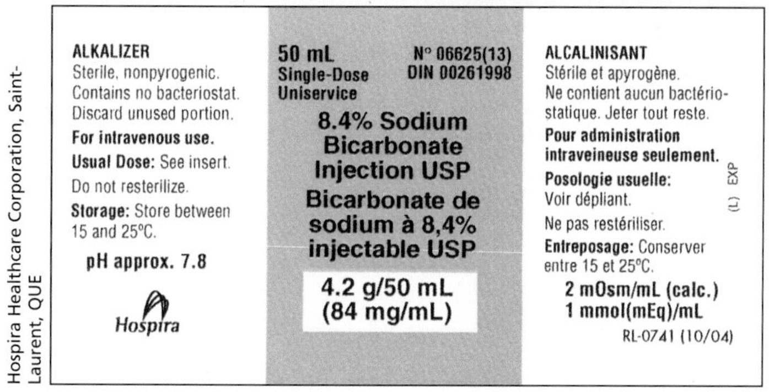
Hospira Healthcare Corporation, Saint-Laurent, QUE
ALKALIZER
Sterile, nonpyrogenic.
Contains no bacteriostat.
Discard unused portion.
For intravenous use.
Usual Dose: See insert.
Do not resterilize.
Storage: Store between 15 and 25°C.
pH approx. 7.8
Hospira
50 mL
N° 06625(13)
DIN 00261998
Single-Dose
Uniservice
8.4% Sodium Bicarbonate Injection USP
Bicarbonate de sodium à 8,4% injectable USP
4.2 g/50 mL
(84 mg/mL)
ALCALINISANT
Stérile et apyrogène.
Ne contient aucun bactériostatique. Jeter tout reste.
Pour administration intraveineuse seulement.
Posologie usuelle:
Voir dépliant.
Ne pas restériliser.
Entreposage: Conserver entre 15 et 25°C.
2 mOsm/mL (calc.)
1 mmol(mEq)/mL
RL-0741 (10/04)
(L) EXP

A

Label B:

4. The generic name of the drug is Cefixime.
5. The reconstitution instruction to mix a supply dosage of 100 mg per 5 mL for oral suspension is ________.
6. The manufacturer of the drug is Sanofi aventis.

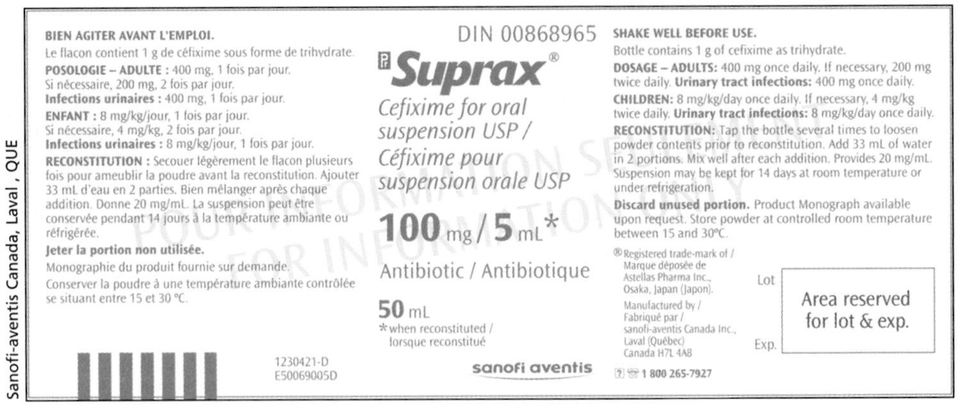
BIEN AGITER AVANT L'EMPLOI.
Le flacon contient 1 g de céfixime sous forme de trihydrate.
POSOLOGIE – ADULTE : 400 mg, 1 fois par jour. Si nécessaire, 200 mg, 2 fois par jour. Infections urinaires : 400 mg, 1 fois par jour.
ENFANT : 8 mg/kg/jour, 1 fois par jour. Si nécessaire, 4 mg/kg, 2 fois par jour. Infections urinaires : 8 mg/kg/jour, 1 fois par jour.
RECONSTITUTION : Secouer légèrement le flacon plusieurs fois pour ameublir la poudre avant la reconstitution. Ajouter 33 mL d'eau en 2 parties. Bien mélanger après chaque addition. Donne 20 mg/mL. La suspension peut être conservée pendant 14 jours à la température ambiante ou réfrigérée.
Jeter la portion non utilisée.
Monographie du produit fournie sur demande.
Conserver la poudre à une température ambiante contrôlée se situant entre 15 et 30 °C.
DIN 00868965
Suprax®
Cefixime for oral suspension USP / Céfixime pour suspension orale USP
100 mg / 5 mL*
Antibiotic / Antibiotique
50 mL
*when reconstituted / lorsque reconstitué
POUR INFORMATION SEULEMENT / FOR INFORMATION ONLY
SHAKE WELL BEFORE USE.
Bottle contains 1 g of cefixime as trihydrate.
DOSAGE – ADULTS: 400 mg once daily. If necessary, 200 mg twice daily. Urinary tract infections: 400 mg once daily.
CHILDREN: 8 mg/kg/day once daily. If necessary, 4 mg/kg twice daily. Urinary tract infections: 8 mg/kg/day once daily.
RECONSTITUTION: Tap the bottle several times to loosen powder contents prior to reconstitution. Add 33 mL of water in 2 portions. Mix well after each addition. Provides 20 mg/mL. Suspension may be kept for 14 days at room temperature or under refrigeration.
Discard unused portion. Product Monograph available upon request. Store powder at controlled room temperature between 15 and 30°C.
® Registered trade-mark of / Marque déposée de Astellas Pharma Inc., Osaka, Japan (Japon).
Manufactured by / Fabriqué par / sanofi-aventis Canada Inc., Laval (Québec) Canada H7L 4A8
Lot
Exp.
Area reserved for lot & exp.
1230421-D
E50069005D
sanofi aventis
1 800 265-7927
Sanofi-aventis Canada, Laval, QUE

B

Label C: C

7. The total volume of the medication container is 2mL.
8. The supply dosage is 50mg / 2mL.
9. How much will you administer to the patient per dose for the order *Methotrexate 25 mg IV stat?*________.

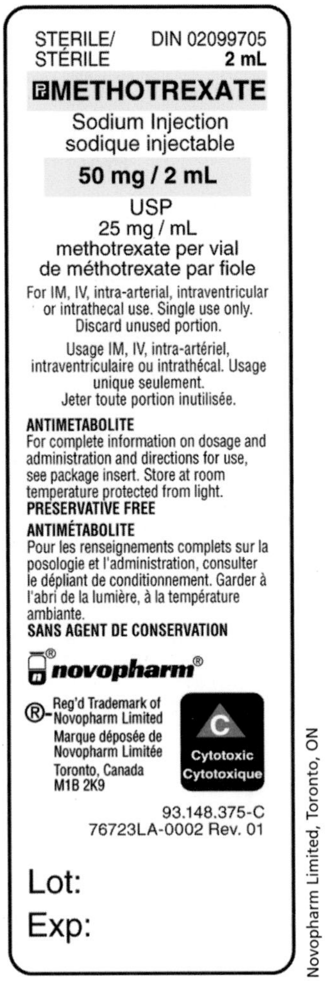
STERILE/ STÉRILE
DIN 02099705
2 mL
METHOTREXATE
Sodium Injection
sodique injectable
50 mg / 2 mL
USP
25 mg / mL
methotrexate per vial
de méthotrexate par fiole
For IM, IV, intra-arterial, intraventricular or intrathecal use. Single use only. Discard unused portion.
Usage IM, IV, intra-artériel, intraventriculaire ou intrathécal. Usage unique seulement. Jeter toute portion inutilisée.
ANTIMETABOLITE
For complete information on dosage and administration and directions for use, see package insert. Store at room temperature protected from light.
PRESERVATIVE FREE
ANTIMÉTABOLITE
Pour les renseignements complets sur la posologie et l'administration, consulter le dépliant de conditionnement. Garder à l'abri de la lumière, à la température ambiante.
SANS AGENT DE CONSERVATION
novopharm®
Reg'd Trademark of Novopharm Limited
Marque déposée de Novopharm Limitée
Toronto, Canada M1B 2K9
C
Cytotoxic
Cytotoxique
93.148.375-C
76723LA-0002 Rev. 01
Lot:
Exp:
Novopharm Limited, Toronto, ON

Label D:

10. The number of doses supplied by this vial is/are ________.
11. The generic name is tobramycin.
12. The Drug Identification Number of the drug is 00533688.

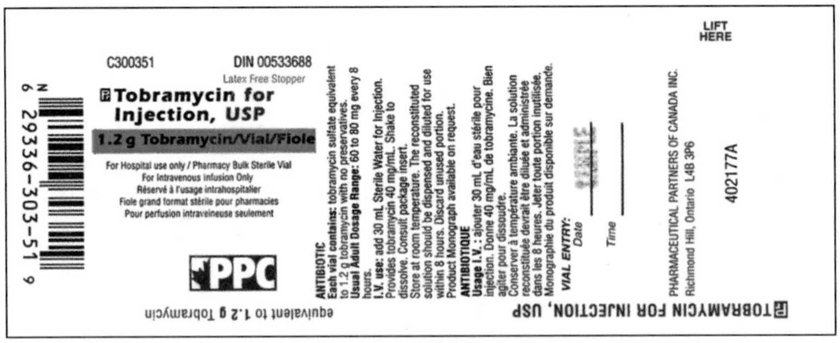
LIFT HERE
C300351
DIN 00533688
Latex Free Stopper
Tobramycin for Injection, USP
1.2 g Tobramycin/Vial/Fiole
For Hospital use only / Pharmacy Bulk Sterile Vial
For Intravenous Infusion Only
Réservé à l'usage intrahospitalier
Fiole grand format stérile pour pharmacies
Pour perfusion intraveineuse seulement
PPC
N 6 29336-303-51 9
ANTIBIOTIC
Each vial contains: tobramycin sulfate equivalent to 1.2 g tobramycin with no preservatives.
Usual Adult Dosage Range: 60 to 80 mg every 8 hours.
I.V. use: add 30 mL Sterile Water for Injection. Provides tobramycin 40 mg/mL. Shake to dissolve. Consult package insert. Store at room temperature. The reconstituted solution should be dispensed and diluted for use within 8 hours. Discard unused portion. Product Monograph available on request.
ANTIBIOTIQUE
Usage I.V. : ajouter 30 mL d'eau stérile pour injection. Donne 40 mg/mL de tobramycine. Bien agiter pour dissoudre. Conserver à température ambiante. La solution reconstituée doit être diluée et administrée dans les 8 heures. Jeter toute portion inutilisée. Monographie du produit disponible sur demande.
VIAL ENTRY: Date Time
PHARMACEUTICAL PARTNERS OF CANADA INC.
Richmond Hill, Ontario L4B 3P6
402177A
TOBRAMYCIN FOR INJECTION, USP
equivalent to 1.2 g Tobramycin

Pharmaceutical Partners of Canada Inc., Richmond Hill, ON

D

Label E:

13. The form of the drug is injection.
14. The total volume of the drug container is 1mL.
15. The administration route is Intramusclar.

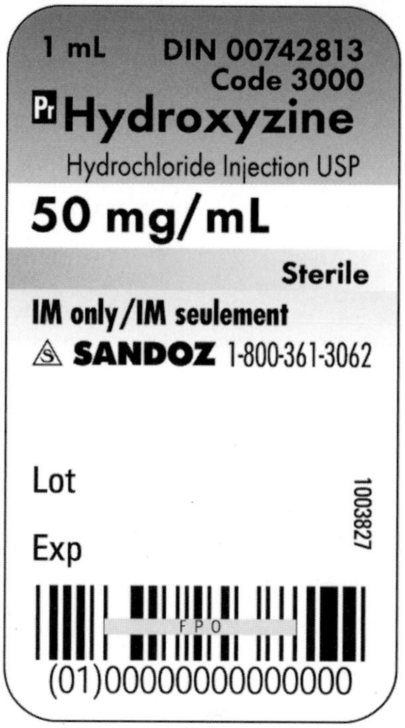
1 mL
DIN 00742813
Code 3000
Pr Hydroxyzine
Hydrochloride Injection USP
50 mg/mL
Sterile
IM only/IM seulement
SANDOZ 1-800-361-3062
Lot
Exp
1003827
FPO
(01)00000000000000

E

Label F:

16. The name of the drug manufacturer is Novopharm.
17. The form of the drug is tablets.
18. The appropriate temperature for storage of this drug is 15-25C.

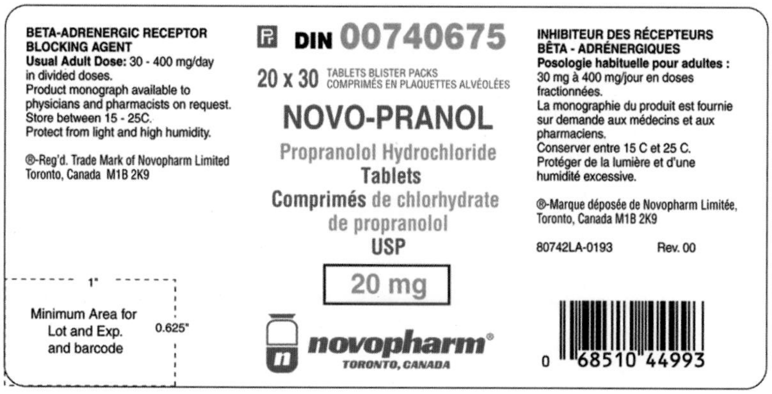
BETA-ADRENERGIC RECEPTOR BLOCKING AGENT
Usual Adult Dose: 30 - 400 mg/day in divided doses.
Product monograph available to physicians and pharmacists on request.
Store between 15 - 25C.
Protect from light and high humidity.
®-Reg'd. Trade Mark of Novopharm Limited Toronto, Canada M1B 2K9
1"
Minimum Area for Lot and Exp. and barcode
0.625"
Pr DIN 00740675
20 x 30 TABLETS BLISTER PACKS COMPRIMÉS EN PLAQUETTES ALVÉOLÉES
NOVO-PRANOL
Propranolol Hydrochloride
Tablets
Comprimés de chlorhydrate de propranolol
USP
20 mg
novopharm®
TORONTO, CANADA
INHIBITEUR DES RÉCEPTEURS BÊTA - ADRÉNERGIQUES
Posologie habituelle pour adultes : 30 mg à 400 mg/jour en doses fractionnées.
La monographie du produit est fournie sur demande aux médecins et aux pharmaciens.
Conserver entre 15 C et 25 C.
Protéger de la lumière et d'une humidité excessive.
®-Marque déposée de Novopharm Limitée, Toronto, Canada M1B 2K9
80742LA-0193
Rev. 00
0 68510 44993

Novopharm Limited, Toronto, ON

F

Label G:

19. The expiration date of the drug is 07/08.
20. The dosage strength of the drug is 20 mEq/10 mL.

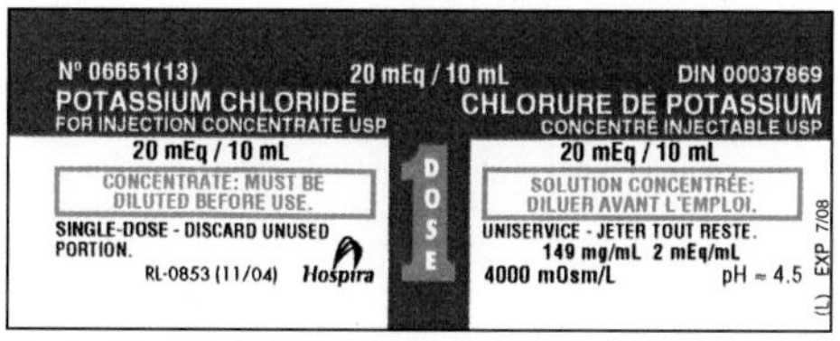
Nº 06651(13)
20 mEq / 10 mL
DIN 00037869
POTASSIUM CHLORIDE
FOR INJECTION CONCENTRATE USP
CHLORURE DE POTASSIUM
CONCENTRÉ INJECTABLE USP
20 mEq / 10 mL
CONCENTRATE: MUST BE DILUTED BEFORE USE.
SINGLE-DOSE - DISCARD UNUSED PORTION.
RL-0853 (11/04)
Hospira
1 DOSE
20 mEq / 10 mL
SOLUTION CONCENTRÉE: DILUER AVANT L'EMPLOI.
UNISERVICE - JETER TOUT RESTE.
149 mg/mL 2 mEq/mL
4000 mOsm/L
pH = 4.5
(L) EXP 7/08

Hospira Healthcare Corporation, Saint-Laurent, QUE

G

Match label H or I with the correct descriptive statement.

21. This label represents a unit- or single-dose drug. ________
22. This label represents a combination drug. ________
23. This label represents a drug usually ordered by the number of tablets or capsules to be administered rather than the dosage strength. ________
24. The administration route for the drug labelled H is ________.
25. The lot number for the drug labelled I is ________.

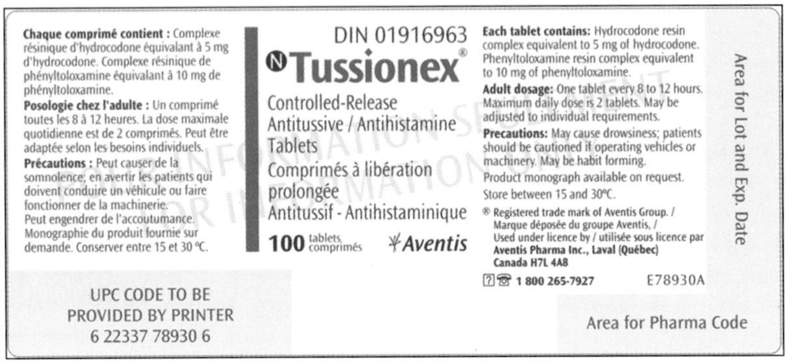

H

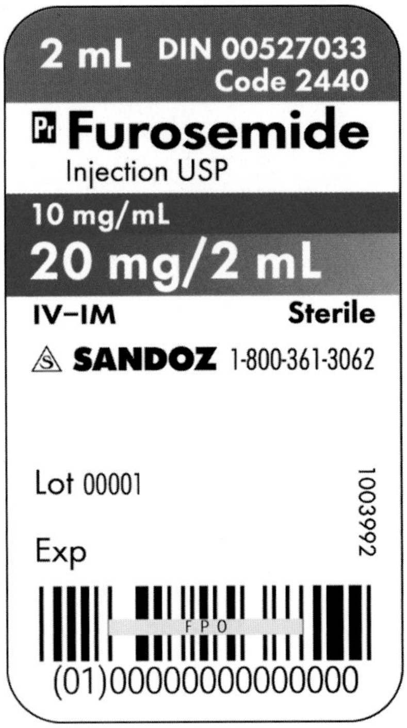

I

Label J:

26. Expressed as a percentage, the supply dosage of the drug is ________.
27. The supply dosage is equivalent to ________ g per ________ mL or ________ mg/mL.

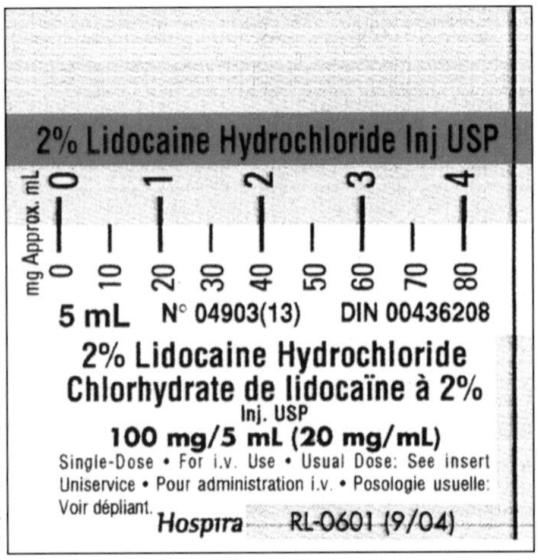

J

28. Critical Thinking Skill: Describe the strategy you would implement to prevent this medication error.

possible scenario

Suppose a physician wrote the order *Celebrex 100 mg PO q12h* (anti-inflammatory to treat rheumatoid arthritis pain), but the order was difficult to read. The unit nurse, processing the order, and pharmacy interpreted the order as *Celexa* (antidepressant), a medication with a similar spelling. Celexa was written on the MAR.

potential outcome

The nurse administered the Celexa for several days, and the patient began complaining of severe knee and hip pain from rheumatoid arthritis. Also, the patient experienced side effects of Celexa, including drowsiness and tremors. A medication error occurred because several healthcare professionals misinterpreted the order.

prevention

What should have alerted the nurse that something was wrong? What should have been considered to prevent this error?

____

____

After completing these problems, see page 466 in the answer section to check your answers.

SECTION 2 SELF-EVALUATION

Directions:

1. Round decimals to two places.
2. Reduce fractions to their lowest terms.

Chapter 5: Equipment Used in Dosage Measurement

Draw an arrow to demonstrate the correct measurement of the doses given.

1. 1.5 mL

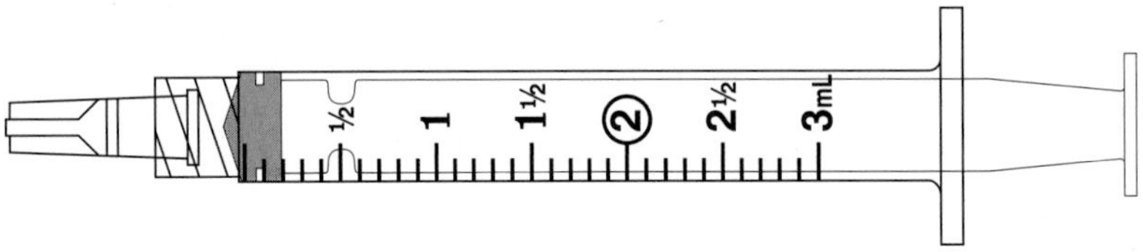

2. 0.33 mL

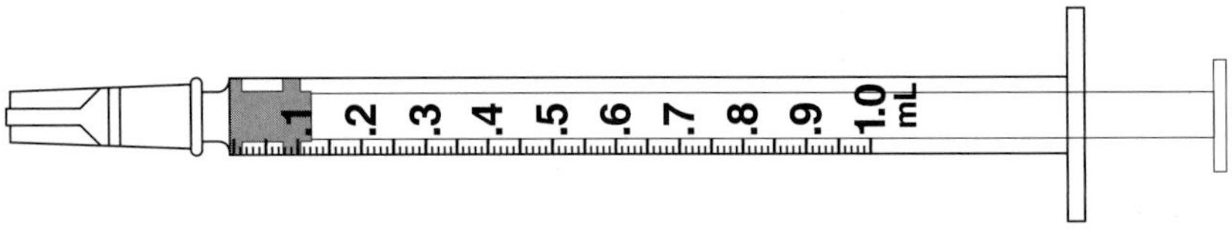

3. 44 units of 100-unit insulin

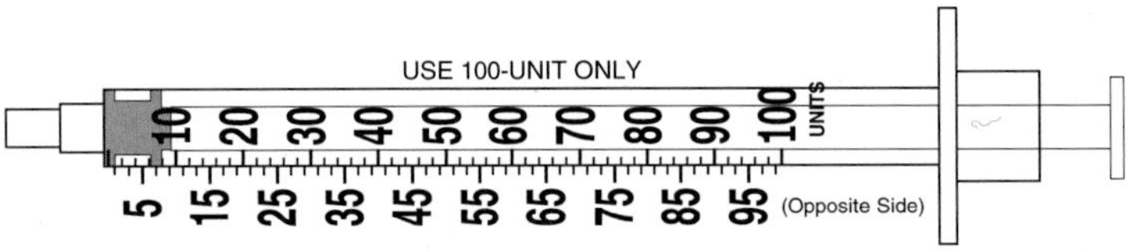

4. 37 units of 100-unit insulin

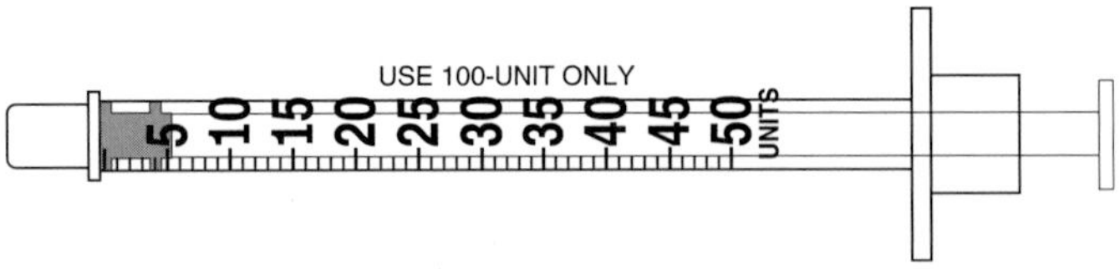

5. 7.5 mL

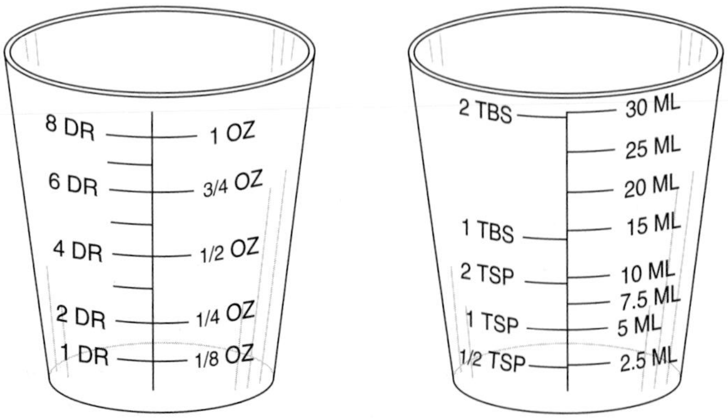

Chapters 6 and 7: Interpreting Drug Orders and Understanding Drug Labels

Use label A to identify the information requested for questions 6 through 9.

6. The generic name is ______________________________.
7. This drug is an otic solution and is intended for ______________________.
8. The total volume of this container is ______________________.
9. Interpret: *Cortisporin Otic Solution 2 gtt both ears q15 min × 3* ______________

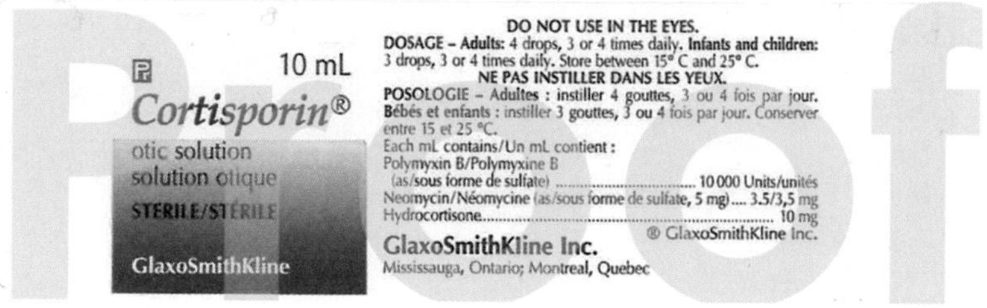

Use label B to identify the information requested for questions 10 through 12.

10. The supply dosage is __________.
11. The Drug Identification Number is __________.
12. Interpret: *heparin sodium 3750 units subcutaneous q8h* __________.

____

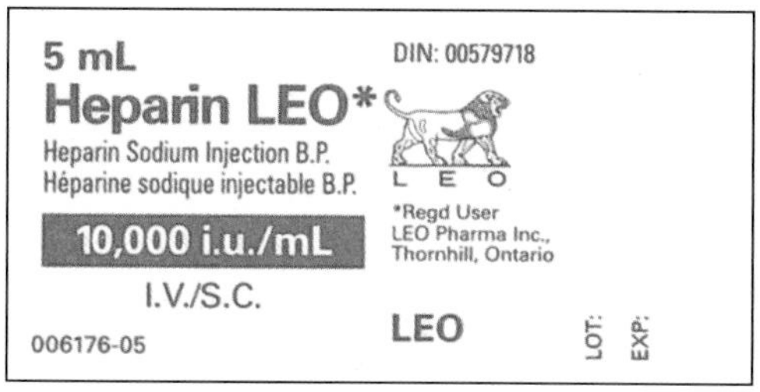

Use label C to identify the information requested for questions 13 through 15.

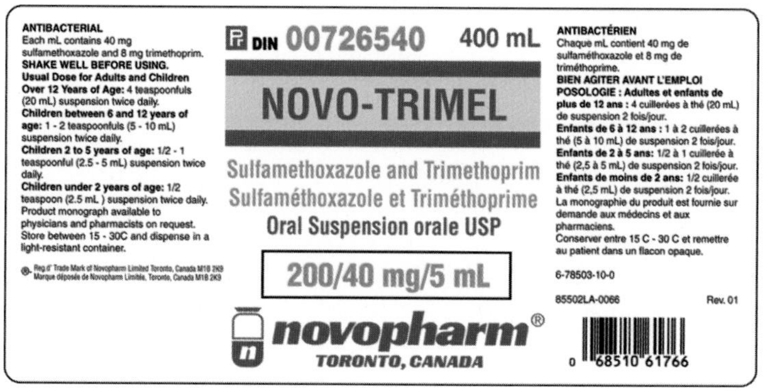

13. The trade name is ______________________________.
14. The supply dosage is ____________.

15. What amount would be given for one dose if the drug order is for a child under 2 years of age?

    a. __________ mL

    b. Draw an arrow on the medicine cup to demonstrate the dose volume.

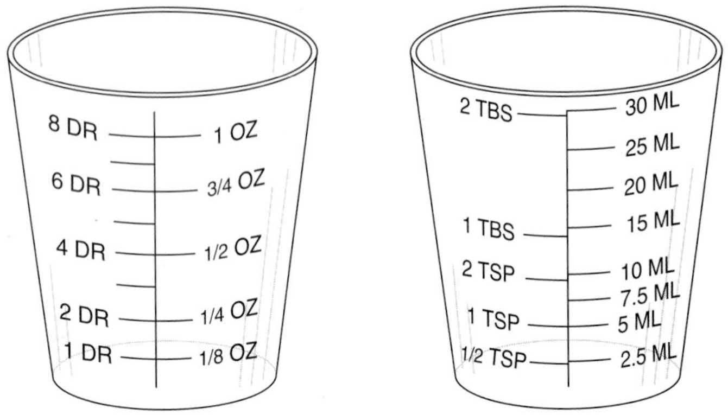

16. Interpret: *Amoxil 250 mg PO TID* ______________________________.

After completing these problems, see pages 466–467 to check your answers.

Perfect score = 100 My score = ________

Mastery score = 86 or higher (14 correct)

SECTION

3

Drug Dosage Calculations

CHAPTER

8

Oral Dosage of Drugs

LEARNING OBJECTIVES

1. Calculate oral dosages of drugs.
2. Convert all units of measurement to the same size units.
3. Estimate the reasonable amount of the drug to be administered.
4. Use the formula $\frac{D}{H} \times Q = X$ to calculate drug dosage.
5. Calculate the number of tablets or capsules that are contained in prescribed dosages.
6. Calculate the volume of liquid per dose when the prescribed dosage is in solution form.

Medications for oral administration are supplied in a variety of forms, such as tablets, capsules, and liquids. They are usually ordered to be administered by mouth, or *PO*, which is an abbreviation for the Latin phrase *"per os."*

When a liquid form of a drug is unavailable, children and many older patients may need to have a tablet crushed or a capsule opened and mixed with a small amount of food or fluid to enable them to swallow the medication. Many of these crushed medications and oral liquids also may be ordered to be given enterally, or into the gastrointestinal tract, via a specially placed tube. Such tubes and their associated enteral routes include the *nasogastric* (NG) tube from nares to stomach; the *nasojejunal* (NJ) tube from nares to jejunum; the *gastrostomy tube* (GT) placed directly through the abdomen into the stomach; and the *percutaneous endoscopic gastrostomy* (PEG) tube.

It is important to recognize that some solid-form medications are intended to be given whole to achieve a specific effect in the body. For example, enteric-coated medications protect the stomach by dissolving in the duodenum. Sustained-release capsules allow for gradual release of medication over time and should be swallowed whole. Consult a drug reference or the pharmacist if you are in doubt about the safety of crushing tablets or opening capsules.

TABLETS AND CAPSULES

Medications prepared in tablet and capsule form are supplied in the strengths or dosages in which they are commonly prescribed (Figure 8-1). It is desirable to obtain the drug in the same strength as the dosage ordered or in multiples of that dosage. When necessary, scored tablets (those marked for division) can be divided into halves or quarters. **Only scored tablets are intended to be divided.**

CAUTION

It is safest and most accurate to give the fewest number of whole, undivided tablets possible.

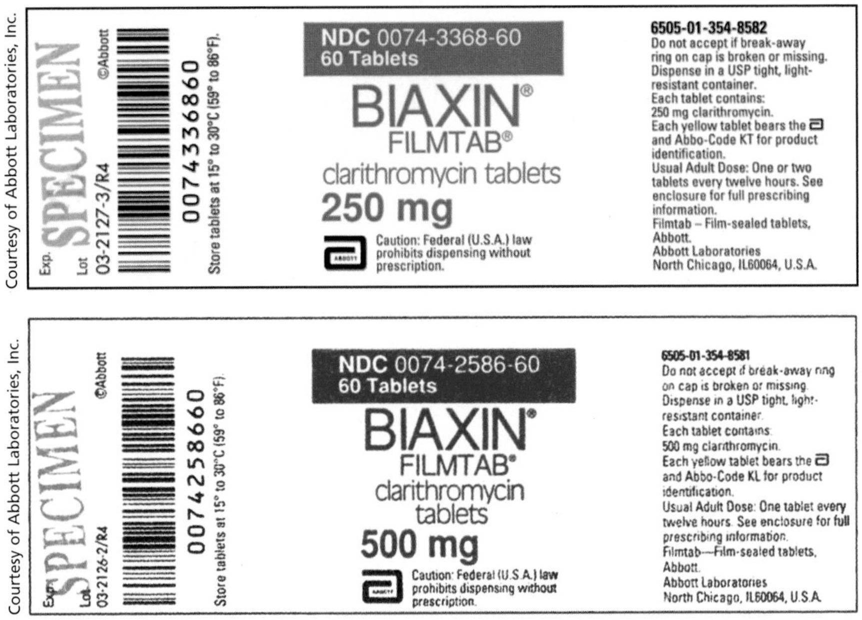

FIGURE 8-1 Clarithromycin 250-mg and 500-mg tablets

Example 1:

The patient care order reads: *clarithromycin 500 mg PO q12h.*

Clarithromycin comes in tablet strengths of 250 milligrams per tablet and 500 milligrams per tablet. When both strengths are available, the nurse should select the 500-milligram strength, and give 1 whole tablet for each dose.

Example 2:

The patient care order reads: *lorazepam 1.5 mg PO TID*

Lorazepam comes in strengths of 0.5-mg, 1-mg, and 2-mg tablets (Figure 8-2). When the three strengths are available, the nurse should select one 1-mg tablet and one 0.5-mg tablet (1 mg + 0.5 mg = 1.5 mg). This provides the ordered dosage of 1.5 mg and is the least number of tablets (2 tablets total) for the patient to swallow.

You might want to halve the 2-mg tablet to obtain two 1-mg parts and pair one-half with a 0.5 mg tablet. This would also equal 1.5 mg and give you $1\frac{1}{2}$ tablets. However, cutting any tablet in half may produce slightly unequal halves. Your patient may not get the ordered dose as a result. It is preferable to give whole, undivided tablets, when they are available.

If the medication is received as a pre-packaged unit dose blister pack from the pharmacy, the unit dose package will be filled with 3 of the 0.5 mg tablets per dose.

THREE-STEP APPROACH TO DOSAGE CALCULATIONS

Now you are ready to learn to solve dosage problems. The following simple three-step method has been proved to reduce anxiety about calculations and ensure that your results are accurate. Take notice that you will be asked to think or estimate before you apply a formula. Learn and memorize this simple three-step approach and use it for every dosage calculation every time.

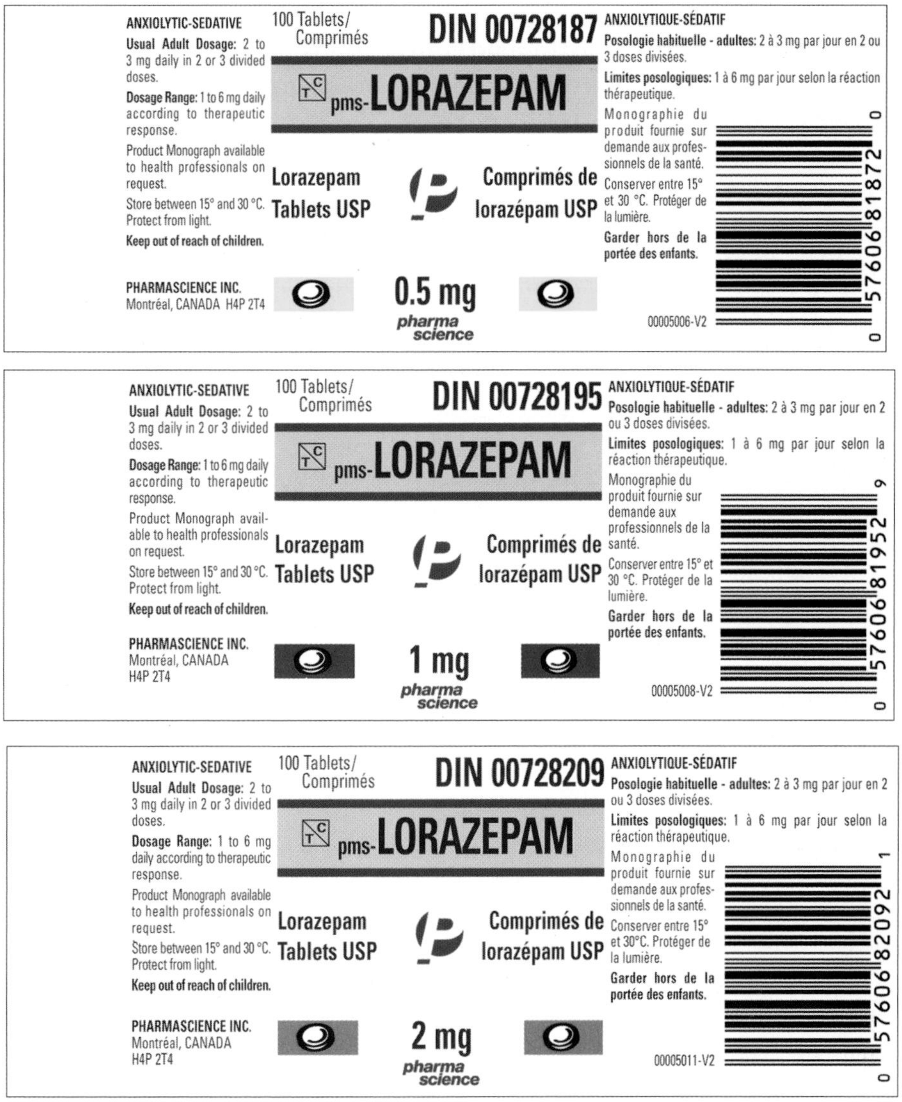

Pharmascience Inc., Montreal, Que

FIGURE 8-2 Lorazepam 0.5-mg, 1-mg, and 2-mg tablets

REMEMBER

Three-Step Approach to Dosage Calculations

Step 1	**Convert**	Ensure that all measurements are in the same size unit of measurement. If not, convert before proceeding.
Step 2	**Think**	Estimate what is a *reasonable amount* of the drug to administer.
Step 3	**Calculate**	Apply the formula: $\frac{D}{H} \times Q = X$

$$\frac{\text{D(desired)}}{\text{H(have)}} \times \text{Q (quantity)} = \text{X (amount)}$$

Let us carefully examine each of the three steps as essential and consecutive rules of accurate dosage calculation.

RULE

Step 1	**Convert**	Be sure that all measurements are in units of the same size, converting when necessary.

Many medications are both ordered and supplied in the same size unit of measurement. This makes dosage calculation easy, because no conversion is necessary. When this is not the case, you must convert to the same size units. Let's look at two examples where conversion is a necessary first step in dosage calculation.

Example 1:

The drug order reads: *cephalexin 0.5 g PO q6h*. The supply dosage (what is available on hand) is labelled *Novo-Lexin (cephalexin) 500 mg per capsule*. This is an example of a medication order written and supplied in the same system (metric), but in different size units (grams and milligrams). A drug order written in grams but supplied in milligrams will have to be converted to the same size unit.

RATIONALE FOR PRACTICE

In most cases, it is more practical to change to the smaller unit (such as grams to milligrams). This requires multiplication and usually eliminates the decimal or fraction, keeping the calculation in whole numbers.

To continue with Example 1, you should convert 0.5 gram to milligrams. Notice that milligrams is the smaller unit and converting eliminates the decimal fraction.

Equivalent: 1 g = 1000 mg

Remember: You are converting from a larger to a smaller unit. Therefore, you will multiply by the conversion factor of 1000, or move the decimal point three places to the right.

$0.5 \text{ g} = 0.5 \times 1000 = 500 \text{ mg}$ or $0.5 \text{ g} = 0.500. = 500 \text{ mg}$

Order: *cephalexin 500 mg PO q6h*

Supply: *cephalexin 500 mg per capsule*

You would give the patient 1 cephalexin 500-mg capsule by mouth every 6 hours.

Example 2:

The patient care order reads: *levothyroxine sodium 75 mcg PO daily*. The supply dosage (what you have available on hand) is labelled *levothyroxine sodium 0.15 mg, scored tablets.* This is an example of the medication ordered and supplied in differently sized units. The order is in micrograms, the smaller unit, but the medication is supplied in milligrams, the larger unit.

Equivalent: 1 mg = 1000 mcg

Remember: You are converting from a larger to a smaller unit. Therefore you will multiply by a conversion factor of 1000.

$0.15 \text{ mg} \times 1000 = 150 \text{ mcg}$

Now the problem looks like this:

Order: *levothyroxine sodium 75 mcg PO daily*

Supply: *levothyroxine sodium 150 mcg, scored tablets*

Now you can probably solve this problem in your head. That's what Step 2 is about.

RULE

Step 2	Think	Carefully consider what is the reasonable amount of the drug that should be administered.

Once you have converted all units to the same size, Step 2 asks you to logically conclude what amount should be given. Before you go on to Step 3, you may be able to picture in your mind a reasonable amount of medication to be administered, as was demonstrated in the previous example. At least you should be able to estimate a very close approximation, such as more or less than 1 tablet (or capsule or millilitre). Basically, Step 2 asks you to *stop and think before you go any farther.*

In the levothyroxine example, you estimate that the patient should receive less than 1 tablet. In fact, you realize that you would administer $\frac{1}{2}$ of the 150-mcg tablet to fill the order for 75 mcg.

RULE

Step 3	**Calculate**	Apply the dosage calculation formula: $\frac{D}{H} \times Q = X$

Always double-check your estimated amount from Step 2 with the simple formula $\frac{D}{H} \times Q = X$.

In this formula, *D* represents the *desired* dosage or the dosage ordered. You will find this in the patient care order. *H* represents the dosage you *have* on hand per a *quantity, Q*. Both *H* and *Q* constitute the *supply dosage* found on the label of the drug available.

RATIONALE FOR PRACTICE

When solving dosage problems for drugs supplied in tablets or capsules, Q (quantity) is always 1, because the supply dosage is per one tablet or capsule. Therefore, Q = 1 tablet or capsule.

Let's use the $\frac{D}{H} \times Q = X$ formula to double-check our thinking, and calculate the dosages for the previous levothyroxine sodium example.

Order: *levothyroxine sodium 75 mcg PO daily*

Supply: *levothyroxine sodium 0.15 mg, converted to levothyroxine 150 mcg*

D = desired = 75 mcg

H = have = 150 mcg

Q = quantity = 1 tablet

$$\frac{D}{H} \times Q = \frac{75 \text{ mcg}}{150 \text{ mcg}} \times 1 \text{ tablet}$$

$$\frac{\overset{1}{\cancel{75}\ \cancel{\text{mcg}}}}{\underset{2}{\cancel{150}\ \cancel{\text{mcg}}}} \times 1 \text{ tablet} = \frac{1}{2} \times 1 \text{ tablet} = \frac{1}{2} \text{ or } 0.5 \text{ tablet}$$ (Notice that mcg cancels out.)

Give $\frac{1}{2}$ (0.5) of the levothyroxine sodium 0.15 mg tablets orally once a day. The calculations verify your estimate from Step 2.

It is wise to get in the habit of always inserting the *quantity* value in the formula, even when Q is 1. Then you will be prepared to accurately calculate dosages for oral liquid or parenteral injection drugs that may be supplied in a solution strength quantity of more or less than 1 (mL).

Notice that the formula is set up with *D* (*desired dosage*) as the numerator and *H* (dosage *strength* you *have* on hand) as the denominator of a fraction. You are calculating for some portion of *Q* (*quantity* you have on hand). You can see that setting up a dosage calculation like this makes sense. Let's look at two more examples to reinforce this concept.

Example 3:

Order: *furosemide 10 mg PO BID*

Supply: *furosemide 20 mg per tablet*

$$\frac{D}{H} \times Q = \frac{10 \text{ mg}}{20 \text{ mg}} \times 1 \text{ tablet}$$

$$\frac{\overset{1}{\cancel{10 \text{ mg}}}}{\underset{2}{\cancel{20 \text{ mg}}}} \times 1 \text{ tablet} = \frac{1}{2} \times 1 \text{ tablet} = \frac{1}{2} \text{ tablet}$$

Notice that you want to give $\frac{1}{2}$ of the Q (quantity of the supply dosage you have on hand, which in this case is 1 tablet). Therefore, you want to give $\frac{1}{2}$ tablet of furosemide 20 mg tablets orally twice daily.

Example 4:

Order: *acetaminophen 650 mg PO q3–4h prn for headache*

Supply: *acetaminophen 325 mg per tablet*

$$\frac{D}{H} \times Q = \frac{650 \text{ mg}}{325 \text{ mg}} \times 1 \text{ tablet}$$

$$\frac{\overset{2}{\cancel{650 \text{ mg}}}}{\underset{1}{\cancel{325 \text{ mg}}}} \times 1 \text{ tablet} = 2 \times 1 \text{ tablet} = 2 \text{ tablet}$$

Notice that you want to give 2 times the amount of Q; that is, you want to give 2 of the acetaminophen 325 mg tablets orally every 3–4 hours as needed for headache.

Now you are ready to apply all three steps of this logical approach to dosage calculations. The same three steps will be used to solve both oral and parenteral dosage calculation problems. It is most important that you develop the ability to reason for the answer or estimate before you apply the $\frac{D}{H} \times Q = X$ formula.

Note to Learner

Healthcare professionals can unknowingly make errors if they rely solely on a formula rather than first asking themselves what the answer should be. As a nurse or allied health professional, you are expected to be able to reason sensibly, problem solve, and justify your judgments rationally. With these same skills you gained admission to your educational program and to your profession. While you sharpen your math skills, your ability to think and estimate are your best resources for avoiding errors. Use the formula as a calculation tool to validate the dose amount you anticipate should be given, rather than the reverse. If your reasoning is sound, you will find the dosages you compute make sense and are accurate. For example, question any calculation that directs you to administer 15 tablets of any medication.

CAUTION

Recheck your calculation if a single dose seems unreasonable. Although not impossible, amounts less than $\frac{1}{2}$ tablet or greater than 3 tablets or capsules are uncommon and should be reassessed.

Let's examine more examples of oral dosages supplied in capsules and tablets to reinforce the three basic steps. Then you will be ready to solve problems like these on your own.

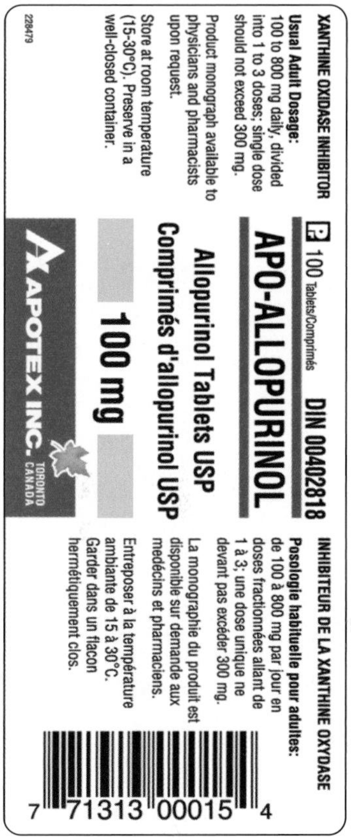

Apotex Inc., Weston, ON

Example 1:

The patient care order reads: *allopurinol 200 mg PO BID*. The medicine container is labelled *allopurinol 100 mg per tablet.* Calculate one dose.

Step 1 Convert No conversion is necessary. The units are in the same system (metric) and the same size (milligrams).

Step 2 Think You want to administer 200 milligrams, and you have 100 milligrams in each tablet. You want to give twice the equivalent of each tablet, or you want to administer 2 tablets per dose.

Step 3 Calculate $\frac{D}{H} \times Q = \frac{200 \text{ mg}}{100 \text{ mg}} \times 1 \text{ tablet}$

$$\frac{\overset{2}{\cancel{200 \text{ mg}}}}{\underset{1}{\cancel{100 \text{ mg}}}} \times 1 \text{ tablet} = 2 \times 1 \text{ tablet} = 2 \text{ tablets; given orally twice daily}$$

Double-check to be sure your calculated dosage matches your *reasonable* dosage from Step 2. If, for example, you had calculated to give more or less than 2 tablets of allopurinol, you would suspect a calculation error.

Example 2:

The physician prescribes *amoxicillin 0.5 g PO QID*. The dosage available is *amoxicillin 250 mg per capsule.* How many capsules should the nurse give to the patient per dose?

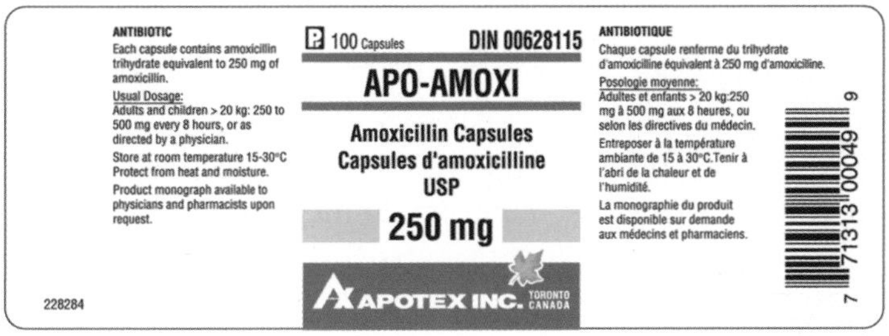

Apotex Inc., Weston, ON

Step 1 Convert To the same size units. Convert 0.5 grams to milligrams. Remember the math tip: Convert larger unit (g) to the smaller unit (mg).

Equivalent: 1 g = 1000 mg. Conversion factor is 1000.

Larger → Smaller: (×)

0.5 g = 0.5 × 1000 = 0.500. = 500 mg

Now you have the order and supply measured in the same size units.

Order: *amoxicillin 0.5 g = 500 mg*

Supply: *amoxicillin 250 mg capsule*

By now you probably can do conversions like this from memory.

Step 2 Think 500 mg is twice as much as 250 mg. You want to give 2 capsules.

Step 3 Calculate $\frac{D}{H} \times Q = \frac{500 \text{ mg}}{250 \text{ mg}} \times 1 \text{ capsule}$

$$\frac{\overset{2}{\cancel{500}\ \cancel{\text{mg}}}}{\underset{1}{\cancel{250}\ \cancel{\text{mg}}}} \times 1 \text{ capsule} = 2 \times 1 \text{ capsule} = 2 \text{ capsules; given orally 4 times daily}$$

Example 3:

The order is *levothyroxine sodium 0.05 mg PO daily*. *Levothyroxine sodium 25 mcg tablets* are available. How many tablets will you give?

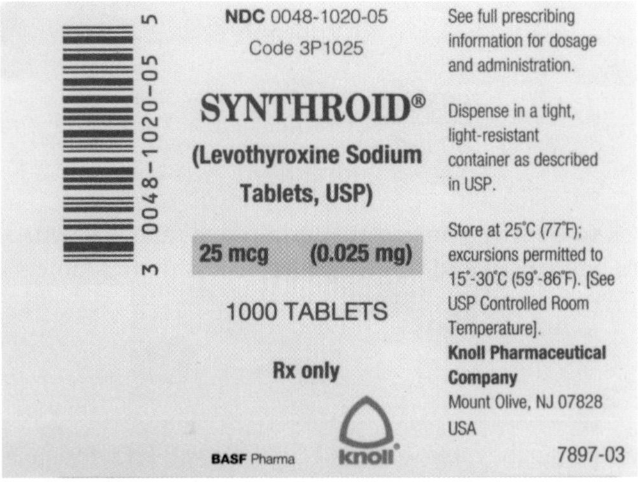

3 0048-1020-05 5
NDC 0048-1020-05
Code 3P1025
SYNTHROID®
(Levothyroxine Sodium
Tablets, USP)
25 mcg (0.025 mg)
1000 TABLETS
Rx only
BASF Pharma
knoll
See full prescribing information for dosage and administration.
Dispense in a tight, light-resistant container as described in USP.
Store at 25°C (77°F); excursions permitted to 15°-30°C (59°-86°F). [See USP Controlled Room Temperature].
Knoll Pharmaceutical Company
Mount Olive, NJ 07828
USA
7897-03

Courtesy Knoll Pharmaceutical Company

Step 1 Convert To same size units. Remember: Convert larger unit (mg) to smaller unit (mcg).

Approximate equivalent: 1 mg = 1000 mcg. Conversion factor is 1000.

Larger → Smaller: (×)

0.05 mg = 0.05 × 1000 = 0.050. = 50 mcg

Order: *levothyroxine sodium 0.05 mg = 50 mcg*

Supply: *levothyroxine sodium 25 mcg tablets*

Step 2 Think As soon as you convert the ordered dosage of levothyroxine sodium 0.05 mg to levothyroxine sodium 50 mcg, you realize that you want to give more than 1 tablet for each dose. In fact, you want to give twice the supply dosage, which is the same as 2 tablets.

Avoid getting confused by the way the original problem is presented. Be sure that you recognize which is the dosage ordered (*D*—desired) and which is the supply dosage (*H*—have on hand) per the quantity on hand (*Q*). A common error is to misread the information and mix up the calculations in Step 3. This demonstrates the importance of thinking (Step 2) before you calculate.

Step 3 Calculate $\frac{D}{H} \times Q = \frac{50 \text{ mcg}}{25 \text{ mcg}} \times 1 \text{ tablet}$

$$\frac{\overset{2}{\cancel{50}\ \cancel{\text{mcg}}}}{\underset{1}{\cancel{25}\ \cancel{\text{mcg}}}} \times 1 \text{ tablet} = 2 \times 1 \text{ tablet} = 2 \text{ tablets; given orally once a day}$$

Example 4:

Your patient is to receive *hydrochlorothiazide 37.5 mg PO each morning*. The label on the available Apo-Hydro (hydrochlorothiazide) bottle tells you that each tablet provides 25 mg. How much will you give your patient?

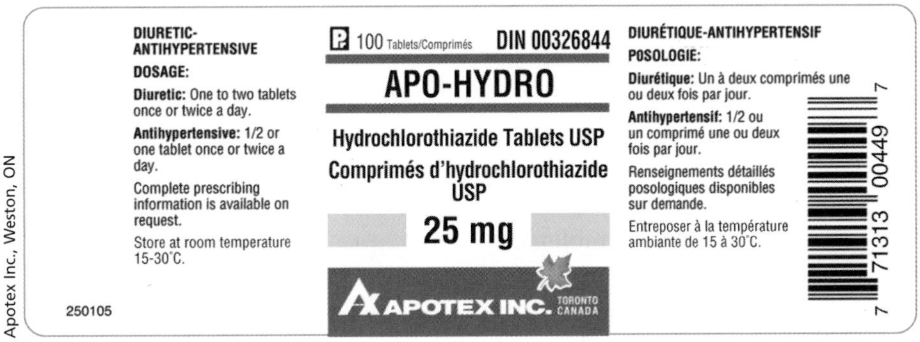

Step 1 Convert Recognize desired dose and supply dose are in same units. No conversion required.

Step 2 Think Look at the supply dosage and compare the ordered dosage of 37.5 mg with the supply dosage of 25 mg per tablet. You can reason that you want to give more than 1 tablet. Further, you can see that if you move decimal point to make numbers whole, you want to give $\frac{1}{2}$ tablet. Check your reasoning in Step 3.

Step 3 Calculate Move decimal point to make *D* a whole number. Move decimal point similarly in *H* by adding "0" (as per Chapter 1).

$$\frac{D}{H} \times Q = \frac{37.5 \text{ mg}}{25 \text{ mg}} \times 1 \text{ tablet}$$

$$\frac{\overset{3}{\cancel{375}\ \cancel{\text{mg}}}}{\underset{2}{\cancel{250}\ \cancel{\text{mg}}}} \times 1 \text{ tablet} = 1\tfrac{1}{2} \text{ tablets given orally each morning}$$

QUICK REVIEW

Simple Three-Step Approach to Dosage Calculations

Step 1	**Convert**	To units of the same system and the same size.
Step 2	**Think**	Estimate for a reasonable amount to give.
Step 3	**Calculate**	$\frac{D}{H} \times Q = X$

$$\frac{\text{D (desired)}}{\text{H (have)}} \times \text{Q (quantity)} = \text{X (amount)}$$

- For most dosage calculation problems:
  - Convert to smaller size unit. Example: g → mg
- Consider the reasonableness of the calculated amount to give. Example: You would question giving less than $\frac{1}{2}$ tablet or more than 3 tablets or capsules per dose for oral administration.

REVIEW SET 20

Calculate the correct number of tablets or capsules to be administered per dose. Tablets are scored.

1. The physician writes an order for *nitrofurantoin 0.1 g PO QID*. The drug container label reads *nitrofurantoin 100 mg tablets.*

   Give: ________ tablet(s)

2. cephalexin 500 mg tablets available. The order is for *cephalexin 0.5 g PO BID*

   Give: ________ tablet(s)

3. bethanechol chloride 10 mg tablets available. Order: *bethanechol chloride 15 mg PO TID*

   Give: ________ tablet(s)

4. Order: *hydrochlorothiazide 12.5 mg PO TID.* Available: hydrochlorothiazide 25 mg tablets.

   Give: ________ tablet(s)

5. Order: *digoxin 0.125 mg PO daily*

   Supply: digoxin 0.25 mg tablets

   Give: ________ tablet(s)

6. Order: *ibuprofen 600 mg PO BID*

   Supply: ibuprofen 300 mg tablets

   Give: ________ tablet(s)

7. Order: *potassium chloride 16 mEq PO stat*

   Supply: potassium chloride 8 mEq tablets

   Give: ________ tablet(s)

8. cyclophosphamide 25 mg tablets available. Order: *cyclophosphamide 50 mg PO daily*

   Give: ________ tablet(s)

9. metolazone 5 mg tablets available. Order: *metolazone 7.5 mg PO BID*

   Give: ________ tablet(s)

10. *warfarin sodium 5 mg PO daily* ordered. Warfarin sodium 2.5 mg tablets available.

    Give: ________ tablet(s)

11. levofloxacin is available in 500-mg tablets. Ordered dose is *levofloxacin 0.5 g PO daily.*

    Give ________ tablet(s)

12. Order: *labetalol hydrochloride 150 mg PO BID*

    Supply: labetalol hydrochloride 300 mg tablets

    Give: ________ tablet(s)

13. Order: *cephalexin 1 g PO BID*

    Supply: cephalexin 500 mg capsules

    Give: ________ capsule(s)

14. levothyroxine sodium 50 mcg tablets available. Order: *levothyroxine sodium 0.1 mg PO daily.*

    Give: ________ tablet(s)

15. *clorazepate dipotassium 7.5 mg PO QID* is ordered and you have 3.75 mg clorazepate *dipotassium* capsules available.

    Give: ________ capsule(s)

16. Order: *atenolol 100 mg BID*

    Supply: atenolol 50 mg tablets

    Give: ________

17. The doctor orders *minoxidil 7.5 mg PO stat* and you have available minoxidil 10 mg and 2.5-mg scored tablets. Select ________ mg tablets and give ________ tablet(s).

18. Order: *metoclopramide 15 mg PO 1 h ac and at bedtime.* You have available metoclopramide 10 mg and metoclopramide 5 mg scored tablets. Select ________ mg tablets and give ________ tablet(s). How many doses of metoclopramide will the patient receive in 24 hours? ________ dose(s)

19. Order: *phenobarbital sodium 45 mg PO daily*

    Supply: phenobarbital *sodium* 30 mg and 60 mg scored tablets.

    Select ________ mg tablets and give ________ tablet(s).

20. Order: *acetaminophen 300 mg/codeine 60 mg PO q4h prn for pain*

    Supply: acetaminophen 300 mg with codeine 7.5 mg, 15 mg, 30 mg, and 60 mg tablets.

    Select ________ mg tablets and give ________ tablet(s).

Calculate one dose for each of the medication orders 21 through 28. The labels lettered A through H are the drugs you have available. Indicate the letter corresponding to the label you select.

21. Order: *verapamil hydrochloride sustained release 240 mg PO daily*

    Select: ________

    Give: ________

22. Order: *carbamazepine 0.2 g PO TID*

    Select: ________

    Give: ________

23. Order: *metoprolol 50 mg PO BID*

    Select: ________

    Give: ________

24. Order: *potassium chloride 16 mEq PO daily*

    Select: ________

    Give: ________

25. Order: *procainamide hydrochloride 750 mg PO q6h*

    Select: ________

    Give: ________

26. Order: *cephalexin 0.5 g PO QID*

    Select: ________

    Give: ________

27. Order: *levothyroxine sodium 0.2 mg PO daily*

    Select: ________

    Give: ________

28. Order: *allopurinol 0.1 g PO TID*

    Select: ________

    Give: ________

After completing these problems, see page 467–468 in the answer section to check your answers.

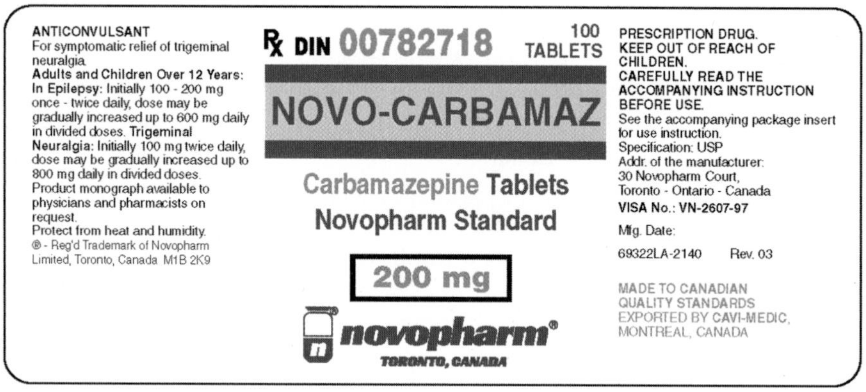

Novopharm Limited, Toronto, ON

A

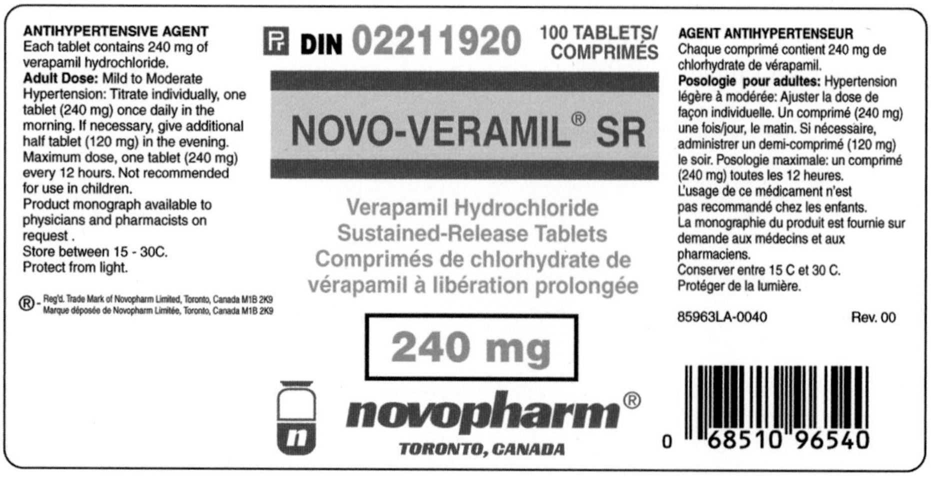

Novopharm Limited, Toronto, ON

B

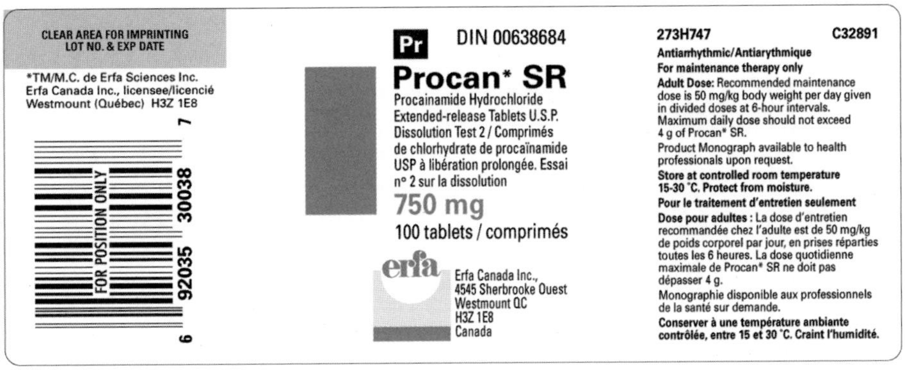
CLEAR AREA FOR IMPRINTING LOT NO. & EXP DATE
*TM/M.C. de Erfa Sciences Inc.
Erfa Canada Inc., licensee/licencié
Westmount (Québec) H3Z 1E8
FOR POSITION ONLY
6 92035 30038 7
Pr DIN 00638684
Procan* SR
Procainamide Hydrochloride Extended-release Tablets U.S.P. Dissolution Test 2 / Comprimés de chlorhydrate de procaïnamide USP à libération prolongée. Essai n° 2 sur la dissolution
750 mg
100 tablets / comprimés
erfa
Erfa Canada Inc., 4545 Sherbrooke Ouest Westmount QC H3Z 1E8 Canada
273H747
C32891
Antiarrhythmic/Antiarythmique
For maintenance therapy only
Adult Dose: Recommended maintenance dose is 50 mg/kg body weight per day given in divided doses at 6-hour intervals. Maximum daily dose should not exceed 4 g of Procan* SR.
Product Monograph available to health professionals upon request.
Store at controlled room temperature 15-30 °C. Protect from moisture.
Pour le traitement d'entretien seulement
Dose pour adultes : La dose d'entretien recommandée chez l'adulte est de 50 mg/kg de poids corporel par jour, en prises réparties toutes les 6 heures. La dose quotidienne maximale de Procan* SR ne doit pas dépasser 4 g.
Monographie disponible aux professionnels de la santé sur demande.
Conserver à une température ambiante contrôlée, entre 15 et 30 °C. Craint l'humidité.

Erfa Canada Inc., Westmount, QUE

C

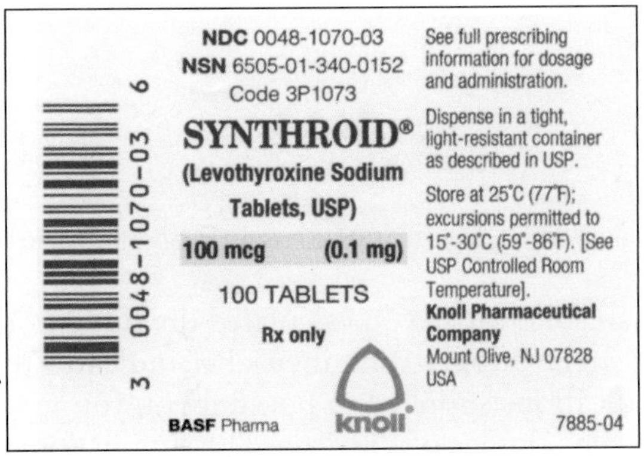
3 0048-1070-03 6
NDC 0048-1070-03
NSN 6505-01-340-0152
Code 3P1073
SYNTHROID®
(Levothyroxine Sodium Tablets, USP)
100 mcg (0.1 mg)
100 TABLETS
Rx only
BASF Pharma
knoll
See full prescribing information for dosage and administration.
Dispense in a tight, light-resistant container as described in USP.
Store at 25°C (77°F); excursions permitted to 15°-30°C (59°-86°F). [See USP Controlled Room Temperature].
Knoll Pharmaceutical Company
Mount Olive, NJ 07828 USA
7885-04

Courtesy of Abbott Laboratories, Inc.

D

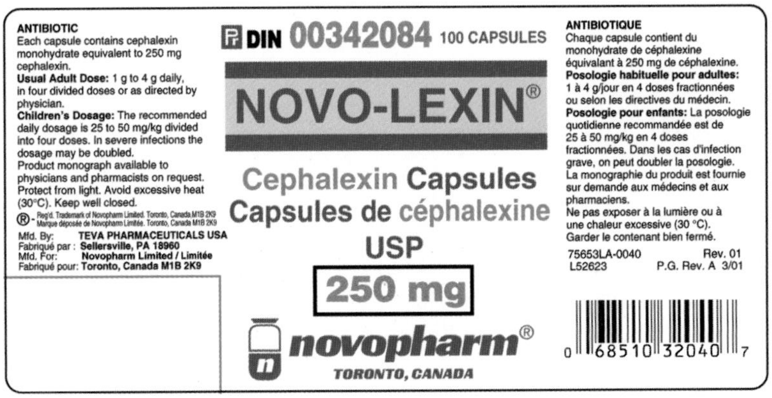
ANTIBIOTIC
Each capsule contains cephalexin monohydrate equivalent to 250 mg cephalexin.
Usual Adult Dose: 1 g to 4 g daily, in four divided doses or as directed by physician.
Children's Dosage: The recommended daily dosage is 25 to 50 mg/kg divided into four doses. In severe infections the dosage may be doubled.
Product monograph available to physicians and pharmacists on request. Protect from light. Avoid excessive heat (30°C). Keep well closed.
Mfd. By: TEVA PHARMACEUTICALS USA
Fabriqué par : Sellersville, PA 18960
Mfd. For: Novopharm Limited / Limitée
Fabriqué pour: Toronto, Canada M1B 2K9
DIN 00342084 100 CAPSULES
NOVO-LEXIN®
Cephalexin Capsules
Capsules de céphalexine
USP
250 mg
novopharm®
TORONTO, CANADA
ANTIBIOTIQUE
Chaque capsule contient du monohydrate de céphalexine équivalant à 250 mg de céphalexine.
Posologie habituelle pour adultes: 1 à 4 g/jour en 4 doses fractionnées ou selon les directives du médecin.
Posologie pour enfants: La posologie quotidienne recommandée est de 25 à 50 mg/kg en 4 doses fractionnées. Dans les cas d'infection grave, on peut doubler la posologie.
La monographie du produit est fournie sur demande aux médecins et aux pharmaciens.
Ne pas exposer à la lumière ou à une chaleur excessive (30 °C). Garder le contenant bien fermé.
75653LA-0040 Rev. 01
L52623 P.G. Rev. A 3/01
0 68510 32040 7

Novopharm Limited, Toronto, ON

E

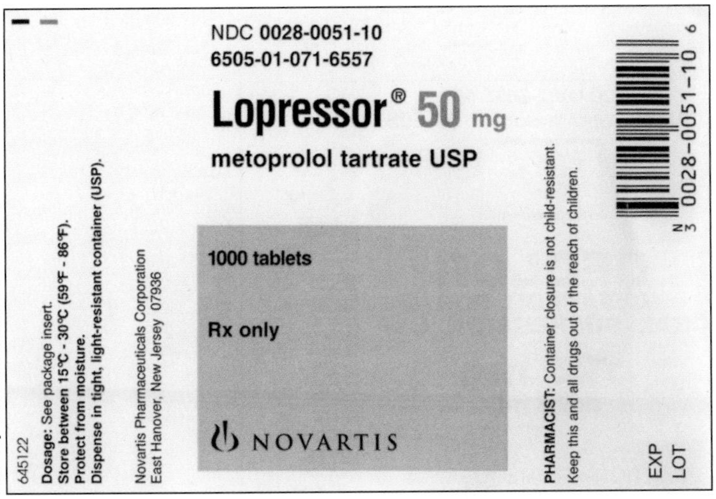
645122
Dosage: See package insert.
Store between 15°C - 30°C (59°F - 86°F).
Protect from moisture.
Dispense in tight, light-resistant container (USP).
Novartis Pharmaceuticals Corporation
East Hanover, New Jersey 07936
NDC 0028-0051-10
6505-01-071-6557
Lopressor® 50 mg
metoprolol tartrate USP
1000 tablets
Rx only
NOVARTIS
PHARMACIST: Container closure is not child-resistant.
Keep this and all drugs out of the reach of children.
N 3 0028-0051-10 6
EXP
LOT

Courtesy Novartis Pharmaceuticals Corporation

F

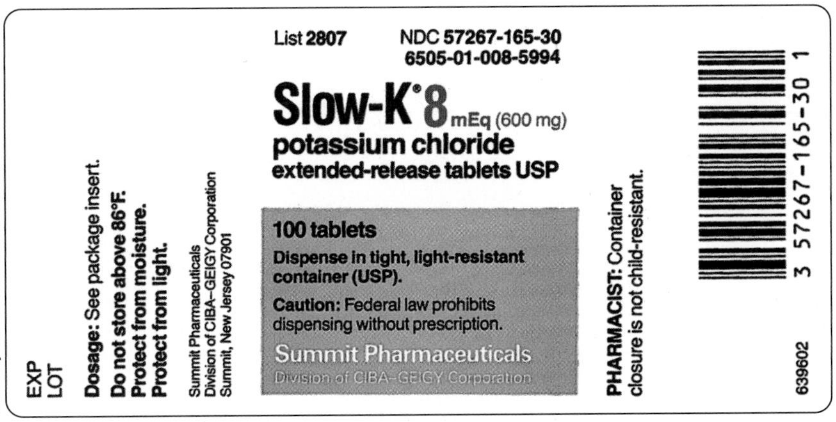
EXP
LOT
Dosage: See package insert.
Do not store above 86°F.
Protect from moisture.
Protect from light.
Summit Pharmaceuticals
Division of CIBA-GEIGY Corporation
Summit, New Jersey 07901
List 2807
NDC 57267-165-30
6505-01-008-5994
Slow-K® 8 mEq (600 mg)
potassium chloride
extended-release tablets USP
100 tablets
Dispense in tight, light-resistant container (USP).
Caution: Federal law prohibits dispensing without prescription.
Summit Pharmaceuticals
Division of CIBA-GEIGY Corporation
PHARMACIST: Container closure is not child-resistant.
3 57267-165-30 1
639602

Courtesy Summit Pharmaceuticals

G

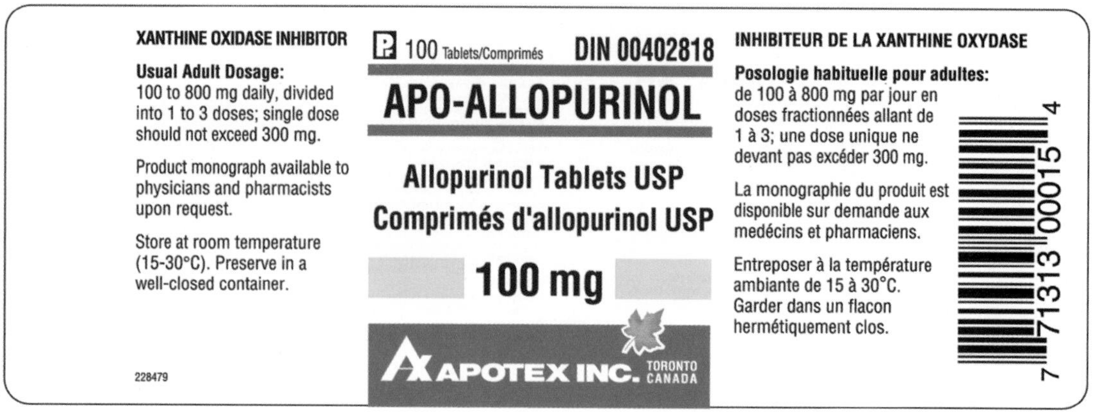
XANTHINE OXIDASE INHIBITOR
Usual Adult Dosage:
100 to 800 mg daily, divided into 1 to 3 doses; single dose should not exceed 300 mg.
Product monograph available to physicians and pharmacists upon request.
Store at room temperature (15-30°C). Preserve in a well-closed container.
228479
100 Tablets/Comprimés DIN 00402818
APO-ALLOPURINOL
Allopurinol Tablets USP
Comprimés d'allopurinol USP
100 mg
APOTEX INC. TORONTO CANADA
INHIBITEUR DE LA XANTHINE OXYDASE
Posologie habituelle pour adultes:
de 100 à 800 mg par jour en doses fractionnées allant de 1 à 3; une dose unique ne devant pas excéder 300 mg.
La monographie du produit est disponible sur demande aux medécins et pharmaciens.
Entreposer à la température ambiante de 15 à 30°C. Garder dans un flacon hermétiquement clos.
7 71313 00015 4

Apotex Inc., Weston, ON

H

ORAL LIQUIDS

Oral liquids are supplied in solution form and contain a specific amount of drug in a given amount of solution as stated on the label (Figures 8-3A through C).

In solving dosage problems when the drug is supplied in solid form, you calculated the number of tablets or capsules that contained the prescribed dosage. The supply container label indicates the amount of medication per 1 tablet or 1 capsule. For medications supplied in liquid form, you must calculate the volume of the liquid that contains the prescribed dosage of the drug. The supply dosage noted on the label may indicate the amount of drug per 1 millilitre or per multiple millilitres of solution, such as 10 mg per 2 mL, 125 mg per 5 mL, or 1.2 g per 30 mL.

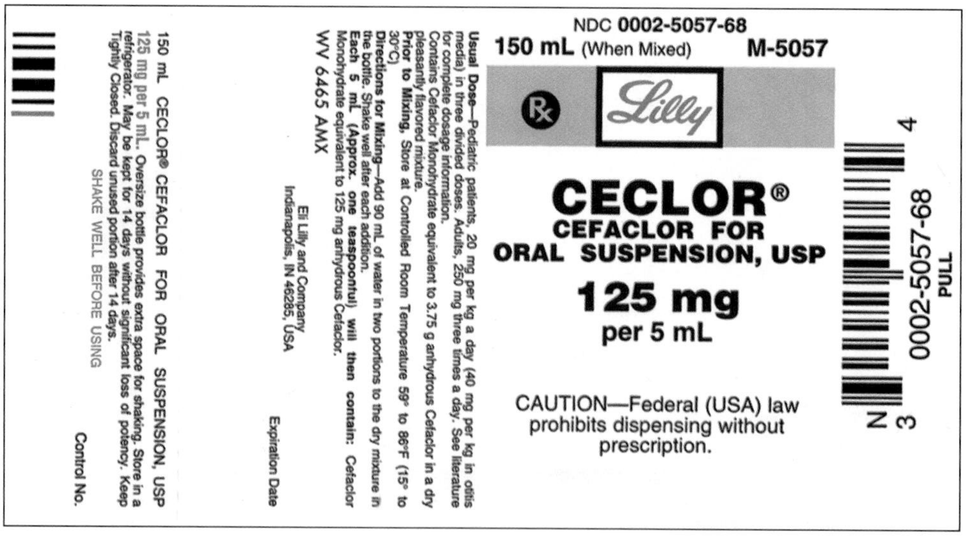
NDC 0002-5057-68
150 mL (When Mixed)
M-5057
Lilly
CECLOR®
CEFACLOR FOR
ORAL SUSPENSION, USP
125 mg
per 5 mL
CAUTION—Federal (USA) law prohibits dispensing without prescription.
150 mL CECLOR® CEFACLOR FOR ORAL SUSPENSION, USP
SHAKE WELL BEFORE USING
Control No.
Eli Lilly and Company
Indianapolis, IN 46285, USA
Expiration Date
WV 6465 AMX
N 3 0002-5057-68 4
PULL

Courtesy of Eli Lilly and Company

FIGURE 8-3(A) Oral Liquid: Ceclor 125 mg per 5 mL

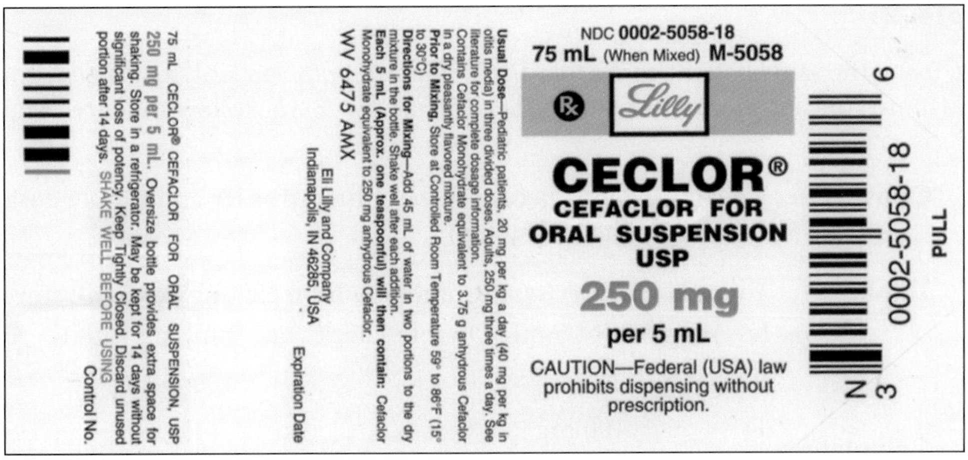

Courtesy of Eli Lilly and Company

FIGURE 8-3(B) Oral Liquid: Ceclor 250 mg per 5 mL

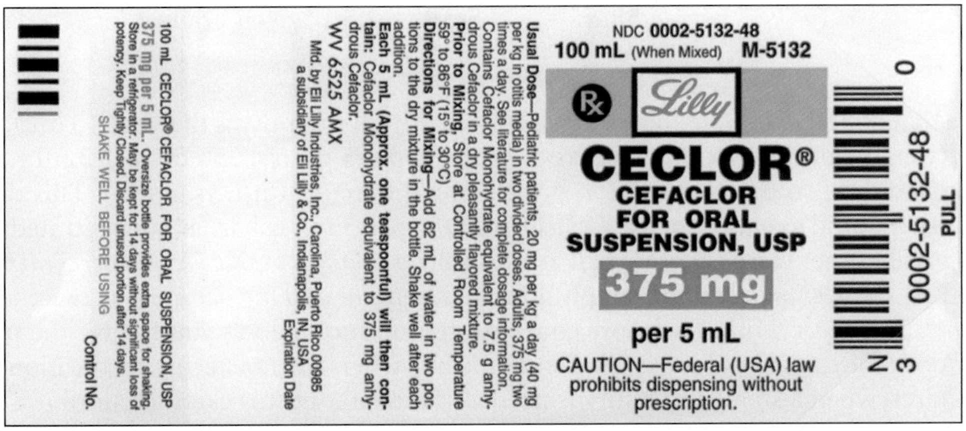

Courtesy of Eli Lilly and Company

FIGURE 8-3(C) Oral Liquid: Ceclor 375 mg per 5 mL

Steps 1, 2, and 3 can be used to solve liquid oral dosage calculations in the same way that solid-form oral dosages are calculated. Let us apply the three steps to dosage calculations in a few examples.

Example 1:

The doctor orders *cefaclor 100 mg PO QID*. Look at the labels of cefaclor available in Figure 8-3. You choose *cefaclor 125 mg per 5 mL*. Follow the three steps to dosage calculations.

Step 1 Convert No conversion is necessary, because the order and supply dosage are both in the same units.

Step 2 Think You want to give less than 125 mg, so you want to give less than 5 mL. Double-check your thinking with the $\frac{D}{H} \times Q = X$ formula.

Step 3 Calculate $\frac{D}{H} \times Q = \frac{100 \text{ mg}}{125 \text{ mg}} \times 5 \text{ mL}$

$$\frac{\overset{4}{\cancel{100}} \cancel{\text{mg}}}{\underset{5}{\cancel{125}} \cancel{\text{mg}}} \times 5 \text{ mL} = \frac{4}{\cancel{5}} \times \overset{1}{\cancel{5}} \text{ mL} = 4 \text{ mL; given orally 4 times a day}$$

You will give 4 mL of the cefaclor with the dosage strength of 125 mg per 5 mL. Double-check to be sure your calculated dosage is consistent with your *reasonable* dosage from Step 2. If, for instance, you calculate to give *more* than 5 mL, then you should suspect a calculation error.

Example 2:

Suppose, using the same patient care order in Example 1, *cefaclor 100 mg PO QID*, you choose a stronger (more concentrated) solution, *cefaclor 250 mg per 5 mL*. Follow the three steps to dosage calculations.

Step 1 Convert No conversion is necessary, because the order and supply dosage are both in the same units and system.

Step 2 Think You want to give 100 mg, and you have 250 mg per 5 mL so you will give less than half of 5 mL. Double-check your thinking with the $\frac{D}{H} \times Q = X$ formula.

Step 3 Calculate $\frac{D}{H} \times Q = \frac{100 \text{ mg}}{250 \text{ mg}} \times 5 \text{ mL}$

$$\frac{\overset{2}{\cancel{100}\ \cancel{\text{mg}}}}{\underset{5}{\cancel{250}\ \cancel{\text{mg}}}} \times 5 \text{ mL} = \frac{2}{\cancel{5}} \times \overset{1}{\cancel{5}}\text{mL} = 2 \text{ mL; given orally 4 times a day}$$

Notice that in both Example 1 and Example 2, the supply quantity is the same (5 mL), but the dosage strength (weight) of medication is different (125 mg per 5 mL vs. 250 mg per 5 mL). This results in the calculated dose volume (amount to give) being different (4 mL vs. 2 mL). This difference is the result of each liquid's *concentration*. *Cefaclor 125 mg per 5 mL* is half as concentrated as *cefaclor 250 mg per 5 mL*. In other words, there is half as much drug in 5 mL of the *125 mg per 5 mL* supply as there is in 5 mL of the *250 mg per 5 mL* supply. Likewise, *cefaclor 250 mg per 5 mL* is twice as concentrated as *cefaclor 125 mg per 5 mL*. The more concentrated solution allows you to give the patient less volume per dose for the same dosage. This is significant when administering medication to infants and small children when a smaller quantity is needed. Think about this carefully until it is clear.

> **CAUTION**
>
> Think before you calculate. It is important to estimate before you apply any formula. In this way, if you make a careless error in math or if you set up the problem incorrectly, your thinking will alert you to *try again*.

Example 3:

The doctor orders *potassium chloride 40 mEq PO daily*. The label on the package reads *potassium chloride 20 mEq per 15 mL*. How many mL should you administer?

Step 1 Convert No conversion is necessary.

Step 2 Think You want to give more than 15 mL. In fact, you want to give exactly twice as much as 15 mL. You know this is true because 40 mEq is twice as much as 20 mEq. Therefore, it will take 2 × 15 mL, or 30 mL, to give 40 mEq. Continue to Step 3 to double-check your thinking.

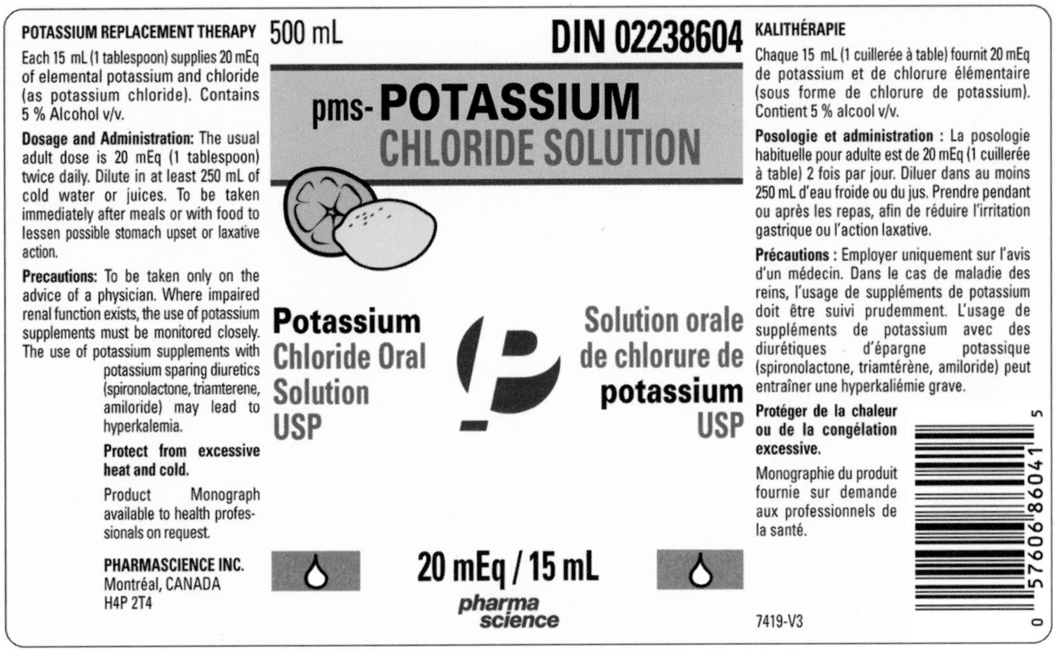
POTASSIUM REPLACEMENT THERAPY
Each 15 mL (1 tablespoon) supplies 20 mEq of elemental potassium and chloride (as potassium chloride). Contains 5 % Alcohol v/v.
Dosage and Administration: The usual adult dose is 20 mEq (1 tablespoon) twice daily. Dilute in at least 250 mL of cold water or juices. To be taken immediately after meals or with food to lessen possible stomach upset or laxative action.
Precautions: To be taken only on the advice of a physician. Where impaired renal function exists, the use of potassium supplements must be monitored closely. The use of potassium supplements with potassium sparing diuretics (spironolactone, triamterene, amiloride) may lead to hyperkalemia.
Protect from excessive heat and cold.
Product Monograph available to health professionals on request.
PHARMASCIENCE INC.
Montréal, CANADA
H4P 2T4
500 mL
DIN 02238604
pms-POTASSIUM
CHLORIDE SOLUTION
Potassium Chloride Oral Solution USP
Solution orale de chlorure de potassium USP
20 mEq / 15 mL
pharma science
KALITHÉRAPIE
Chaque 15 mL (1 cuillerée à table) fournit 20 mEq de potassium et de chlorure élémentaire (sous forme de chlorure de potassium). Contient 5 % alcool v/v.
Posologie et administration : La posologie habituelle pour adulte est de 20 mEq (1 cuillerée à table) 2 fois par jour. Diluer dans au moins 250 mL d'eau froide ou du jus. Prendre pendant ou après les repas, afin de réduire l'irritation gastrique ou l'action laxative.
Précautions : Employer uniquement sur l'avis d'un médecin. Dans le cas de maladie des reins, l'usage de suppléments de potassium doit être suivi prudemment. L'usage de suppléments de potassium avec des diurétiques d'épargne potassique (spironolactone, triamtérène, amiloride) peut entraîner une hyperkaliémie grave.
Protéger de la chaleur ou de la congélation excessive.
Monographie du produit fournie sur demande aux professionnels de la santé.
7419-V3
0 57606 86041 5

Pharmascience Inc., Montreal, Que

Step 3 **Calculate** $\frac{D}{H} \times Q = \frac{\overset{2}{\cancel{40}\ \cancel{mEq}}}{\underset{1}{\cancel{20}\ \cancel{mEq}}} \times 15\text{ mL} = 30\text{ mL}$; given orally once a day

Many oral medications are measured using a calibrated medication cup as was described in Chapter 5. Due to surface tension of the liquid against the sides of the container, the top of the poured solution will have a U-shaped or concave curve, called a *meniscus* (Figure 8-4). To read the amount, hold the container at eye level and note the level at the bottom of the curve.

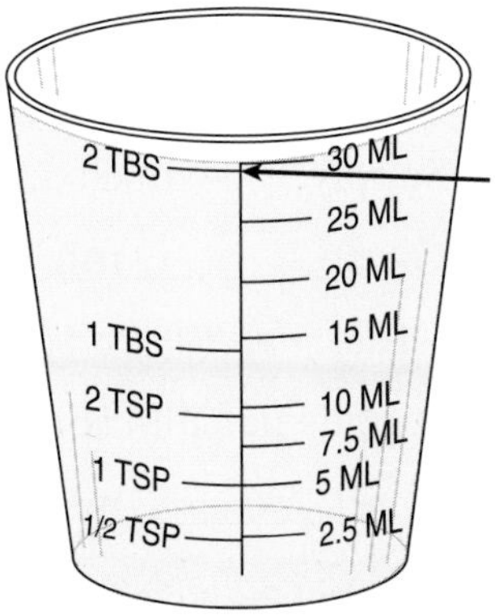
2 TBS
30 ML
25 ML
20 ML
1 TBS
15 ML
2 TSP
10 ML
7.5 ML
1 TSP
5 ML
1/2 TSP
2.5 ML

FIGURE 8-4 Calibrated Medication Cup Showing Meniscus

QUICK REVIEW

Look again at steps 1 through 3 as a valuable dosage calculation checklist.

Step 1 **Convert** Be sure that all measurements are in the same system, and all units are in the same size.

Step 2 **Think** Carefully estimate the reasonable amount of the drug that you should administer.

Step 3 **Calculate** $\frac{D}{H} \times Q = X \quad \frac{D\text{ (desired)}}{H\text{ (have)}} \times Q\text{ (quantity)} = X\text{ (amount)}$

REVIEW SET 21

Calculate one dose of the drugs ordered.

1. Order: *meperidine syrup 75 mg PO q4h prn for pain*

   Supply: meperidine syrup 50 mg per 5 mL

   Give: ________ mL

2. Order: *lorazepam 1.5 mg SL stat*

   Supply: lorazepam sublingual tablets 0.5 mg, 1 mg, 2 mg

   Give: ________ tablets of ________ mg

3. Order: *penicillin v potassium 1 g PO 1h pre-op dental surgery*

   Supply: penicillin v potassium suspension 300 mg (500 000 units) per 5 mL

   Give: ________ mL

4. Order: *amoxicillin 100 mg PO QID*

   Supply: 80 mL bottle of amoxicillin oral pediatric suspension 125 mg per 5 mL

   Give: ________ mL

5. Order: *acetaminophen 0.16 g PO q4h prn for pain*

   Supply: acetaminophen 160 mg/5 mL

   Give: ________ mL

6. Order: *Apo-Amoxi Clav 25 mg PO q6h*

   Supply: Apo-Amoxi Clav 62.5 mg/5 mL

   Give: ________ mL

7. Order: *perphenazine 4 mg PO q8h*

   Supply: perphenazine concentrate 3.2 mg/mL

   Give: ________ mL

8. Order: *erythromycin suspension 600 mg PO q6h*

   Supply: erythromycin 400 mg/5 mL

   Give: ________ mL

9. Order: *cefaclor suspension 225 mg PO BID*

   Supply: cefaclor suspension 375 mg per 5 mL

   Give: ________ mL

10. Order: *Septra-DS suspension 200 mg PO BID*

    Supply: Septra-DS suspension 400 mg per 5 mL

    Give: ________ mL

11. Order: *theophylline liquid 0.24 g PO stat*

    Supply: theophylline liquid 80 mg/7.5 mL

    Give: ________ mL

12. Order: *ampicillin suspension 750 mg PO TID*

    Supply: ampicillin suspension 250 mg/5 mL

    Give: ________ mL

13. Order: *hydrochlorothiazide solution 100 mg PO BID*

    Supply: hydrochlorothiazide solution 10 mg/mL

    Give: ________ mL

14. Order: *magnesium 20 mg PO QID*

    Supply: Ratio-Magnesium (magnesium glucoheptonate) 5 mg/5 mL

    Give: ________ mL

15. Order: *digoxin elixir 0.25 mg PO daily*

    Supply: digoxin elixir 50 mcg/mL

    Give: ________ mL

16. Order: *nafcillin sodium 0.75 g PO q6h*

    Supply: nafcillin sodium 250 mg/5 mL

    Give: ________ mL

17. Order: *cephalexin 375 mg PO TID*

    Supply: cephalexin 250 mg/5 mL

    Give: ________ mL

18. Order: *lactulose 20 g via gastric tube BID today*

    Supply: lactulose 10 g/15 mL

    Give: ________ mL

19. Order: *erythromycin 1.2 g PO q8h*

    Supply: erythromycin 400 mg/5 mL

    Give: ________ mL

20. Order: *oxacillin sodium 0.25 g PO q8h*

    Supply: oxacillin sodium 125 mg/2.5 mL

    Give: ________ mL

21. Order: *amoxicillin suspension 100 mg PO q6h*

    Supply: amoxicillin suspension 250 mg/5 mL

    Give: ________ mL

Use the labels A, B, and C below to calculate one dose of the following orders (22, 23, and 24). Indicate the letter corresponding to the label you select.

22. Order: *erythromycin 125 mg PO TID*

    Select: ________

    Give: ________

23. Order: *cephalexin 50 mg PO q6h*

    Select: ________

    Give: ________

24. Order: *hydroxyzine 10 mg PO QID*

    Select: ________

    Give: ________

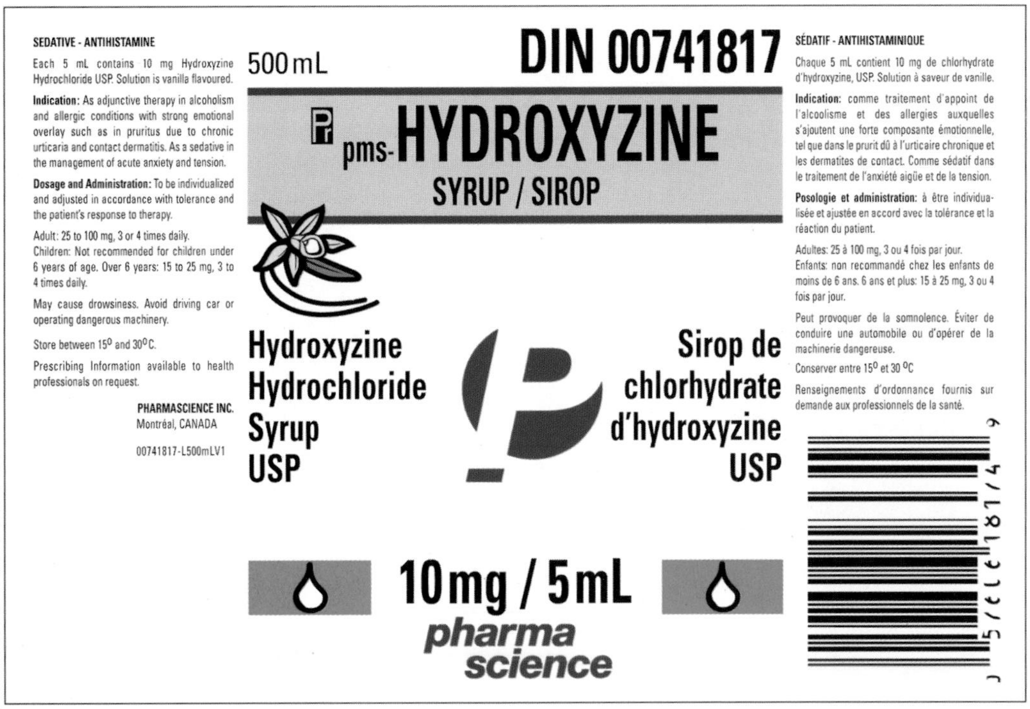
SEDATIVE - ANTIHISTAMINE
Each 5 mL contains 10 mg Hydroxyzine Hydrochloride USP. Solution is vanilla flavoured.
Indication: As adjunctive therapy in alcoholism and allergic conditions with strong emotional overlay such as in pruritus due to chronic urticaria and contact dermatitis. As a sedative in the management of acute anxiety and tension.
Dosage and Administration: To be individualized and adjusted in accordance with tolerance and the patient's response to therapy.
Adult: 25 to 100 mg, 3 or 4 times daily.
Children: Not recommended for children under 6 years of age. Over 6 years: 15 to 25 mg, 3 to 4 times daily.
May cause drowsiness. Avoid driving car or operating dangerous machinery.
Store between 15° and 30°C.
Prescribing Information available to health professionals on request.
PHARMASCIENCE INC.
Montréal, CANADA
00741817-L500mLV1
500 mL
DIN 00741817
pms-HYDROXYZINE
SYRUP / SIROP
Hydroxyzine Hydrochloride Syrup USP
Sirop de chlorhydrate d'hydroxyzine USP
10 mg / 5 mL
pharma science
SÉDATIF - ANTIHISTAMINIQUE
Chaque 5 mL contient 10 mg de chlorhydrate d'hydroxyzine, USP. Solution à saveur de vanille.
Indication: comme traitement d'appoint de l'alcoolisme et des allergies auxquelles s'ajoutent une forte composante émotionnelle, tel que dans le prurit dû à l'urticaire chronique et les dermatites de contact. Comme sédatif dans le traitement de l'anxiété aigüe et de la tension.
Posologie et administration: à être individualisée et ajustée en accord avec la tolérance et la réaction du patient.
Adultes: 25 à 100 mg, 3 ou 4 fois par jour.
Enfants: non recommandé chez les enfants de moins de 6 ans. 6 ans et plus: 15 à 25 mg, 3 ou 4 fois par jour.
Peut provoquer de la somnolence. Éviter de conduire une automobile ou d'opérer de la machinerie dangereuse.
Conserver entre 15° et 30 °C
Renseignements d'ordonnance fournis sur demande aux professionnels de la santé.

Pharmascience Inc., Montreal, Que

A

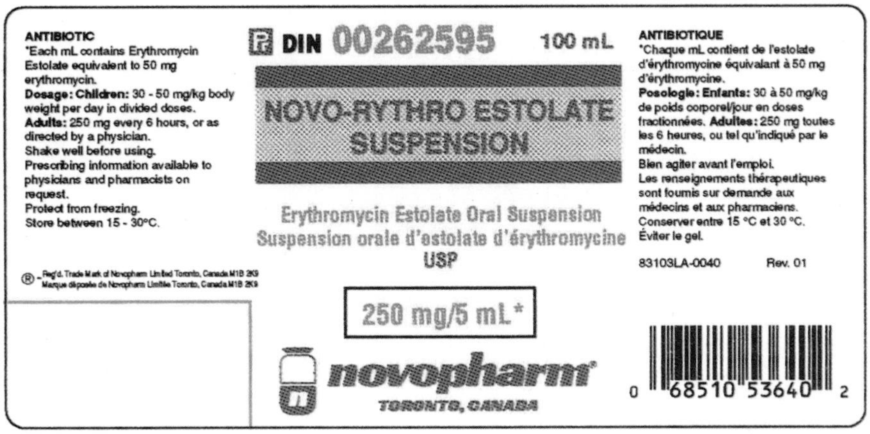
ANTIBIOTIC
*Each mL contains Erythromycin Estolate equivalent to 50 mg erythromycin.
Dosage: Children: 30 - 50 mg/kg body weight per day in divided doses.
Adults: 250 mg every 6 hours, or as directed by a physician.
Shake well before using.
Prescribing information available to physicians and pharmacists on request.
Protect from freezing.
Store between 15 - 30°C.
DIN 00262595
100 mL
NOVO-RYTHRO ESTOLATE SUSPENSION
Erythromycin Estolate Oral Suspension
Suspension orale d'estolate d'érythromycine
USP
250 mg/5 mL*
novopharm
TORONTO, CANADA
ANTIBIOTIQUE
*Chaque mL contient de l'estolate d'érythromycine équivalant à 50 mg d'érythromycine.
Posologie: Enfants: 30 à 50 mg/kg de poids corporel/jour en doses fractionnées. Adultes: 250 mg toutes les 6 heures, ou tel qu'indiqué par le médecin.
Bien agiter avant l'emploi.
Les renseignements thérapeutiques sont fournis sur demande aux médecins et aux pharmaciens.
Conserver entre 15 °C et 30 °C.
Éviter le gel.
83103LA-0040
Rev. 01
0 68510 53640 2

Novopharm Limited, Toronto, ON

B

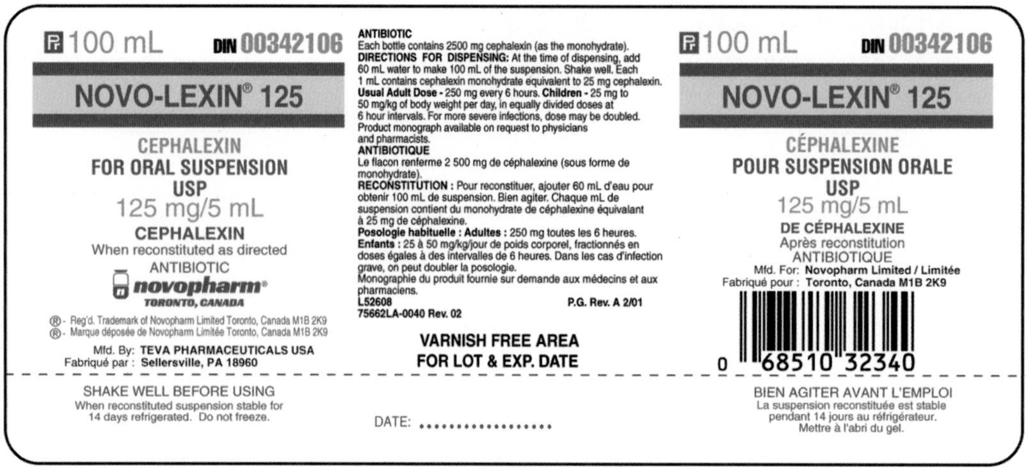

Novopharm Limited, Toronto, ON

C

Calculate the information requested based on the drugs ordered. The labels provided are the drugs available.

25. Order: *furosemide oral solution 40 mg PO TID*

    Give: ________ mL

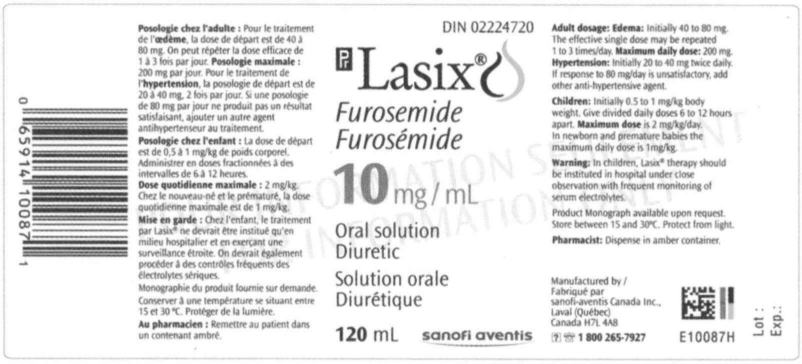

Sanofi-aventis Canada, Laval, QUE

26. Order: *morphine hydrochloride (oral solution concentrate) 15 mg PO q6h prn for pain*

    Give: ________ mL

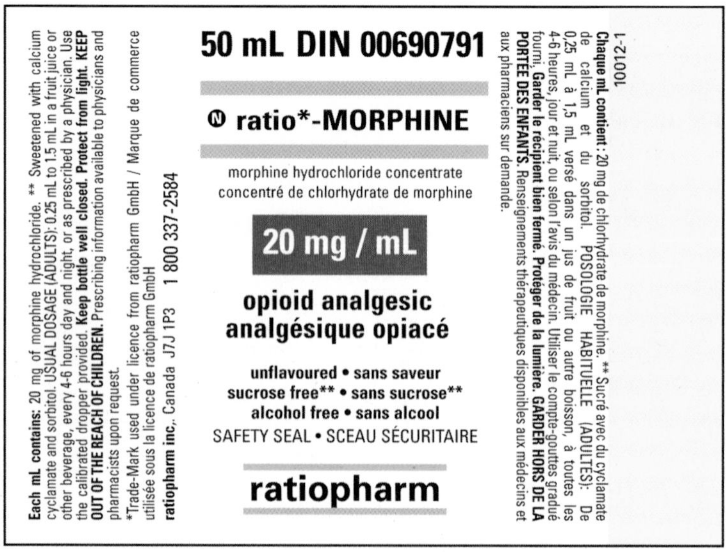

Ratiopharm Inc., Mirabel, QUE

27. Order: *valproic acid 0.5 g PO TID*

    Give: ________ mL

    How many full doses are available in this bottle?

    ________ full doses

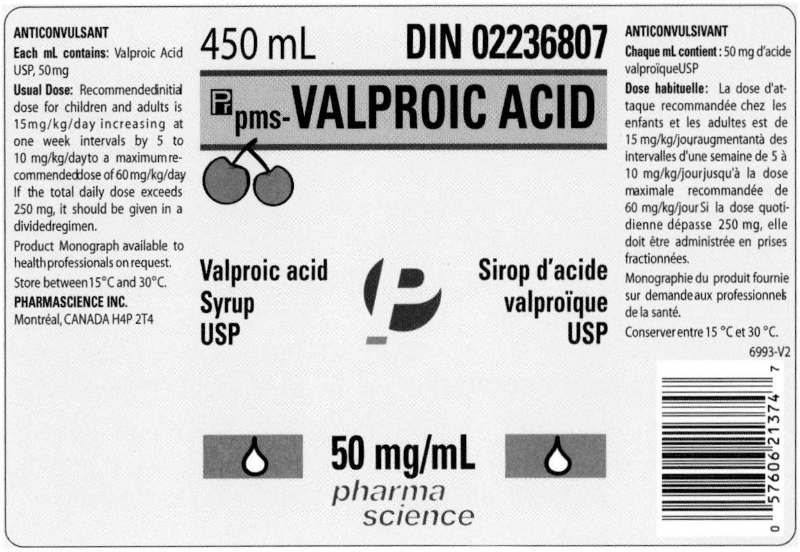

Pharmascience Inc., Montreal, Que

28. Order: *clarithromycin 75 mg PO q12h*

    Give: ________ mL

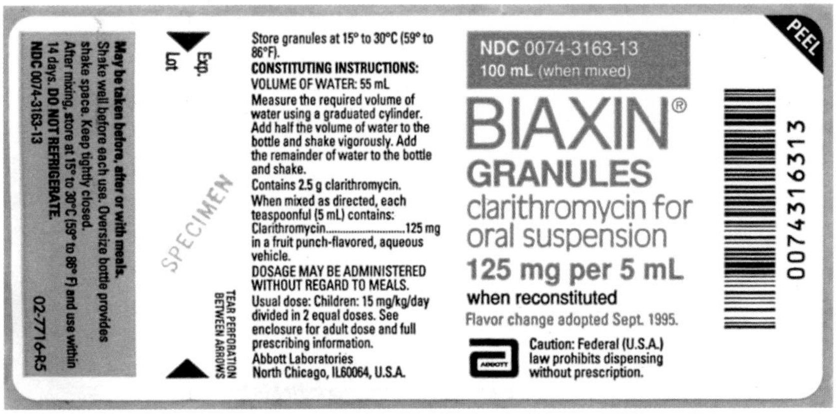

Courtesy of Abbott Laboratories, Inc.

After completing these problems, see page 468 to check your answers.

SUMMARY

Let us examine where you are in mastering the skill of dosage calculations. You have learned to convert equivalent units within systems of measurements. You have also applied this conversion skill to the calculation of oral dosages—both solid and liquid forms. By now, you know that solving dosage problems requires that all units of measurement first be expressed in the same size.

Next, you learned to think through the dosage ordered and dosage supplied to estimate the amount to be given. *To minimize medication errors, it is essential that you consider the reasonableness of the amount before applying a calculation method or formula.*

Finally, you have learned the formula method $\frac{D}{H} \times Q = X$ (*desired* over *have* times *quantity = amount to give*). This method is so simple and easy to recall that it will stick with you throughout your career.

Review the Critical Thinking Skills and work the practice problems for Chapter 8. If you are having difficulty, get help from an instructor before proceeding to Chapter 9. Continue to concentrate on accuracy. Keep in mind that one error can be a serious mistake when you are calculating the dosages of medicines. Medication administration is a *legal responsibility*. Remember, when you give a medication, you are legally responsible for your action.

CRITICAL THINKING SKILLS

Inaccuracy in dosage calculation is often attributed to errors in calculating the dosage. By first asking the question, "What is the reasonable amount to give?" many medication errors can be avoided.

error

Incorrect calculation and not assessing the reasonableness of the calculation before administering the medication.

possible scenario

The physician ordered *phenobarbital 60 mg PO BID* for a patient with seizures. The pharmacy supplied *phenobarbital 30 mg per tablet*. The nurse did not use Step 2 to think about the reasonable dosage, and calculated the dosage this way:

$$\frac{\textbf{DESIRED}}{\textbf{HAVE}} \times \textbf{QUANTITY} = \textbf{AMOUNT}$$

$$\frac{60 \text{ mg}}{30 \text{ mg}} \times 1 \text{ tab} = 20 \text{ tab (incorrect)}$$

Suppose the nurse then gave the patient 20 tablets of the 30 mg per tablet of phenobarbital. The patient would have received 600 mg of phenobarbital, or 10 times the correct dosage. This is a very serious error.

potential outcome

The patient would likely develop signs of phenobarbital toxicity, such as nystagmus (rapid eye movement), ataxia (lack of coordination), central nervous system depression, respiratory depression, hypothermia, and hypotension. When the error was caught and the physician notified, the patient would likely be given doses of charcoal to hasten elimination of the drug. Depending on the severity of the symptoms, the patient would likely be moved to the intensive care unit for monitoring of respiratory and neurological status.

prevention

This medication error could have been prevented if the nurse had used the three-step method and estimated for the reasonable dosage of the drug to give. The order is for 60 mg of phenobarbital and the available drug has 30 mg per tablet, so the nurse should give 2 tablets. The incorrect calculation that indicated such a large amount of tablets to give per dose should have alerted the nurse to a possible error. The formula $\frac{D}{H} \times Q = X$ should be used to verify thinking about the *reasonable* dosage. Further, the nurse should double-check the math to find the error.

$$\frac{\textbf{D}}{\textbf{H}} \times \textbf{Q} = \frac{60 \text{ mg}}{30 \text{ mg}} \times 1 \text{ tablet}$$

$$\frac{\overset{2}{\cancel{60}} \text{ mg}}{\underset{1}{\cancel{30}} \text{ mg}} \times 1 \text{ tablet} = 2 \text{ tablets, not } 20 \text{ tablets}$$

PRACTICE PROBLEMS—CHAPTER 8

Calculate one dose of the following drug orders. The tablets are scored in half.

1. Order: *metformin 250 mg PO BID*

   Supply: metformin 0.5 g tablets

   Give: ________ tablet(s)

2. Order: *codeine 45 mg PO q4h prn for pain*

   Supply: codeine 15 mg tablets

   Give: ________ tablet(s)

3. Order: *levothyroxine sodium 0.075 mg PO daily*

   Supply: levothyroxine sodium 150 mcg tablets

   Give: ________ tablet(s)

4. Order: *largactil 15 mg PO TID*

   Supply: largactil drops 40 mg/mL

   Give: ________ mL

5. Order: *cephalexin 500 mg PO QID*

   Supply: cephalexin 250 mg per 5 mL

   Give: ________ mL

6. Order: *propranolol hydrochloride 20 mg PO QID*

   Supply: propranolol hydrochloride 10 mg tablets

   Give: ________ tablet(s)

7. Order: *amoxicillin 400 mg PO q6h*

   Supply: amoxicillin 250 mg per 5 mL

   Give: ________ mL

8. Order: *gliclazide 120 mg PO BID*

   Supply: (gliclazide 80 mg tablets

   Give: ________ tablet(s)

9. Order: *acetylsalicylic acid (Aspirin) 650 mg PO daily*

   Supply: acetylsalicylic acid 325 mg tablets

   Give: ________ tablet(s)

10. Order: *codeine 15 mg PO daily*

    Supply: codeine 30 mg tablets

    Give: ________ tablet(s)

11. Order: *propranolol hydrochloride 30 mg PO QID*

    Supply: propranolol hydrochloride 20 mg tablets

    Give: ________ tablet(s)

12. Order: *levothyroxine sodium 300 mcg PO daily*

    Supply: levothyroxine sodium 0.3 mg tablets

    Give: ________ tablet(s)

13. Order: *furosemide 60 mg PO daily*

    Supply: furosemide 40 mg tablets

    Give: ________ tablet(s)

14. Order: *penicillin V potassium 400 000 units PO QID*

    Supply: penicillin V potassium 250 mg (400 000 units) tablets

    Give: ________ tablet(s)

15. Order: *enalapril maleate 7.5 mg PO daily*

    Supply: enalapril maleate 5 mg and 10 mg tablets

    Select: ________ mg tablets

    and give ________ tablet(s)

16. Order: *penicillin v potassium 300 000 units PO QID*

    Supply: penicillin v potassium 200 000 units/5 mL

    Give: ________ mL

17. Order: *pyrazinamide 0.75 g PO BID*

    Supply: pyrazinamide 500 mg tablets

    Give: ________ tablet(s)

18. Order: *triazolam 0.25 mg PO at bedtime*

    Supply: triazolam 0.125 mg tablets

    Give: ________ tablet(s)

19. Order: *morphine 5 mg PO q3-4h for pain*

    Supply: morphine 10 mg/5 mL

    Give: ________ mL

20. Order: *dexamethasone 750 mcg PO BID*

    Supply: dexamethasone 0.75 mg and 1.5 mg tablets

    Select: ________ mg tablets

    Give: ________ tablet(s)

21. Order: *eethacrynic acid 12.5 mg PO BID*

    Supply: eethacrynic acid 25 mg tablets

    Give: ________ tablet(s)

22. Order: *bethanechol chloride 50 mg PO TID*

    Supply: bethanechol chloride 25 mg tablets

    Give: ________ tablet(s)

23. Order: *erythromycin 0.5 g PO q12h*

    Supply: erythromycin 250 mg tablets

    Give: ________ tablet(s)

24. Order: *glyburide 2.5 mg PO daily*

    Supply: glyburide 1.25 mg tablets

    Give: ________ tablet(s)

25. Order: *clorazepate dipotassium 7.5 mg PO qAM*

    Supply: clorazepate dipotassium 3.75 mg capsules

    Give: ________ capsules

26. Order: *oxazepam 45 mg PO at bedtime*

    Supply: oxazepam 10 mg, 15 mg, 30 mg scored tablets

    Which strength of tablet(s) would you select, and how much would you give?

    Select: ________ mg tablets

    Give: ________ tablet(s)

27. Order: *acetaminophen 240 mg PO q4h prn for pain or T greater than 38.5°C*

    Supply: acetaminophen drops 80 mg per 1 mL

    Give: ________ mL

28. Order: *acetaminophen 160 mg PO q4h prn for pain or T greater than 38.5°C*

    Supply: acetaminophen liquid 100 mg per mL

    Give: ________ mL

29. Order: *warfarin 7.5 mg PO daily*

    Supply: warfarin 2.5 mg tablets

    Give: ________ tablet(s)

See the three medication administration records and accompanying labels on the following pages for questions 30 through 42.

Calculate one dose of each of the drugs prescribed. Labels A–O provided on pages 176–180 are the drugs you have available. Indicate the letter corresponding to the label you select.

PAGE ____ of ____

MEDICATION ADMINISTRATION RECORD

	ORIGINAL ORDER DATE	DATE STARTED / RENEWED	MEDICATION - DOSAGE	ROUTE	SCHEDULE 23-07	SCHEDULE 07-15	SCHEDULE 15-23	DATE 1/5/xx 23-07	DATE 1/5/xx 07-15	DATE 1/5/xx 15-23	DATE 23-07	DATE 07-15	DATE 15-23	DATE 23-07	DATE 07-15	DATE 15-23	DATE 23-07	DATE 07-15	DATE 15-23
30.	1/5/xx	1/5	carbamezipine 200 mg BID	PO		09	21		09 GP	21 MS									
31.	1/5/xx	1/5	fexofenadine HCl 60 mg BID	PO		09	21		09 GP	21 MS									
32.	1/5/xx	1/5	sucralfate 1000 mg BID	PO		09	21		09 GP	21 MS									
33.	1/5/xx	1/5	naproxen 0.5 g QID	PO		09 13			09 GP 13 GP	17 MS 21 MS									

PRN

PRINTED BY STANDARD REGISTER U.S.A. ZIPSET ®

INJECTION SITES: B - RIGHT ARM; C - RIGHT ABDOMEN; D - RIGHT ANTERIOR THIGH; G - LEFT ARM; H - LEFT ABDOMEN; J - LEFT ANTERIOR THIGH; L - LEFT BUTTOCKS; M - RIGHT BUTTOCKS

DATE GIVEN	TIME	INT.	ONE - TIME MEDICATION - DOSAGE	RT.

SIGNATURE OF NURSE ADMINISTERING MEDICATIONS	DATE 1/5/xx	DATE	DATE	DATE
23-07	GP G. Pickar, RN			
07-15	MS M. Smith, RN			
15-23				

DATE GIVEN	TIME	INT.	MEDICATION-DOSAGE-CONT.	RT.
			RECOPIED BY:	
			CHECKED BY:	

LITHO IN U.S.A. K6508 (7-92) D395538

Patient, Mary Q.

ALLERGIES: NKA

602-31 (7-XX) (MPC# 1355)

1 ORIGINAL COPY

30. Select: ________

Give: ________

31. Select: ________

Give: ________

32. Select: ________

Give: ________

33. Select: ________

Give: ________

PAGE ____ of ____

MEDICATION ADMINISTRATION RECORD

	ORIGINAL ORDER DATE	DATE STARTED / RENEWED	MEDICATION - DOSAGE	ROUTE	SCHEDULE 23-07	SCHEDULE 07-15	SCHEDULE 15-23	DATE 1/5/xx 23-07	DATE 1/5/xx 07-15	DATE 1/5/xx 15-23	DATE 23-07	DATE 07-15	DATE 15-23	DATE 23-07	DATE 07-15	DATE 15-23	DATE 23-07	DATE 07-15	DATE 15-23
34.	1/5/xx	1/5	sucralfate 1000 mg	PO		09			GP 09										
35.	1/5/xx	1/5	glyburide 5 mg daily	PO		09			GP 09										
36.	1/5/xx	1/5	erythromycin 0.6 g q12h	PO	24 06	12	18		GP 12	MS 18									
37.	1/5/xx	1/5	spironolactone 0.1 g daily	PO		09	21		GP 09	MS 21									

PRN

INJECTION SITES: B - RIGHT ARM; C - RIGHT ABDOMEN; D - RIGHT ANTERIOR THIGH; G - LEFT ARM; H - LEFT ABDOMEN; J - LEFT ANTERIOR THIGH; L - LEFT BUTTOCKS; M - RIGHT BUTTOCKS

DATE GIVEN	TIME	INT.	ONE - TIME MEDICATION - DOSAGE	RT.

SIGNATURE OF NURSE ADMINISTERING MEDICATIONS	DATE 1/5/xx	DATE	DATE	DATE
23-07				
07-15	GP G. Pickar, RN			
15-23	MS M. Smith, RN			

DATE GIVEN	TIME	INT.	MEDICATION-DOSAGE-CONT.	RT.
			RECOPIED BY:	
			CHECKED BY:	

Patient, John Q.

ALLERGIES:

602-31 (7-XX) (MPC# 1355)

1 ORIGINAL COPY

PRINTED BY STANDARD REGISTER U.S.A. ZIPSET ® LITHO IN U.S.A. K6508 (7-92) D395538

34. Select: ________

Give: ________

35. Select: ________

Give: ________

36. Select: ________

Give: ________

37. Select: ________

Give: ________

PAGE ____ of ____

MEDICATION ADMINISTRATION RECORD

PRINTED BY STANDARD REGISTER U.S.A. ZIPSET ®

	ORIGINAL ORDER DATE	DATE STARTED / RENEWED	MEDICATION - DOSAGE	ROUTE	SCHEDULE 23-07	SCHEDULE 07-15	SCHEDULE 15-23	DATE 1/5/xx 23-07	DATE 1/5/xx 07-15	DATE 1/5/xx 15-23
38.	1/5/xx	1/5	synthroid 50 mcg daily	PO		09			09 GP	
39.	1/5/xx	1/5	potassium chloride 40 mEq c̄ 120 mL of juice BID	PO		08 09	21		09 GP	21 MS
40.	1/5/xx	1/5	gemfibrozil 0.6 g BID ac	PO		07^{30}	16^{30}		07^{30} GP	16^{30} MS
41.	1/5/xx	1/5	furosemide 40 mg daily	PO		09			09 GP	
			PRN							
42.	1/5/xx	1/5	oxycodone HCl 5 mg acetaminophen 325 mg	PO					07^{30}GP 11^{30}GP	

PRN

INJECTION SITES

B - RIGHT ARM
C - RIGHT ABDOMEN
D - RIGHT ANTERIOR THIGH
G - LEFT ARM
H - LEFT ABDOMEN
J - LEFT ANTERIOR THIGH
L - LEFT BUTTOCKS
M - RIGHT BUTTOCKS

DATE GIVEN	TIME	INT.	ONE - TIME MEDICATION - DOSAGE	RT.

SIGNATURE OF NURSE ADMINISTERING MEDICATIONS	DATE 1/5/xx	DATE	DATE	DATE
23-07				
07-15	GP G. Pickar RN			
15-23	MS M. Smith, RN			

DATE GIVEN	TIME	INT.	MEDICATION-DOSAGE-CONT.	RT.
			RECOPIED BY:	
			CHECKED BY:	

LITHO IN U.S.A. K6508 (7-92) D395538

Doe, Jane Q.

ALLERGIES: NKA

602-31 (7-xx) (MPC# 1355)

1 ORIGINAL COPY

38. Select:________
    Give:________
39. Select:________
    Give:________
40. Select:________
    Give:________
41. Select:________
    Give:________
42. Select:________
    Give:________

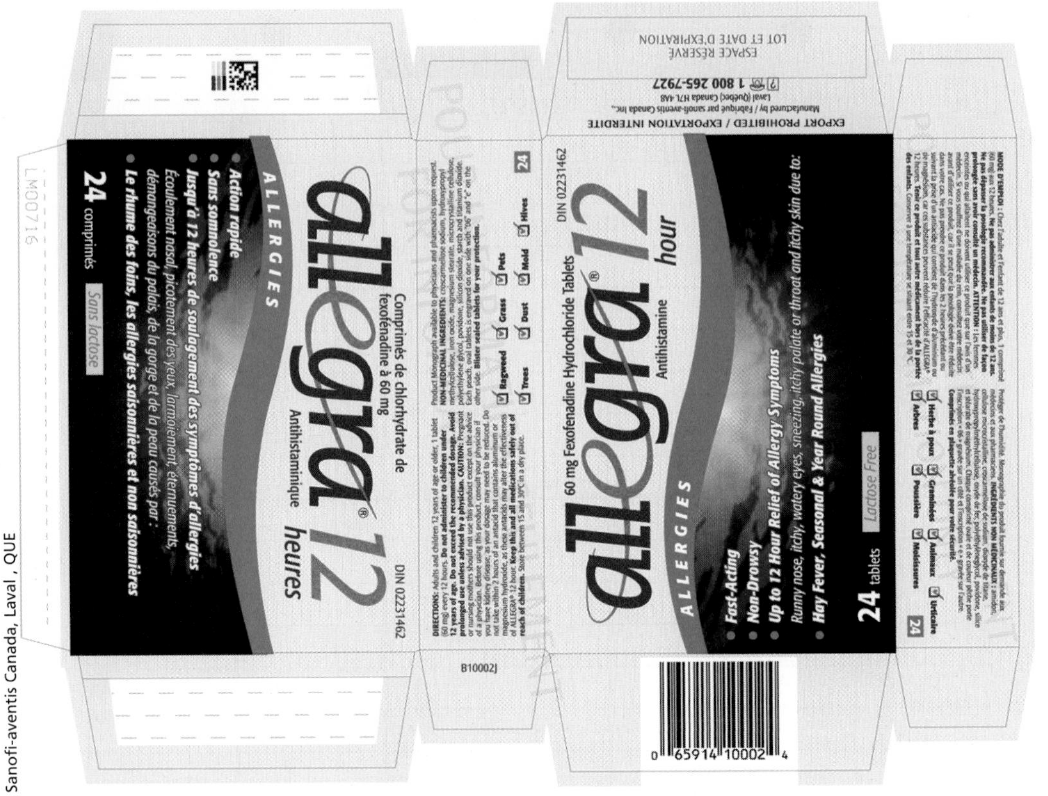

Sanofi-aventis Canada, Laval , QUE

A

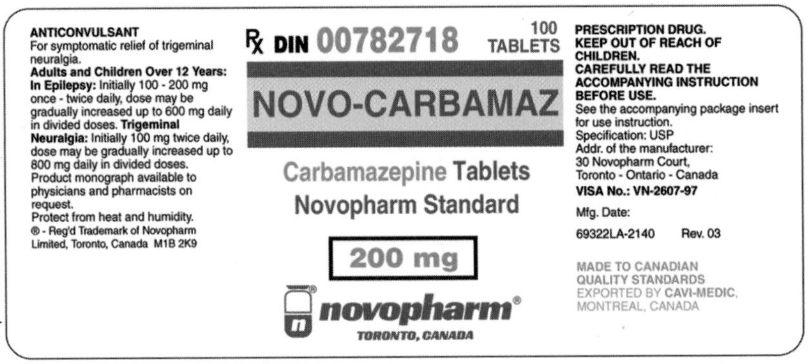

Novopharm Limited, Toronto, ON

B

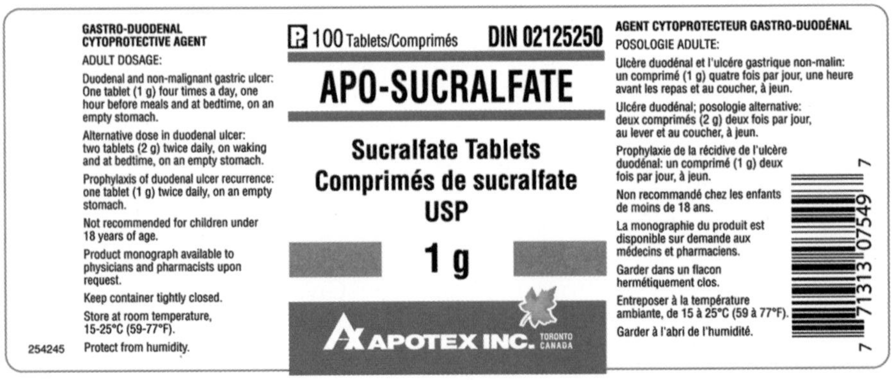

Apotex Inc., Weston, ON

C

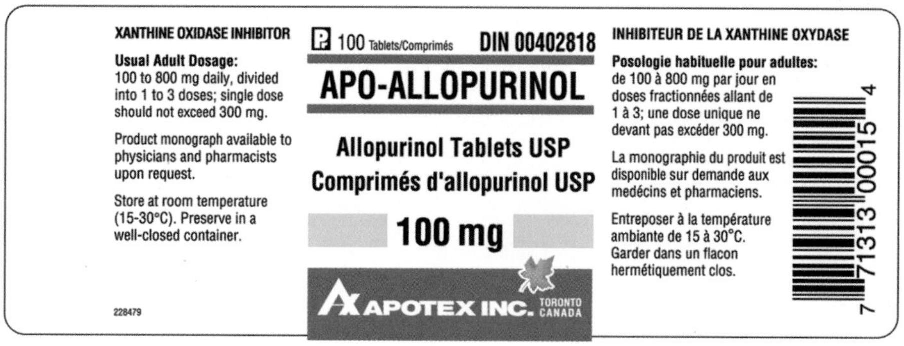
XANTHINE OXIDASE INHIBITOR
Usual Adult Dosage:
100 to 800 mg daily, divided into 1 to 3 doses; single dose should not exceed 300 mg.
Product monograph available to physicians and pharmacists upon request.
Store at room temperature (15-30°C). Preserve in a well-closed container.
228479
100 Tablets/Comprimés
DIN 00402818
APO-ALLOPURINOL
Allopurinol Tablets USP
Comprimés d'allopurinol USP
100 mg
APOTEX INC. TORONTO CANADA
INHIBITEUR DE LA XANTHINE OXYDASE
Posologie habituelle pour adultes:
de 100 à 800 mg par jour en doses fractionnées allant de 1 à 3; une dose unique ne devant pas excéder 300 mg.
La monographie du produit est disponible sur demande aux medécins et pharmaciens.
Entreposer à la température ambiante de 15 à 30°C. Garder dans un flacon hermétiquement clos.
7 71313 00015 4

Apotex Inc., Weston, ON

D

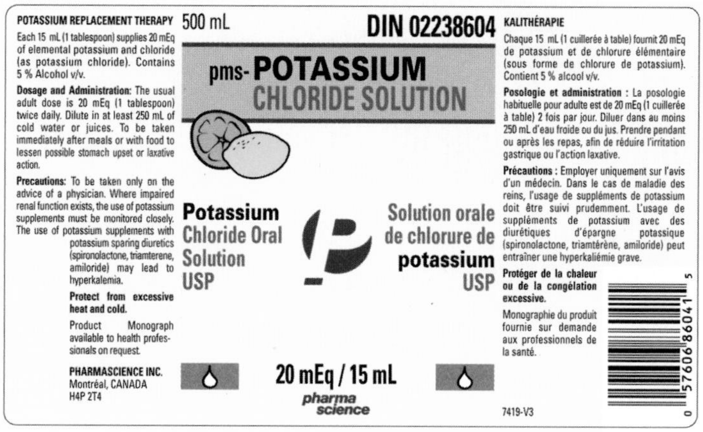
POTASSIUM REPLACEMENT THERAPY
Each 15 mL (1 tablespoon) supplies 20 mEq of elemental potassium and chloride (as potassium chloride). Contains 5 % Alcohol v/v.
Dosage and Administration: The usual adult dose is 20 mEq (1 tablespoon) twice daily. Dilute in at least 250 mL of cold water or juices. To be taken immediately after meals or with food to lessen possible stomach upset or laxative action.
Precautions: To be taken only on the advice of a physician. Where impaired renal function exists, the use of potassium supplements must be monitored closely. The use of potassium supplements with potassium sparing diuretics (spironolactone, triamterene, amiloride) may lead to hyperkalemia.
Protect from excessive heat and cold.
Product Monograph available to health professionals on request.
PHARMASCIENCE INC.
Montréal, CANADA
H4P 2T4
500 mL
DIN 02238604
pms-POTASSIUM CHLORIDE SOLUTION
Potassium Chloride Oral Solution USP
Solution orale de chlorure de potassium USP
20 mEq / 15 mL
pharma science
KALITHÉRAPIE
Chaque 15 mL (1 cuillerée à table) fournit 20 mEq de potassium et de chlorure élémentaire (sous forme de chlorure de potassium). Contient 5 % alcool v/v.
Posologie et administration : La posologie habituelle pour adulte est de 20 mEq (1 cuillerée à table) 2 fois par jour. Diluer dans au moins 250 mL d'eau froide ou du jus. Prendre pendant ou après les repas, afin de réduire l'irritation gastrique ou l'action laxative.
Précautions : Employer uniquement sur l'avis d'un médecin. Dans le cas de maladie des reins, l'usage de suppléments de potassium doit être suivi prudemment. L'usage de suppléments de potassium avec des diurétiques d'épargne potassique (spironolactone, triamtérène, amiloride) peut entraîner une hyperkaliémie grave.
Protéger de la chaleur ou de la congélation excessive.
Monographie du produit fournie sur demande aux professionnels de la santé.
7419-V3
0 57606 86041 5

Pharmascience Inc., Montreal, Que

E

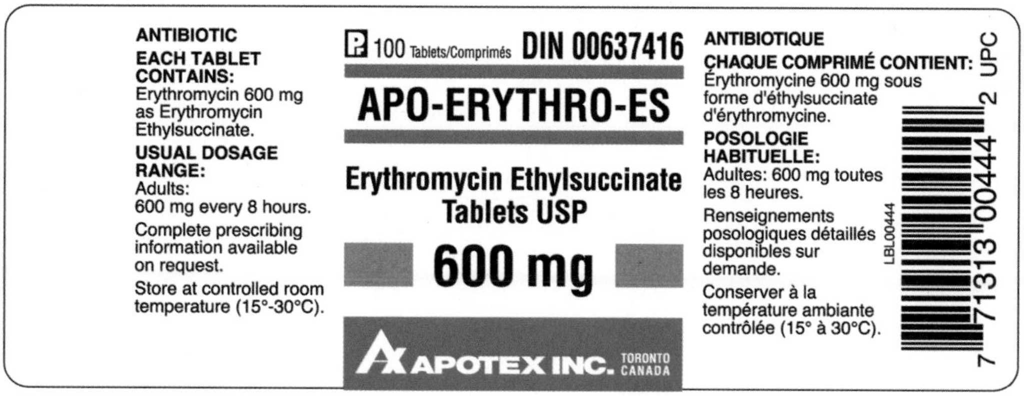
ANTIBIOTIC
EACH TABLET CONTAINS:
Erythromycin 600 mg as Erythromycin Ethylsuccinate.
USUAL DOSAGE RANGE:
Adults:
600 mg every 8 hours.
Complete prescribing information available on request.
Store at controlled room temperature (15°-30°C).
100 Tablets/Comprimés
DIN 00637416
APO-ERYTHRO-ES
Erythromycin Ethylsuccinate Tablets USP
600 mg
APOTEX INC. TORONTO CANADA
ANTIBIOTIQUE
CHAQUE COMPRIMÉ CONTIENT:
Érythromycine 600 mg sous forme d'éthylsuccinate d'érythromycine.
POSOLOGIE HABITUELLE:
Adultes: 600 mg toutes les 8 heures.
Renseignements posologiques détaillés disponibles sur demande.
Conserver à la température ambiante contrôlée (15° à 30°C).
LBL00444
7 71313 00444 2 UPC

Apotex Inc., Weston, ON

F

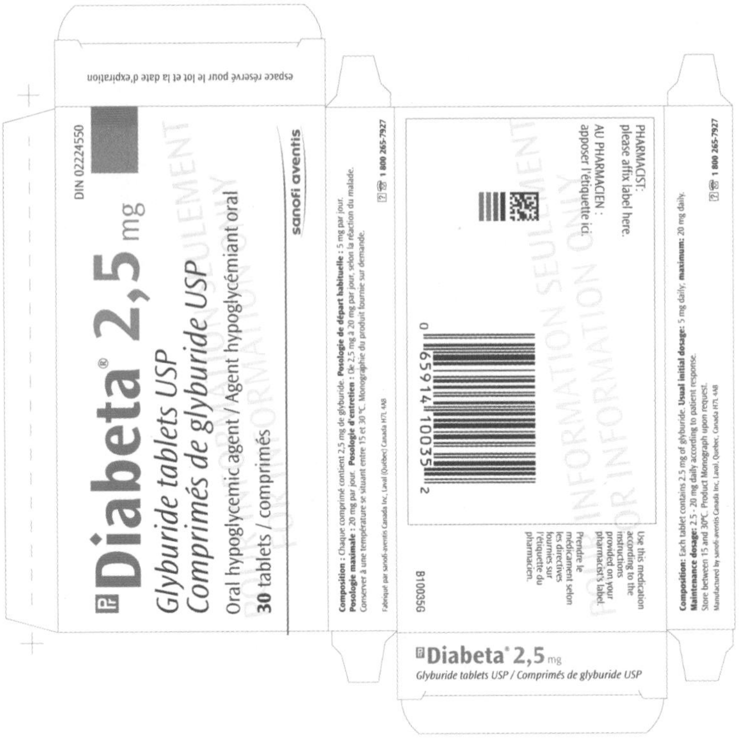

Sanofi-aventis Canada, Laval, QUE

G

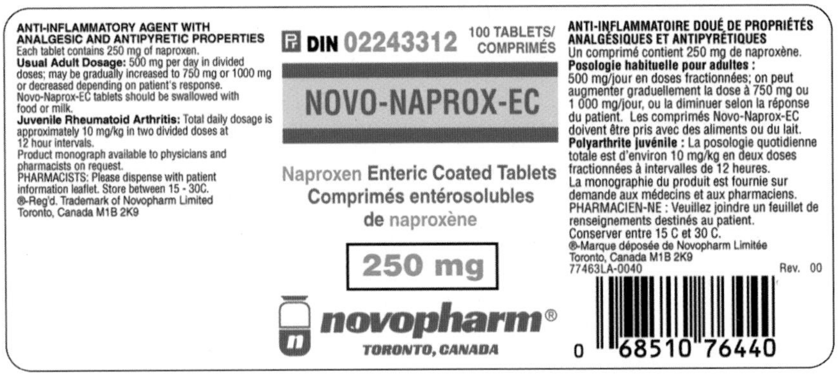

Novopharm Limited, Toronto, ON

H

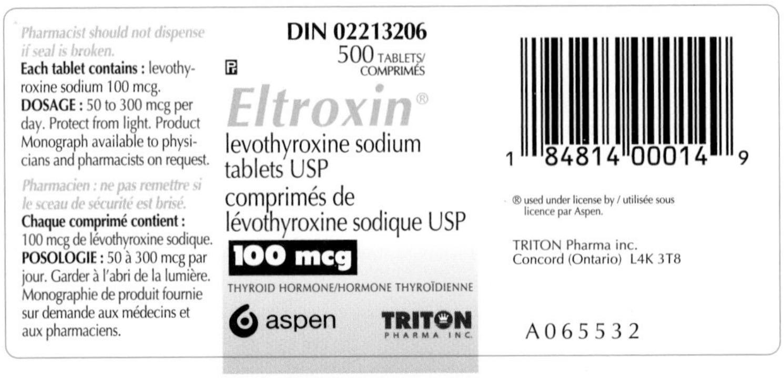

Triton Pharma Inc., Concord, ON

I

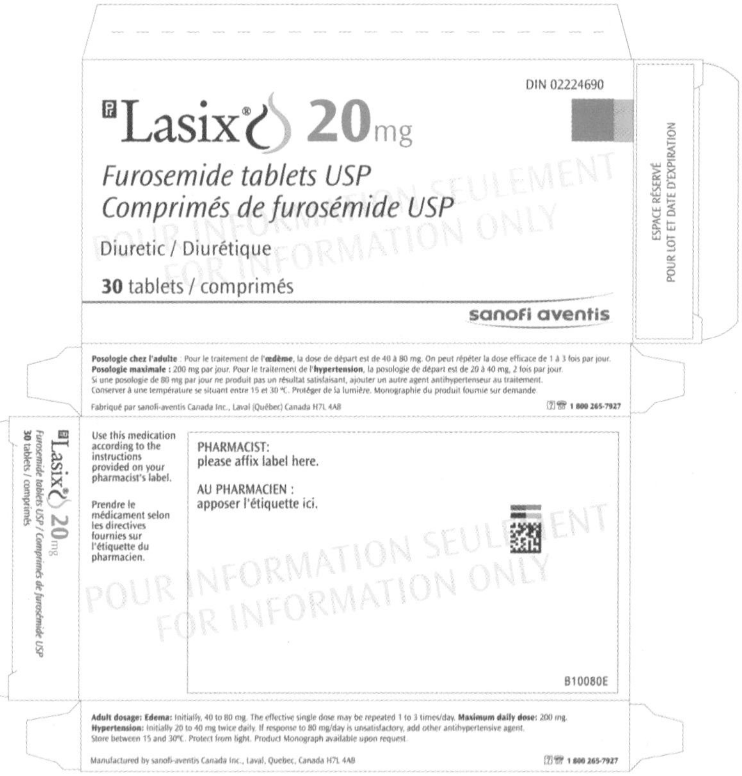

Sanofi-aventis Canada, Laval, QUE

J

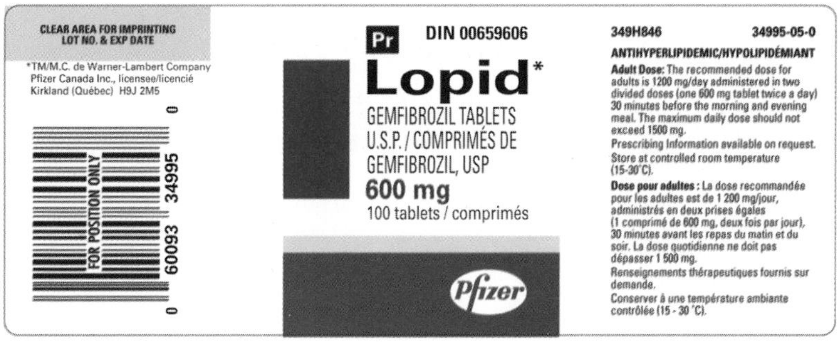

©Pfizer Canada Inc., Kirkland, Que

K

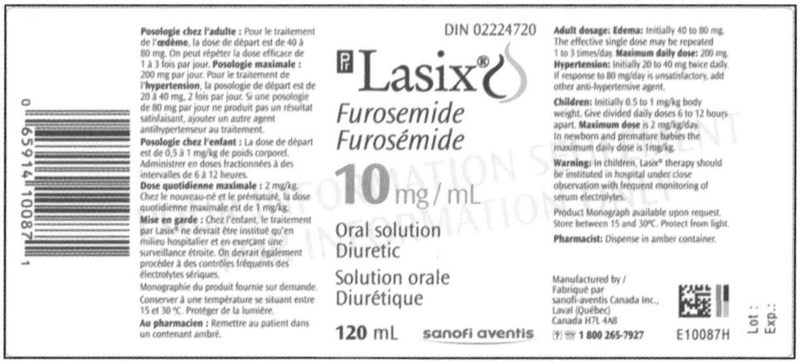

Sanofi-aventis Canada, Laval, QUE

L

©Pfizer Canada Inc., Kirkland, Que

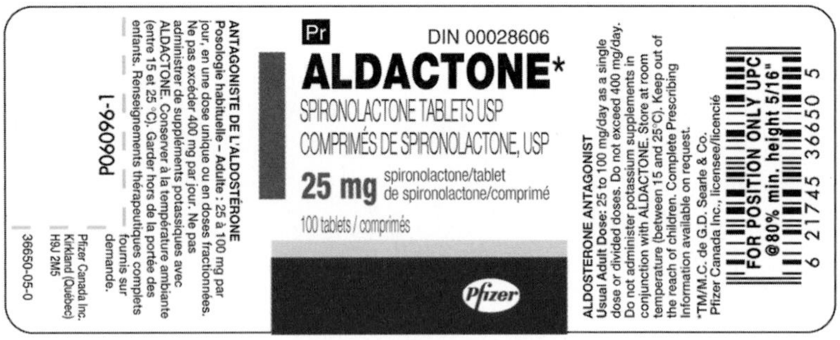

M

©Pfizer Canada Inc., Kirkland, Que

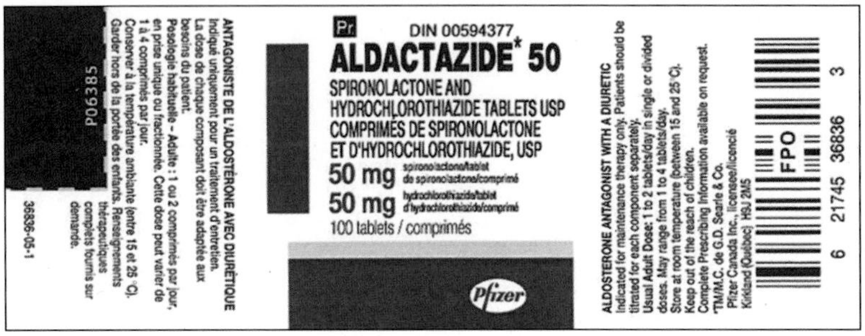

N

Bristol-Myers Squibb, Montreal, QUE

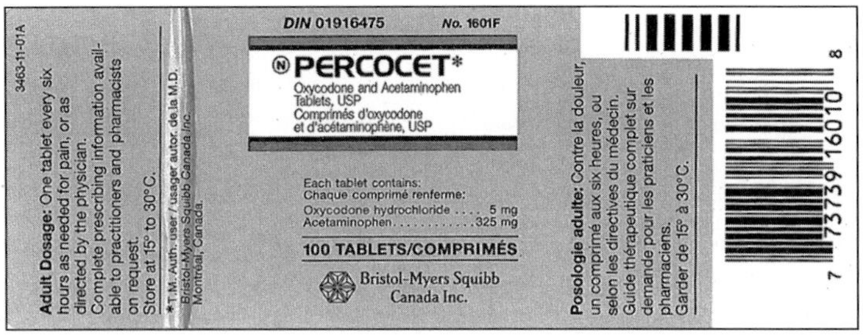

O

Calculate one dose of the medications indicated on the medication administration record that follows. Labels P–S provided on the following pages are the drugs available. Indicate the letter corresponding to the label you select.

43. Select: ________

Give: ________

44. Select: ________

Give: ________

45. Select: ________

Give: ________

46. Select: ________

Give: ________

PAGE ____ of ____

MEDICATION ADMINISTRATION RECORD

	ORIGINAL ORDER DATE	DATE STARTED / RENEWED	MEDICATION - DOSAGE	ROUTE	SCHEDULE 23-07	SCHEDULE 07-15	SCHEDULE 15-23	DATE 3/8/xx 23-07	07-15	15-23	DATE 23-07	07-15	15-23	DATE 23-07	07-15	15-23	DATE 23-07	07-15	15-23
43.	3/8/xx	3-8	ranitidine HCl 300 mg bedtime	PO			22			22 MS									
44.	3/8/xx	3-8	propranolol HCl 80 mg BID	PO		09	21		09 GP	21 MS									
45.	3/8/xx	3-8	furosemide 20 mg BID	PO		09	21		09 GP	21 MS									
46.	3/8/xx	3-8	potassium chloride 600 mg daily	PO		09			09 GP										

PRN

PRINTED BY STANDARD REGISTER U.S.A. ZIPSET ®

INJECTION SITES
B - RIGHT ARM
C - RIGHT ABDOMEN
D - RIGHT ANTERIOR THIGH
G - LEFT ARM
H - LEFT ABDOMEN
J - LEFT ANTERIOR THIGH
L - LEFT BUTTOCKS
M - RIGHT BUTTOCKS

DATE GIVEN	TIME	INT.	ONE - TIME MEDICATION - DOSAGE	RT.

SIGNATURE OF NURSE ADMINISTERING MEDICATIONS	DATE	DATE	DATE	DATE
23-07	GP G. Pickar RN			
07-15	MS M. Smith, RN			
15-23				

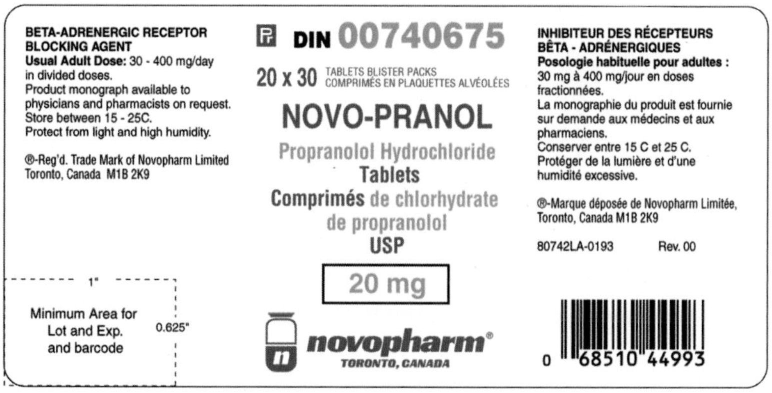

BETA-ADRENERGIC RECEPTOR BLOCKING AGENT
Usual Adult Dose: 30 - 400 mg/day in divided doses.
Product monograph available to physicians and pharmacists on request.
Store between 15 - 25C.
Protect from light and high humidity.
®-Reg'd. Trade Mark of Novopharm Limited Toronto, Canada M1B 2K9
Minimum Area for Lot and Exp. and barcode
1"
0.625"
DIN 00740675
20 x 30 TABLETS BLISTER PACKS COMPRIMÉS EN PLAQUETTES ALVÉOLÉES
NOVO-PRANOL
Propranolol Hydrochloride Tablets
Comprimés de chlorhydrate de propranolol
USP
20 mg
novopharm® TORONTO, CANADA
INHIBITEUR DES RÉCEPTEURS BÊTA - ADRÉNERGIQUES
Posologie habituelle pour adultes : 30 mg à 400 mg/jour en doses fractionnées.
La monographie du produit est fournie sur demande aux médecins et aux pharmaciens.
Conserver entre 15 C et 25 C.
Protéger de la lumière et d'une humidité excessive.
®-Marque déposée de Novopharm Limitée, Toronto, Canada M1B 2K9
80742LA-0193 Rev. 00
0 68510 44993

P

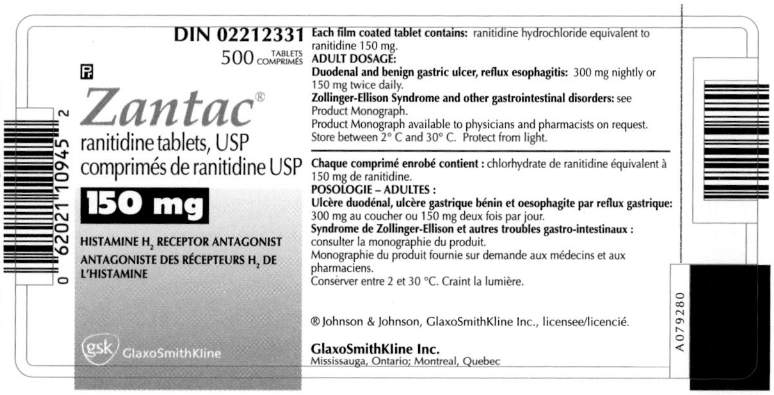

DIN 02212331
500 TABLETS COMPRIMÉS
Zantac®
ranitidine tablets, USP
comprimés de ranitidine USP
150 mg
HISTAMINE H2 RECEPTOR ANTAGONIST
ANTAGONISTE DES RÉCEPTEURS H2 DE L'HISTAMINE
GlaxoSmithKline
Each film coated tablet contains: ranitidine hydrochloride equivalent to ranitidine 150 mg.
ADULT DOSAGE:
Duodenal and benign gastric ulcer, reflux esophagitis: 300 mg nightly or 150 mg twice daily.
Zollinger-Ellison Syndrome and other gastrointestinal disorders: see Product Monograph.
Product Monograph available to physicians and pharmacists on request.
Store between 2° C and 30° C. Protect from light.
Chaque comprimé enrobé contient : chlorhydrate de ranitidine équivalent à 150 mg de ranitidine.
POSOLOGIE – ADULTES :
Ulcère duodénal, ulcère gastrique bénin et oesophagite par reflux gastrique: 300 mg au coucher ou 150 mg deux fois par jour.
Syndrome de Zollinger-Ellison et autres troubles gastro-intestinaux : consulter la monographie du produit.
Monographie du produit fournie sur demande aux médecins et aux pharmaciens.
Conserver entre 2 et 30 °C. Craint la lumière.
® Johnson & Johnson, GlaxoSmithKline Inc., licensee/licencié.
GlaxoSmithKline Inc.
Mississauga, Ontario; Montreal, Quebec
0 62021 10945 2
A079280

Q

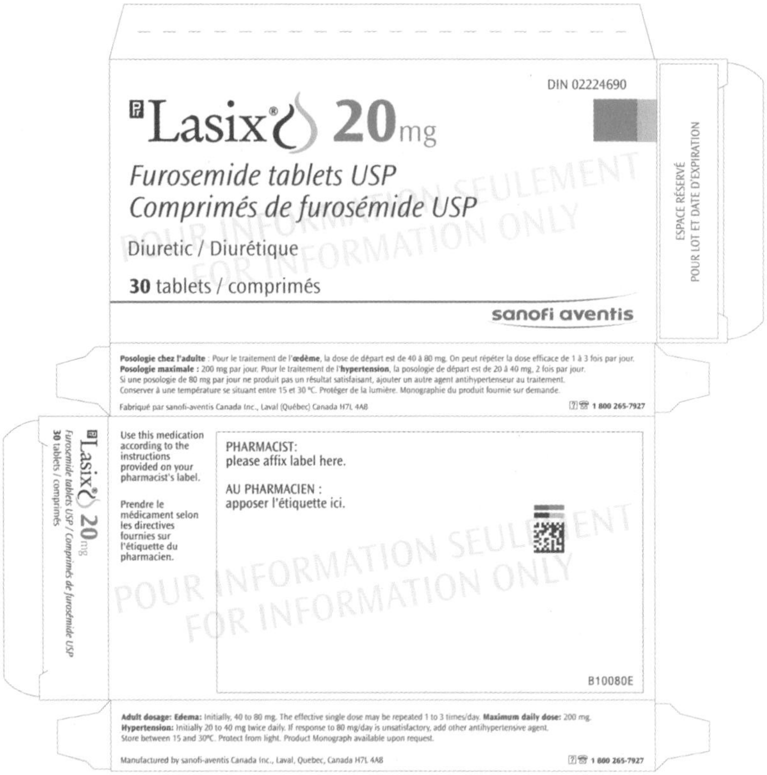

R

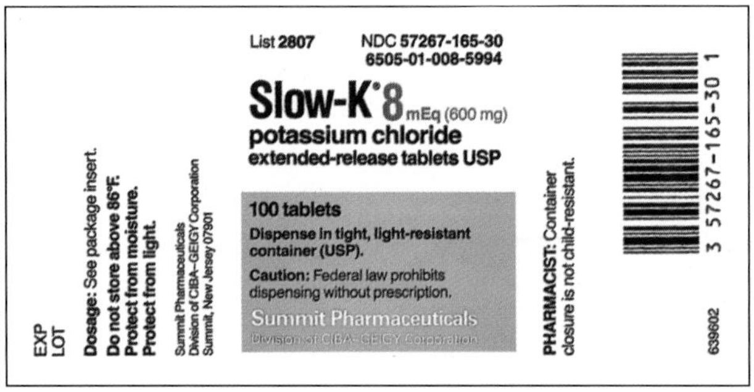

S

47. Critical Thinking Skill: Describe the strategy to prevent this medication error.

possible scenario

Suppose the physician ordered *penicillin V potassium 5 mL (250 mg) PO QID* for a patient with an upper respiratory tract infection. The pharmacy supplied *penicillin V potassium 125 mg per 5 mL*. In a rush to administer the medication on time, the nurse read the order as "penicillin V potassium 5 mL," checked the label for penicillin V potassium and poured that amount and administered the drug. In a hurry, the nurse failed to recognize that 5 mL of the supply dosage of 125 mg per 5 mL did not provide the ordered dosage of 250 mg and underdosed the patient.

potential outcome

The patient received one-half of the ordered dosage of antibiotic needed to treat the respiratory infection. If this error was not caught, the patient's infection would not be halted. This would add to the patient's illness time and might lead to a more severe infection. Additional tests might be required to determine why the patient was not responding to the medication.

prevention

____

____

After completing these problems, see page 469 to check your answers.

CHAPTER 9

Parenteral Dosage of Drugs

LEARNING OBJECTIVES

1. Apply the three steps for parenteral dosage calculations: convert, think, and calculate.
2. Use the formula $\frac{D}{H} \times Q = X$ to calculate the amount to give.
3. Measure insulin in a matching insulin syringe.
4. Compare the calibration of 100-unit insulin syringe units to millilitres (100 units = 1 mL).

The term *parenteral* is used to designate routes of administration other than gastrointestinal, such as the injection routes of intramuscular (IM), subcutaneous, intradermal (ID), and intravenous (IV). In this chapter IM, subcutaneous, and IV injections will be emphasized. IV flow-rate calculations are discussed in Chapters 12–14.

Intramuscular indicates an injection given into a muscle, such as meperidine hydrochloride (Demerol) given IM for pain. *Subcutaneous* means an injection given into the subcutaneous tissue, such as an insulin injection for the management of diabetes. *Intravenous* refers to an injection given directly into a vein, either by direct injection (IV push) or diluted in a larger volume of IV fluid and administered as part of an IV infusion. When a patient has an IV site or IV infusing, the IV injection route is frequently used to administer parenteral drugs rather than the IM route. *Intradermal* means an injection given under the skin, such as an allergy test or tuberculin skin test.

INJECTABLE SOLUTIONS

Most parenteral medications are prepared in liquid or solution form, and packaged in dosage vials, ampules, or prefilled syringes (Figure 9-1). Injectable drugs are measured in syringes.

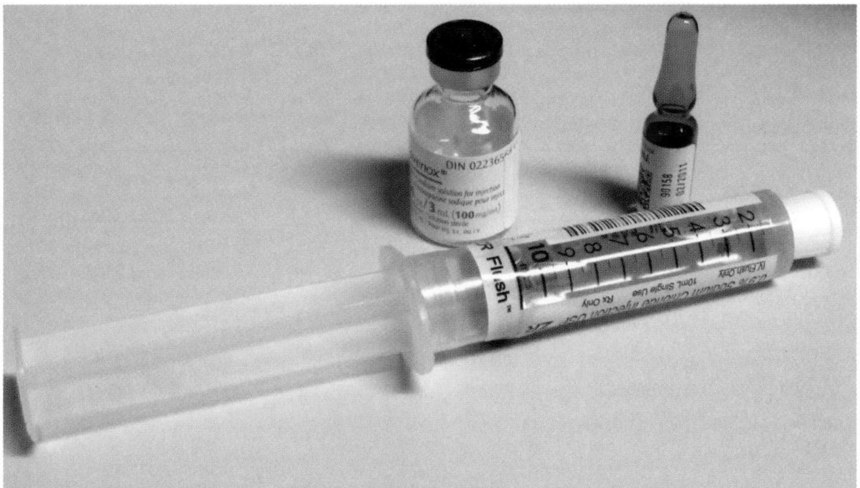
Catherine Thomson

FIGURE 9-1 Examples of vial, ampule, and prefilled syringe for parenteral medications

In general, the nurse must follow the institutional policy for maximum dosage volume to be administered. For example, the condition of the patient and choice of injection site must be considered. It may be necessary to divide the dose into two injections. For example, 5 mL of solution would not be safe to administer in the deltoid muscle of an average size adult; however, 5 mL may be tolerated in the ventrogluteal muscle. See Table 9-1 for recommended maximum volume, usual site, angle, needle size and gauge, and length for administering injections. More often, the parenteral route of administration is the preferred choice over the IM route. *Adults or children who have decreased muscle mass or poor circulation may not be able to tolerate the maximum dosage volumes.*

TABLE 9-1 Recommended Maximum Volume, Usual Site, Angle, Needle Size and Gauge, and Length for Administering Injections

Type of Injection	Maximum Volume	Usual Site	Angle	Type and Gauge of Syringe	Length
Intradermal All ages	0.1 mL	Anterior surface of the forearm or upper back	5° to 15°	1 mL tuberculin; 25 to 27	10–16 mm
Subcutaneous All ages	2.5 mL	Slightly lateral to the insertion of the deltoid and abdomen although other sites are acceptable	90° or 45°	3 mL: 25	12–16 mm
Intramuscular Children (older than 1 year) Adolescents and adults	Children (older than 1 year): 1 mL Adults: 2 mL	Deltoid	90°	3 mL: 22 to 27 (oil-based or more viscous medication require 18 to 25)	Children: 16–25 mm Adult: 25–38 mm
Intramuscular Infants under 12 months Children and adults (only if necessary	Infants (birth to 1 year): 0.5 mL. Children (1–2 years): 1 mL Children 2–12 years: 2 mL Adults: 5 mL	Vastus lateralis	90°	3–5 mL: 22 to 25	Children: 16–25 mm Adult: 25–38 mm
Intramuscular	Infants (older than 7 months): 1 mL. Children (1–2 years): 2 mL Children (3 years and older): 3 mL Adolescents (older than 12 years): 5 mL Adult: 5 mL	Ventrogluteal (do not use for immunizations)	90°	3–5 mL: 22 to 25	Children: 16–25 mm Adult: 25–38 mm

Note: The above are recommended sites, ages, and doses. Always check the institutional policy before administering any injection.

REMEMBER

Step 1	**Convert**	All units of measurement to the same system, and all units to the same size.
Step 2	**Think**	Estimate the logical amount.
Step 3	**Calculate**	$\frac{\textbf{D}\text{ (desired)}}{\textbf{H}\text{ (have)}} \times \textbf{Q}\text{ (quantity)} = \textbf{X}\text{ (amount)}$

Use the following recommendations to help you decide which size syringe to select to administer parenteral dosages.

RECOMMENDED SYRINGE SIZES

As you calculate parenteral dosages:

1. **Round the amount to be administered (X) to tenths if the amount is greater than 1 mL, and measure it in a 3-mL syringe.**
2. **Measure amounts of less than 1 mL rounded to hundredths, and all amounts less than 0.5 mL, in a 1-mL syringe.**
3. **Amounts of 0.5 to 1 mL, calculated in tenths, can be accurately measured in either a 1-mL or 3-mL syringe.**

Let us now examine some examples of appropriate syringe selections for the dosages to be measured and review how to read the calibrations. Refer to Chapter 5, *Equipment Used in Dosage Measurement,* regarding how to measure medication in a syringe. To review, the top black ring should align with the desired calibration, not the raised midsection and not the bottom ring. Look carefully at the illustrations that follow.

Example 1:

Measure 0.33 mL in a 1-mL syringe.

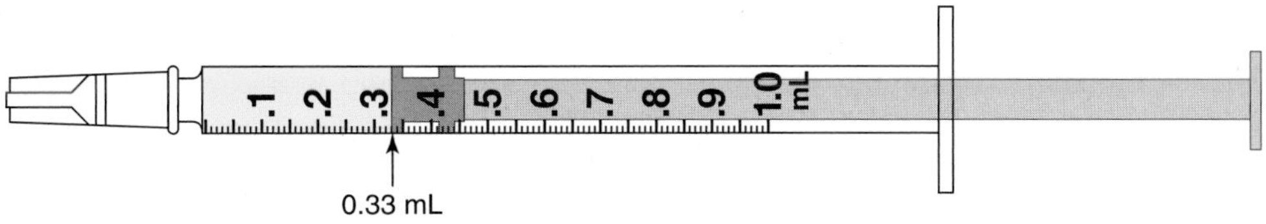

Example 2:

Round 1.33 mL to 1.3 mL, and measure in a 3-mL syringe.

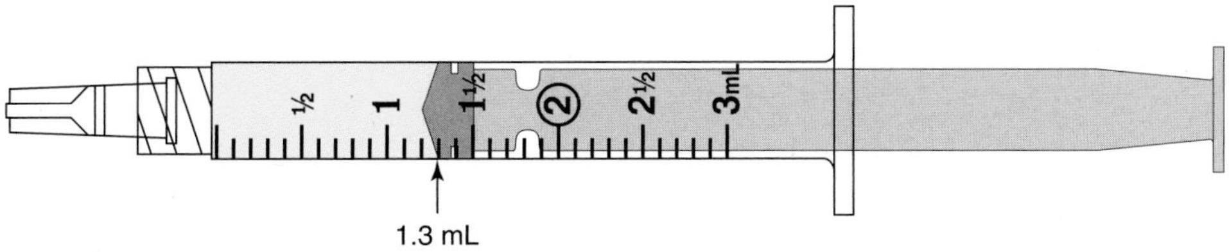

Example 3:

Measure 0.6 mL in either a 1-mL or 3-mL syringe. (Notice that the amount is measured in tenths so the 3-mL syringe would be preferable.)

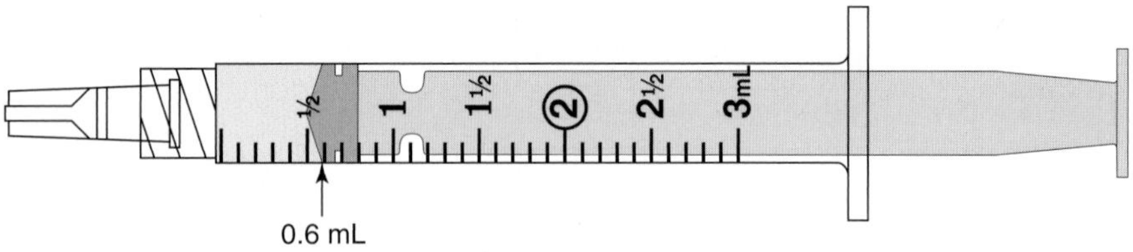
½
1
1½
2
2½
3mL
0.6 mL

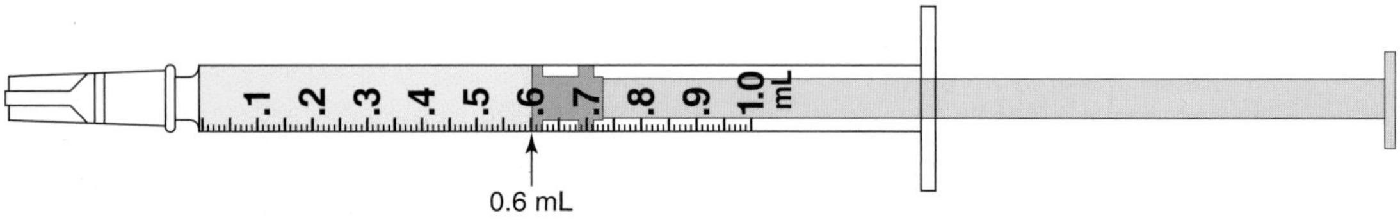
.1 .2 .3 .4 .5 .6 .7 .8 .9 1.0 mL
0.6 mL

Example 4:

Measure 0.65 mL in a 1-mL syringe. (Notice that the amount is measured in hundredths and is less than 1 mL.)

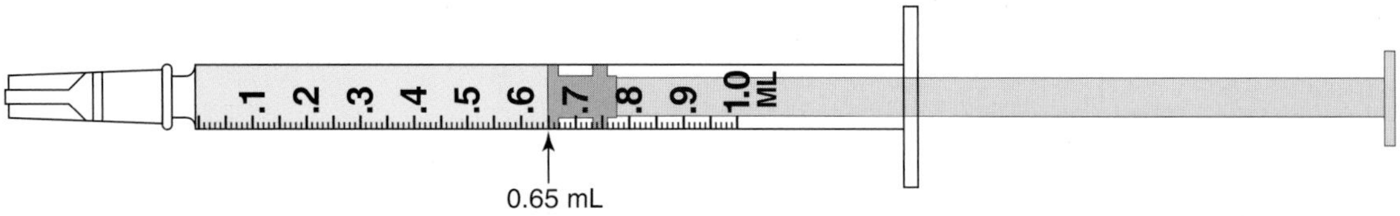
.1 .2 .3 .4 .5 .6 .7 .8 .9 1.0 ML
0.65 mL

An amber colour has been added to selected syringe drawings throughout the text *to simulate a specific amount of medication*, as indicated in the example or problem. Because the colour used may not correspond to the actual colour of the medications named, **it must not be used as a reference for identifying medications.**

Let us look at some examples of parenteral dosage calculations.

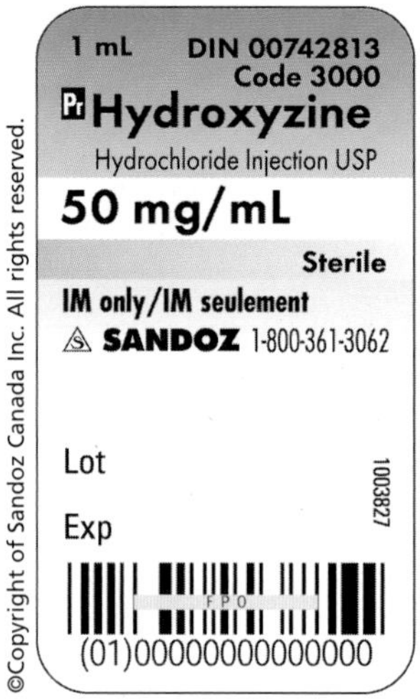
1 mL DIN 00742813
Code 3000
Pr Hydroxyzine
Hydrochloride Injection USP
50 mg/mL
Sterile
IM only/IM seulement
SANDOZ 1-800-361-3062
Lot
Exp
1003827
(01)00000000000000

Example 1:

The patient care order reads *hydroxyzine hydrochloride 100 mg IM stat.* Available is *hydroxyzine hydrochloride for injection 50 mg/mL* in a 1-mL vial. How many millilitres should be administered to the patient?

Step 1 Convert No conversion is necessary.

Step 2 Think You want to give more than 1 mL. In fact, you want to give twice as much, because 100 mg is twice as much as 50 mg.

Step 3 Calculate

$$\frac{D}{H} \times Q = \frac{\overset{2}{\cancel{20}\ \cancel{mg}}}{\underset{1}{\cancel{10}\ \cancel{mg}}} \times 1\text{ mL} = 2\text{ mL}$$

given intramuscularly immediately

Select a *3-mL syringe and measure 2 mL* of hydroxyzine hydrochloride 50 mg/mL. Look carefully at the illustration to clearly identify the part of the black rubber stopper that measures the exact dosage.

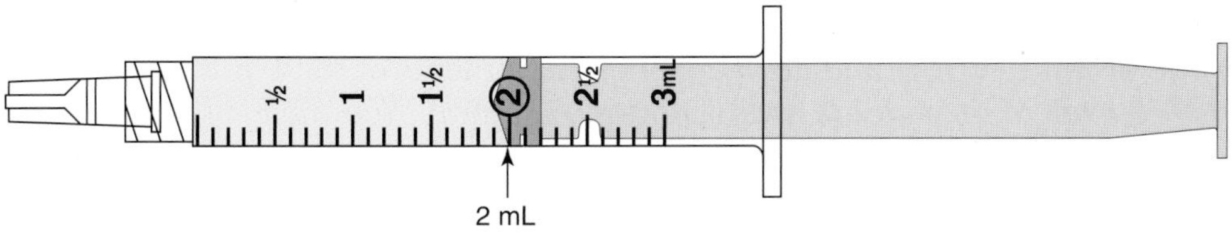
½
1
1½
2
2½
3mL
2 mL

Example 2:

The patient care order reads *nalbuphine hydrochloride 5 mg subcutaneous q3h prn for pain.* The 1-mL unit dose vial is labelled *nalbuphine hydrochloride 10 mg per mL injection.*

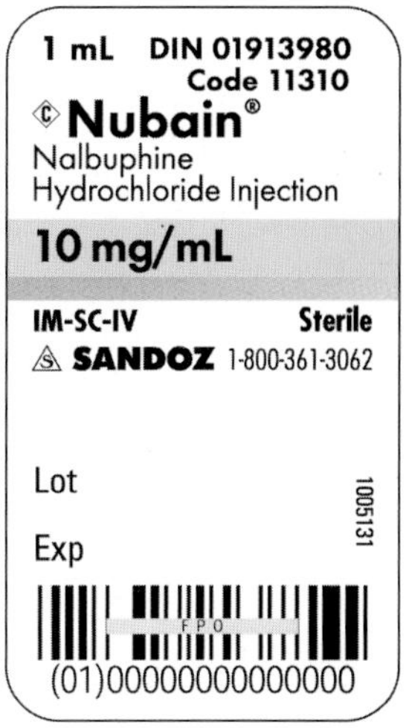
1 mL DIN 01913980
Code 11310
Nubain®
Nalbuphine
Hydrochloride Injection
10 mg/mL
IM-SC-IV Sterile
SANDOZ 1-800-361-3062
Lot
Exp
1005131
(01)00000000000000

Step 1 Convert No conversion necessary.

Step 2 Think You want to give less than 1 mL. Actually you want to give $\frac{1}{2}$ or 0.5 of a mL.

Step 3 Calculate $\frac{D}{H} \times Q = \frac{\overset{1}{\cancel{5}\ \cancel{\text{mg}}}}{\underset{2}{\cancel{10}\ \cancel{\text{mg}}}} \times 1\text{ mL} = \frac{1}{2}\text{ mL} = 0.5\text{ mL}$

given subcutaneously as needed for pain every 3 hours

> **KEY POINT**
>
> **Dosages measured in hundredths (such as 0.25 mL) and all amounts less than 0.5 mL should be prepared in a 1-mL syringe, which is calibrated in hundredths. However, if the route is IM, you may need to change needles to a more appropriate length.**

Select a *1-mL syringe and measure 0.5 mL* of nalbuphine hydrochloride 10 mg/mL. Look carefully at the illustration to clearly identify the part of the black rubber stopper that measures the exact dosage.

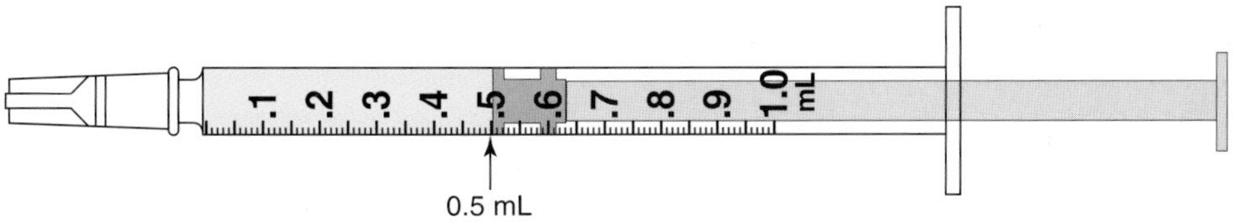
.1
.2
.3
.4
.5
.6
.7
.8
.9
1.0 mL
0.5 mL

Example 3:

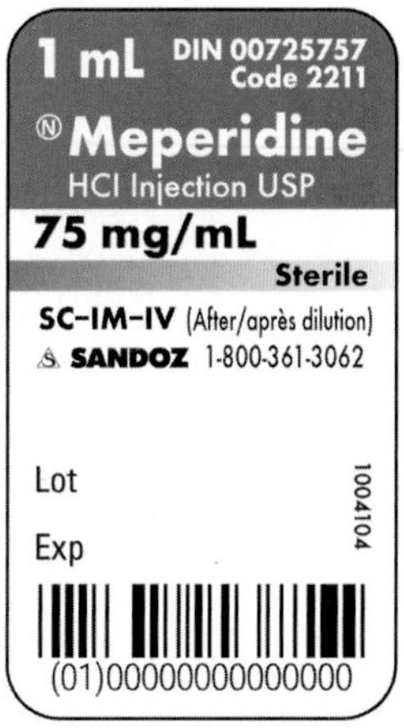
1 mL DIN 00725757
Code 2211
Meperidine
HCl Injection USP
75 mg/mL
Sterile
SC-IM-IV (After/après dilution)
SANDOZ 1-800-361-3062
Lot
Exp
1004104
(01)00000000000000

Order: *meperidine hydrochloride 60 mg IM q4h prn for pain*

Supply: meperidine hydrochloride injection 75 mg/mL

Step 1 Convert No conversion is necessary.

Step 2 Think You want to give less than 1 mL but more than 0.5 mL.

Step 3 Calculate $\frac{D}{H} \times Q = \frac{\overset{4}{\cancel{60\text{ mg}}}}{\underset{5}{\cancel{75\text{ mg}}}} \times 1\text{ mL} = \frac{4}{5}\text{ mL} = 0.8\text{ mL}$

given intramuscularly every 4 hours as needed for pain

Select a 1-mL or 3-mL syringe and draw up all of the contents of the 1-mL vial. Then *discard 0.2 mL to administer 0.8 mL* of meperidine hydrochloride 75 mg/mL. You must discard the 0.2 mL in the presence of another nurse because meperidine hydrochloride is a controlled substance. As it is a controlled substance, you cannot just leave 0.2 mL in the single dosette vial.

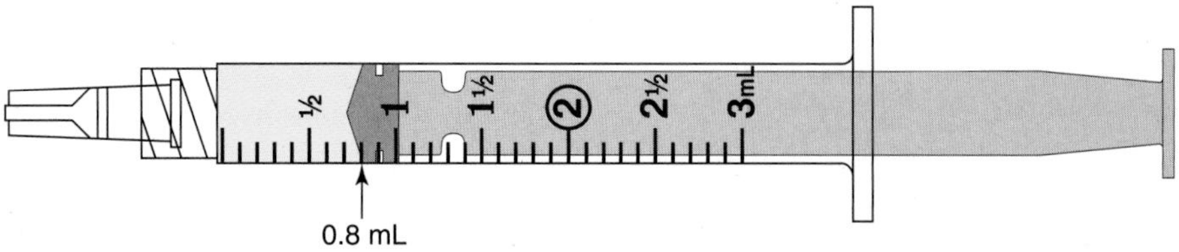
½
1
1½
2
2½
3mL
0.8 mL

Example 4:

Order: *heparin sodium 8000 units subcutaneous BID*

Supply: A vial of heparin sodium injection 10 000 units/mL

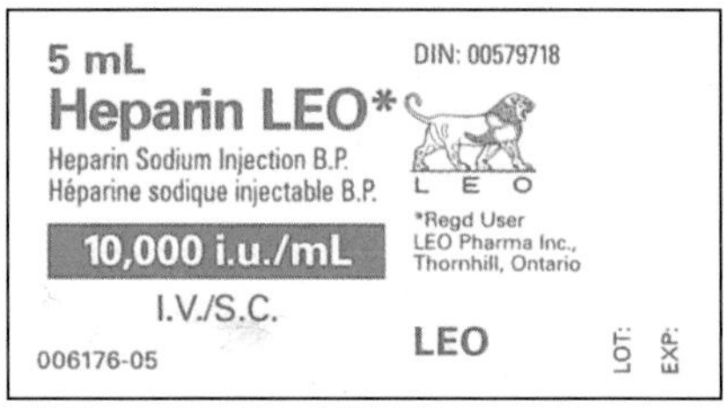
5 mL
DIN: 00579718
Heparin LEO*
Heparin Sodium Injection B.P.
Héparine sodique injectable B.P.
L E O
10,000 i.u./mL
*Regd User
LEO Pharma Inc.,
Thornhill, Ontario
I.V./S.C.
006176-05
LEO
LOT:
EXP:

LEO Pharma Inc., Thornhill, ON

Step 1 Convert No conversion is necessary.

Step 2 Think You want to give less than 1 mL but more than 0.5 mL.

Step 3 Calculate $\frac{D}{H} \times Q = \frac{8000\text{ units}}{10\,000\text{ units}} \times 1\text{ mL} = \frac{8}{10}\text{ mL} = 0.8\text{ mL}$

given subcutaneously twice daily

Select a *1-mL* or a *3-mL syringe and measure 0.8 mL* of heparin sodium 10 000 units/mL. Heparin sodium is a potent anticoagulant drug. It is safest to measure it in a 1-mL syringe.

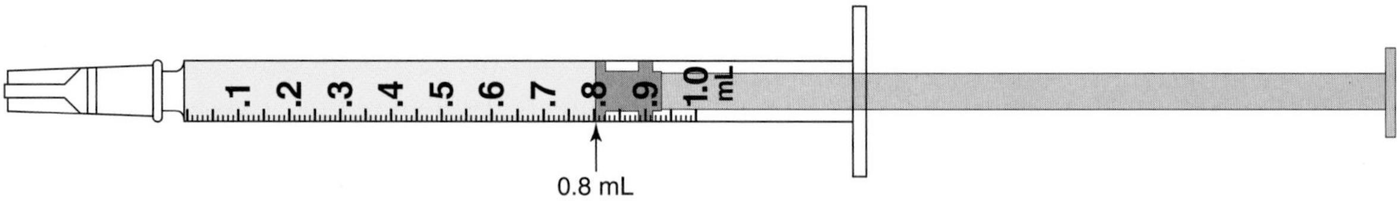
.1
.2
.3
.4
.5
.6
.7
.8
.9
1.0 mL
0.8 mL

Example 5:

Order: *clindamycin 150 mg IM q12h*

Supply: clindamycin injection 300 mg/2 mL

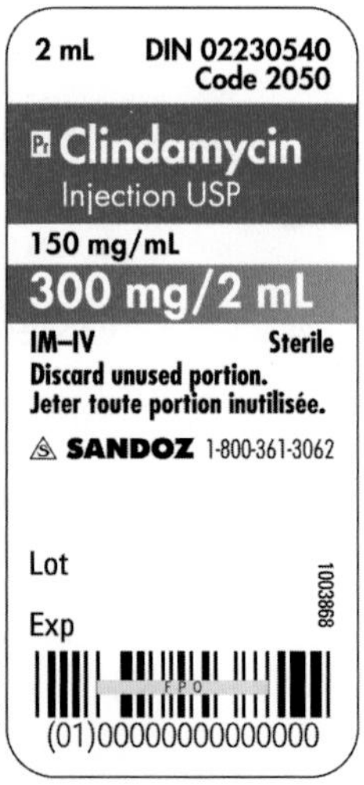
2 mL
DIN 02230540
Code 2050
Clindamycin
Injection USP
150 mg/mL
300 mg/2 mL
IM–IV
Sterile
Discard unused portion.
Jeter toute portion inutilisée.
SANDOZ 1-800-361-3062
Lot
Exp
(01)00000000000000

Step 1 Convert No conversion is necessary.

Step 2 Think You want to give less than 2 mL. Actually, you want to give 150 mg, which is $\frac{1}{2}$ of 300 mg and $\frac{1}{2}$ of 2 mL, or 1 mL. Calculate to double-check your estimate.

Step 3 Calculate $\frac{D}{H} \times Q = \frac{\overset{1}{\cancel{150\text{ mg}}}}{\underset{2}{\cancel{300\text{ mg}}}} \times 2\text{ mL} = \frac{\overset{1}{\cancel{2}}}{\underset{1}{\cancel{2}}}\text{ mL} = 1\text{ mL}$

given intramuscularly every 12 hours

Select a *1-mL syringe, and measure 1 mL* of clindamycin injection 300 mg/2 mL. A 3-mL syringe could also be safely used to withdraw 1 mL of clindamycin injection.

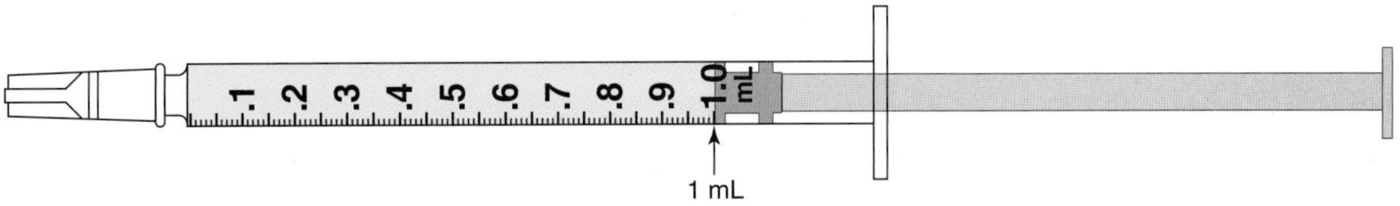

.1 .2 .3 .4 .5 .6 .7 .8 .9 1.0 mL
1 mL

Example 6:

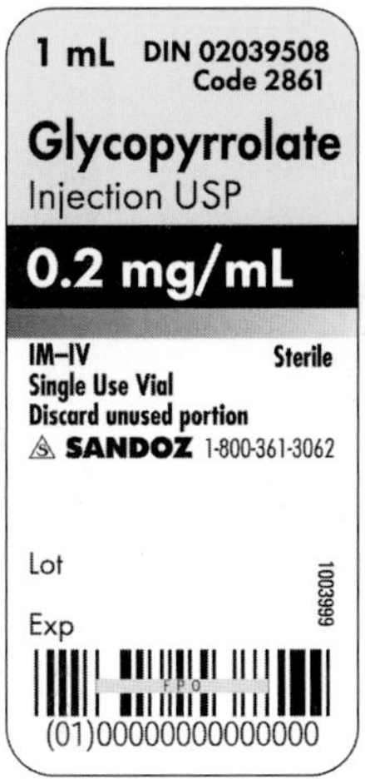

1 mL DIN 02039508
Code 2861
Glycopyrrolate
Injection USP
0.2 mg/mL
IM–IV
Sterile
Single Use Vial
Discard unused portion
SANDOZ 1-800-361-3062
Lot
Exp
1003993
(01)00000000000000

Order: *glycopyrrolate 150 mcg IM stat*

Supply: glycopyrrolate 0.2 mg/mL

Step 1 Convert Order: *glycopyrrolate 150 mcg*

Supply: glycopyrrolate 0.2 mg $= 0.2 \times 1000 = 200$ mcg

Equivalent: 1 mg $=$ 1000 mcg

Step 2 Think You want to give less than 1 mL but more than 0.5 mL. Be careful with the units and decimals. Do not be fooled into thinking 0.2 mg is less than 150 mcg. After conversion you can clearly see that 0.2 mg is more than 150 mcg because 0.2 mg $=$ 200 mcg, which is more than 150 mcg.

Step 3 Calculate $\frac{D}{H} \times Q = \frac{\overset{3}{\cancel{150}}\ \cancel{\text{mg}}}{\underset{4}{\cancel{200}}\ \cancel{\text{mg}}} \times 1\text{ mL} = \frac{3}{4}\text{ mL} = 0.75\text{ mL}$

given intramuscularly immediately

Select a *1-mL syringe, and measure 0.75 mL* of glycopyrrolate 0.2 mg/mL. You may have to change needles, as this is an IM injection and the needle gauge on a 1-mL syringe is insufficient for an IM injection.

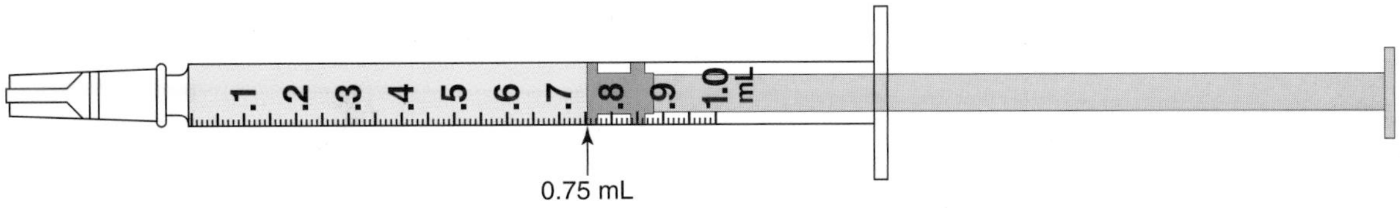

.1 .2 .3 .4 .5 .6 .7 .8 .9 1.0 mL
0.75 mL

Example 7:

The patient care is for *morphine sulfate 10 mg IM q4h prn for pain,* and the label on the vial states *morphine sulfate 25 mg/mL.*

Step 1 Convert No conversion is necessary.

Supply: morphine sulfate 25 mg/mL

Step 2 Think You want to give less than 1 mL. Actually you want to give 0.4 mL.

Step 3 Calculate $\frac{D}{H} \times Q = \frac{10 \text{ mg}}{25 \text{ mg}} \times 1 \text{ mL} = 0.4 \text{ mL}$

given intramuscularly every 4 hours as needed for pain

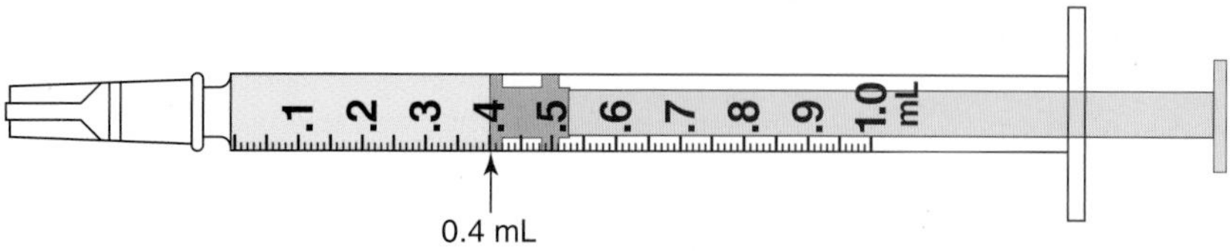

QUICK REVIEW

- To solve parenteral dosage problems, apply the three steps to dosage calculations:
  Step 1 **Convert**
  Step 2 **Think**
  Step 3 **Calculate** $\frac{\text{D (desired)}}{\text{H (have)}} \times \text{Q (quantity)} = \text{X (amount)}$
- Prepare a maximum of 5 mL per IM ventrogluteal injection site for an average-size adult, 2 mL per site for children age 2 through 12, 1 mL for children older than 7 months to 2 years, and 0.5 mL for infants less than 7 months old. Refer to Table 9-1 for recommendations for the vastus lateralis and deltoid injecton sites.
- Calculate dose volumes and prepare injectable fractional doses in a syringe using these guidelines:
  - Standard doses more than 1 mL: Round to *tenths* and measure in a 3-mL syringe. The 3-mL syringe is calibrated to 0.1-mL increments. Example: 1.53 mL is rounded to 1.5 mL and drawn up in a 3-mL syringe.
  - Small (less than 0.5 mL) doses: Round to *hundredths* and measure in a 1-mL syringe. Critical care and children's doses less than 1 mL calculated in hundredths should also be measured in a 1-mL syringe. The 1-mL syringe is calibrated in 0.01-mL increments. Example: 0.257 mL is rounded to 0.26 mL and drawn up in a 1-mL syringe.
  - Amounts of 0.5–1 mL, calculated in tenths, can be accurately measured in either a 1-mL or 3-mL syringe.

REVIEW SET 22

Calculate the amount you will prepare for each dose. The labels provided represent the drugs available. Draw an arrow to the syringe calibration that corresponds to the amount you will administer. Indicate doses that have to be divided.

1. Order: *medroxyprogesterone acetate 100 mg IM every 2 weeks*

   Give: _________ mL

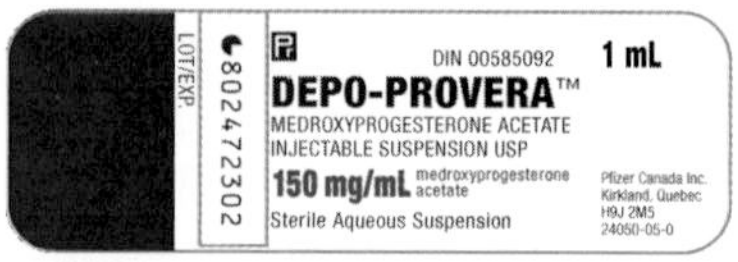

©Pfizer Canada Inc., Kirkland, Que

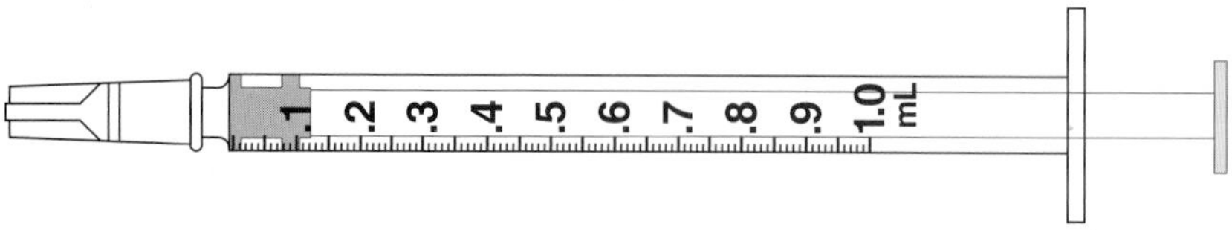

2. Order: *penicillin G sodium 2 400 000 units IV stat*

   Give: ________ mL

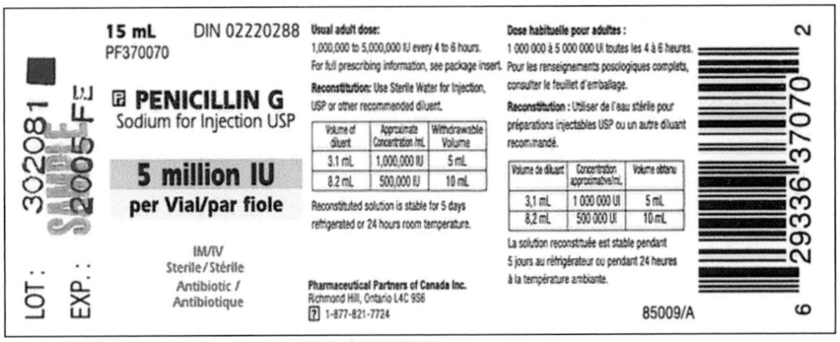

Pharmaceutical Partners of Canada Inc., Richmond Hill, ON

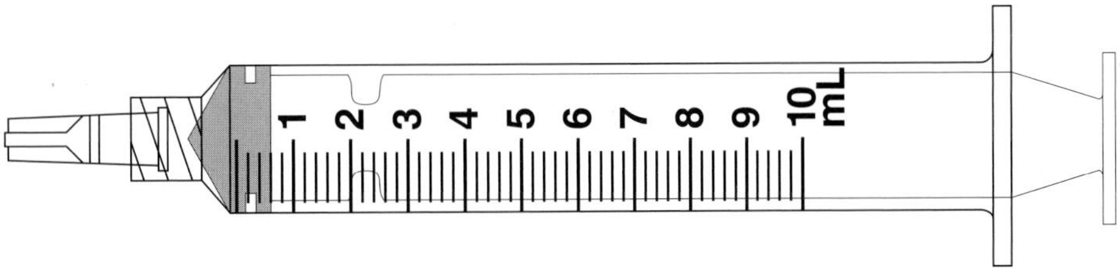

3. Order: *haloperidol 2 mg IV stat*

   Give: ________ mL

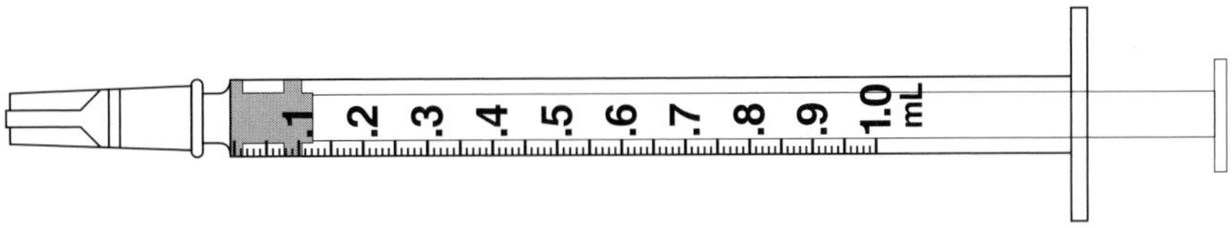

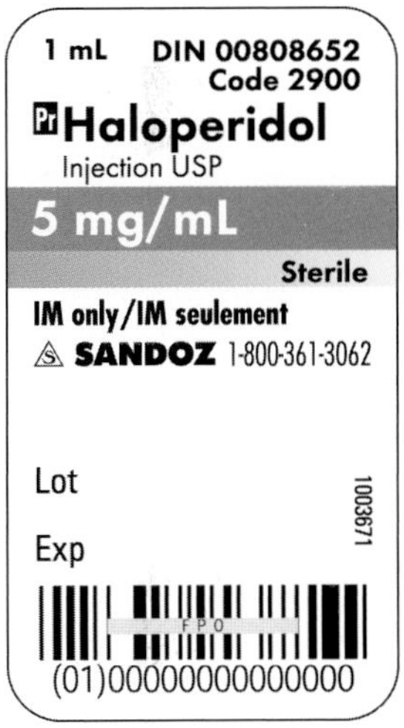

4. Order: *dexamethasone sodium phosphate 1.5 mg IM q12h*

   Give: ________ mL

Pharmascience Inc., Montreal, Que

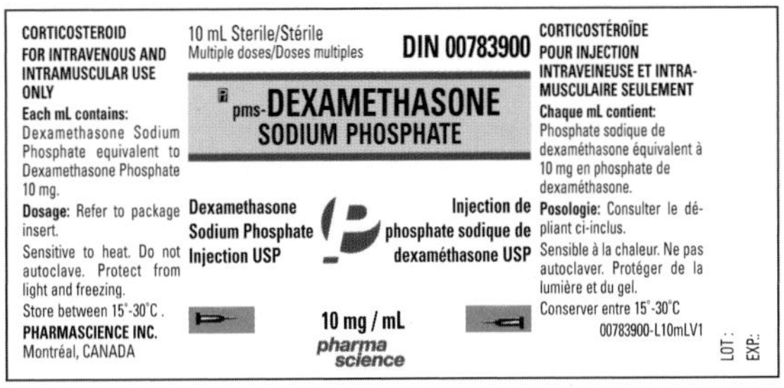

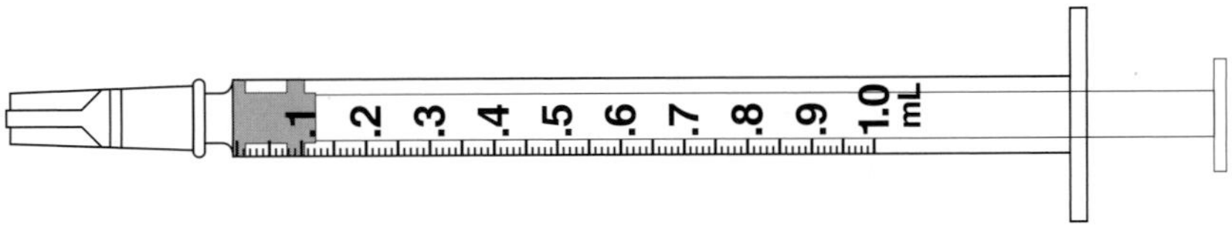

5. Order: *ondansetron hydrochloride dihydrate (Zofran) 4 mg IV stat for nausea*

   Give: ________ mL stat

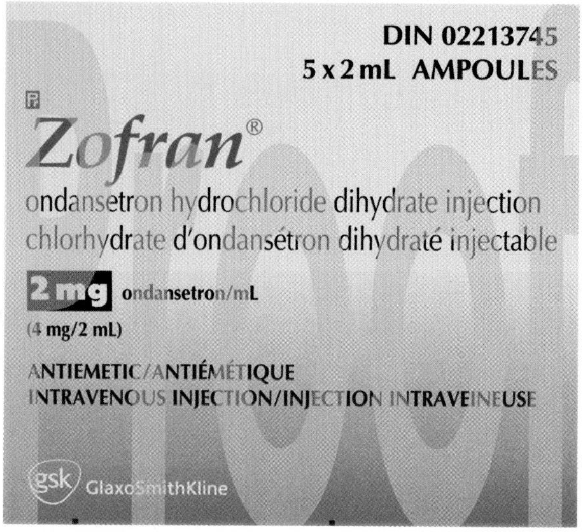
DIN 02213745
5 x 2 mL AMPOULES
Zofran®
ondansetron hydrochloride dihydrate injection
chlorhydrate d'ondansétron dihydraté injectable
2 mg ondansetron/mL
(4 mg/2 mL)
ANTIEMETIC/ANTIÉMÉTIQUE
INTRAVENOUS INJECTION/INJECTION INTRAVEINEUSE
gsk GlaxoSmithKline

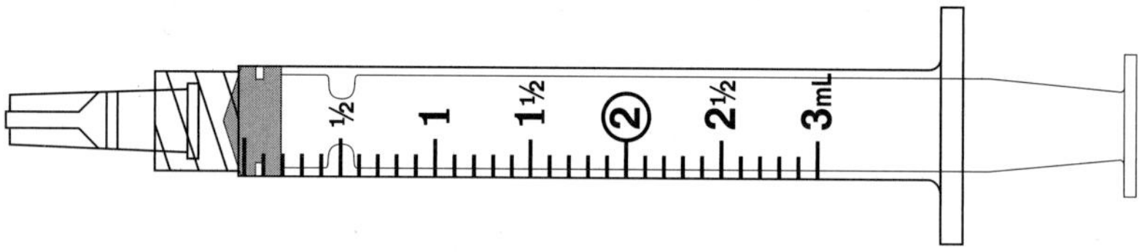
½
1
1½
2
2½
3mL

6. Order: *heparin sodium 3500 units subcutaneous q8h*

   Give: ________ mL

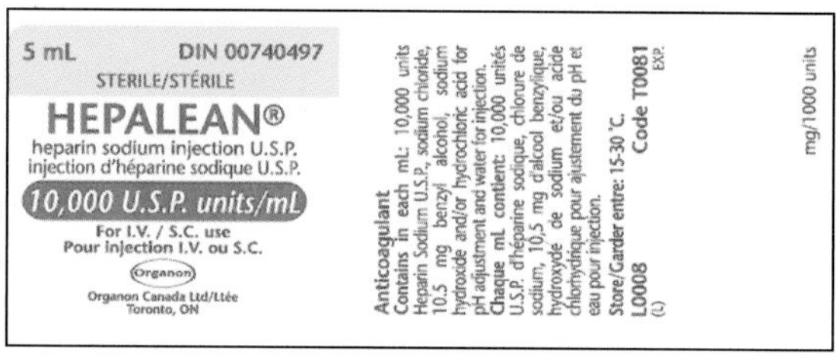
5 mL
DIN 00740497
STERILE/STÉRILE
HEPALEAN®
heparin sodium injection U.S.P.
injection d'héparine sodique U.S.P.
10,000 U.S.P. units/mL
For I.V. / S.C. use
Pour injection I.V. ou S.C.
Organon
Organon Canada Ltd/Ltée
Toronto, ON

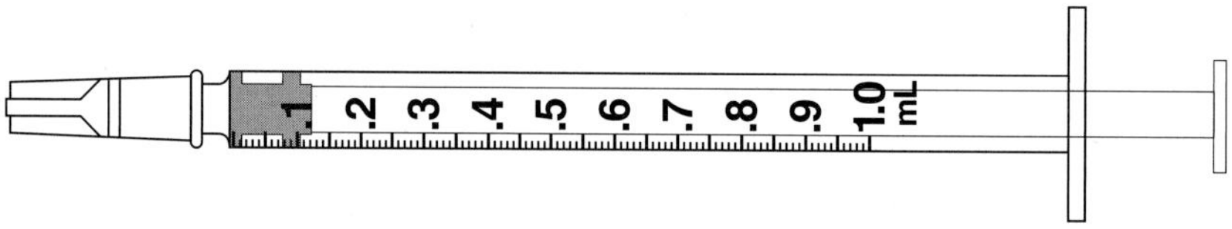
.1
.2
.3
.4
.5
.6
.7
.8
.9
1.0
mL

7. Order: *ketorolac tromethamine 15 mg IM q6h*

   Give: ________ mL

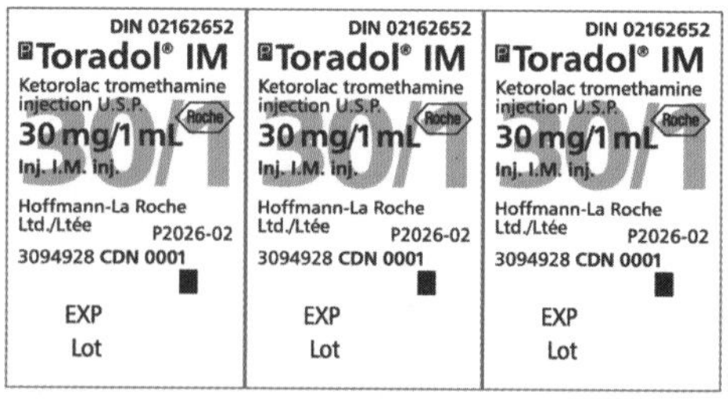
DIN 02162652
Toradol® IM
Ketorolac tromethamine
injection U.S.P.
30 mg/1 mL
Inj. I.M. inj.
Hoffmann-La Roche
Ltd./Ltée
P2026-02
3094928 CDN 0001
EXP
Lot

Label submitted by manufacturer for general information and may change; please always refer to the latest product monograph/label. ©Copyright 2007, Hoffman-LaRoche Limited.

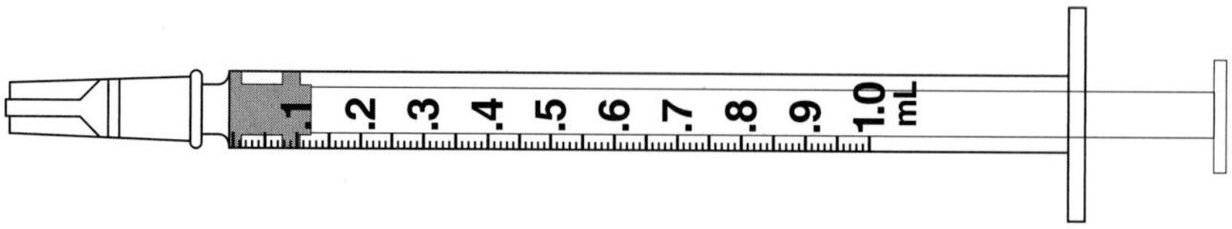
.1
.2
.3
.4
.5
.6
.7
.8
.9
1.0
mL

8. Order: *meperidine hydrochloride 35 mg IM for pain*

Give: _________ mL

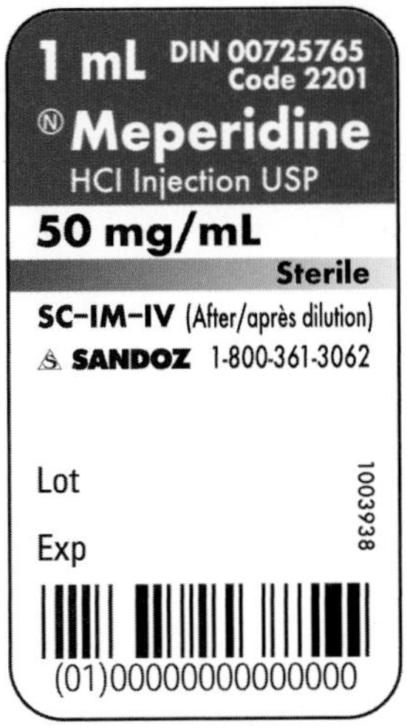
1 mL DIN 00725765
Code 2201
Ⓝ Meperidine
HCl Injection USP
50 mg/mL
Sterile
SC-IM-IV (After/après dilution)
SANDOZ 1-800-361-3062
Lot
Exp
1003938
(01)00000000000000

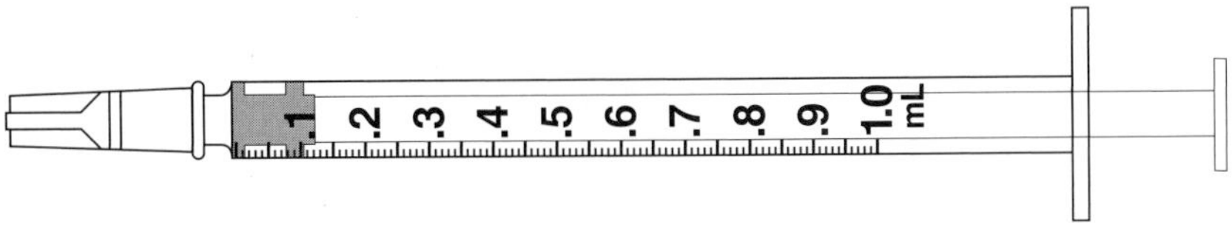
.1 .2 .3 .4 .5 .6 .7 .8 .9 1.0 mL

9. Order: *furosemide 40 mg IV bolus stat*

Give: _________ mL

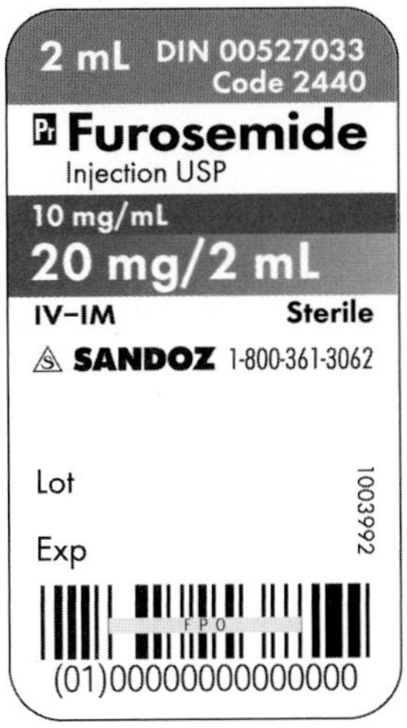
2 mL DIN 00527033
Code 2440
Pr Furosemide
Injection USP
10 mg/mL
20 mg/2 mL
IV-IM
Sterile
SANDOZ 1-800-361-3062
Lot
Exp
1003992
FPO
(01)00000000000000

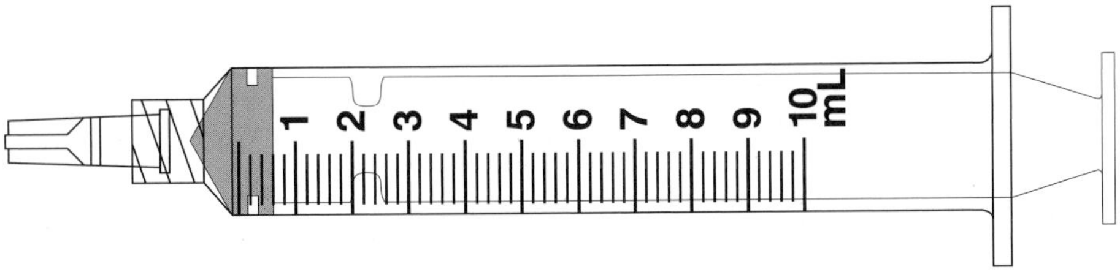
1 2 3 4 5 6 7 8 9 10 mL

10. Order: *morphine sulfate 15 mg IM q3h prn for pain*

Give: _________ mL

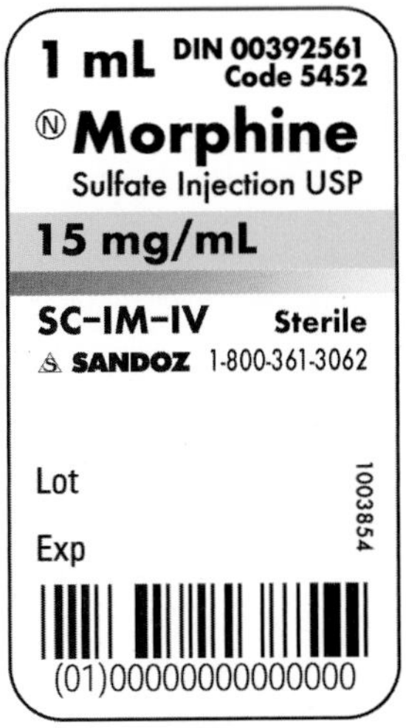
1 mL DIN 00392561
Code 5452
Ⓝ Morphine
Sulfate Injection USP
15 mg/mL
SC-IM-IV
Sterile
SANDOZ 1-800-361-3062
Lot
Exp
1003854
(01)00000000000000

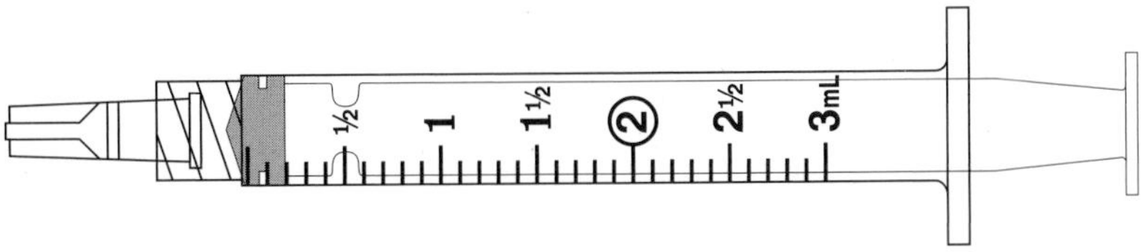
½ 1 1½ 2 2½ 3mL

11. Order: *methotrexate sodium 30 mg IV day 1 and day 8*

Give: ________ mL

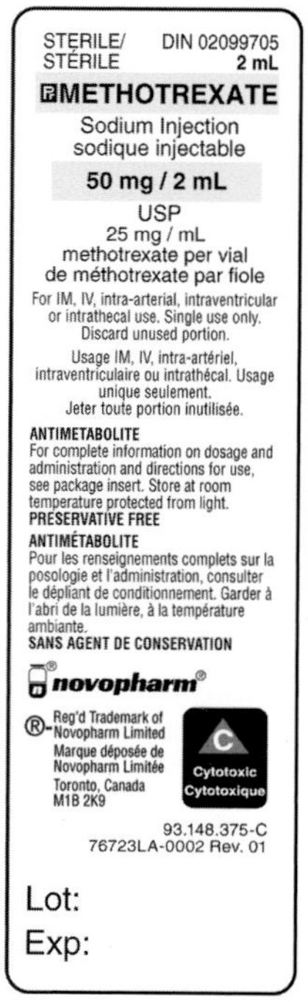
STERILE/ STÉRILE
DIN 02099705
2 mL
METHOTREXATE
Sodium Injection
sodique injectable
50 mg / 2 mL
USP
25 mg / mL
methotrexate per vial
de méthotrexate par fiole
For IM, IV, intra-arterial, intraventricular or intrathecal use. Single use only. Discard unused portion.
Usage IM, IV, intra-artériel, intraventriculaire ou intrathécal. Usage unique seulement. Jeter toute portion inutilisée.
ANTIMETABOLITE
For complete information on dosage and administration and directions for use, see package insert. Store at room temperature protected from light.
PRESERVATIVE FREE
ANTIMÉTABOLITE
Pour les renseignements complets sur la posologie et l'administration, consulter le dépliant de conditionnement. Garder à l'abri de la lumière, à la température ambiante.
SANS AGENT DE CONSERVATION
novopharm
Reg'd Trademark of Novopharm Limited
Marque déposée de Novopharm Limitée
Toronto, Canada M1B 2K9
Cytotoxic
Cytotoxique
93.148.375-C
76723LA-0002 Rev. 01
Lot:
Exp:

Novopharm Limited, Toronto, ON

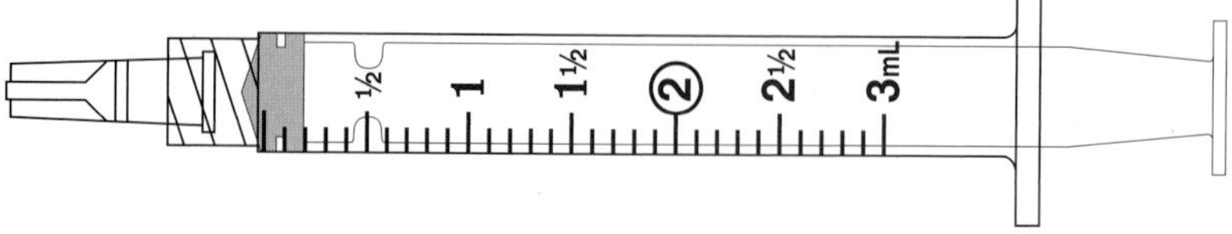
½
1
1½
2
2½
3mL

12. Order: *enoxaparin sodium 40 mg subcutaneous daily*

Give: ________ mL

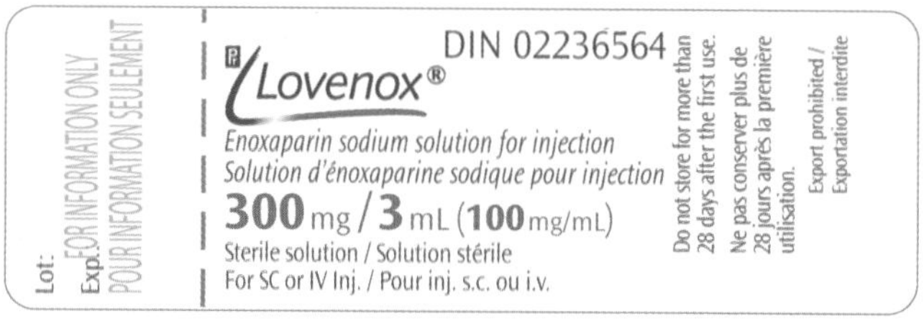
Lot:
Exp.
FOR INFORMATION ONLY
POUR INFORMATION SEULEMENT
DIN 02236564
Lovenox®
Enoxaparin sodium solution for injection
Solution d'énoxaparine sodique pour injection
300 mg / 3 mL (100 mg/mL)
Sterile solution / Solution stérile
For SC or IV Inj. / Pour inj. s.c. ou i.v.
Do not store for more than 28 days after the first use.
Ne pas conserver plus de 28 jours après la première utilisation.
Export prohibited / Exportation interdite

Sanofi-aventis Canada, Laval, QUE

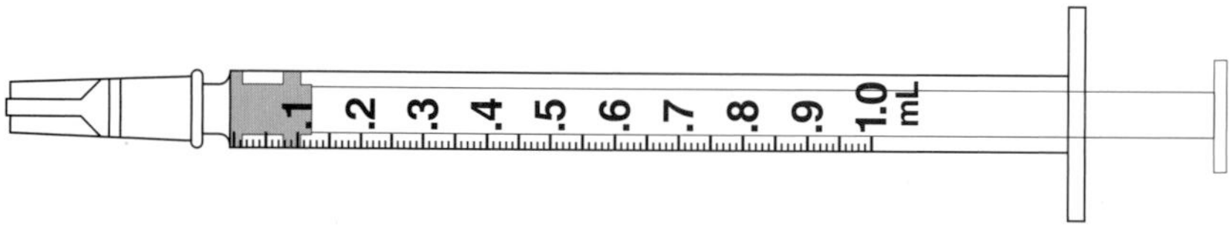
.1
.2
.3
.4
.5
.6
.7
.8
.9
1.0 mL

13. Order: *midazolam 2.5 mg IM 30 min preoperatively*

Give: ________ mL

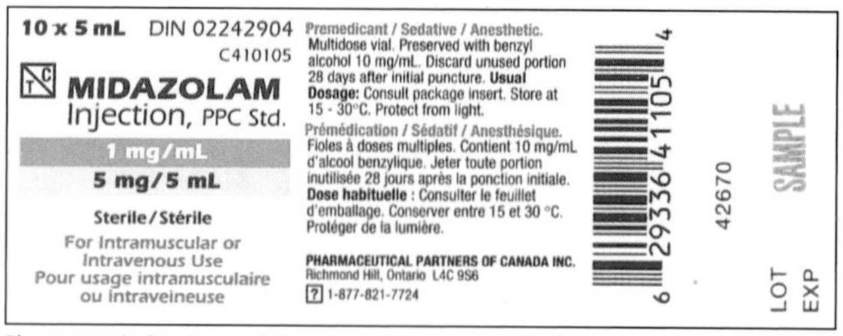
10 x 5 mL
DIN 02242904
C410105
MIDAZOLAM
Injection, PPC Std.
1 mg/mL
5 mg/5 mL
Sterile/Stérile
For Intramuscular or Intravenous Use
Pour usage intramusculaire ou intraveineuse
Premedicant / Sedative / Anesthetic.
Multidose vial. Preserved with benzyl alcohol 10 mg/mL. Discard unused portion 28 days after initial puncture. Usual Dosage: Consult package insert. Store at 15 - 30°C. Protect from light.
Prémédication / Sédatif / Anesthésique.
Fioles à doses multiples. Contient 10 mg/mL d'alcool benzylique. Jeter toute portion inutilisée 28 jours après la ponction initiale. Dose habituelle : Consulter le feuillet d'emballage. Conserver entre 15 et 30 °C. Protéger de la lumière.
PHARMACEUTICAL PARTNERS OF CANADA INC.
Richmond Hill, Ontario L4C 9S6
1-877-821-7724
6 29336 41105 4
42670
SAMPLE
LOT
EXP

Pharmaceutical Partners of Canada Inc., Richmond Hill, ON

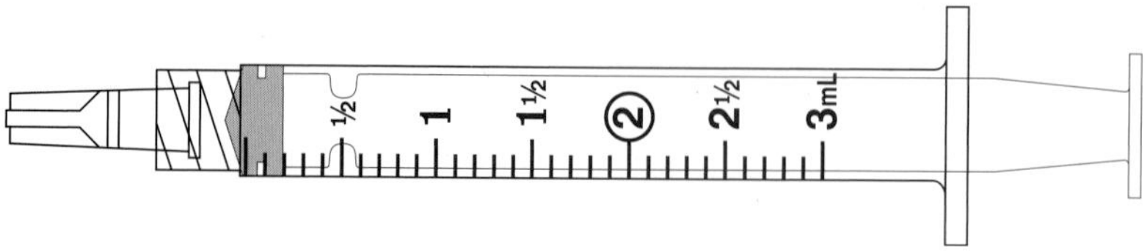
½
1
1½
2
2½
3mL

14. Order: *hydroxyzine hydrochloride 25 mg IM q4h prn for nausea*

    Give: ________ mL

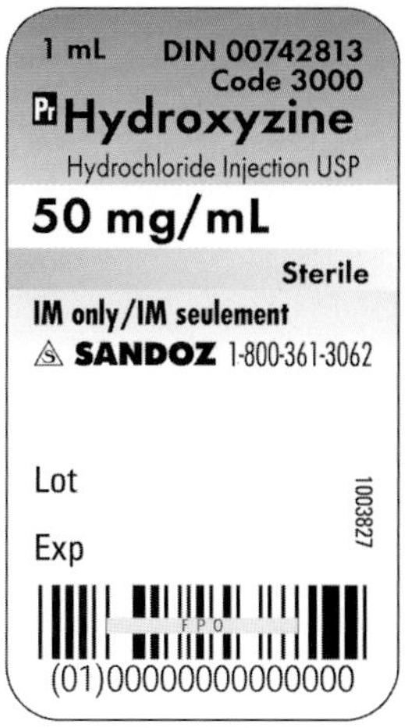

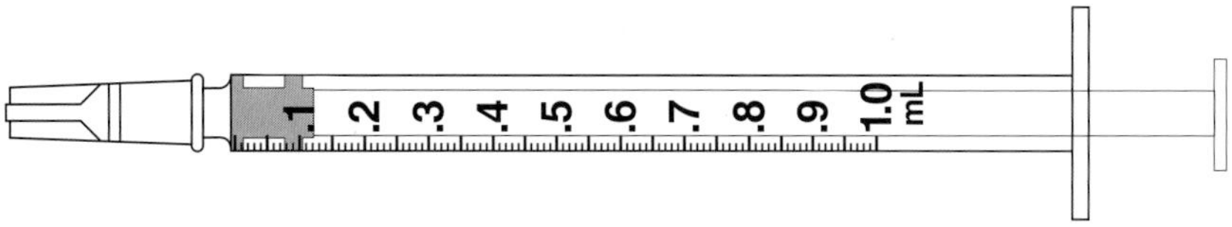

15. Order: *metronidazole 500 mg IV prior to surgery*

    Give: ________ mL

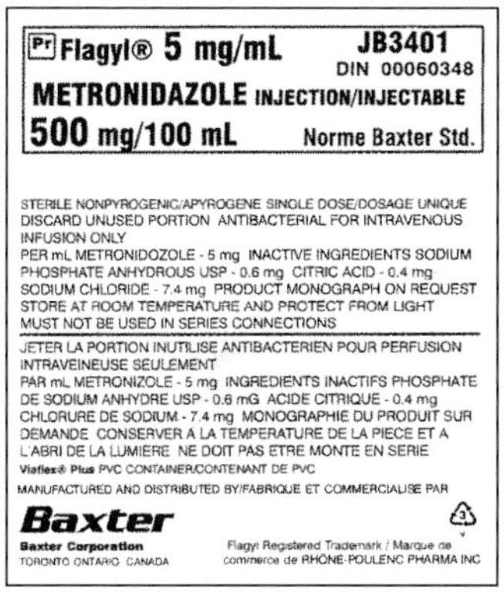

Baxter Corporation, Mississauga, ON

16. Order: *calcitriol 1.5 mcg IV 3 times/week once daily M-W-F*

    Give: ________ mL

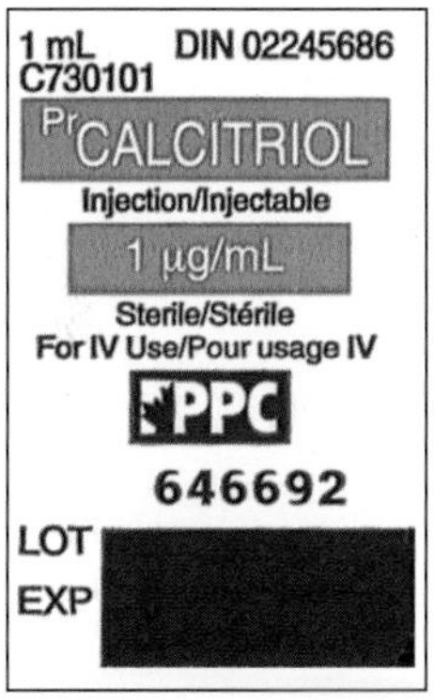

Pharmaceutical Partners of Canada Inc, Richmond Hill, ON

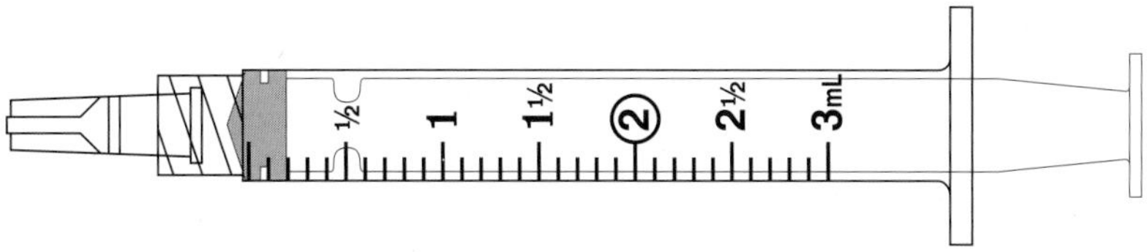

17. Order: *cyanocobalamin 0.5 mg IM once/week*

    Give: ________ mL

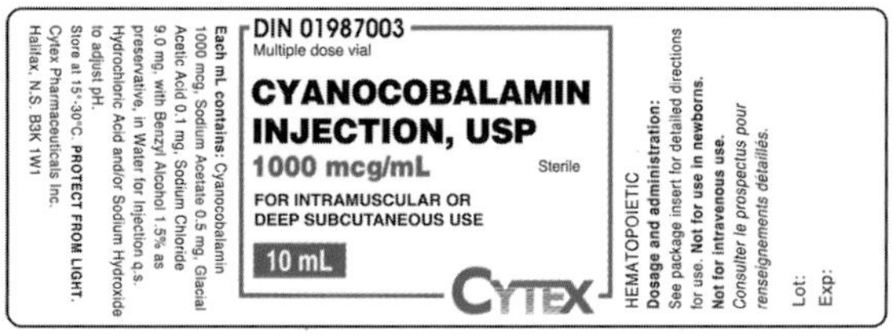

Cytex Pharmaceuticals, Halifax, NS

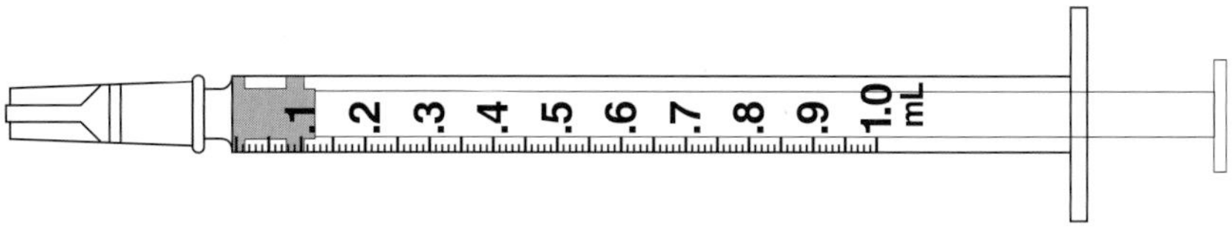

18. Order: *ranitidine hydrochloride 25 mg IV BID*

Give: ________ mL

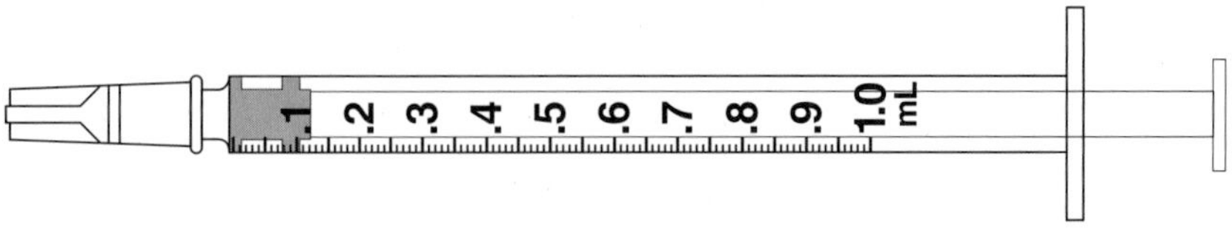

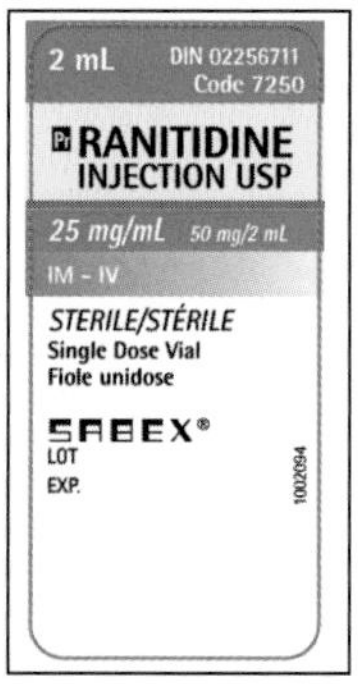

19. Order: *promethazine hydrochloride 12.5 mg IM stat*

Give: ________ mL

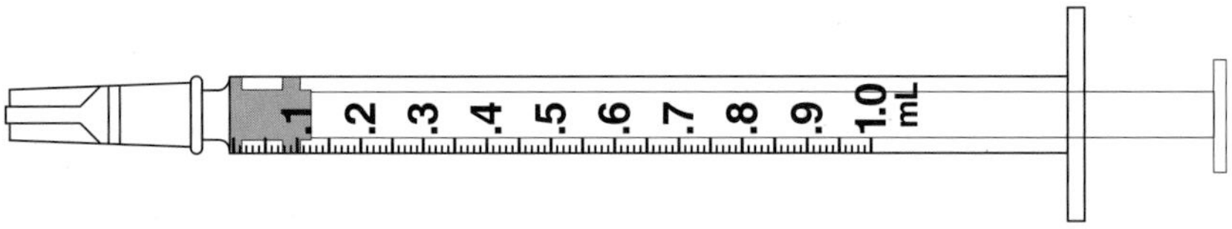

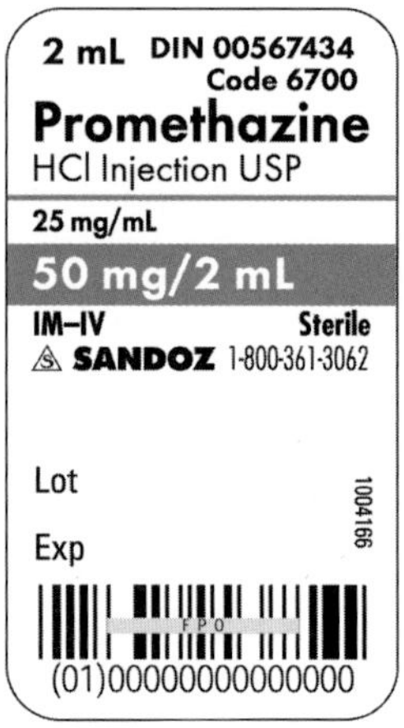

20. Order: *furosemide 15 mg IV daily*

Give: ________ mL

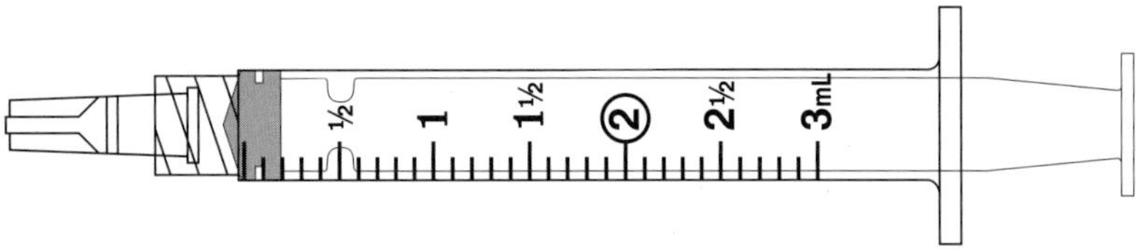

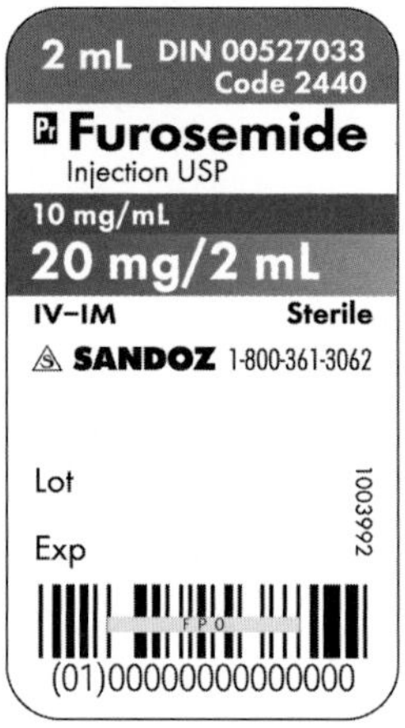

After completing these problems, see pages 469–473 to check your answers.

INSULIN

Insulin, a hormone made in the pancreas, is necessary for the metabolism of glucose, proteins, and fats. Patients who are deficient in insulin are required to take insulin by injection daily. Insulin is a ready-to-use solution that is measured in units. The most common supply dosage is *100 units per mL.*

MATH TIP

The supply dosage of insulin is **100 units per mL** (which is abbreviated on some labels as **U-100**). Think: U-100 = 100 units per mL.

> **CAUTION**
>
> Accuracy in insulin preparation and administration is critical. Inaccuracy is potentially life-threatening. It is essential for nurses to *understand the information on the insulin label*, to correctly *interpret the insulin order*, and to *select the correct syringe* to measure insulin for administration.

Insulin Label

Figure 9-2 identifies the essential components of insulin labels. The insulin label includes important information. For example, the *trade and generic names*, the *supply dosage* or *concentration*, and the *storage* instructions are details commonly found on most parenteral drug labels. Chapter 7 explains these and other typical drug label components. Let us look closely at different insulin types classified by the insulin *action times* and insulin *species*, which are critical identifiers of this important hormone supplement.

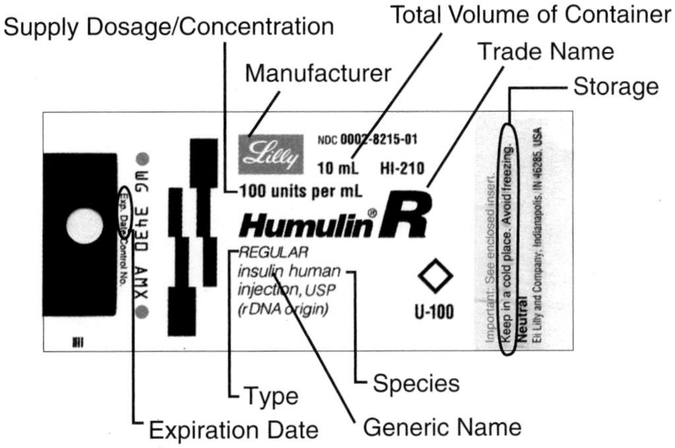

FIGURE 9-2 Insulin Label

Insulin Action Times

Insulins vary in onset, peak, and duration of action. See Table 9-2 for a comparison of the onset, peak, and duration of action according to the classification of insulin. Figure 9-3, on page 199, shows a sampling of insulin labels arranged by the four action times: rapid-acting, short-acting, intermediate-acting, and long-acting. Notice the uppercase, bold letters on the regular and neutral protamine Hagedorn (NPH) insulin labels: **R** for **R**egular insulin and **N** for **N**PH insulin. A short-acting insulin or a rapid-acting insulin analogue is usually administered at each meal and for continuous subcutaneous insulin infusions, while an intermediate-acting insulin or a long-acting insulin analogue is administered once or twice daily to manage normal daily blood glucose fluctuations. Intermediate insulins (Humulin N and Novolin ge NPH) are crystalline zinc suspensions of human regular insulin combined with the polypeptide protamine (protein taken from salmon) in a phosphate buffer and have a milky white or cloudy appearance. The protamine delays the onset of NPH insulin.

An analogue is defined as a chemical compound that is structurally similar to another compound, but differs slightly in composition. Insulin analogues are produced by recombinant DNA technology by altering the amino acid sequencing on the A and B chains of the human insulin. Such structural changes can influence the pharmacokinetics (absorption, distribution, metabolism, and excretion) of the drug. For example, insulin lispro (Humalog), insulin aspart (NovoRapid), and insulin glulisine (Aprida) are rapid-acting insulin analogues. The rapid-acting analogues have a faster onset of action and shorter duration time. Insulin glargine (Lantus) and detemer (Levemir) are long-acting insulin analogues. Glargine and detemer are released steadily and continuously over 24 hours with no peak of action after once-daily subcutaneous administration. They should be administered at the same time each day. They are an alternative to the use of NPH insulin. Long-acting insulins are not mixed with any other insulin. You should be aware that the long-acting insulins are clear and colourless and should not be confused with rapid- or short-acting insulins that are also clear.

TABLE 9-2

Insulin Type (Trade name)	Onset	Peak	Duration
Prandial (bolus) Insulin			
Rapid-acting insulin analogues (clear)			
• Insulin aspart (NovoRapid)	10–15 min	1–1.5 h	3–5 h
• Insulin lispro (Humalog)	10–15 min	1–2 h	3.5–4.75 h
• Insulin glulisine (Apidra)	10–15 min	1–1.5 h	3–5 h
Short-acting insulins (clear)			
• Humulin R	30 min	2–3 h	6.5 h
• Novolin ge Toronto			
Inhaled insulin	10–20 min	2 h	6 h
Basal Insulins			
Intermediate-acting (cloudy)			
• Humulin N	1–3 h	5–8 h	up to 18 h
• Novolin ge NPH			
Long-acting basal insulin analogues (clear)			
• Insulin detemir (Levemir) • Insulin glargine (Lantus)	90 min	Not applicable	Up to 24 h (glargine 24h, detemir 16–24 h)
Premixed Insulin			
Premixed regular insulin—NPH (cloudy)			
• Humulin 30/70			
• Novolin ge 30/70, 40/60, 50/50	A single vial or cartridge contains a fixed ratio of insulin (% of rapid-acting or short-acting insulin to % of intermediate-acting insulin)		
Premixed insulin analogues (cloudy)			
• Biphasic insulin aspart (NovoMix 30)			
• Insulin lispro/lispro protamine (Humalog Mix25 and Mix50)			
Prandial—at mealtimes			
Basal—continuous delivery of insulin			

Reprinted with permission from Canadian Diabetes Association 2008 Clinical Practice Guidelines for the Prevention and Management of Diabetes in Canada. Can J Diabetes. 2008;32 (suppl 1): S1-201

CAUTION

Do not confuse trade names for aspart (NovoRapid) and lispro (Humalog) with the trade names for regular insulins (Humulin R, Novolin ge).

Species of Insulin

Human biosynthetic insulin is the most commonly used insulin. It is also called *recombinant* or *DNA-derived.* It is made from bacteria such as *Escherichia coli* or yeast cells that are genetically altered to create human insulin. Beef insulin was withdrawn from the Canadian market in 1999 although it can still be purchased through international sources. Pork insulin was discontinued in April 2006 by the

Rapid-Acting

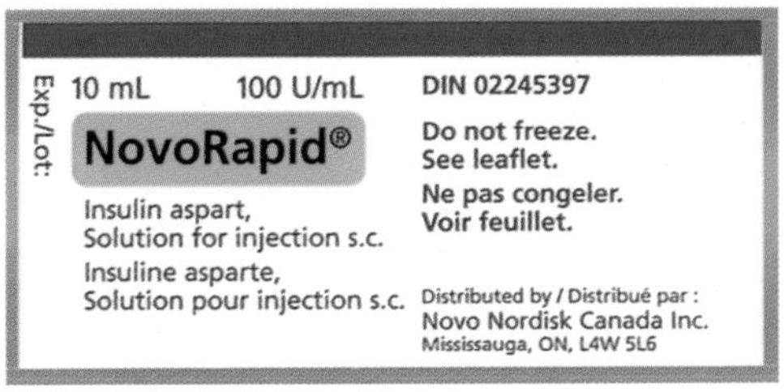
Exp./Lot:
10 mL
100 U/mL
DIN 02245397
NovoRapid®
Insulin aspart,
Solution for injection s.c.
Insuline asparte,
Solution pour injection s.c.
Do not freeze.
See leaflet.
Ne pas congeler.
Voir feuillet.
Distributed by / Distribué par :
Novo Nordisk Canada Inc.
Mississauga, ON, L4W 5L6

A

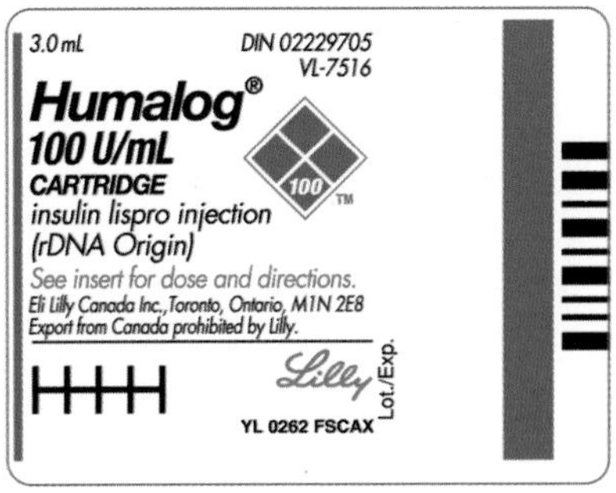
3.0 mL
DIN 02229705
VL-7516
Humalog®
100 U/mL
CARTRIDGE
insulin lispro injection
(rDNA Origin)
See insert for dose and directions.
Eli Lilly Canada Inc., Toronto, Ontario, M1N 2E8
Export from Canada prohibited by Lilly.
Lilly
Lot/Exp.
YL 0262 FSCAX

B

Short-Acting

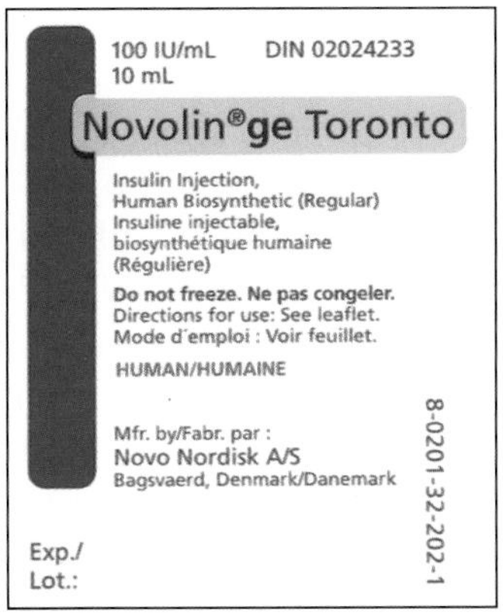
100 IU/mL
DIN 02024233
10 mL
Novolin®ge Toronto
Insulin Injection,
Human Biosynthetic (Regular)
Insuline injectable,
biosynthétique humaine
(Régulière)
Do not freeze. Ne pas congeler.
Directions for use: See leaflet.
Mode d'emploi : Voir feuillet.
HUMAN/HUMAINE
Mfr. by/Fabr. par :
Novo Nordisk A/S
Bagsvaerd, Denmark/Danemark
Exp./
Lot.:
8-0201-32-202-1

C

Intermediate-Acting

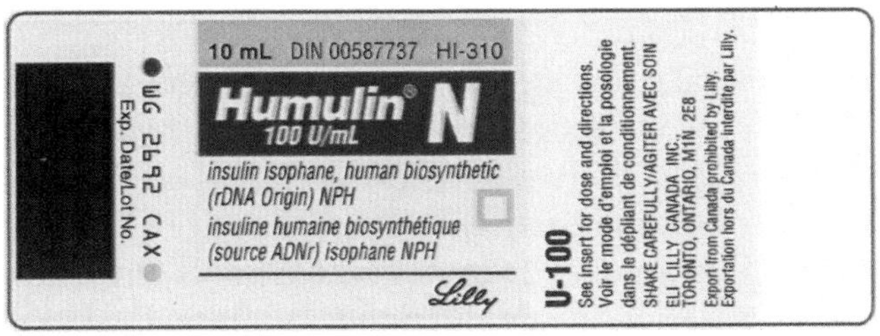
10 mL DIN 00587737 HI-310
Humulin® N
100 U/mL
insulin isophane, human biosynthetic
(rDNA Origin) NPH
insuline humaine biosynthétique
(source ADNr) isophane NPH
Lilly
Exp. Date/Lot No.
U-100
See insert for dose and directions.
Voir le mode d'emploi et la posologie
dans le dépliant de conditionnement.
SHAKE CAREFULLY/AGITER AVEC SOIN
ELI LILLY CANADA INC.
TORONTO, ONTARIO, M1N 2E8
Export from Canada prohibited by Lilly.
Exportation hors du Canada interdite par Lilly.

D

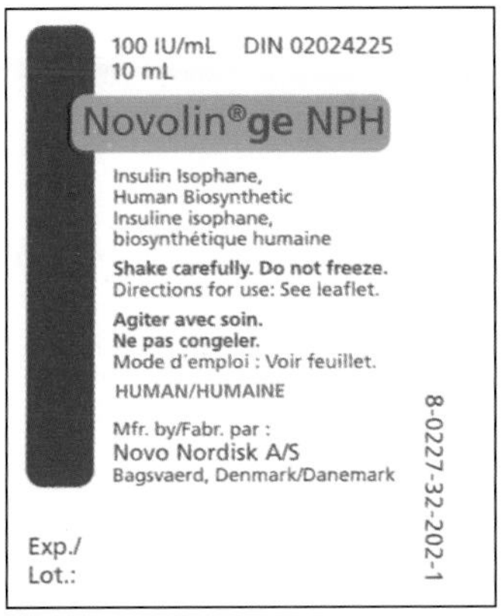
100 IU/mL
DIN 02024225
10 mL
Novolin®ge NPH
Insulin Isophane,
Human Biosynthetic
Insuline isophane,
biosynthétique humaine
Shake carefully. Do not freeze.
Directions for use: See leaflet.
Agiter avec soin.
Ne pas congeler.
Mode d'emploi : Voir feuillet.
HUMAN/HUMAINE
Mfr. by/Fabr. par :
Novo Nordisk A/S
Bagsvaerd, Denmark/Danemark
Exp./
Lot.:
8-0227-32-202-1

E

Long-Acting

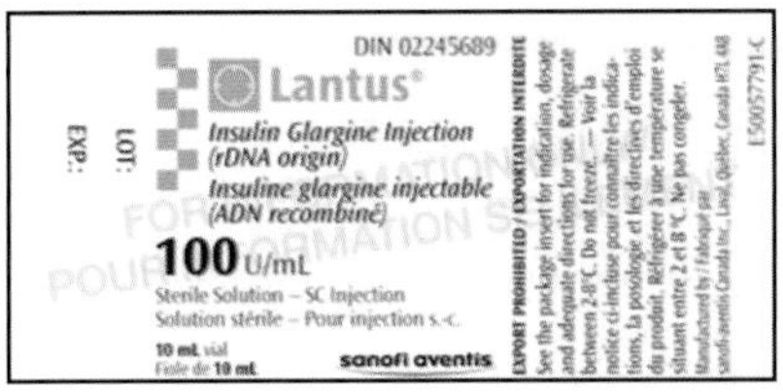
DIN 02245689
Lantus®
Insulin Glargine Injection
(rDNA origin)
Insuline glargine injectable
(ADN recombiné)
100 U/mL
Sterile Solution – SC Injection
Solution stérile – Pour injection s.-c.
10 mL vial
Fiole de 10 mL
sanofi aventis
LOT:
EXP.:

F

FIGURE 9-3 Examples of Labels for Insulin Types Grouped by Action Times distributor Eli Lilly but will still be available through a British distributor. Beef and pork insulins are made from the pancreas of cattle and pigs, respectively.

> **CAUTION**
>
> Avoid a potentially life-threatening medication error. Carefully read the label, and compare it to the drug order to ensure that you select the correct action time and species of insulin.

Fixed Combination Insulin

Premixed insulin combinations that are commercially available contain a combination of a rapid- or short-acting and an intermediate-acting insulin in fixed proportions (Figure 9-4). These product combinations eliminate the visual, manual, or cognitive difficulty some patients encounter to mix insulins. Several different premixed combinations containing 10% to 50% short-acting insulin and 70% to 50% intermediate-acting insulin are available. One example is the 30/70-unit combination insulin. The 30/70-insulin concentration means that there is 30% short-acting insulin and 70% intermediate-acting insulin in each unit. Therefore, if the physician orders 10 units of 30/70 insulin, the patient would receive 3 units of short-acting insulin (30% or 0.3×10 units $= 3$ units) and 7 units of intermediate-acting insulin (70% or 0.7×10 units $= 7$ units). If the physician orders 20 units of 30/70 insulin, the patient would receive 6 units of short-acting insulin ($0.3 \times 20 = 6$) and 14 units ($0.7 \times 20 = 14$) of intermediate-acting insulin.

The 50/50 insulin concentration means that there is 50% NPH insulin and 50% regular insulin in each unit. Therefore, if the physician prescribes 12 units of 50/50 insulin, the patient would receive 6 units of NPH insulin (50% or 0.5×12 units $= 6$ units) and 6 units of regular insulin (50% or $0.5 \times$ 12 units 5 6 units).

Insulin is usually administered by syringe but more frequently the use of a pen or pump (continuous subcutaneous insulin infusion [CSII]) is recommended and encouraged to be used. Insulin pen devices consist of prefilled pens and pens that take replaceable insulin cartridges that facilitate the use of multiple injections of insulin. CSII therapy is considered a safe and effective strategy to deliver intensive insulin therapy for select patients that may provide some advantages over other methods of intensive therapy. The pump is usually worn on a belt and resembles a standard pager. It is preprogrammed to deliver a continuous flow of short-acting insulin over 24 hours with a bolus amount at meal times. The pump is attached to a catheter in the subcutaneous tissue in the abdominal wall through a small plastic tube. Insulin mixes are not used in pumps.

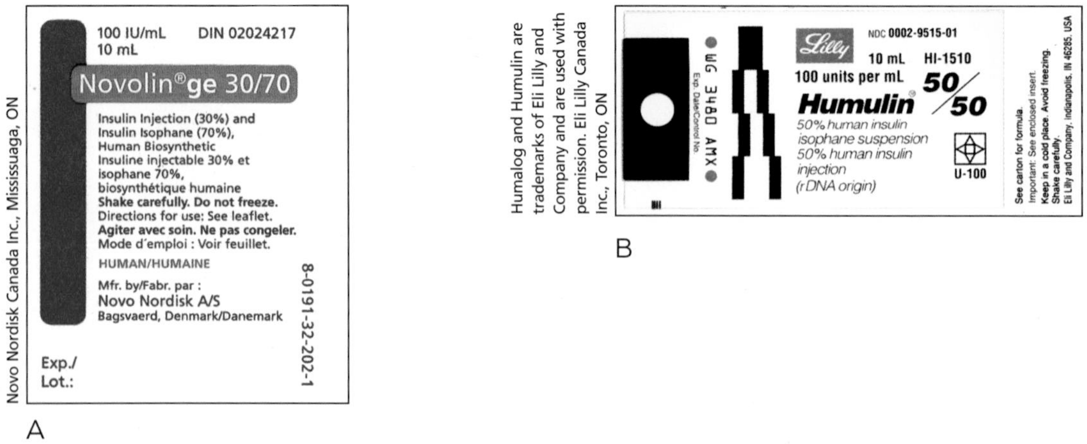
Novo Nordisk Canada Inc., Mississauga, ON
100 IU/mL DIN 02024217
10 mL
Novolin®ge 30/70
Insulin Injection (30%) and Insulin Isophane (70%), Human Biosynthetic
Insuline injectable 30% et isophane 70%, biosynthétique humaine
Shake carefully. Do not freeze.
Directions for use: See leaflet.
Agiter avec soin. Ne pas congeler.
Mode d'emploi : Voir feuillet.
HUMAN/HUMAINE
Mfr. by/Fabr. par :
Novo Nordisk A/S
Bagsvaerd, Denmark/Danemark
Exp./
Lot.:
8-0191-32-202-1
A
Humalog and Humulin are trademarks of Eli Lilly and Company and are used with permission. Eli Lilly Canada Inc., Toronto, ON
Lilly
NDC 0002-9515-01
10 mL HI-1510
100 units per mL
Humulin 50/50
50% human insulin isophane suspension
50% human insulin injection
(rDNA origin)
U-100
B

FIGURE 9-4 Examples of Premixed Combination Insulins

Interpreting the Insulin Order

Insulin orders must be written clearly and contain specific information to ensure correct administration and prevent errors. An insulin order should contain the following:

1. The *trade name, including the species and action time.* Patients are instructed to stay with the same manufacturer's trade-name insulin and species. Slight variations between trade names can affect an individual's response. Verify both the usual trade name used and the actual insulin supplied with the patient before administration. Different species of insulin may cause allergy-like symptoms in some patients, so check carefully. Look for one of the four action times: rapid-acting (lispro, aspart, glulisine), short-acting (Novolin ge Toronto, Humulin R), intermediate-acting (Humulin N, Novolin ge NPH), and long-acting (insulin glargine, insulin detemir).
2. The *supply dosage (concentration) and number of units* to be given; for example, 100-unit insulin 40 units.
3. The *route* of administration and *time or frequency.* All insulin may be administered by the subcutaneous route, and regular insulin may additionally be administered IV for management of ketoacidosis, intensive control of glucose in critical care, and treatment of hyperkalemia.

Examples:

Humulin R 100-unit insulin 14 units subcutaneous stat

Humulin N NPH 100-unit insulin 24 units subcutaneous 30 min before breakfast

Insulin Coverage—The "Sliding Scale"

A special insulin order is sometimes needed to "cover" a patient's increasing blood sugar level that is not yet regulated. A sliding scale consists of scheduled insulin plus supplemental insulin. Capillary blood glucose is checked QID for patients on insulin, 30 minutes prior to meals and at bed time (around 2130–2200). For patients who are on nothing by mouth (NPO), blood glucose is checked q4h (0400, 0800, 1200, 1600, 2000, 2400). *Only* regular insulin is used, because of its rapid action. The physician will specify the amount of insulin in units, which "slide" up or down based on the specific blood sugar level range. Sliding scales are individualized for each patient. The goal is to use as little sliding-scale insulin as possible. A sliding scale is not used during ketoacidosis or if a patient is on IV insulin. Following is an example of a sliding-scale order:

Example:

Order: *Humulin R 100-unit insulin subcutaneously based on glucose reading at 1600*

If the patient's blood glucose is 15 mmol/L, the nurse would administer 6 units of Humulin R 100-unit insulin.

Insulin Dose	Glucose Reading* mmol/L
No coverage	Glucose less than 8
2 units	10.1–12
4 units	12.1–14
6 units	14.1–16
8 units	16.1–18
10 units	18.1–20

*Glucose more than 20: Hold insulin; call MD stat.

Measuring Insulin in an Insulin Syringe

The insulin syringe and measurement of insulin were introduced in Chapter 5. This critical skill warrants attention again. Once you understand how insulin is packaged and how to use the insulin syringe, you will find insulin dosage simple.

> **RATIONALE FOR PRACTICE**
>
> - **Measure insulin in an insulin syringe only. Do not use a 3-mL or 1-mL syringe to measure insulin.**
> - **Use 100-unit insulin syringes to measure 100-unit insulin only. Do not measure other drugs supplied in units in an insulin syringe.**

Measuring insulin with the insulin syringe is simple. The insulin syringe makes it possible to obtain a correct dosage without mathematical calculation. Let us look at three different insulin syringes. They are the *standard* (100-unit) capacity and the *lo dose* (50-unit and 30-unit) capacity.

Standard 100-unit Insulin Syringe

Example:

The standard 100-unit insulin syringe in Figure 9-5 is a dual-scale syringe with 100-unit/mL capacity. It is calibrated on one side in *even*-numbered, 2-unit increments (2, 4, 6, . . .) with every 10 units labelled (10, 20, 30, . . .). It is calibrated on the reverse side in *odd*-numbered, 2-unit increments (1, 3, 5, . . .) with every 10 units labelled (5, 15, 25, . . .). The measurement of 73 units of 100-unit insulin is illustrated in Figure 9-5.

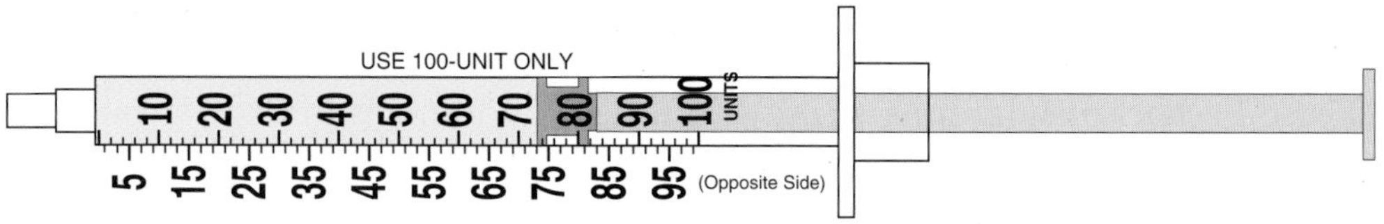

FIGURE 9-5 Standard 100-unit Insulin Syringe Measuring 73 units

> **CAUTION**
>
> Look carefully at the increments on the dual scale. The volume from one mark to the next (on either side) is 2 units. You are probably comfortable counting by 2s for even numbers. Pay close attention when counting by 2s with odd numbers.

Lo Dose 100-unit Insulin Syringes

Example 1:

The lo-dose 100-unit insulin syringe in Figure 9-6 is a single-scale syringe with 50-unit/0.5 mL capacity. It is calibrated in 1-unit increments with every 5 units (5, 10, 15, . . .) labelled up to 50 units. The enlarged 50-unit calibration of this syringe makes it easy to read and use to measure low dosages of insulin. To measure 32 units, withdraw 100-unit insulin to the 32-unit mark (Figure 9-6).

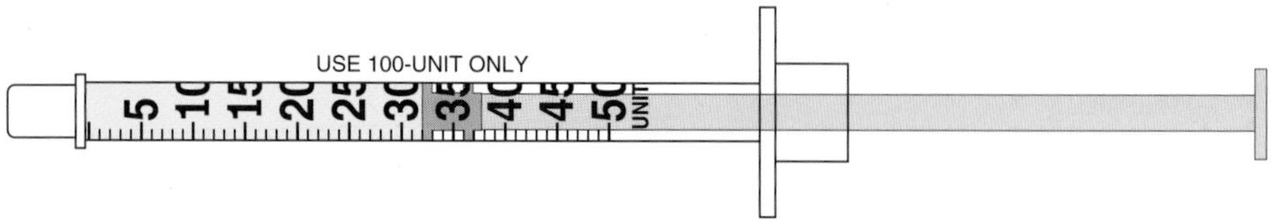

FIGURE 9-6 Fifty-unit Lo-dose 100-unit Insulin Syringe Measuring 32 Units

Example 2:

The lo-dose 100-unit insulin syringe in Figure 9-7 is a single-scale syringe with 30-unit/0.3 mL capacity. It is calibrated in 1-unit increments with every 5 units (5, 10, 15, . . .) labelled up to 30 units. The enlarged 30-unit calibration accurately measures very small amounts of insulin, such as for children. To measure 12 units, withdraw 100-unit insulin to the 12-unit mark (Figure 9-7).

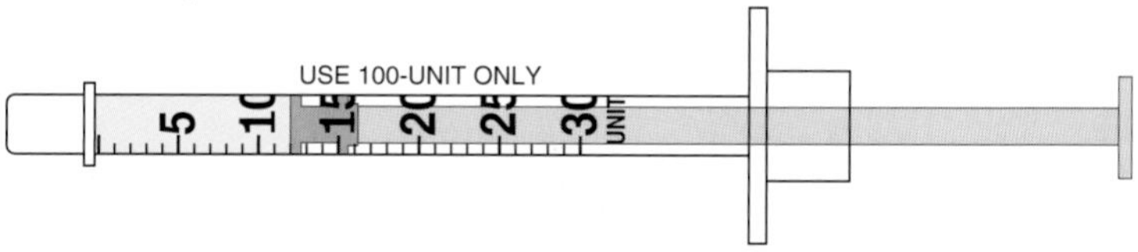

FIGURE 9-7 Thirty-unit Lo-dose 100-unit Insulin Syringe Measuring 12 Units

> **CAUTION**
>
> Always choose the *smallest*-capacity insulin syringe available for accurate insulin measurement. Use standard and lo-dose 100-unit syringes to measure 100-unit insulin *only*. Although the lo-dose 100-unit insulin syringes only measure a maximum of 30 or 50 units, they are still intended for the measurement of 100-unit insulin only.

Be cautious when measuring. The lo-dose 100-unit syringe is calibrated in 1-unit increments; the standard 100-unit insulin syringe is calibrated in 2-unit increments on the even and odd scales.

Combination Insulin Dosage

The patient may have two types of insulin prescribed to be administered at the same time. To avoid injecting the patient twice, it is common practice to draw up both insulins in the same syringe.

> **RATIONALE FOR PRACTICE**
>
> 1. **Draw up *clear insulin first*, then draw up cloudy insulin.**
> 2. **Regular insulin is clear. NPH insulin is cloudy.**
> 3. **Think:** ***First clear, then cloudy.*** **Think:** ***First short-acting regular, then NPH.***

Example 1:

Order: *Novolin ge Toronto 100-unit insulin 12 units with Novolin ge NPH 100-unit insulin 40 units subcutaneous before breakfast*

To accurately draw up both insulins into the same syringe, you will need to know the total units of both insulins: $12 + 40 = 52$ units. Withdraw 12 units of the short-acting Novolin ge Toronto 100-unit insulin (clear) and then withdraw 40 more units of the Novolin ge NPH 100-unit insulin (cloudy) up to the 52-unit mark (Figure 9-8). In this case, the smallest-capacity syringe you can use is the standard 100-unit insulin syringe. Notice that the NPH insulin is drawn up last and is closest to the needle in the diagram. In reality, the drugs mix right away.

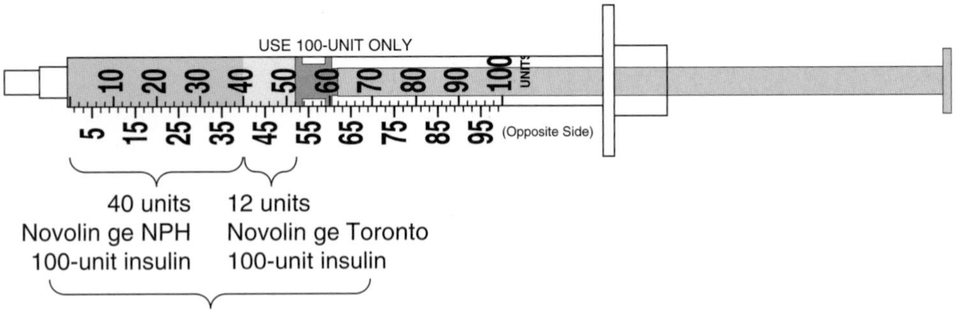

FIGURE 9-8 Combination Insulin Dosage

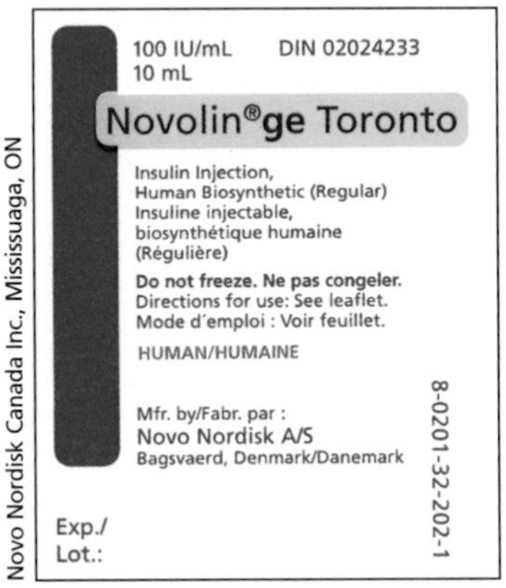

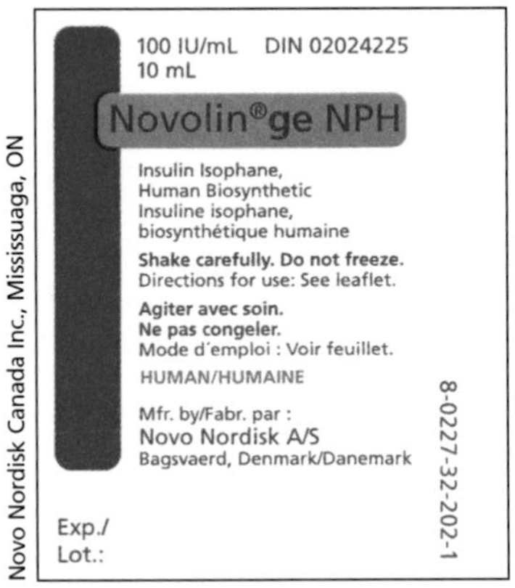

Example 2:

The physician orders *Novolin ge Toronto 100-unit insulin 10 units with Novolin ge NPH 100-unit insulin 30 units subcutaneous 30 min before dinner.*

This example gives step-by-step directions for this procedure. Look closely at Figures 9-9 and 9-10, which demonstrate the procedure below. Notice that to withdraw Novolin ge Toronto insulin (clear) first and then Novolin ge NPH insulin (cloudy), you must inject the dose amount of air into the Novolin ge NPH insulin *before* you inject the dose amount of air into the regular insulin.

1. Draw back and inject 30 units of air into the Novolin ge NPH insulin vial (cloudy liquid). Remove needle.
2. Roll the vial of the NPH insulin in your hands to mix; do not shake it. Draw back and inject 10 units of air into the Novolin ge Toronto insulin vial (clear liquid) and leave the needle in the vial.
3. Turn the vial of Novolin ge Toronto insulin upside down, and draw out the insulin to the 10-unit mark on the syringe. Make sure all air bubbles are removed.
4. Insert the needle into the Novolin ge NPH insulin vial, turn the vial upside down, and slowly draw back to the 40-unit mark, being careful not to exceed the 40-unit calibration. If more NPH insulin is withdrawn, discard and begin again with a new syringe. The cloudy solution contaminates the regular insulin and an accurate amount cannot be determined. Ten units of Novolin ge Toronto + 30 units of Novolin ge NPH = 40 units of insulin total (Figure 9-10).

CAUTION

If you withdraw too much of the cloudy insulin (Novolin ge NPH), you must discard the entire medication and start over. Recommended best practice is to double-check with another nurse when mixing insulin in a syringe. With a combined insulin medication, the nurse must be present to view steps 1–4 of the procedure.

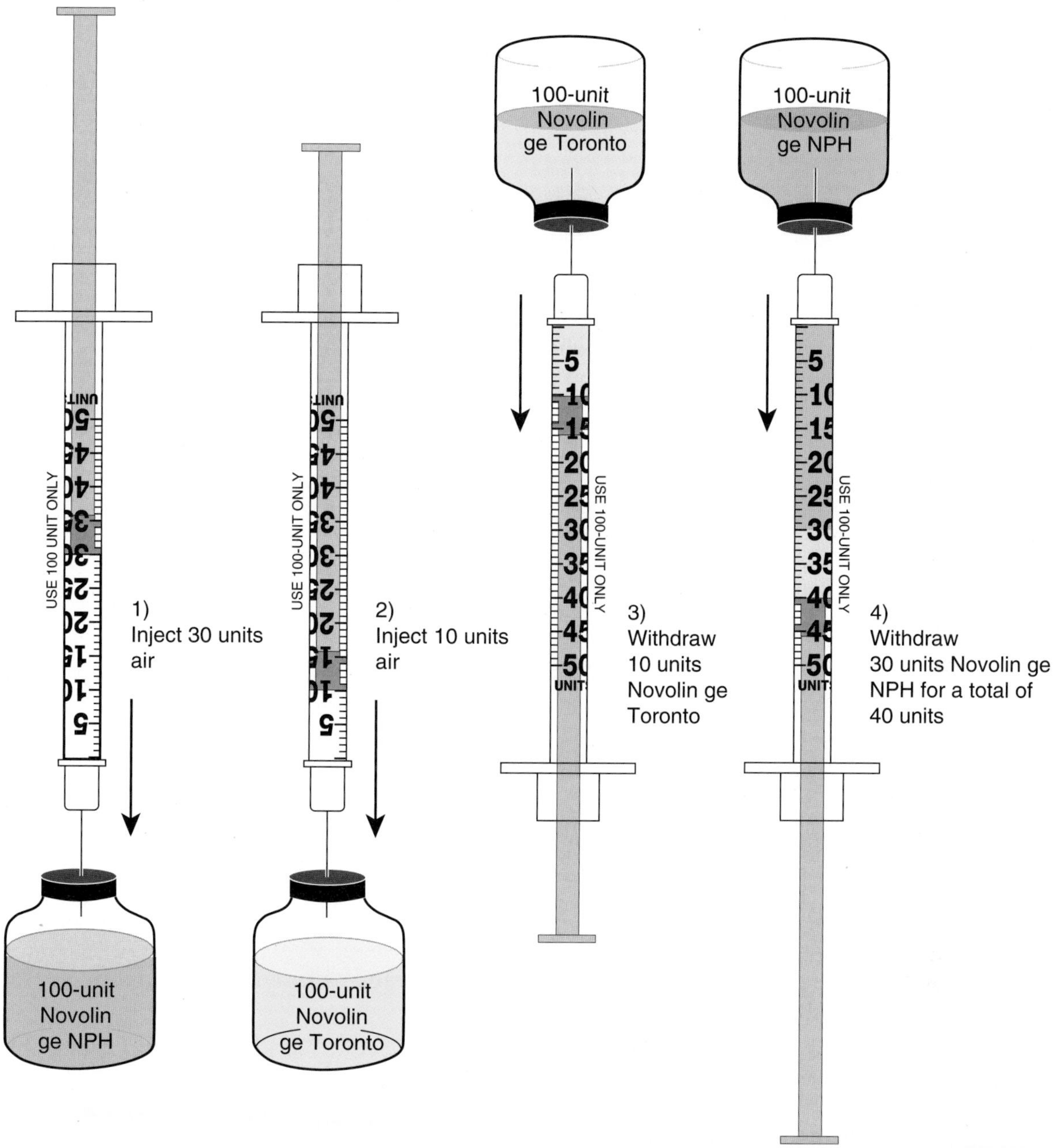

FIGURE 9-9 Procedure for Drawing Up Combination Insulin Dosage: 10 Units Novolin ge Toronto (short-acting) 100-unit Insulin with 30 Units Novolin ge NPH (intermediate-acting) 100-unit Insulin

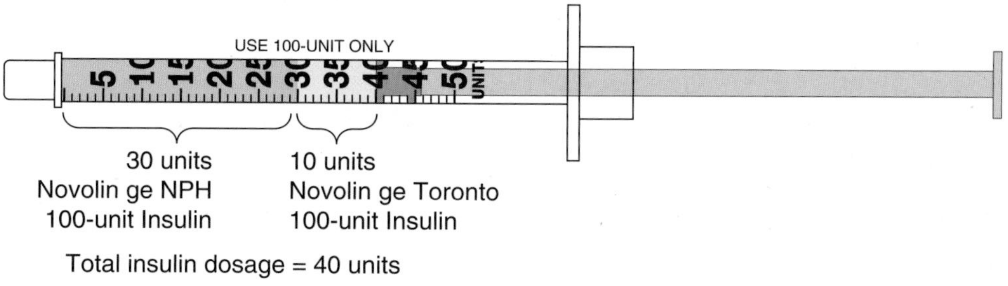

FIGURE 9-10 Combination Insulin Dosage

Avoiding Insulin Dosage Errors

Insulin dosage errors are serious and, unfortunately, too common. They can be avoided by following three important rules.

RATIONALE FOR PRACTICE

1. **Best practice recommendations are that two nurses check insulin dosages to prevent errors.**
2. **When combination dosages are prepared, best practice is that two nurses verify each step of the process.**
3. **In the community setting when a second nurse is not available, an alert patient or family member may do the second independent check.**

QUICK REVIEW

- Carefully read the patient care order, and match the supply dosage for type and species of insulin.
- Always measure insulin in an insulin syringe.
- An insulin syringe is used to measure insulin *only*. Insulin syringes must not be used to measure other medications measured in units.
- Use the smallest-capacity insulin syringe possible to most accurately measure insulin doses.
- When drawing up combination insulin doses, think *clear first, then cloudy*.
- Avoid insulin dosage errors. It is recommended that the insulin dosage should be checked by two nurses.
- There are 100 units per mL for 100-unit insulin.

REVIEW SET 23

Read the following labels. Identify the insulin brand name and its action time (rapid-acting, short-acting, intermediate-acting, or long-acting).

1. Insulin brand name ________

   Action time ________

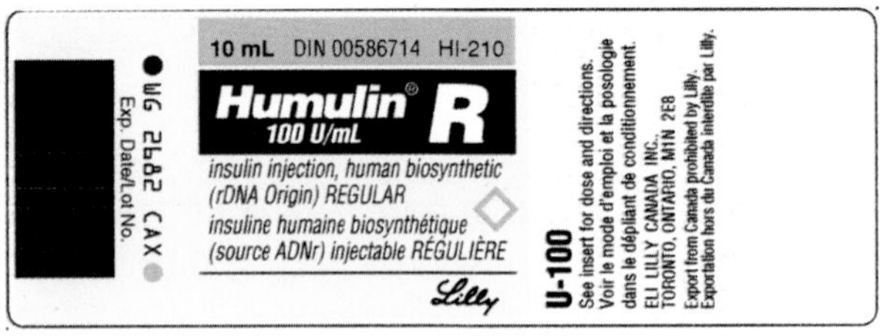
10 mL DIN 00586714 HI-210
Humulin® R
100 U/mL
insulin injection, human biosynthetic
(rDNA Origin) REGULAR
insuline humaine biosynthétique
(source ADNr) injectable RÉGULIÈRE
Lilly
U-100
Exp. Date/Lot No.

Humalog and Humulin are trademarks of Eli Lilly and Company and are used with permission. Eli Lilly Canada Inc., Toronto, ON

2. Insulin brand name ________

   Action time ________

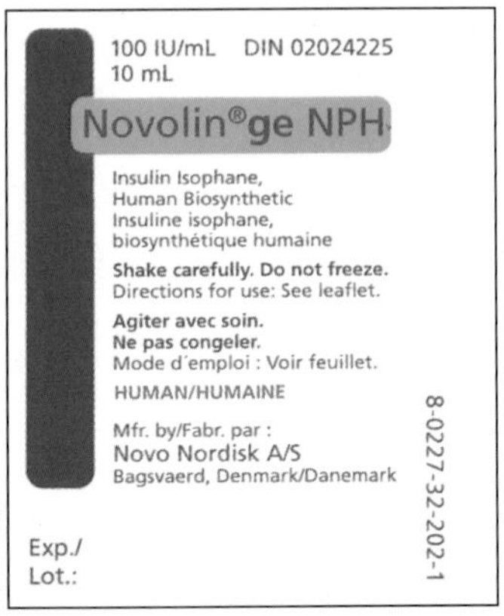
100 IU/mL DIN 02024225
10 mL
Novolin®ge NPH
Insulin Isophane,
Human Biosynthetic
Insuline isophane,
biosynthétique humaine
Shake carefully. Do not freeze.
Directions for use: See leaflet.
Agiter avec soin.
Ne pas congeler.
Mode d'emploi : Voir feuillet.
HUMAN/HUMAINE
Mfr. by/Fabr. par :
Novo Nordisk A/S
Bagsvaerd, Denmark/Danemark
Exp./
Lot.:
8-0227-32-202-1

Novo Nordisk Canada Inc., Mississauga, ON

3. Insulin brand name ________

   Action time ________

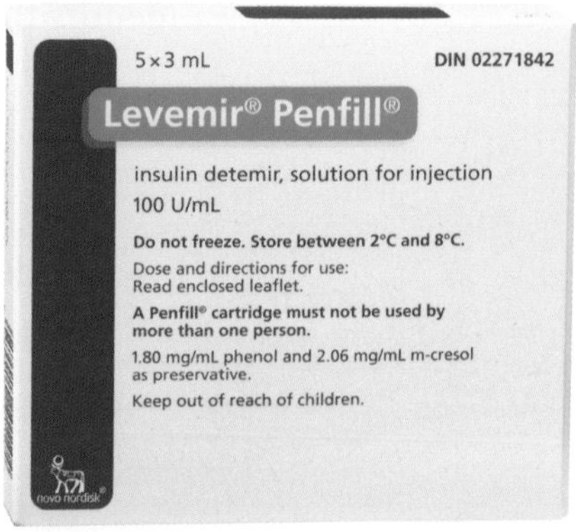
5 × 3 mL
DIN 02271842
Levemir® Penfill®
insulin detemir, solution for injection
100 U/mL
Do not freeze. Store between 2°C and 8°C.
Dose and directions for use:
Read enclosed leaflet.
A Penfill® cartridge must not be used by more than one person.
1.80 mg/mL phenol and 2.06 mg/mL m-cresol as preservative.
Keep out of reach of children.
novo nordisk

Novo Nordisk Canada Inc., Mississuaga, ON

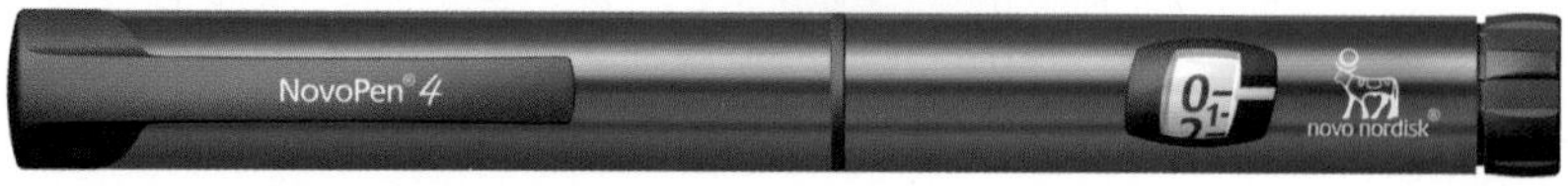
NovoPen® 4
novo nordisk®

Novo Nordisk Canada Inc., Mississuaga, ON

4. Insulin brand name ________

   Action time ________

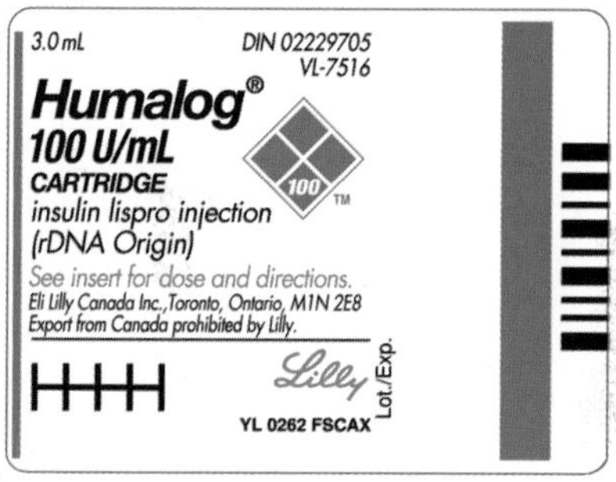
3.0 mL
DIN 02229705
VL-7516
Humalog®
100 U/mL
CARTRIDGE
insulin lispro injection
(rDNA Origin)
100
TM
See insert for dose and directions.
Eli Lilly Canada Inc., Toronto, Ontario, M1N 2E8
Export from Canada prohibited by Lilly.
Lilly
YL 0262 FSCAX
Lot./Exp.

Humalog and Humulin are trademarks of Eli Lilly and Company and are used with permission. Eli Lilly Canada Inc., Toronto, ON

5. Insulin brand name ________

   Action time ________

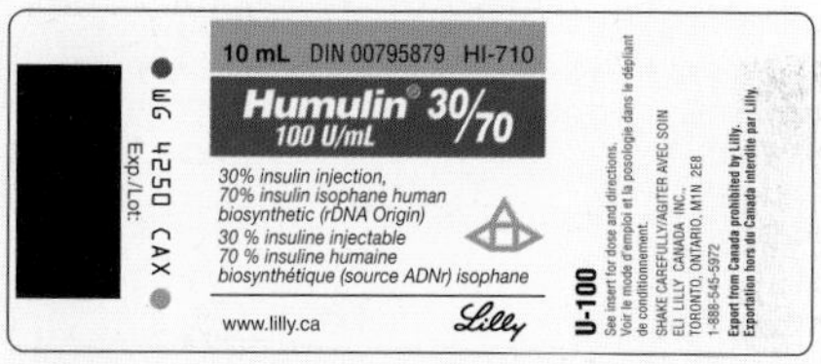
10 mL DIN 00795879 HI-710
Humulin® 30/70
100 U/mL
30% insulin injection,
70% insulin isophane human biosynthetic (rDNA Origin)
30 % insuline injectable
70 % insuline humaine biosynthétique (source ADNr) isophane
www.lilly.ca
Lilly
U-100
Exp./Lot:

Humalog and Humulin are trademarks of Eli Lilly and Company and are used with permission. Eli Lilly Canada Inc., Toronto, ON

6. Describe the three syringes available to measure 100-unit insulin. ____________________

   ____

7. What would be your preferred syringe choice to measure 24 units of 100-unit insulin?

   ____

8. What would be your preferred syringe choice to measure 35 units of 100-unit insulin?

   ____

9. There are 60 units of 100-unit insulin per ________ mL.

10. There are 25 units of 100-unit insulin per ________ mL.

11. Sixty-five units of 100-unit insulin should be measured in a(n) ________ syringe.

12. The 50 unit lo dose 100-unit insulin syringe is intended to measure 50-unit insulin only. ________ (True) (False)

Identify the 100-unit insulin dosage indicated by the coloured area of the syringe.

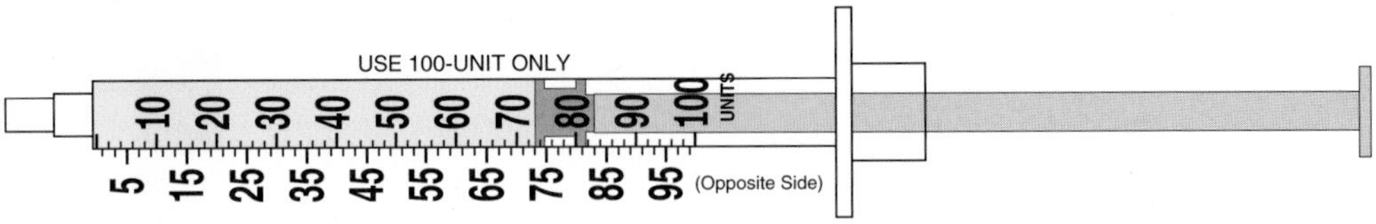

13. ________ units

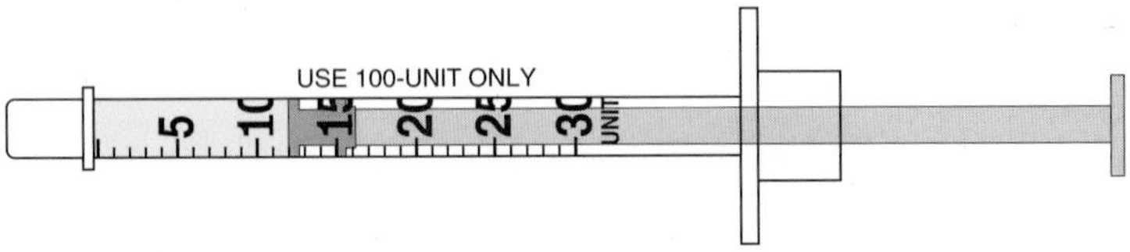

14. ________ units

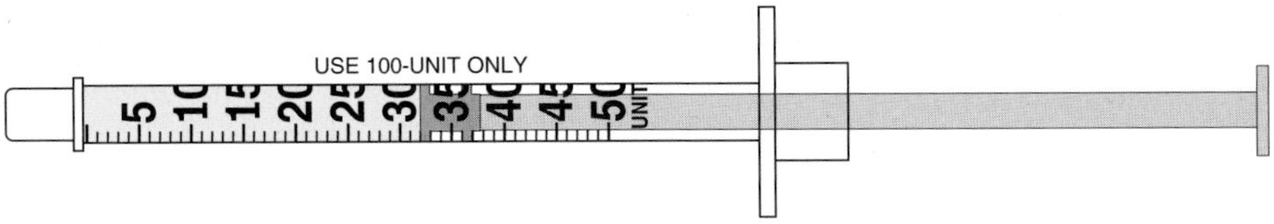

15. ________ units

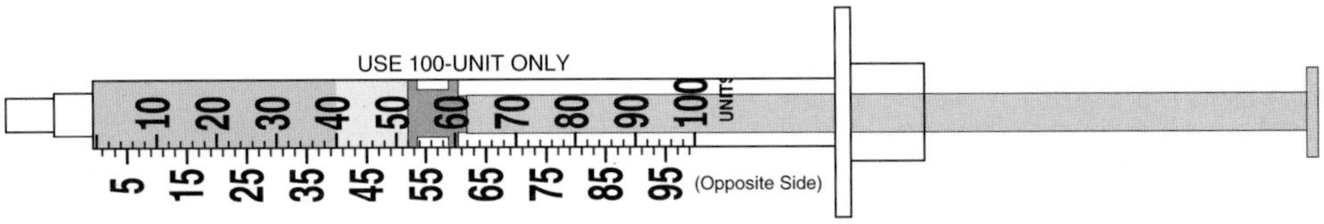

16. ________ units

Draw an arrow on the syringe to identify the given dosages.

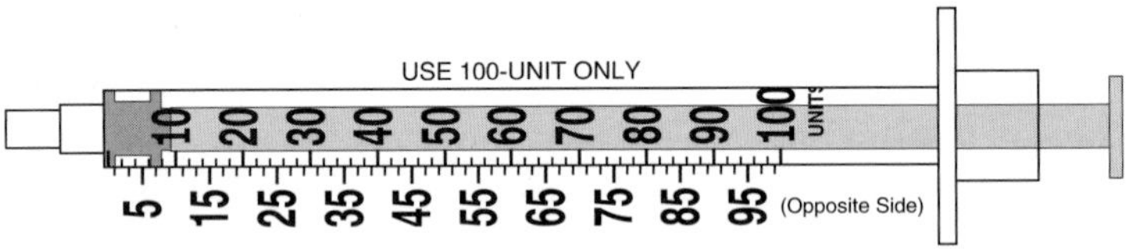

17. 80 units 100-unit insulin

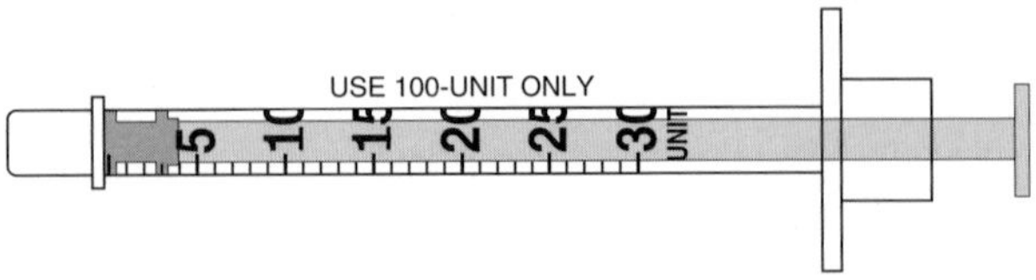

18. 15 units 100-unit insulin

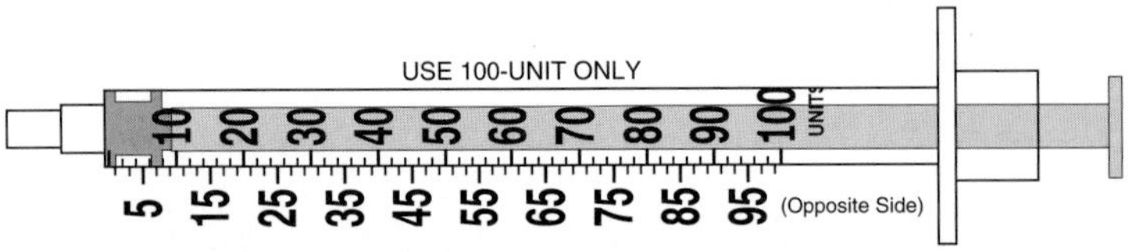

19. 66 units 100-unit insulin

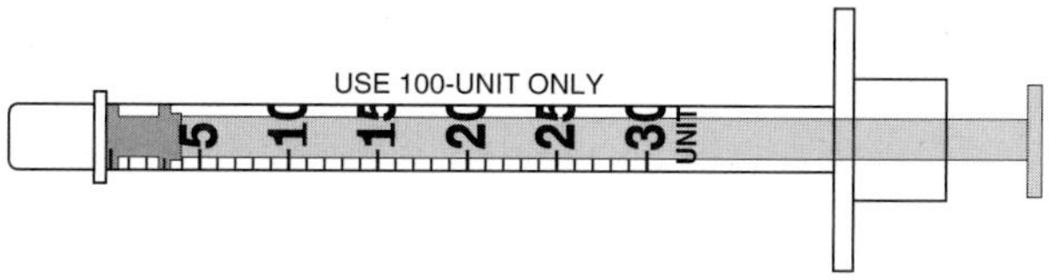

20. 16 units 100-unit insulin

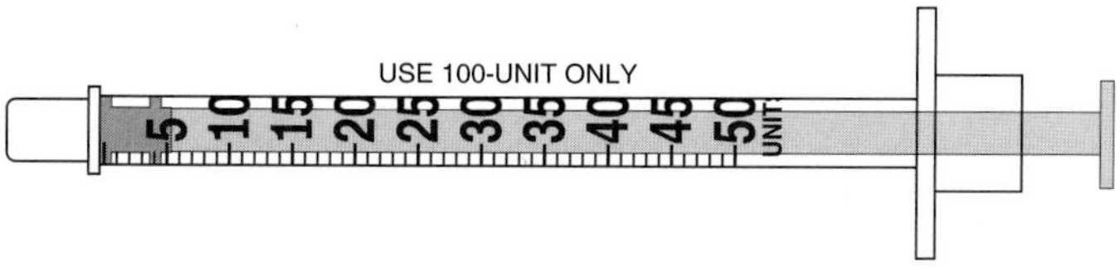

21. 32 units of 100-unit insulin

Draw arrows, and label the dosage for each of the combination insulin orders to be measured in the same syringe. Label and measure the insulins in the correct order, indicating which insulin will be drawn up first.

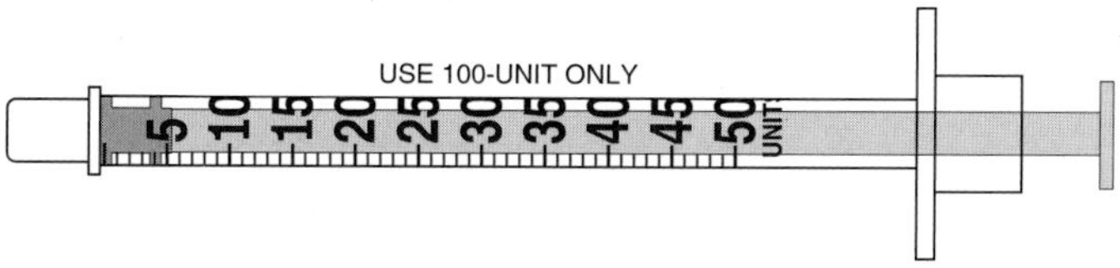

22. *Humulin R 100-unit insulin 21 units with Humulin N NPH 100-unit insulin 15 units subcutaneous stat*

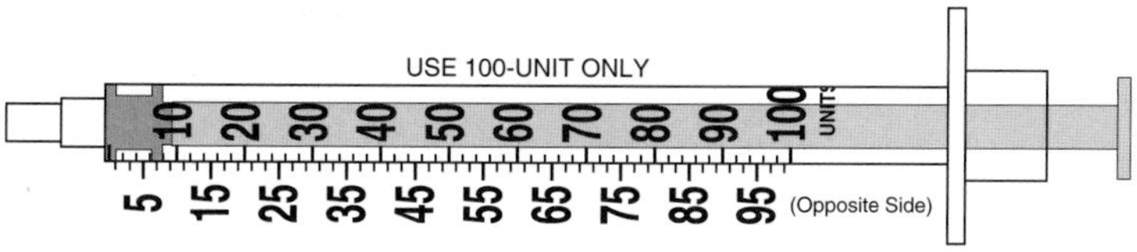

23. *NovoRapid 100-unit insulin 16 units with Novolin ge NPH 100-unit insulin 42 units subcutaneous stat*

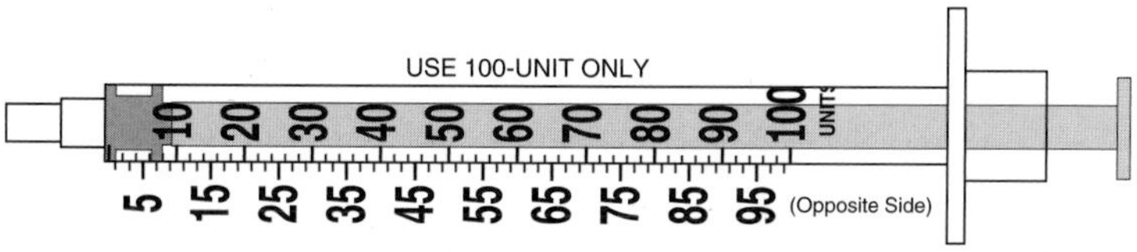

24. *Humulin R 100-unit insulin 32 units with Humulin N NPH 100-unit insulin 40 units subcutaneous before dinner*

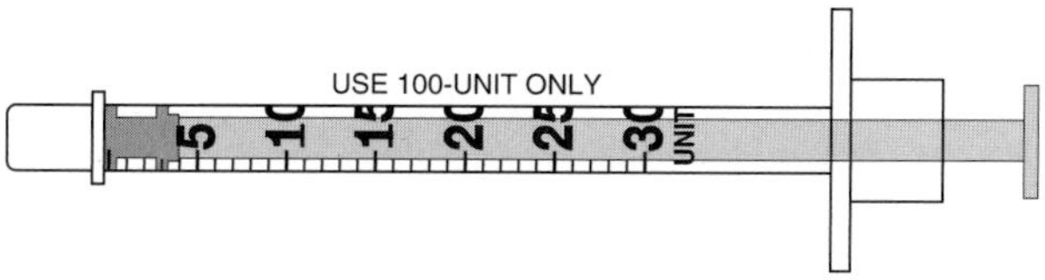

25. *Novolin ge Toronto 100-unit insulin 8 units with Novolin ge NPH 100-unit insulin 12 units subcutaneous stat*

Use the following insulin sliding scale and medication order to answer questions 26 through 30.

Insulin Sliding Scale

Insulin Dose	Glucose Reading* mmol/L
No coverage	Glucose less than 8
2 units	8.1–12
4 units	12.1–14
6 units	14.1–16
8 units	16.1–18
10 units	18.1–20

*Glucose more than 20: Hold insulin; call MD stat.

Order: *Humulin R 100-unit insulin subcutaneous before meals per sliding scale*

26. When will the nurse check the patient's blood glucose level to determine the amount of insulin to give? ______
27. At what range of blood glucose levels will the nurse administer insulin? ______
28. The patient's blood glucose level before breakfast is 13 mmol/L. What should the nurse do? ______
29. The patient's blood glucose level before lunch is 7.5 mmol/L. How much insulin should the nurse give now? ______
30. The patient's blood glucose level before dinner is 18.2 mmol/L. What should the nurse do now? ______

After completing these problems, see pages 473–474 to check your answers.

CRITICAL THINKING SKILLS

Many insulin errors occur when the nurse fails to clarify an incomplete order. Let us look at an example of an insulin error when the order did not include the type of insulin to be given.

error

Failing to clarify an insulin order when the type of insulin is not specified.

possible scenario

Suppose the physician wrote an insulin order this way:

Humulin 100-unit insulin 50 units before breakfast

Because the physician did not specify the type of insulin, the nurse assumed it was short-acting insulin and noted that on the medication administration record. Suppose the patient was given the short-acting insulin for 3 days. On the morning of the third day, the patient developed signs of hypoglycemia (low blood glucose), including shakiness, tremors, confusion, and sweating.

(continues)

(continued)

potential outcome

A stat blood glucose would likely reveal a dangerously low glucose level. The patient would be given a glucose infusion to increase the blood sugar. The nurse may not realize the error until she and the doctor check the original order and find that the incomplete order was filled in by the nurse. When the doctor did not specify the type of insulin, the nurse assumed the physician meant regular, which is short-acting, when in fact intermediate-acting NPH insulin was desired.

prevention

This error could have been avoided by remembering all the essential components of an insulin order: species, type of insulin (such as short-acting or NPH), supply dosage, the amount to give in units, and the frequency. When the nurse fills in an incomplete order, the nurse is essentially practising medicine outside the scope of practice. This would be a clear error of execution. It does not make sense to put you and your patient in such jeopardy. Communicating with the physician verbally or by phone would clarify the situation for everyone involved. Further, the nurse should have double-checked the dosage with another registered healthcare practitioner. Had the nurse done so, the error could have been discovered prior to administration.

SUMMARY

You are now prepared to solve many of the dosage calculations you will encounter in your healthcare career. Oral and parenteral drug orders, written in the forms presented thus far, account for a large percentage of prescriptions. You have learned to think through the process from order to supply to amount administered, and to apply the formula $\frac{D}{H} \times Q = X$.

Work the practice problems for Chapter 9. After completing the practice problems, you should feel comfortable and confident working dosage calculations. If not, seek additional instruction. Concentrate on accuracy. Remember, one error in dosage calculation can be a serious mistake for your patient.

PRACTICE PROBLEMS—CHAPTER 9

Calculate the amount you will prepare for one dose. Indicate the syringe you will select to measure the medication.

1. Order: *meperidine hydrochloride 20 mg IM q3h prn for pain*

   Supply: meperidine hydrochloride 50 mg/mL

   Give: ________ mL Select ________ syringe

2. Order: *morphine sulfate 15 mg IM stat*

   Supply: morphine sulfate 10 mg/mL

   Give: ________ mL Select ________ syringe

3. Order: *haloperidol 2.5 mg IV stat*

   Supply: haloperidol 5 mg/mL

   Give: ________ mL Select ________ syringe

4. Order: *hydroxyzine hydrochloride 20 mg IM stat*

   Supply: hydroxyzine hydrochloride 50 mg/mL

   Give: ________ mL Select ________ syringe

5. Order: *clindamycin 300 mg IM QID*

   Supply: clindamycin 150 mg/mL

   Give: ________ mL Select ________ syringe

6. Order: *naloxolone hydrochloride 0.3 mg IM stat*

   Supply: naloxolone hydrochloride 0.4 mg/mL

   Give: ________ mL Select ________ syringe

7. Order: *ketorolac tromethamine 20 mg IM q4h prn for pain*

   Supply: ketorolac tromethamine 30 mg/mL

   Give: ________ mL Select ________ syringe

8. Order: *midazolam 5 mg IM q4h prn for agitation*

   Supply: midazolam 5 mg/mL

   Give: ________ mL Select ________ syringe

9. Order: *ondansetron 8 mg IV over 15 min given 30 min prior to chemotherapy*

   Supply: ondansetron 2 mg/mL

   Give: ________ mL Select ________ syringe

10. Order: *chlorpromazine hydrochloride 25 mg IM stat*

    Supply: chlorpromazine hydrochloride 25 mg/mL

    Give: ________ mL Select ________ syringe

11. Order: *atropine sulfate 0.6 mg IM on call to the operating room*

    Supply: atropine sulfate 0.6 mg/mL

    Give: ________ mL Select ________ syringe

12. Order: *midazolam 3 mg IV stat*

    Supply: midazolam 10 mg/2 mL

    Give: ________ mL Select ________ syringe

13. Order: *heparin sodium 6000 units subcutaneous q12h*

    Supply: heparin sodium 10 000 units/mL vial

    Give: ________ mL Select ________ syringe

14. Order: *tobramycin sulfate 75 mg IM q8h*

    Supply: tobramycin sulfate 80 mg/2 mL

    Give: ________ mL Select ________ syringe

15. Order: *loxapine hydrochloride 12.5 mg q6h*

    Supply: loxapine hydrochloride, 50 mg/mL

    Give: ________ mL Select ________ syringe

16. Order: *atropine sulfate 0.4 mg IM on call to the operating room*

    Supply: atropine sulfate 0.4 mg/mL

    Give: ________ mL Select ________ syringe

17. Order: *enoxaparin sodium 40 mg subcutaneously BID*

    Supply: enoxaparin sodium 300 mg/mL multidose vial

    Give: ________ mL Select ________ syringe

18. Order: *penicillin G sodium 4 000 000 units stat*

    Supply: penicillinG sodium 5 000 000 units/mL

    Give: ________ mL Select ________ syringe

19. Order: *meperidine hydrochloride 60 mg IM q3h prn for pain*

    Supply: meperidine hydrochloride 75 mg/1.5 mL

    Give: ________ mL Select ________ syringe

20. Order: *dalteparin sodium 5000 units subcutaneously, preoperatively*

    Supply: dalteparin sodium 25 000 units/mL in a 3.8-mL, multi-dose vial

    Give: ________ mL Select: ________ syringe

21. Order: *cyanocobalamin 0.75 mg IM daily*

    Supply: cyanocobalamin 1000 mcg/mL

    Give: ________ mL Select ________ syringe

22. Order: *phytomenadione 15 mg IM stat*

    Supply: phytomenadione 10 mg per mL

    Give: ________ mL Select ________ syringe

23. Order: *promethazine hydrochloride 35 mg IM q4h prn for nausea and vomiting*

    Supply: promethazine hydrochloride 50 mg/1 mL

    Give: ________ mL Select ________ syringe

24. Order: *magnesium sulfate 500 mg IM stat*

    Supply: magnesium sulfate 1 g/2 mL

    Give: ________ mL Select ________ syringe

25. Order: *methylprednisolone acetate, 60 mg IM, daily for 1 week*

    Supply: methylprednisolone acetate 80 mg/mL

    Give: ________ mL Select ________ syringe

26. Order: *haloperidol 2.5 mg IV stat*

    Supply: haloperidol 5 mg/mL

    Give: ________ mL Select ________ syringe

27. Order: *furosemide 60 mg IV stat*

    Supply: furosemide 10 mg/mL

    Give: ________ mL Select ________ syringe

28. Order: *heparin sodium 4000 units subcutaneous q6h*

    Supply: heparin sodium 5000 units/mL

    Give: ________ mL Select ________ syringe

29. Order: *hydralazine hydrochloride 30 mg IV q6h*

    Supply: hydralazine hydrochloride 20 mg/mL

    Give: ________ mL Select ________ syringe

30. Order: *lidocaine hydrochloride 2% 50 mg IV stat*

    Supply: lidocaine hydrochloride 2% 20 mg/mL

    Give: ________ mL Select ________ syringe

31. Order: *verapamil hydrochloride 2.5 mg IV push stat*

    Supply: verapamil hydrochloride 5 mg/2 mL

    Give: ________ mL Select ________ syringe

32. Order: *phenytoin sodium 100 mg IV stat*

    Supply: phenytoin sodium 50 mg/mL

    Give: ________ mL Select ________ syringe

33. Order: *neostigmine methylsulfate 0.5 mg IM TID*

    Supply: neostigmine methylsulfate 1 mg/mL

    Give: ________ mL Select ________ syringe

34. Order: *amikacin sulfate 125 mg IV BID*

    Supply: amikacin sulfate 250 mg/mL

    Give: ________ mL Select ________ syringe

35. Order: *Humulin R 100-unit insulin 16 units subcutaneous*

    Supply: Humulin R 100-unit insulin, with standard 100-unit and lo dose 30 unit 100-unit insulin syringes

    Give: ________ units Select ________ syringe

36. Order: *Novolin ge NPH 100-unit insulin 25 units subcutaneous before breakfast*

    Supply: Novolin ge NPH 100-unit insulin with standard 100-unit and lo dose 50 units 100-unit insulin syringes

    Give: ________ units Select ________ syringe

Calculate one dose of each of the drug orders numbered 37 through 48. Draw an arrow on the syringe indicating the calibration line that corresponds to the dose to be administered. The labels are the medications you have available. Indicate dosages that must be divided.

37. *haloperidol 1.5 mg IM q8h*

Give: ________ mL

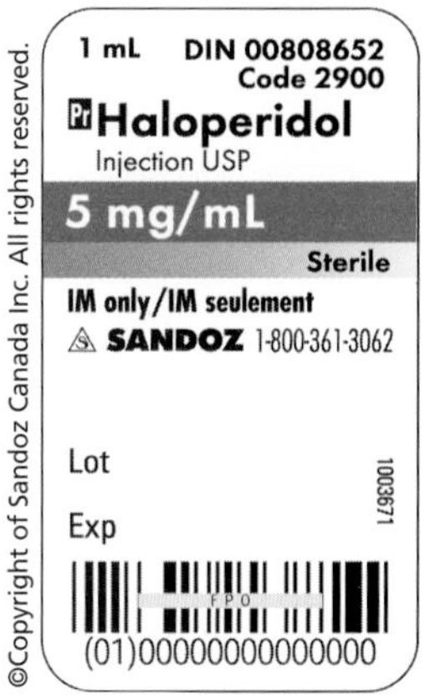

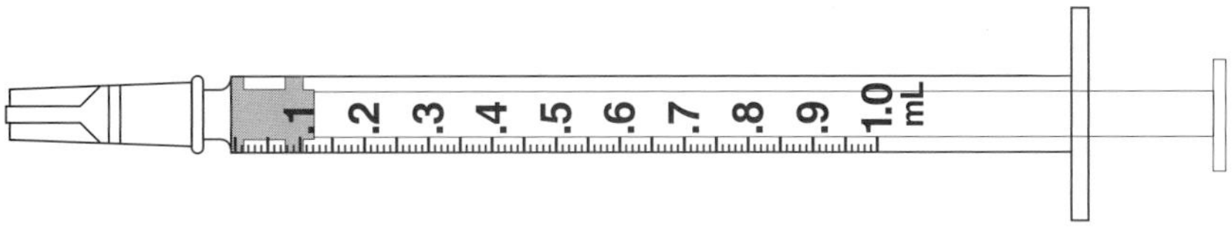

38. *chlorpromazine hydrochloride 40 mg IM q6h*

Give: ________ mL

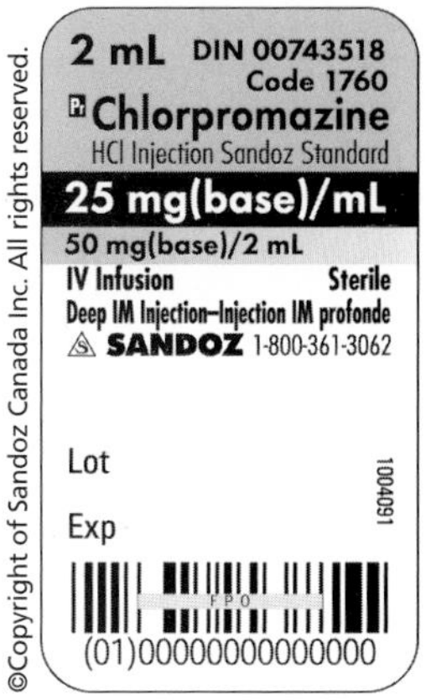

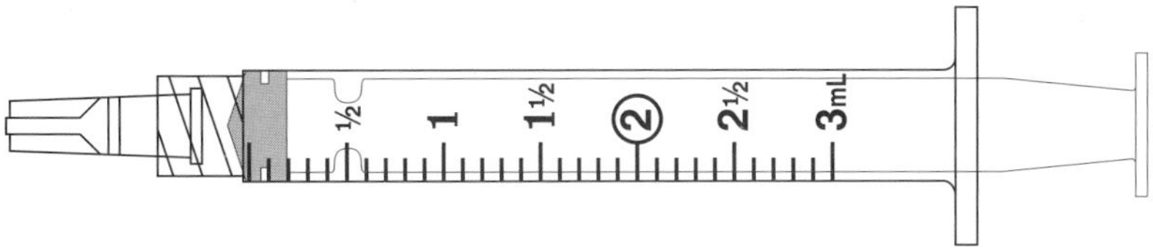

39. *midazolam 1 mg IV stat*

Give: ________ mL

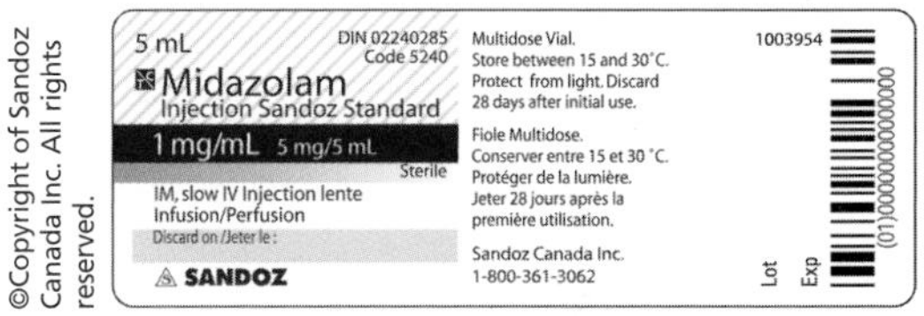

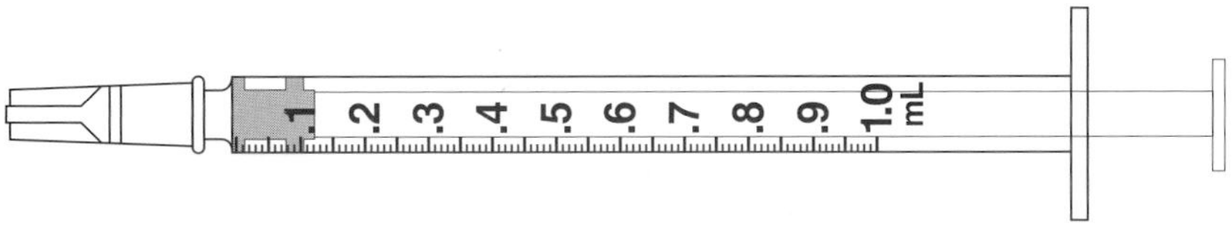

40. *tobramycin 80 mg IM q8h*

Give: ________ mL

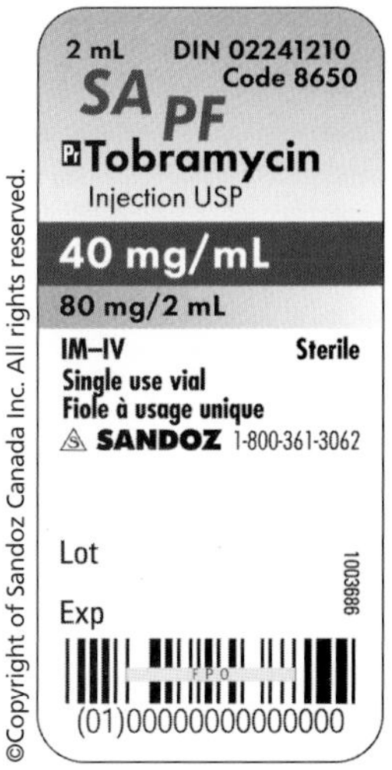

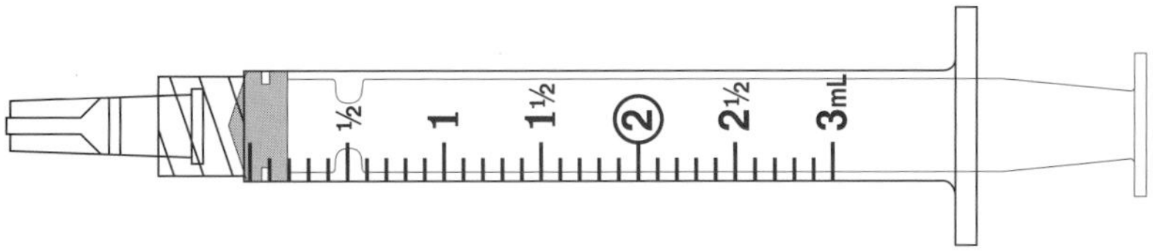

41. *epoetin alfa 12 000 units subcutaneous daily × 10 days*

Give: ________ mL

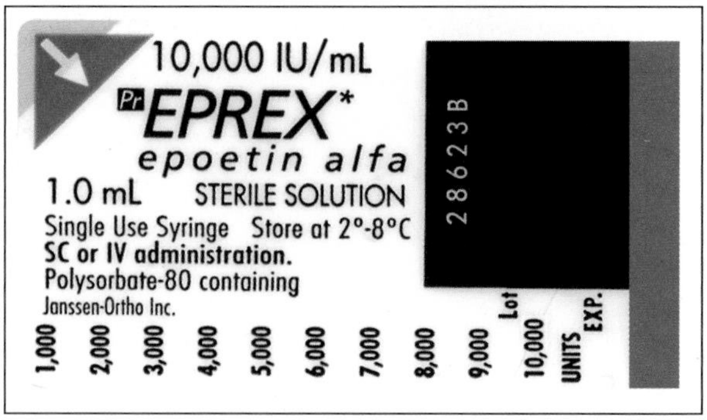
10,000 IU/mL
Pr EPREX*
epoetin alfa
1.0 mL STERILE SOLUTION
Single Use Syringe Store at 2°-8°C
SC or IV administration.
Polysorbate-80 containing
Janssen-Ortho Inc.
28623B
Lot
EXP.
1,000 2,000 3,000 4,000 5,000 6,000 7,000 8,000 9,000 10,000 UNITS

Janssen-Ortho Inc., Toronto, ON

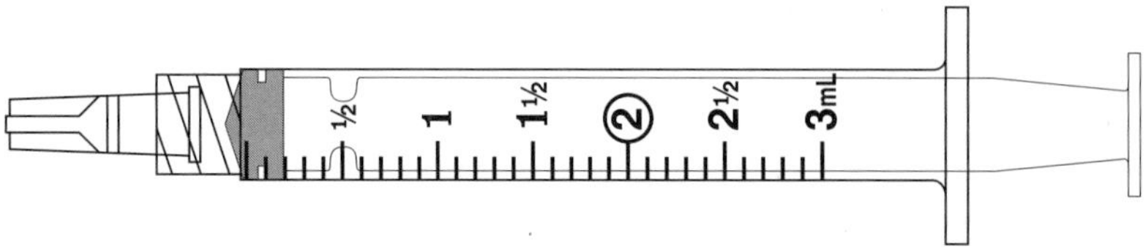
½ 1 1½ 2 2½ 3mL

42. *Humulin R 100-unit insulin 22 units subcutaneous stat*

Give: ________ units

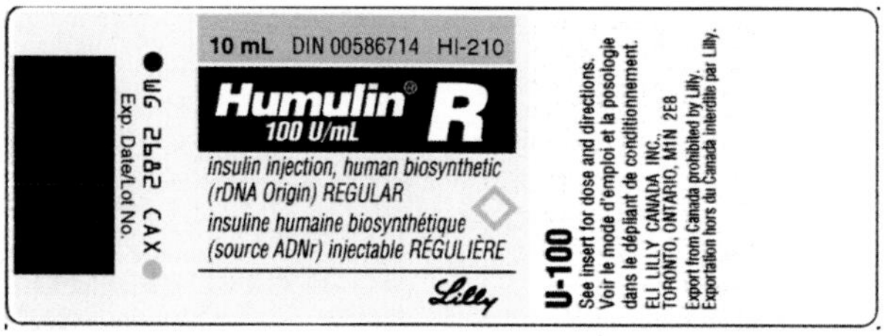
10 mL DIN 00586714 HI-210
Humulin® R
100 U/mL
insulin injection, human biosynthetic (rDNA Origin) REGULAR
insuline humaine biosynthétique (source ADNr) injectable RÉGULIÈRE
Lilly
Exp. Date/Lot No.
U-100
See insert for dose and directions.
Voir le mode d'emploi et la posologie dans le dépliant de conditionnement.
ELI LILLY CANADA INC. TORONTO, ONTARIO, M1N 2E8
Export from Canada prohibited by Lilly.
Exportation hors du Canada interdite par Lilly.

Humalog and Humulin are trademarks of Eli Lilly and Company and are used with permission. Eli Lilly Canada Inc., Toronto, ON

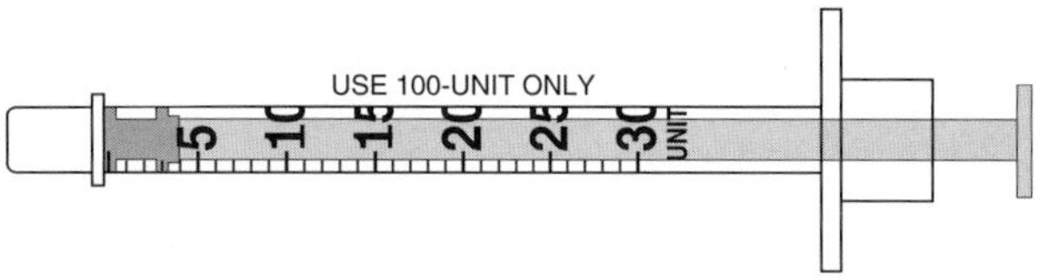
USE 100-UNIT ONLY
5 10 15 20 25 30 UNIT

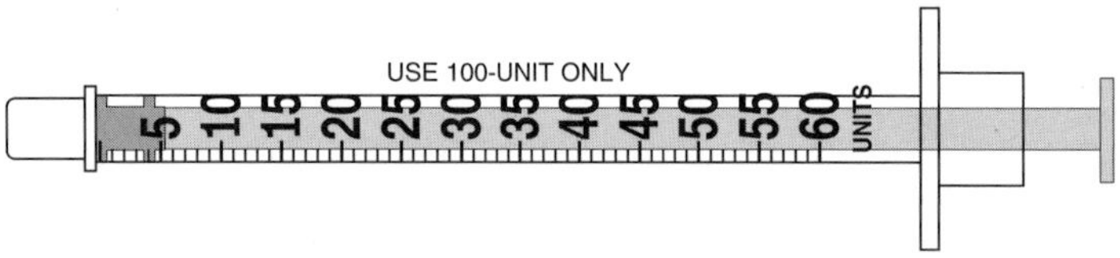
USE 100-UNIT ONLY
5 10 15 20 25 30 35 40 45 50 55 60 UNITS

43. *meperidine hydrochloride 60 mg IM q4h prn for pain*

Give:________ mL

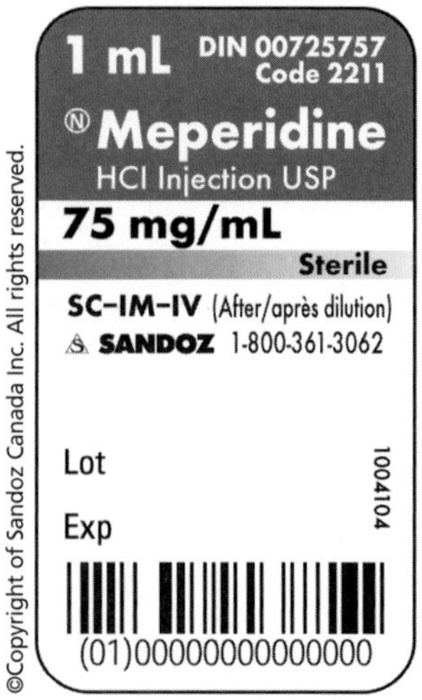
1 mL DIN 00725757 Code 2211
Ⓝ Meperidine
HCl Injection USP
75 mg/mL
Sterile
SC-IM-IV (After/après dilution)
SANDOZ 1-800-361-3062
Lot
Exp
1004104
(01)00000000000000
©Copyright of Sandoz Canada Inc. All rights reserved.

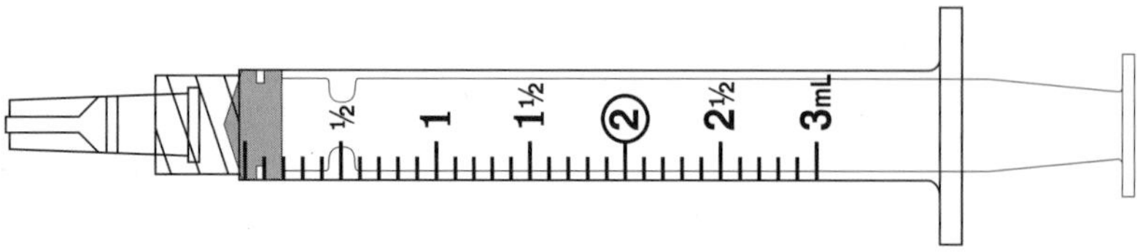
½ 1 1½ 2 2½ 3mL

44. *promethazine hydrochloride 15 mg IM q4h prn for nausea and vomiting*

Give: ________ mL

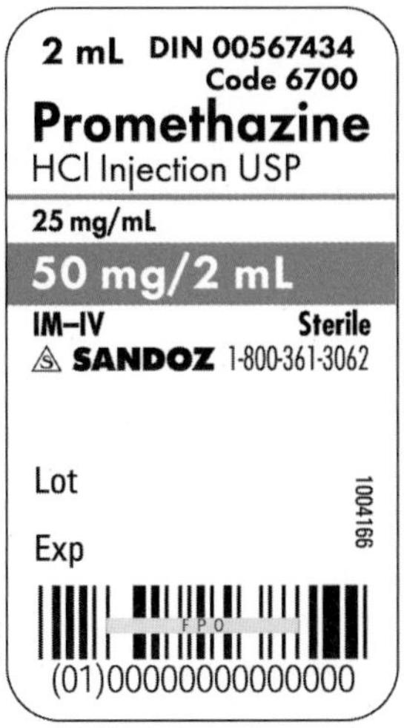

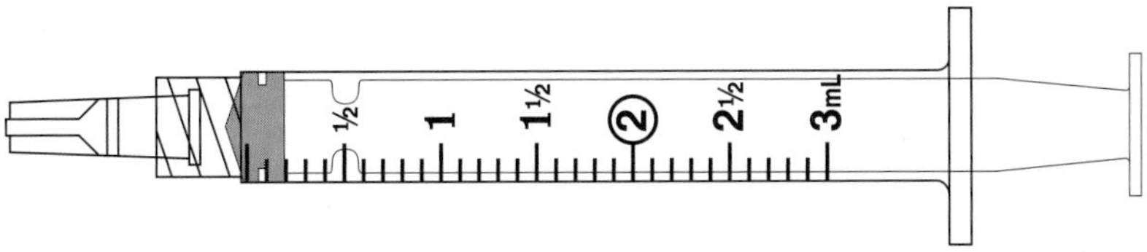

45. *metoclopramide hydrochloride 7 mg IM stat*

Give: ________ mL

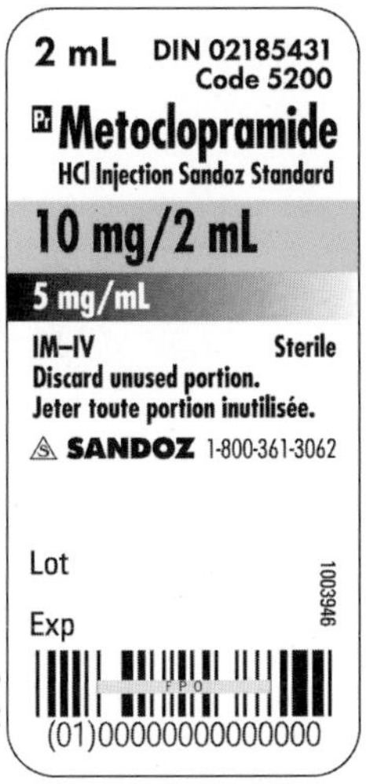

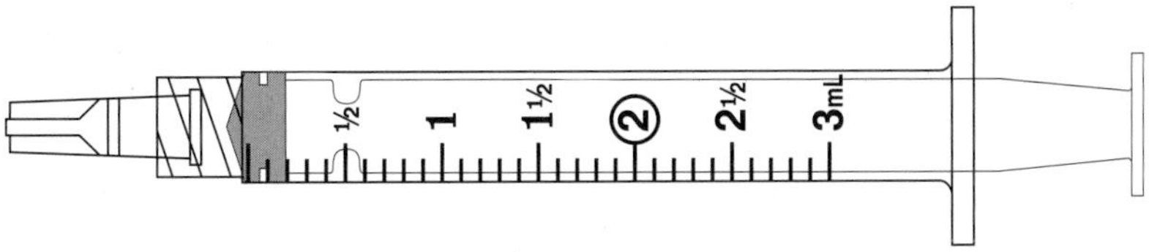

46. *filgrastim 225 mcg subcutaneous daily × 2 weeks*

Give: ________ mL

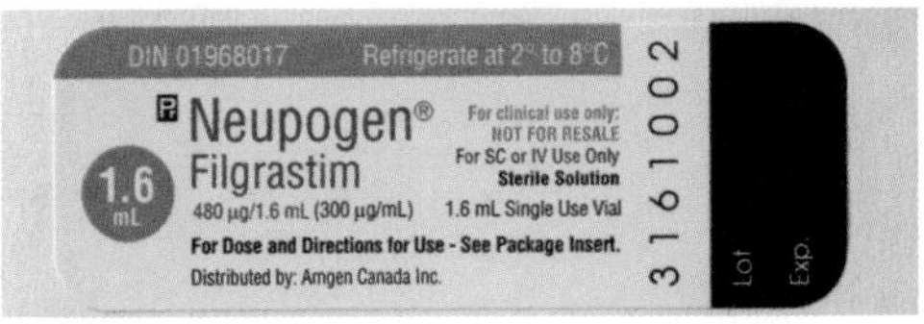

Amgen Canada Inc., Mississauga, ON

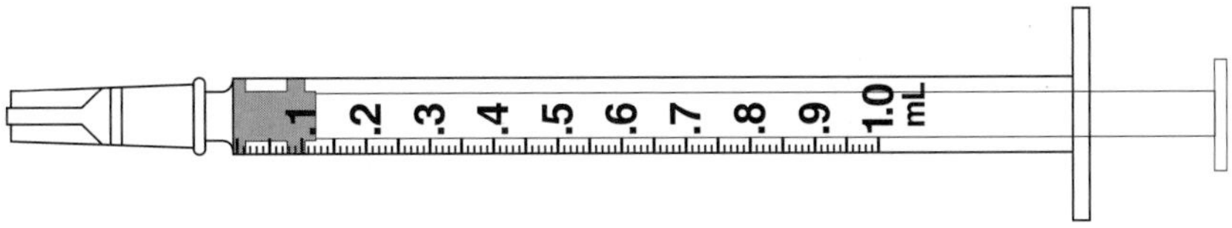

47. *Novolin ge Toronto 100-unit insulin 32 units with Novolin ge NPH 100-unit insulin 54 units subcutaneous before breakfast*

Give: ________ total units

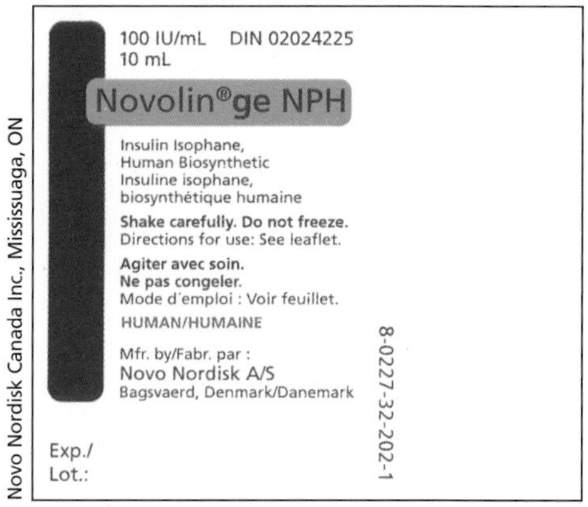

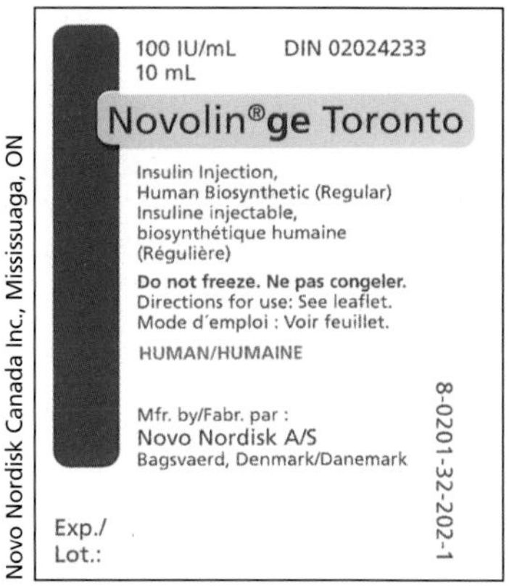

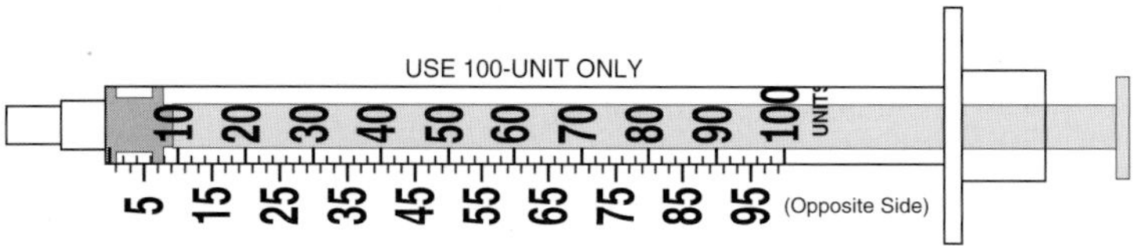

48. *Novolin ge 30/70 100-unit insulin 46 units subcutaneous before dinner*

Give: ________ units

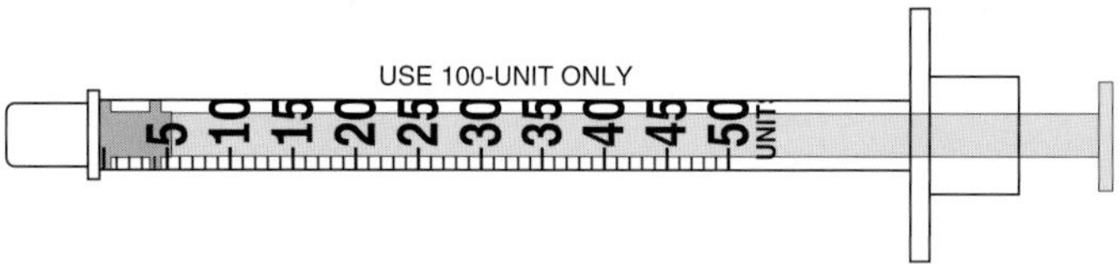

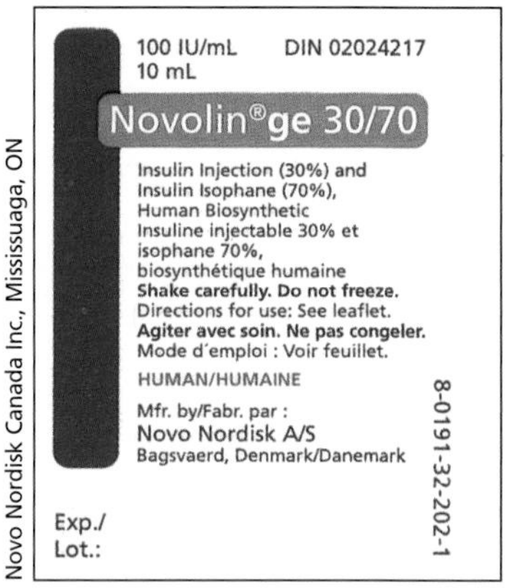

49. Critical Thinking Skill: Describe the strategy you would implement to prevent this medication error.

possible scenario

Suppose the physician ordered Humulin R 100-unit insulin 20 units mixed with Humulin N 100-unit insulin 40 units to be administered subcutaneously before breakfast. The nurse selected the vials of Humulin R and Humulin N 100-unit insulin from the medication drawer and injected 20 units of air in the Humulin N vial and 40 units of air in the Humulin R vial, drew up 40 units of Humulin R, and then drew up 20 units of Humulin N.

potential outcome

The patient received the incorrect dosage of insulin because the nurse drew up 40 units of Humulin R and 20 units of Humulin N instead of the dosage that was ordered: 20 units of Humulin R and 40 units of Humulin N. Because the patient received too much short-acting insulin (twice the amount ordered), the patient would likely show signs of hypoglycemia, such as shakiness, confusion, and diaphoresis.

prevention

____

____

50. Critical Thinking Skill: Describe the strategy you would implement to prevent this medication error.

possible scenario

Suppose the physician ordered 10 units of Novolin ge Toronto 100-unit insulin subcutaneous stat for a patient with a blood glucose of 17 mmol/L. The nurse selected the Novolin ge Toronto 100-unit insulin from the patient's medication drawer and selected a 1-mL syringe to administer the dose. The nurse looked at the syringe for the 10-unit mark and was confused as to how much should have been drawn up. The nurse finally decided to draw up 1 mL of insulin into the syringe, administered the dose, and then began to question whether the correct dosage was administered. The nurse called the supervisor for advice.

potential outcome

The patient would have received 10 times the correct dosage of insulin. Because this was a short-acting insulin, the patient would likely show signs of severe hypoglycemia, such as loss of consciousness and seizures.

prevention

____

____

After completing these problems, see pages 475–477 to check your answers.

CHAPTER

10

Reconstitution of Solutions

LEARNING OBJECTIVES

1. Define the terms *solvent*, *solute*, and *solution*.
2. Reconstitute and label medications supplied in powder or dry form.
3. Differentiate between varying directions for reconstitution and select the correct set to prepare the dosage ordered.
4. Calculate the amount of solute and solvent needed to prepare a desired strength and quantity of an irrigating solution or enteral feeding.

Some parenteral and oral medications are unstable in liquid form for long periods of time and are thus supplied in powder form to be mixed with a diluent or solvent before administration. As more healthcare is provided in the home setting, nurses and other healthcare workers will also need to dilute topical irrigants, soaks, and nutritional feedings that are available in both liquid concentrate and powder form. The process of adding a solvent or diluent to a medication in a powdered or liquid concentrate form to dissolve and create a solution is referred to as *reconstitution.*

The process of reconstitution is comparable to the preparation of hot chocolate from a powdered mix. Adding the correct amount of hot water (the *solvent* or *diluent*) to the package of powdered, hot chocolate drink mix (the *solute*) results in a tasty, hot beverage (the resulting *solution*).

The properties of solutions are important concepts to learn. These concepts will be applied again with the administration of intravenous solutions.

SOLUTION PROPERTIES

Refer to Figures 10-1 and 10-2 and define the terms of reconstitution.

- *Solute*—a substance to be dissolved or diluted. It can be in solid or liquid form.
- *Solvent*—a substance (liquid) that dissolves another substance to prepare a solution. *Diluent* is a synonymous term.
- *Solution*—the resulting mixture of a solute plus a solvent.

To prepare a therapeutic *solution*, it is necessary to *add a solvent or diluent* (often normal saline or water) *to a solute* (solid substance or concentrated stock solution) to obtain the required strength of a stated volume of a solution. This means that the solid substance or concentrate, the *solute*, is diluted with a *solvent* to obtain a reconstituted *solution* of a weaker strength. However, the amount of the drug that was in the pure solute or concentrated stock solution still equals the amount of pure drug in the diluted solution. Only the solvent has been added to the solute, expanding the total volume.

In Figure 10-1, the amount of pure drug (solute) remains the same in the concentrated form and in the resulting solution. However, in solution, notice the solute particles are dispersed or suspended throughout the resulting weaker solution. The particles evident in Figure 10-1 are for illustration purposes only. In a solution, the solute would be dissolved.

Amoxicillin trihydrate and clavulanic acid (a potassium salt) is an example of a solid solute that is available in a white to off-white powder form that must be reconstituted with purified water to provide an oral suspension. For example, 96 mL (solvent) of purified water is added to the powder (solute) in the 100 mL bottle size. The resulting solution contains 125 mg/31.25 mg per 5 mL concentration of reconstituted solution.

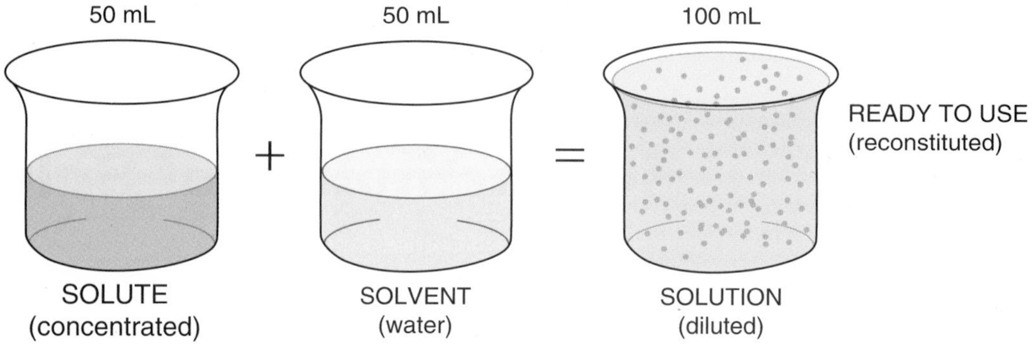

FIGURE 10-1 Concentrated Liquid Solute: 50 mL of concentrated solute is diluted with 50 mL of solvent to make 100 mL of diluted solution

The *strength of a solution* or *concentration* was briefly discussed in Chapters 7 and 8. Solution strength indicates the ratio of solute to solvent. Consider how each of these substances—solute and solvent—contributes a certain number of parts to the total solution.

Look at the azithromycin dihydrate 500 mg label (Figure 10-2). Reconstitution directions may be found on the label. Often, however, the nurse is referred to the package insert for detailed instructions for use. In the azithromycin dihydrate example, reconstitution instructions are found in the insert. The insert directions indicate that 4.8 mL of sterile water (*solvent*) should be added to the powder (*solid solute*) to prepare the reconstituted *solution.* As the label indicates, the resulting supply dosage would be 100 mg of azithromycin dihydrate per 1 mL of solution. It is also important to note that the prepared azithromycin must be further diluted in an appropriate diluent for intravenous administration. This is usual for a medication that is given intermittently using a larger amount of fluid and administered over a longer period of time.

Prepare the initial solution of **Zithromax** for injection by adding 4.8 mL of sterile water for injection to the 500-mg vial. Shake the vial until all of the drug is dissolved. Since the vial is evacuated, it is recommended that a standard 5-mL (non-automated) syringe be used to ensure that the exact volume of 4.8 mL is dispensed. Each mL of reconstituted solution contains azithromycin dihydrate equivalent to 100 mg azithromycin. Reconstituted solution is stable for 24 hours when stored below 30°C. **The reconstituted solution must be further diluted prior to administration.** Dilution of reconstituted solution: To provide azithromycin over a concentration range of 1.0–2.0 mg/mL, transfer 5 mL of the 100 mg/mL azithromycin solution into the appropriate amount of the following diluents:

Final Infusion Concentration (mg/mL)	**Amount of Diluent (mL)**
1.0 mg/mL	500 mL
2.0 mg/mL	250 mL

Appropriate Diluents
0.9% Sodium Chloride Injection
5% Dextrose in Water for Injection
0.45% Sodium Chloride Injection
Lactated Ringer's Injection
5% Dextrose in 0.45% Sodium Chloride Injection with 20 mEq Potassium Chloride
5% Dextrose in Lactated Ringer's Injection
5% Dextrose in 0.3% Sodium Chloride Injection
5% Dextrose in 0.45% Sodium Chloride Injection
Normosol-M in 5% Dextrose

Diluted solutions prepared in this manner are stable for 24 hours at or below room temperature (30°C), or for 72 hours if stored under refrigeration (5°C). As with all parenteral drug products, intravenous admixtures should be inspected visually for clarity, particulate matter, precipitate, discoloration, and leakage prior to administration, whenever solution and container permit. Solutions showing haziness, particulate matter, precipitate, discoloration, or leakage should be discarded.

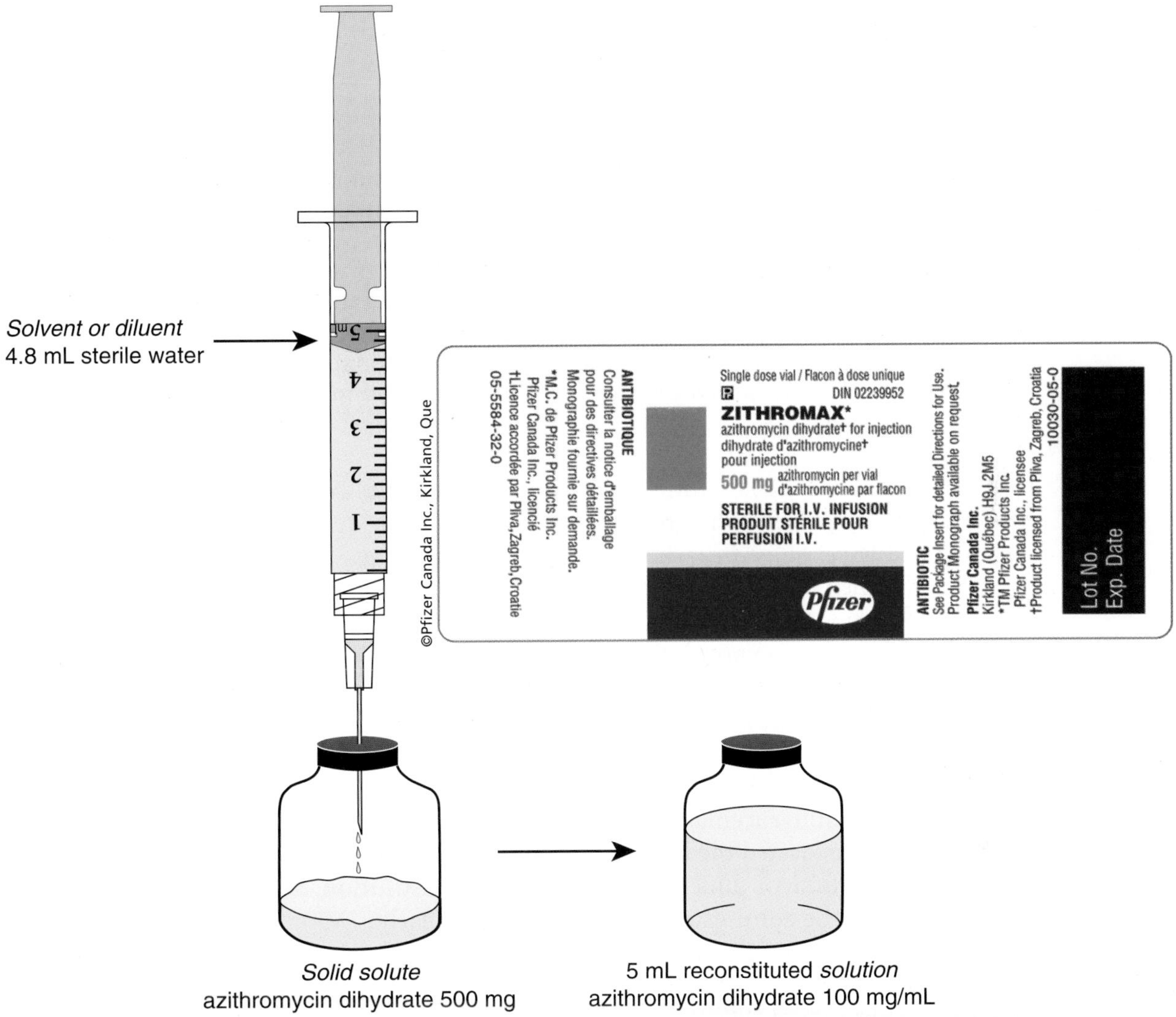

FIGURE 10-2 Solid Solute: The solid powder form of 500 mg of azithromycin dihydrate is reconstituted with 4.8 mL of sterile water as the diluent to make 5 mL of azithromycin dihydrate IV solution with the supply dosage of 100 mg/mL

RECONSTITUTION OF INJECTABLE MEDICATIONS IN POWDER FORM

As already mentioned, some medications are unstable when stored in solution or liquid form. Thus they are packaged in powdered form and must be dissolved or *reconstituted* by a liquid *solvent or diluent* and mixed thoroughly. Reconstitution is a necessary step in medication preparation to create a measurable and usable dosage form. The pharmacist often does this before dispensing liquid medications, for oral as well as parenteral routes. However, nurses need to understand the process of reconstitution. Some medications must be prepared by the nurse just prior to administration, as they become unstable when stored.

CAUTION

Before reconstituting injectable drugs, read and follow the label or package insert directions carefully. Consult a pharmacist with *any* questions.

There are standard principles for reconstituting injectable medications from powder to liquid form. Follow these principles carefully to ensure that the patient receives the intended solution.

RATIONALE FOR PRACTICE

When reconstituting injectable medications, determine both the *type* and *amount* of diluent to be used. Carefully read the instructions for reconstitution on either the drug label or the package insert. The manufacturer of the drug will provide information about the amount of diluent or solvent to be added, as well as the type of diluent. The concentration of the reconstituted drug is also indicated on the label. Lastly, the expiration date or the time the drug remains usable will be provided. Remember that the route of administration may influence the amount of diluent to be used for reconstitution (e.g., a drug may have different concentrations depending on whether it is intended for IV or IM use).

Sterile water and 0.9% sodium chloride (normal saline) prepared for injection are most commonly used as diluents (solvent) in parenteral medications. Both sterile water (Figure 10-3) and normal saline are available *preservative-free* when intended for a single use only, as well as in *bacteriostatic* form with preservative when intended for more than one use. Carefully check the instructions and vial label or drug insert for the appropriate diluent. Some oral powdered medications may be diluted with tap or distilled water. In addition, some powdered medications are packaged by the manufacturer with special diluents for reconstitution (e.g., octreotide acetate [powder] comes with a prefilled syringe of diluent).

Some drugs are available in double-chambered vials with powder in the lower chamber and a diluent in the upper chamber. By pressing the rubber stopper on the top of the container, the rubber is dislodged, releasing the diluent, which mixes with the drug in the lower chamber (e.g., Act-O-Vial system for methylprednisolone sodium succinate).

Once you have located the instructions for reconstitution on the label or insert, you need to identify the type and volume of diluent to be used for reconstitution. Because many reconstituted parenteral medications can be administered either intramuscularly (IM) or intravenously (IV), it is essential to verify the route of administration before reconstituting the medication. Remember that the IM volume of 5 mL or less per injection site is determined by the patient's age and condition and the IM site selected. The directions take this into account by stating the minimum volume or quantity of diluent that should be added to the powdered drug for IM use.

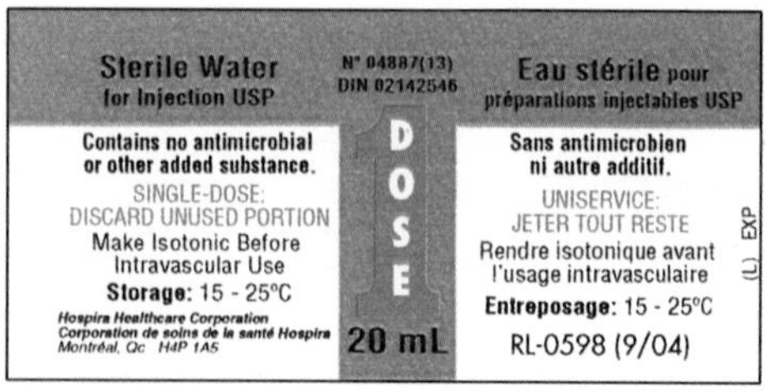

FIGURE 10-3 Reconstitution Diluent for Parenteral Powdered Drugs

RATIONALE FOR PRACTICE

When reconstituting injectable medications, determine the *volume in mL* of diluent to be used for the route as ordered, then reconstitute the drug and *note the resulting supply dosage* on the vial.

Examine the directions on the cefazolin label (Figure 10-4): "Reconstitution: IM: add 2 mL Sterile Water for Injection or 0.9% Sodium Chloride Injection. Provides 225 mg/mL." Note that when 2 mL of diluent is added and the powder is dissolved, the weight of the powder, or powder volume, adds an additional 0.2 mL for a total solution volume of 2.2 mL. (The amount of diluent added will vary with each medication.) Thus, the supply dosage available after reconstitution is *225 mg of cefazolin per mL of solution.* Figure 10-4 demonstrates the reconstitution procedure for cefazolin 500 mg, to fill the order of *cefazolin 225 mg IM q6h.*

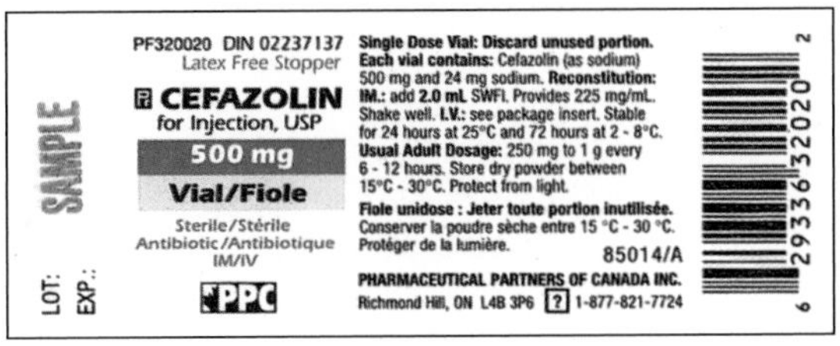

Pharmaceutical Partners of Canada Inc., Richmond Hill, ON

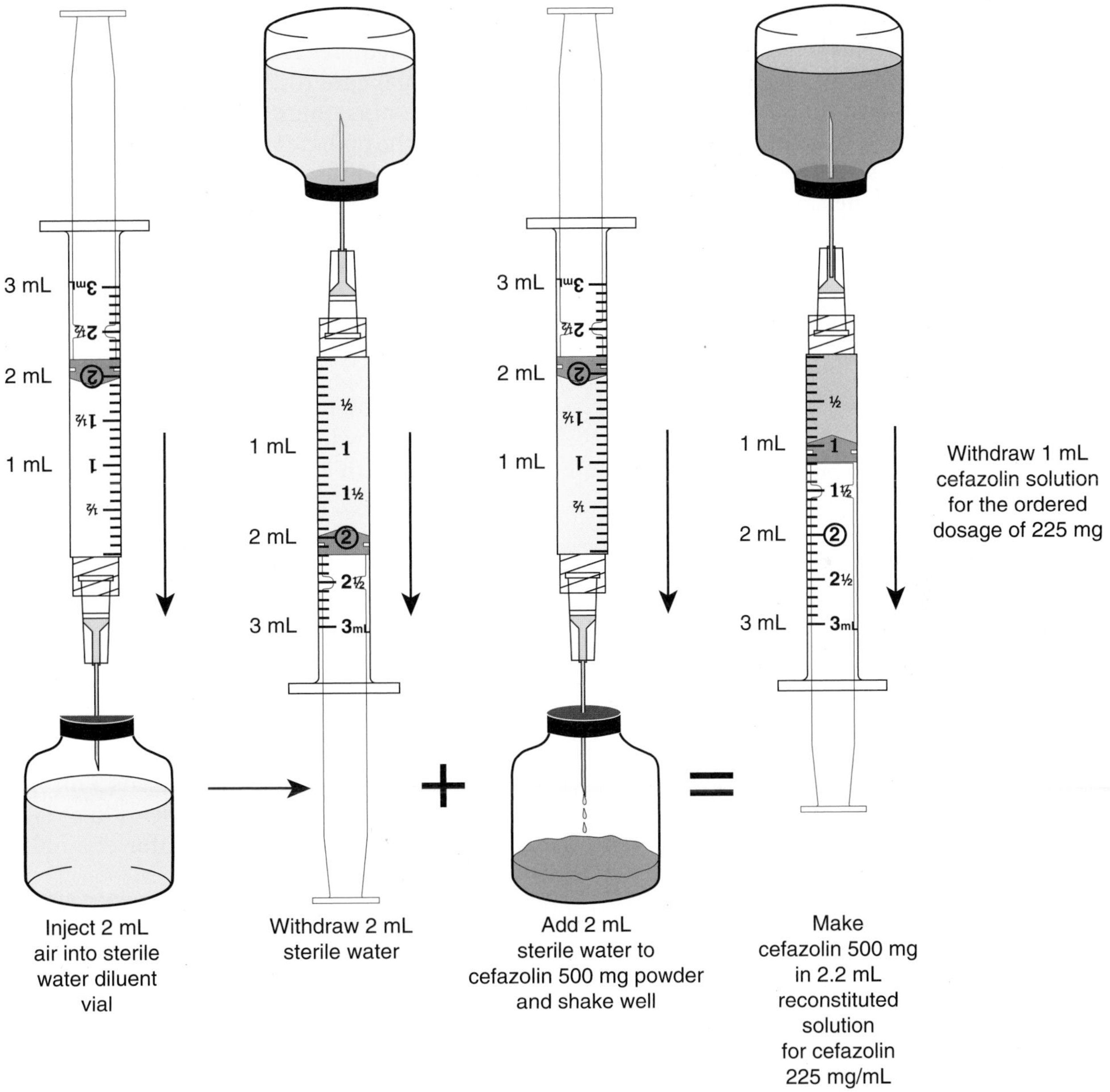

FIGURE 10-4 Cefazolin Reconstitution Procedure to Fill the Order *cefazolin 225 mg IM q6h*

Single-dose vials contain only enough medication for one dose, and the resulting contents are administered after the powder is diluted. But in some cases the nurse also may dilute a powdered medication in a multiple-dose vial that will yield more than one dose. When this is the case, it is important to clearly label the vial after reconstitution. Labelling is discussed in the next section.

TYPES OF RECONSTITUTED PARENTERAL SOLUTIONS

There are two types of reconstituted parenteral solutions: single strength and multiple strength. The simplest type to dilute is a *single-strength* solution. This type usually has the recommended dilution directions and resulting supply dosage printed on the label, such as the cefazolin 500 mg label in Figure 10-4 (page 225) and the azithromycin dihydrate insert in Figure 10-5.

Some medications have several directions for dilution that allow the nurse to select the best supply dosage. This is called a *multiple-strength* solution and requires even more careful reading of the instructions, such as the penicillin G sodium label shown in Figure 10-7 (page 230). Because these directions for reconstitution will not fit on the vial label, the nurse must consult the package insert or other printed instructions to ensure accurate dilution of the parenteral medication.

Let us look at some examples to clarify what the healthcare professional needs to do to correctly reconstitute and calculate dosages of parenteral medications supplied in powder form.

Single-Strength Solution/Single-Dose Vial

Example:

Order: *azithromycin dihydrate 400 mg IV daily × 2 days*

Supply: 500-mg vial of powdered azithromycin dihydrate with directions on package insert as follows: "Reconstitute to 100 mg/mL with 4.8 mL of sterile water for injection" (Figure 10-5).

Carefully sort through and analyze the information provided on the label.

- First, how much and what type of diluent must you add? The directions indicate to *add 4.8 mL of sterile water.*
- Second, what is the resulting supply dosage or concentration? When reconstituted, the *supply dosage is azithromycin dihydrate 100 mg/mL.*
- Third, what is the resulting total volume of the reconstituted solution? The *total volume is 5 mL.* The powder added 0.2 mL to the solution. This is because the supply dosage is 100 mg/mL and you added 4.8 mL of diluent. Therefore, it is only logical that the total volume is 5 mL.
- Finally, to fill the order as prescribed, how many full doses are available in this vial? The order is for 400 mg and the single-dose vial contains 500 mg. This is enough for one full dose, but not enough for two full doses. Two doses would require 800 mg.

Now, let us put it all together.

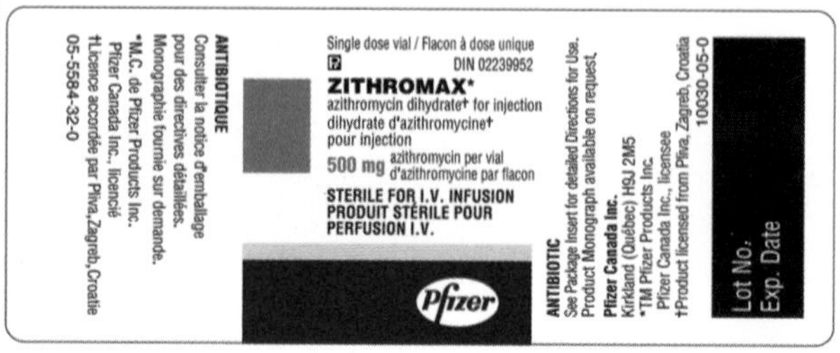

RECONSTITUTION DIRECTIONS

ZITHROMAX for Injection:

RECONSTITUTION OF ZITHROMAX FOR INJECTION				
Strength	Reconstitution Solution	Volume to be Added	Approximate Volume Available	Nominal Concentration
500 mg	Sterile water for injection	4.8 mL	5 mL	100 mg/mL

Prepare the initial solution of **ZITHROMAX** for injection by adding 4.8 mL of sterile water for injection to the 500-mg vial. Shake the vial until all of the drug is dissolved. Since the vial is evacuated, it is recommended that a standard 5-mL (non-automated) syringe be used to ensure that the exact volume of 4.8 mL is dispensed. Each mL of reconstituted solution contains azithromycin dihydrate equivalent to 100 mg azithromycin. Reconstituted solution is stable for 24 hours when stored below 30°C. **The reconstituted solution must be further diluted prior to administration.**

Dilution of reconstituted solution: To provide azithromycin over a concentration range of 1.0–2.0 mg/mL, transfer 5 mL of the 100 mg/mL azithromycin solution into the appropriate amount of the following diluents:

Final Infusion Concentration (mg/mL)	Amount of Diluent (mL)
1.0 mg/mL	500 mL
2.0 mg/mL	250 mL

Appropriate Diluents

0.9% Sodium Chloride Injection
5% Dextrose in Water for Injection
0.45% Sodium Chloride Injection
Lactated Ringer's Injection
5% Dextrose in 0.45% Sodium Chloride Injection with 20 mEq Potassium Chloride
5% Dextrose in Lactated Ringer's Injection
5% Dextrose in 0.3% Sodium Chloride Injection
5% Dextrose in 0.45% Sodium Chloride Injection
Normosol-M in 5% Dextrose

Diluted solutions prepared in this manner are stable for 24 hours at or below room temperature (30°C), or for 72 hours if stored under refrigeration (5°C). As with all parenteral drug products, intravenous admixtures should be inspected visually for clarity, particulate matter, precipitate, discoloration, and leakage prior to administration, whenever solution and container permit. Solutions showing haziness, particulate matter, precipitate, discoloration, or leakage should be discarded.

Only limited data are available on the compatibility of **ZITHROMAX** for injection with other intravenous substances; therefore additives or other medications should not be added to **ZITHROMAX** for injection or infused simultaneously through the same intravenous line. If the same intravenous line is used for sequential infusion of several different drugs, the line should be flushed before and after infusion of **ZITHROMAX** for injection with an infusion solution compatible with **ZITHROMAX** for injection and with any other drug(s) administered via the common line. If **ZITHROMAX** for injection is to be given concomitantly with another drug, each drug should be given separately in accordance with the recommended dosage and route of administration for each drug.

AVAILABILITY OF DOSAGE FORMS

Composition:

ZITHROMAX for injection contains azithromycin dihydrate equivalent 500 mg of azithromycin per vial. The non-medicinal ingredients include the following: 384.6 mg anhydrous citric acid and 198.3 wig sodium hydroxide for pH adjustment. After reconstitution, each mL contains azithromycin dihydrate equivalent to 100 mg azithromycin (see **DOSAGE AND ADMINISTRATION, Reconstitution Directions** section).

Stability and Storage Recommendations:

ZITHROMAX for injection:

Dry powder: Store at controlled room temperature (15–30°C).

Diluted Solution: Stable for 24 hours at or below 30°C, or for 72 hours if stored under refrigeration (5°C). For single-use only. Discard any unused portion after use.

ZITHROMAX for injection 500 mg: Each vial contains azithromycin dihydrate in a lyophilized form equivalent to 500 mg azithromycin for injection. Provides 500 mg/5 mL (100 mg/mL) azithromycin when reconstituted as directed. Cartons of 10 single-dose vials.

FIGURE 10-5 Azithromycin Dihydrate Label and Reconstitution Instructions from the Package Insert

Available is a vial of 500 mg of azithromycin dihydrate to which you will add 4.8 mL of sterile water as the diluent. The powdered drug displaces 0.2 mL. The resulting 5 mL of the solution contains 500 mg of the drug, and there is 100 mg of azithromycin dihydrate in each 1 mL of solution.

After reconstitution, you are ready to apply the same three steps of dosage calculation that you learned in Chapters 8 and 9.

Step 1 Convert No conversion necessary

Order: *azithromycin dihydrate 400 mg IV daily × 2 days*

Supply: 100 mg/mL

Step 2 Think You want to give more than 1 mL. In fact, you want to give four times 1 mL.

Step 3 Calculate $\frac{D}{H} \times Q = \frac{\overset{4}{\cancel{400}}\,\text{mg}}{\underset{1}{\cancel{100}}\,\text{mg}} \times 1\,\text{mL} = \frac{4}{1}\,\text{mL} = 4\,\text{mL}$

Give 4 mL azithromycin dihydrate reconstituted to 100 mg/mL, intravenously each day for 2 days.

This vial of azithromycin dihydrate 500 mg contains only one full ordered dose of reconstituted drug. Any remaining medication is usually discarded. Because this vial provides only one dose, no label or storage of any of the reconstituted drug is required.

CAUTION:

The reconstituted vial must be further diluted prior to administration. The 4 mL prescribed dosage can be withdrawn from the vial of 100 mg/mL azithromycin solution and injected into the appropriate amount (either 250 mL or 500 mL) of the appropriate diluent (see insert) and then infused into the patient over a specified time/rate once daily for 2 days.

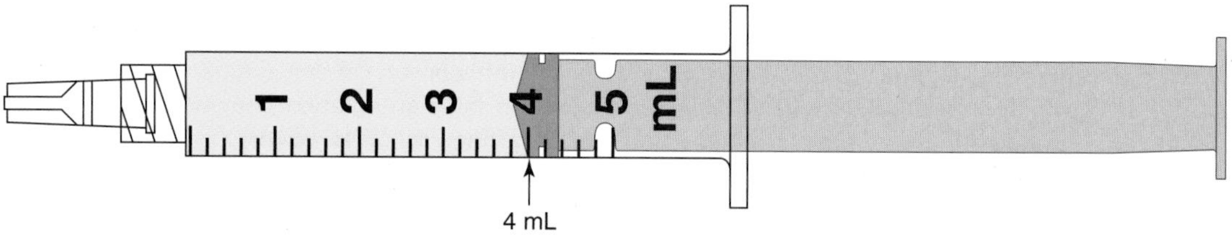

RATIONALE FOR PRACTICE

Single-use vials should only be used for one patient and one procedure, with a new, clean needle and syringe. The vial and syringe should be wasted and discarded at the end of the procedure.

Single-Strength Solution/Multiple-Dose Vial

A multi-dose vial is a bottle of liquid medication (injectable) that contains more than one dose of medication. A multi-dose vial contains antibacterial preservatives and according to manufacturer's instructions can be used more than once. The multiple use of medication vials is limited to products that are known to remain stable and retain potency for at least 24 hours under refrigeration.

Example:

Suppose the drug order reads *azithromycin dihydrate 250 mg IV daily*. Using the same size vial of azithromycin dihydrate and the same dilution instructions as in the previous example, you would now have two full doses of azithromycin dihydrate, or a multiple-dose vial.

$$\frac{D}{H} \times Q = \frac{25\cancel{0}\,\cancel{mg}}{10\cancel{0}\,\cancel{mg}} \times 1\,mL = 2.5\,mL$$

Select a 3-mL syringe and measure 2.5 mL of azithromycin dihydrate reconstituted to 100 mg/mL.

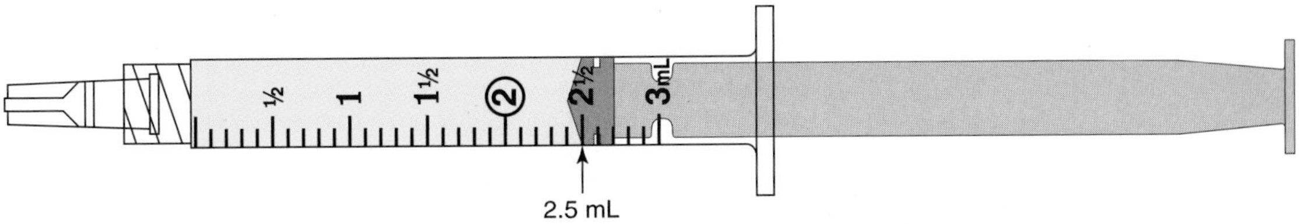

CAUTION:

The reconstituted vial must be further diluted prior to administration. The 2.5 mL prescribed dosage can be withdrawn from the vial of 100 mg/mL azithromycin solution and injected into the appropriate amount (either 250 mL or 500 mL) of the appropriate diluent (see insert) then infused into the patient over a specified time/rate once daily. Also note that the insert states that this vial is for single use only. Discard any unused portion after use. Not intended to be used as a multiple-use vial.

RATIONALE FOR PRACTICE

When reconstituting multiple-dose injectable medications, verify the length of drug potency. Store the reconstituted drug appropriately with a reconstitution label attached.

If multiple doses result from the reconstitution of a powdered drug, the solution must be used in a timely manner. Because the drug potency (or stability) may be several hours to several days, check the drug label, package information sheet, or *Hospital Formulary* for the length of time that the drug may be used after reconstitution. Store the drug appropriately at room temperature or refrigerate according to the manufacturer's instructions.

CAUTION

The length of potency is different from the expiration date. The expiration date is provided by the manufacturer on the label. It indicates the *last* date the drug may be reconstituted and used.

When you reconstitute or mix a multiple-dose vial of medication in powdered form, it is important that the vial be *clearly labelled* with the *date* and *time* of preparation, the strength or *supply dosage* you prepared, *length of potency*, *storage directions*, and your *initials*. Because the medication becomes unstable after storage for long periods, the date and time are especially important. Figure 10-6 is an example of the proper label for the azithromycin dihydrate reconstituted to 100 mg/mL. Because there are two doses of reconstituted drug in this vial, and two doses will be administered 24 hours apart (now at 0800, then again the next day at 0800), this drug should be refrigerated. Refrigeration will protect the potency of the drug in case the second dose is administered slightly later than 0800. Indicate the need for refrigeration on the label.

10/01/xx, 0800, reconstituted as 100 mg/mL. Expires 17/01/xx, 0800. Keep refrigerated. G.D.P.

FIGURE 10-6 Reconstitution Label for Azithromycin Dihydrate

Multiple-Strength Solution/Multiple-Dose Vial

Some parenteral powdered medications have directions for preparing several different solution strengths, to allow you to select a particular dosage strength (Figure 10-7). This results in a reasonable amount to be given to a particular patient.

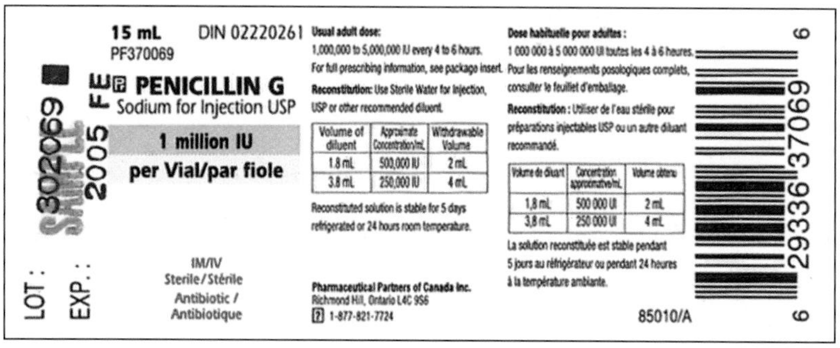

FIGURE 10-7 Penicillin G Sodium Label

Example:

Order: *penicillin G sodium 300 000 units IM QID*

Supply: penicillin G sodium 1 000 000 unit vial

This vial contains a total of 1 000 000 units of penicillin G sodium. The reconstitution instructions are shown on the right side of the label. The instructions detail two different parenteral solution supply dosages or concentrations that are determined by the added diluent volume. Examine each of the two instructions. Notice how these reconstituted concentrations differ and when each might be selected.

Add 1.8 mL Diluent

The first set of directions instructs you to add 1.8 mL diluent for a solution concentration of 500 000 units/mL. Examine this information.

- First, to fulfill the first set of directions, how much and what type of diluent must be added? The directions indicate to add 1.8 mL of diluent. (Check the package insert to determine the type of diluent, as this information is not stated on the label. Use sterile water or normal saline.)
- Second, what is the supply dosage of the reconstituted penicillin G sodium? When adding 1.8 mL of diluent, the supply dosage is 500 000 units/mL.
- Third, what is the resulting total volume of this reconstituted solution? The total volume is 2 mL. This is because the supply dosage is 500 000 units/mL or 1 000 000 units/2 mL. The powder displaces 0.2 mL of the solution. (Notice that this is the most concentrated, or the strongest, of the four concentrations.)
- Finally, how many full doses of penicillin G sodium are available in this vial? The vial contains 1 000 000 units and the order is for 300 000 units. Notice that regardless of the concentration, there are three full doses (plus some extra) in this vial. Prepare a different reconstitution label, as this is a different concentration.

Following the fourth set of directions, add 1.8 mL of diluent to prepare 2 mL of solution with a resulting concentration of 500 000 units of penicillin G sodium in each 1 mL.

Calculate one dose.

Step 1 Convert No conversion necessary

Order: *penicillin G sodium 300 000 units IM QID*

Supply: 500 000 units/mL

Step 2 Think You want to give less than 1 mL.

Step 3 Calculate

$$\frac{D}{H} \times Q = \frac{\overset{3}{\cancel{300\,000}}\,\text{units}}{\underset{5}{\cancel{500\,000}}\,\text{units}} \times 1\,\text{mL} = \frac{3}{5}\,\text{mL} = 0.6\,\text{mL}$$

given intramuscularly four times a day

Because each dose is 0.6 mL and the total volume is 2 mL, you would have enough for two additional full doses. This supply dosage would result in a reasonable volume for an IM injection for an infant, small child, or anyone with wasted muscle mass.

Select a *3-mL syringe, and measure 0.6 mL* of penicillin G sodium reconstituted to 500 000 units/mL.

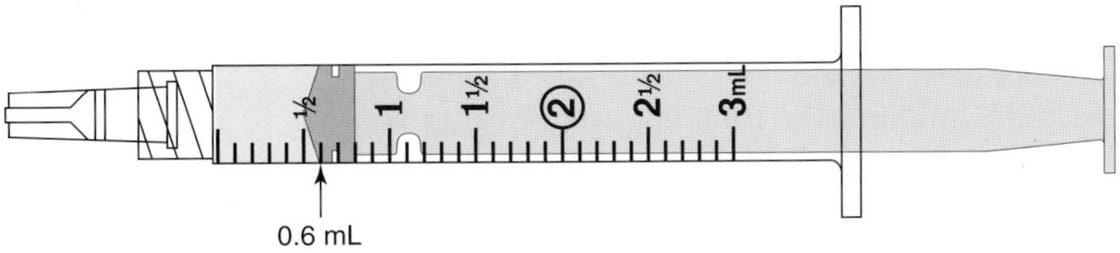

Finally, add the label to the reconstituted penicillin G sodium 500 000-unit/mL vial (Figure 10-9).

30/01/xx, 0800, reconstituted as 500 000 units/mL. Expires 06/02/xx, 0800, keep refrigerated. G.D.P.

FIGURE 10-9 Reconstitution Label for Penicillin G Sodium 1 000 000 Units with 1.8 mL Diluent

Add 3.8 mL Diluent

Refer to the second set of directions on the penicillin label, which indicates to add 3.8 mL of diluent for 250 000 units per millilitre of solution. Would this prepare an appropriate concentration to fill the order?

What is different about this set of directions? Analyze the information provided on the label.

- First, to follow the third set of directions, how much and what type of diluent must be added? The directions indicate to add 3.8 mL of diluent. (Remember, check the package insert to determine the type of diluent, as this information is not stated on the label. The recommendation is for sterile water or normal saline.)
- Second, what is the supply dosage of the reconstituted penicillin G sodium? When adding 3.8 mL of diluent, the supply dosage is 250 000 units/mL.

- Third, what is the resulting total volume of this reconstituted solution? The total volume is 4 mL. This is because the supply dosage is 250 000 units/mL or 1 000 000 units/4 mL. The powder adds 0.2 mL volume to the solution.
- Finally, how many full doses of penicillin are available in this vial? The vial contains 1 000 000 units and the order is for 300 000 units. Regardless of the concentration, there are still three full doses (plus some extra) in this vial. A reconstitution label would be needed.

This means that when 3.8 mL of sterile diluent is added to the vial of powdered penicillin G sodium, the result is 4 mL of solution with 250 000 units of penicillin G sodium per millilitre.

Calculate one dose.

Step 1 Convert No conversion necessary

Order: *penicillin G sodium 300 000 units IM QID*

Supply: 250 000 units/mL

Step 2 Think You want to give more than 1 mL but less than 2 mL.

Step 3 Calculate

$$\frac{D}{H} \times Q = \frac{\overset{6}{\cancel{300\,000}}\,\text{units}}{\underset{5}{\cancel{250\,000}}\,\text{units}} \times 1\,\text{mL} = \frac{6}{5}\,\text{mL} = 1.2\,\text{mL}$$

given intramuscularly four times a day

Because each dose is 1.2 mL and the total volume is 4 mL, you would have enough for two additional full doses. As an IM dose, 5 mL is the maximum volume for a large, adult muscle. This concentration would result in a reasonable volume that would be readily absorbed. This is a good choice of concentration instructions to use to prepare this order.

Select a 3-mL syringe, and measure 1.2 mL of penicillin G sodium reconstituted to 250 000 units/mL.

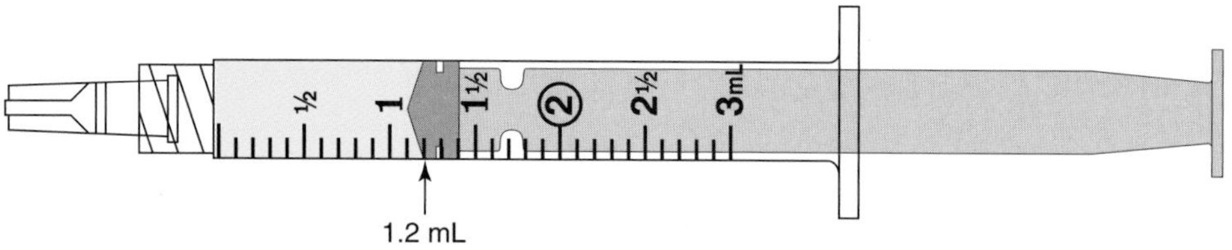

CAUTION

The supply dosage of a reconstituted drug is an essential detail that the preparer must write on the multiple-dose vial label. Once a powdered drug is reconstituted, there is no way to verify how much diluent was actually added, unless it is properly labelled.

Be sure to add a label to the reconstituted penicillin G sodium 250 000-unit/mL vial (Figure 10-8).

30/01/xx, 0800, reconstituted as 250 000 units/mL. Expires 06/02/xx, 0800, keep refrigerated. G.D.P.

FIGURE 10-8 Reconstitution Label for Penicillin G Sodium 1 000 000 Units with 3.8 mL Diluent

As you can see from these possible reconstituted strengths, three full doses are available from this multiple-dose vial in each case. The added diluent volume is the key factor that determines the resulting concentration. The *supply dosage* ultimately determines the *injectable volume per dose.*

> **MATH TIP**
>
> When multiple directions for diluting are given, the *smaller* the amount of diluent added, the *greater* or *stronger* the resulting solution concentration will be.

RECONSTITUTED PARENTERAL SOLUTIONS WITH VARIOUS ROUTES

A variety of drugs are labelled and packaged with reconstitution instructions. Some drugs are for IM use only and some are for IV use only, whereas others may be used for either. Some are even suitable for subcutaneous, IM, or IV administration. Carefully check the route and related reconstitution directions. The following material gives examples of several types of directions you will encounter.

Drugs with Injection Reconstitution Instructions—Either IM or IV

Example:

Order: *methylprednisolone sodium succinate 200 mg IV q6h*

Supply: 500-mg vial of powdered methylprednisolone sodium succinate for IM or IV injection (Figure 10-10) with directions on the left side of the label, "Reconstitution: Add 7.8 mL Sterile Water for Injection and use within 24 hours or 7.8 mL of Bacteriostatic Water for Injection and use within 48 hrs. Each reconstituted vial contains approximately 8 mL. Each mL contains 62.5 mg methylprednisolone."

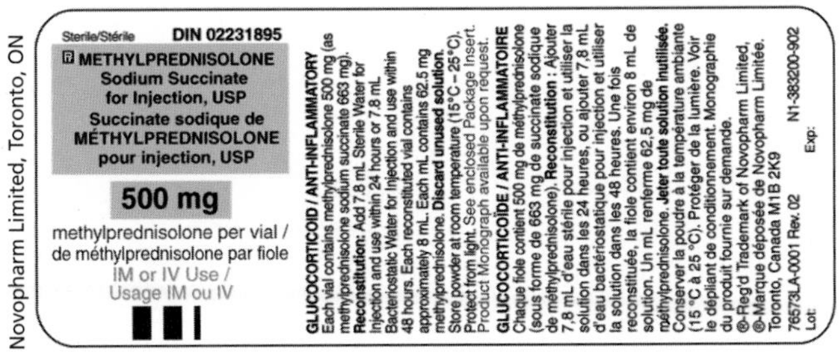

FIGURE 10-10 Methylprednisolone Sodium Succinate 500 mg Label

What is known?

- First, to fill the order, how much and what type of diluent must be added? The directions indicate to add 7.8 mL of bacteriostatic water for injection.
- Second, what is the supply dosage of the reconstituted methylprednisolone? When adding 7.8 mL of diluent, the supply dosage is 62.5 mg/mL.
- Third, what is the resulting total volume of this reconstituted solution? The total volume is 8 mL. You know this because 62.5 mg/mL × 8 mL = 500 mg.
- Finally, how many full doses of methylprednisolone sodium succinate are available in this vial? The vial contains 500 mg and the order is for 200 mg. There are two full doses in the vial. A reconstitution label is needed.

This means that you have available a vial of 500 mg of methylprednisolone sodium succinate to which you will add 8 mL of diluent. The final yield of the solution is 62.5 mg per mL, which is the supply dosage.

Calculate one dose.

Step 1 Convert No conversion necessary

Order: *methylprednisolone sodium succinate 200 mg IV q6h*

Supply: 62.5 mg/mL

Step 2 Think You want to give more than 1 mL. In fact, you want to give more than three times 1 mL.

Step 3 Calculate $\frac{D}{H} \times Q = \frac{200 \cancel{mg}}{62.5 \cancel{mg}} \times 1\,mL = 3.2\,mL$

given intravenously every 6 hours

30/01/xx, 0800, reconstituted as 62.5 mg/mL. Expires 01/02/xx, 0800, store at room temperature 15–25°C. G.D.P.

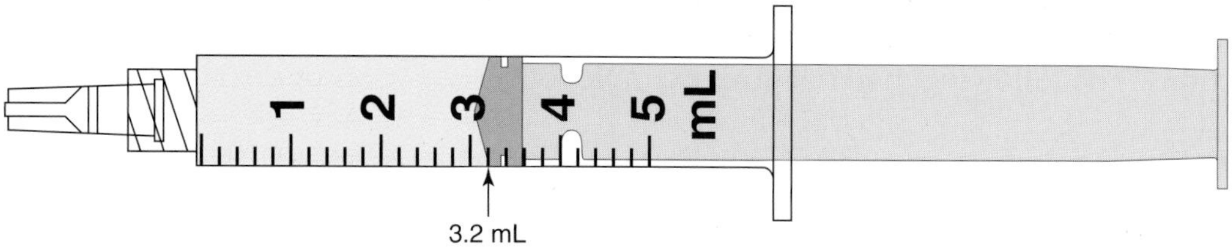

Drugs with Different IM and IV Reconstitution Instructions

Notice that the ceftazidime label (Figure 10-11) has one set of instructions for IM use and another set of instructions for IV administration. The nurse must carefully check the route ordered, and then follow the directions that correspond to that route. In such cases, it is important not to interchange the dilution instructions for IM and IV administrations.

Example 1:

Order: *ceftazidime 250 mg IM q12h*

Supply: 1000-mg vial of powdered ceftazidime (Figure 10-11) with IM reconstitution directions "IM : Add Add 3 mL of sterile water for injection or other approved diluent. SHAKE WELL. Provides ceftazidime approx. 280 mg per mL."

- First, to fill the order, how much and what type of diluent must be added? The directions indicate to add 3 mL of sterile water for injection or another approved diluent. Bacteriostatic water for injection is listed in the package insert as another possible diluent.
- Second, what is the supply dosage of the reconstituted ceftazidime? When adding 3 mL of diluent, the resulting supply dosage is 280 mg/mL.
- Third, how many full doses of ceftazidime are available in this vial? The vial contains 1000 mg and the order is for 250 mg. There are four full doses in the vial. A reconstitution label is needed.
- Finally, what is the resulting total volume of this reconstituted solution? The total volume is 3.6 mL, as indicated on the label for IM reconstitution.

This means that you have available a vial of 1000 mg of ceftazidime to which you will add 3 mL of diluent. The final yield of the solution is 3.6 mL with a supply dosage of 280 mg/mL.

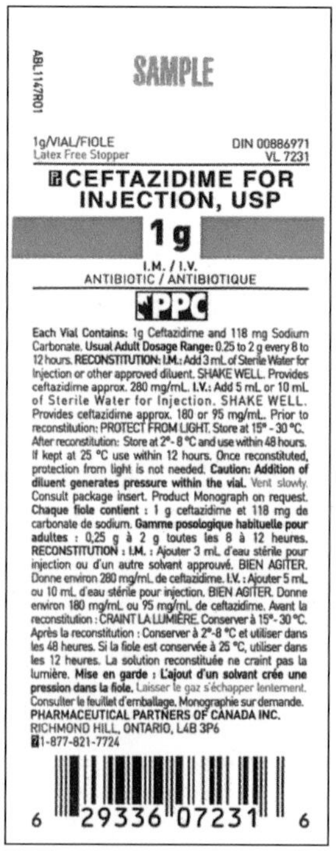

Pharmaceutical Partners of Canada Inc., Richmond Hill, ON

FIGURE 10-11
Ceftazidime Label

Calculate one dose.

Step 1 Convert No conversion necessary

Order: *ceftazidime 250 mg IM q12h*

Supply: 280 mg/mL

Step 2 Think You want to give less than 1 mL.

Step 3 Calculate $\frac{D}{H} \times Q = \frac{25\cancel{0}\,\cancel{mg}}{28\cancel{0}\,\cancel{mg}} \times 1\,mL = 0.9\,mL$

given intramuscularly every 12 hours

30/01/xx, 0800, reconstituted as 280 mg/mL for IM use. Expires 01/02/xx, 0800, store in refrigerator. G.D.P.

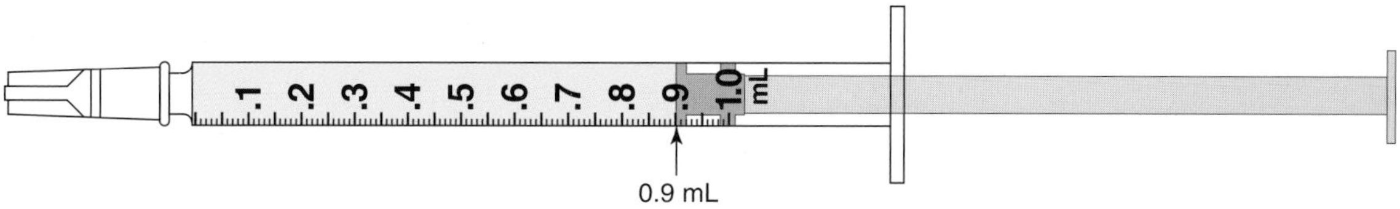

Example 2:

Order: *ceftazidime 400 mg IV q8h*

Supply: 1000-mg vial of powdered ceftazidime with IV reconstitution directions: "IV: Add 5 mL or 10 mL of Sterile Water for Injection. SHAKE WELL. Provides approx. 180 or 95 mg/mL.

- First, to prepare the order, how much and what type of diluent must be added? The directions indicate to add 5 mL or 10 mL of sterile water.
- Second, what is the supply dosage of the reconstituted ceftazidime? When adding 5 mL of diluent, the resulting dosage is 1000 mg/5.6 mL or 180 mg/mL.
- Third, what is the resulting total volume of this reconstituted solution? The total volume is 5.6 mL. Unless indicated otherwise, the solution volume is sufficient to dilute the powder without adding additional volume.
- Finally, how many full doses of ceftazidime are available in this vial? The vial contains 1000 mg and the order is for 400 mg. There are two full doses in the vial. A reconstitution label is needed.

This means that you have available a vial of 1000 mg of ceftazidime to which you will add 5.6 mL of diluent. The final yield of the solution is 5.6 mL with a supply dosage of 180 mg/mL. Most IV antibiotics are then further diluted in an approved IV solution and infused over a specified time period. You will learn more about this in the next section and in Chapter 14.

Calculate 1 dose.

Step 1 Convert No conversion necessary

Order: *ceftazidime 400 mg IV q8h*

Supply: 180 mg/mL

Step 2 Think You want to give more than 1 mL.

Step 3 Calculate $\frac{D}{H} \times Q = \frac{\overset{2.2}{\cancel{400}}\,mg}{\underset{1}{\cancel{180}}\,mg} \times 1 = 2.2\,mL$

given intravenously every 8 hours

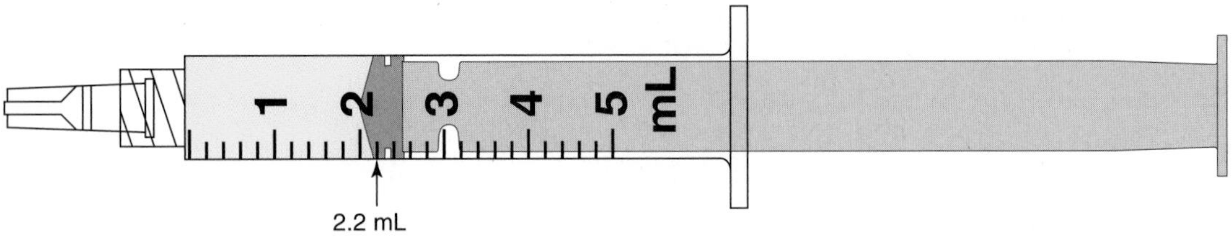

Drugs with Instructions to "See Package Insert" for Dilution and Administration

Some labels only provide the dosage strength contained in the vial and other minimal information that is insufficient to properly reconstitute or safely store the drug. To prepare the powdered medication, examine the package insert. Look at the amphotericin B label (Figure 10-12). There are no instructions for reconstitution on the label so it is important to examine the package insert for specific directions.

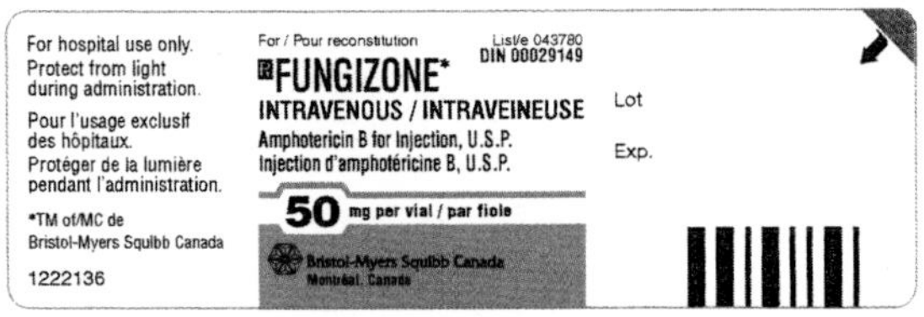

PREPARATION OF SOLUTIONS

Reconstitute as follows: An initial concentrate of 5 mg amphotericin B per mL is first prepared by rapidly expressing 10 mL sterile water for injection, USP *without a bacteriostatic agent* directly into the lyophilized cake, using a sterile needle (minimum diameter: 20 gauge) and syringe. Shake the vial immediately until the colloidal solution is clear. The infusion solution, providing 0.1 mg amphotericin B per mL, is then obtained by further dilution (1:50) with 5% Dextrose injection, USP *of pH above 4.2*. The pH of each container of Dextrose injection should be ascertained before use. Commercial Dextrose Injection usually has a pH above 4.2; however, if it is below 4.2, then 1 or 2 mL of buffer should be added to the Dextrose injection before it is used to dilute the concentrated solution of amphotericin B. The recommended buffer has the following composition

Dibasic sodium phosphate (anhydrous)	1.59 g
Monobasic sodium phosphate (anhydrous)	0.96 g
Water for injection, USP	qs 100.0 mL

The buffer should be sterilized before it is added to the Dextrose injection, either by filtration through a bacterial retentive stone mat or membrane, or by autoclaving for 30 minutes at 15 lb pressure (121°C). **CAUTION: Aseptic technique must be strictly observed in all handling,** since no preservative or bacteriostatic agent is present in the antibiotic or in the materials used to prepare it for administration. **All entries into the vial or into the diluents must be made with a sterile needle. Do not reconstitute with saline solutions. The use of any diluent other than the ones recommended or the presence of a bacteriostatic agent** (e.g., benzyl alcohol) **in the diluent may cause precipitation of the antibiotic. Do not use the initial concentrate or the infusion solution if there is any evidence of precipitation or foreign matter in either one.**

An in-line membrane filter may be used for intravenous infusion of amphotericin B; **however, the mean pore diameter of the filter should not be less than 1.0 micron in order to assure passage of the antibiotic dispersion.**

FIGURE 10-12 Amphotericin B Label and Package Insert Instructions for Reconstitution

Example:

Order: *amphotericin B 37.5 mg IV daily*

Supply: amphotericin B 50 mg

- First, to fill the order, how much and what type of diluent must you add? The directions advise the preparer, for initial reconstitution, to add 10 mL of sterile water for injection without a bacteriostatic agent. The reconstitution needs to be done first before the further dilution is performed.
- Second, what is the supply dosage of the reconstituted amphotericin B? When adding 10 mL of diluent, the supply dosage is 5 mg/mL.

- Third, what is the resulting total volume of this reconstituted solution? The total volume is 10 mL. You know this because the supply dosage is 5 mg/mL.
- Finally, how many full doses of amphotericin B are available in this vial? The vial contains 50 mg and the order is for 37.5 mg. There is enough for one full dose in the vial, but not enough for two full doses. No reconstitution label is needed.

This means that you have available a vial of 50 mg of amphotericin B to which you will add 10 mL of diluents using strict aseptic technique. The final yield of the solution is 5 mg/mL (50 mg/10 mL), which is your supply dosage.

Calculate one dose of the initial concentration (before further dilution).

Step 1 Convert No conversion is necessary.

Order: *amphotericin B 37.5 mg IV daily*

Supply: amphotericin B 5 mg/mL

Step 2 Think You want to give more than 1 mL, but less than 10 mL.

Step 3 Calculate 37.5 mg/5 mg × 1 mL = 7.5 mL given intravenously

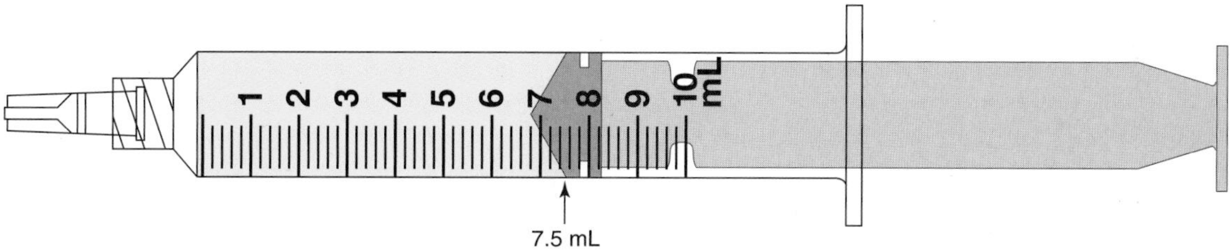

NOTE: Further dilution is required before you can use inject this product.

Using strict aseptic technique, the preparer (usually the pharmacy technician in the hospital pharmacy) will withdraw 7.5 mL of amphotericin B from the reconstituted vial and inject it into a 500-mL IV bag of 5% dextrose solution. The IV bag will then be appropriately labelled as containing 37.5 mg amphotericin B in 500 mL of 5% dextrose (concentration of 37.5 mg/500 mL or 0.75 mg/mL). The IV bag would then be delivered to the appropriate nursing unit to be infused into the patient at a slow infusion rate (over 2 to 6 hours, i.e., 100 mL/h) once daily.

QUICK REVIEW

It is important to remember the following points when reconstituting drugs:

- If any medicine remains for future use after reconstitution, clearly label:
  1. date and time of preparation
  2. strength or concentration per volume
  3. potency expiration
  4. recommended storage
  5. your initials
- Read all instructions carefully. If no instructions accompany the vial, confer with the pharmacist before proceeding.
- When reconstituting multiple-strength parenteral powders, select the dosage strength that is appropriate for the patient's age, size, and condition.
- Carefully select the correct reconstitution directions for IM or IV administration.

REVIEW SET 24

Calculate the amount you will prepare for each dose. The labels provided are the drugs available. Draw an arrow to the syringe calibration that corresponds with the amount you will draw up and prepare a reconstitution label, if needed.

1. Order: *ceftazidime 200 mg IM q12h*

   Reconstitute with __3__ mL diluent for a concentration of __280__ mg/mL.

   Give: __0.7__ mL

   How many full doses are available in this vial? __5__ dose(s).

   Prepare a reconstitution label for the remaining solution.

   Reconstitution Label

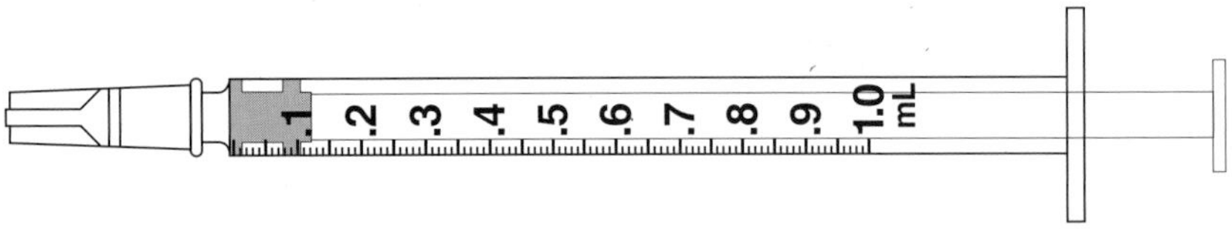

.1
.2
.3
.4
.5
.6
.7
.8
.9
1.0 mL

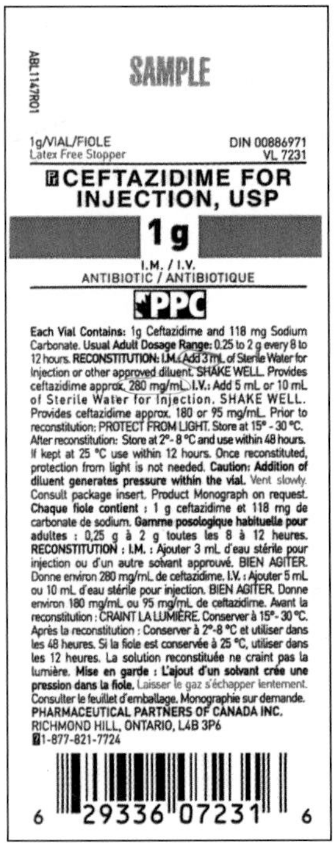

ABL1147R01
SAMPLE
1g/VIAL/FIOLE
Latex Free Stopper
DIN 00886971
VL 7231
CEFTAZIDIME FOR INJECTION, USP
1 g
I.M. / I.V.
ANTIBIOTIC / ANTIBIOTIQUE
PPC
Each Vial Contains: 1g Ceftazidime and 118 mg Sodium Carbonate. Usual Adult Dosage Range: 0.25 to 2 g every 8 to 12 hours. RECONSTITUTION: I.M.: Add 3 mL of Sterile Water for Injection or other approved diluent. SHAKE WELL. Provides ceftazidime approx. 280 mg/mL. I.V.: Add 5 mL or 10 mL of Sterile Water for Injection. SHAKE WELL. Provides ceftazidime approx. 180 or 95 mg/mL. Prior to reconstitution: PROTECT FROM LIGHT. Store at 15° - 30 °C. After reconstitution: Store at 2°- 8 °C and use within 48 hours. If kept at 25 °C use within 12 hours. Once reconstituted, protection from light is not needed. Caution: Addition of diluent generates pressure within the vial. Vent slowly. Consult package insert. Product Monograph on request.
Chaque fiole contient : 1 g ceftazidime et 118 mg de carbonate de sodium. Gamme posologique habituelle pour adultes : 0,25 g à 2 g toutes les 8 à 12 heures. RECONSTITUTION : I.M. : Ajouter 3 mL d'eau stérile pour injection ou d'un autre solvant approuvé. BIEN AGITER. Donne environ 280 mg/mL de ceftazidime. I.V. : Ajouter 5 mL ou 10 mL d'eau stérile pour injection. BIEN AGITER. Donne environ 180 mg/mL ou 95 mg/mL de ceftazidime. Avant la reconstitution : CRAINT LA LUMIÈRE. Conserver à 15°- 30 °C. Après la reconstitution : Conserver à 2°-8 °C et utiliser dans les 48 heures. Si la fiole est conservée à 25 °C, utiliser dans les 12 heures. La solution reconstituée ne craint pas la lumière. Mise en garde : L'ajout d'un solvant crée une pression dans la fiole. Laisser le gaz s'échapper lentement. Consulter le feuillet d'emballage. Monographie sur demande.
PHARMACEUTICAL PARTNERS OF CANADA INC.
RICHMOND HILL, ONTARIO, L4B 3P6
1-877-821-7724
6 29336 07231 6

Pharmaceutical Partners of Canada Inc., Richmond Hill, ON

2. Order: *bacitracin 2500 units IM q12h*

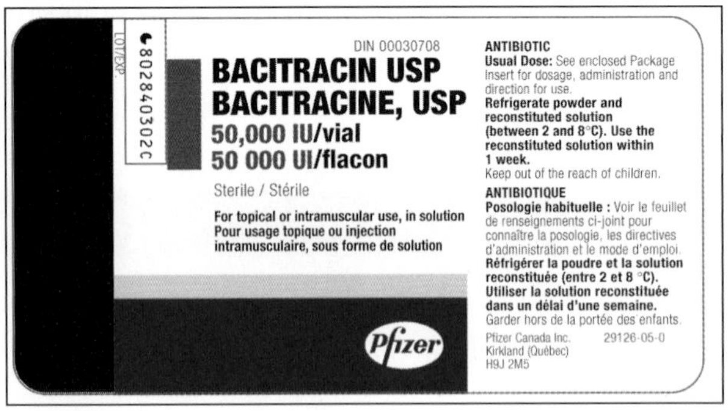

LOT/EXP
8028403O2C
DIN 00030708
BACITRACIN USP
BACITRACINE, USP
50,000 IU/vial
50 000 UI/flacon
Sterile / Stérile
For topical or intramuscular use, in solution
Pour usage topique ou injection intramusculaire, sous forme de solution
ANTIBIOTIC
Usual Dose: See enclosed Package Insert for dosage, administration and direction for use.
Refrigerate powder and reconstituted solution (between 2 and 8 °C). Use the reconstituted solution within 1 week.
Keep out of the reach of children.
ANTIBIOTIQUE
Posologie habituelle : Voir le feuillet de renseignements ci-joint pour connaître la posologie, les directives d'administration et le mode d'emploi.
Réfrigérer la poudre et la solution reconstituée (entre 2 et 8 °C). Utiliser la solution reconstituée dans un délai d'une semaine.
Garder hors de la portée des enfants.
Pfizer
Pfizer Canada Inc. 29126-05-0
Kirkland (Québec)
H9J 2M5

©Pfizer Canada Inc., Kirkland, Que

DOSAGE AND ADMINISTRATION
TO BE ADMINISTERED INTRAMUSCULARLY
Infant dose:
For infants under 2500 grams—900 units/kg/24 hours in two or three divided doses. For infants over 2500 grams—1000 units/kg/24 hours, in two or three divided doses. Intramuscular injections of the solution should be given in the upper outer quadrant of the buttocks, alternating right and left and avoiding multiple injections in the same region because of the transient pain following injection.

Preparation of Solutions:
Should be dissolved in sodium chloride injection containing 2% procaine hydrochloride. The concentration of the antibiotic in the solution should not be less than 5000 units per mL or more than 10 000 units per mL.
Diluents containing parabens should not be used to reconstitute bacitracin; cloudy solutions and precipitate formation have occurred. Reconstitution of the 50 000 unit vial with 9.8 mL of diluent will result in a concentration of 5000 units per mL.

TO BE ADMINISTERED TOPICALLY.
Preparation of Solution:
Solutions for topical application are prepared by dissolving bacitracin in sterile water for injection or sodium chloride injection in amounts to give the following concentrations:

Skin	500 units per mL
Ophthalmic Solutions	500 to 1000 units per mL
Intranasal Therapy	250 units per mL
Aerosol	500 to 1000 units per mL

STABILITY AND STORAGE RECOMMENDATIONS:
Store unreconstituted bacitracin in a refrigerator (between 2 and 8°C). Solutions are rapidly inactivated at room temperature but are stable for 1 week when stored in a refrigerator (between 2 and 8°C).

Reconstitute with __9.8__ mL diluent for a concentration of __5000__ units/mL.

Give: __0.5__ mL

How many full doses are available in this vial? __20__ dose(s).

Prepare a reconstitution label for the remaining solution.

$\frac{2500\,u}{5000\,u} = 0.5$

$\frac{50{,}000\,u}{2500\,u}$

Reconstitution Label

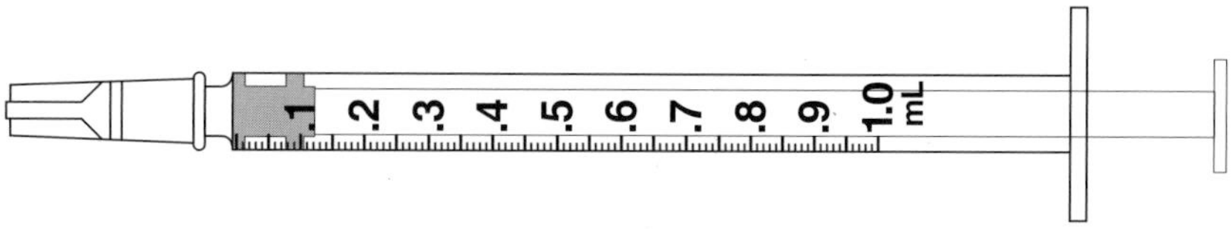

3. Order: *enfuvirtide 90 mg subcutaneous BID*

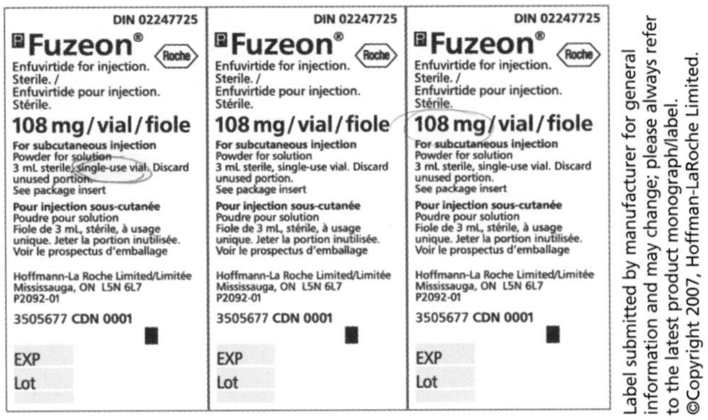

Package insert directions: "Add 1.1 mL Sterile Water supplied diluent to make a total volume of 1.2 mL and a concentration of 90 mg/mL."

Reconstitute with ________ mL diluent for a concentration of ________ mg/________ mL.

Give: ________ mL

How many full doses are available in this vial? ________ dose(s).

Does this reconstituted medication require a reconstitution label? ________

Explain: ____

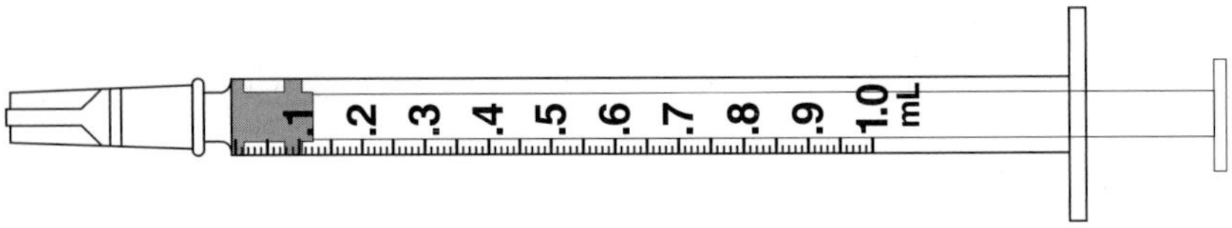

4. Order: *azithromycin dihydrate 0.5 g IV daily*

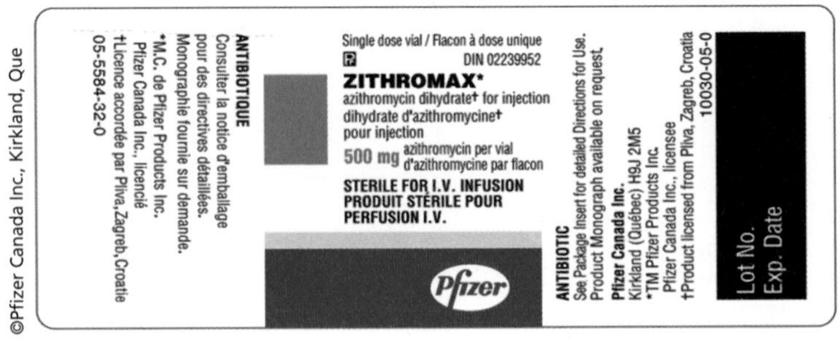

RECONSTITUTION DIRECTIONS

ZITHROMAX for Injection:

RECONSTITUTION OF ZITHROMAX FOR INJECTION

Strength	Reconstitution Solution	Volume to be Added	Approximate Volume Available	Nominal Concentration
500 mg	Sterile Water for Injection	4.8 mL	5 mL	100 mg/mL

Prepare the initial solution of **ZITHROMAX** for injection by adding 4.8 mL of sterile water for injection to the 500-mg vial. Shake the vial until all of the drug is dissolved. Since the vial is evacuated, it is recommended that a standard 5-mL (non-automated) syringe be used to ensure that the exact volume of 4.8 mL is dispensed. Each mL of reconstituted solution contains azithromycin dihydrate equivalent to 100 mg azithromycin. Reconstituted solution is stable for 24 hours when stored below 30°C. **The reconstituted solution must be further diluted prior to administration.**

Dilution of reconstituted solution: To provide azithromycin over a concentration range of 1.0–2.0 mg/mL, transfer 5 mL of the 100 mg/mL azithromycin solution into the appropriate amount of the following diluents:

Final Infusion Concentration (mg/mL)	Amount of Diluent (mL)
1.0 mg/mL	500 mL
2.0 mg/mL	250 mL

Appropriate Diluents

0.9% Sodium Chloride Injection
5% Dextrose in Water for Injection
0.45% Sodium Chloride Injection
Lactated Ringer's Injection
5% Dextrose in 0.45% Sodium Chloride Injection with 20 mEq Potassium Chloride
5% Dextrose in Lactated Ringer's Injection
5% Dextrose in 0.3% Sodium Chloride Injection
5% Dextrose in 0.45% Sodium Chloride Injection
Normosal M in 5% Dextrose

0.5

Diluted solutions prepared in this manner are stable for 24 hours at or below room temperature (30°C), or for 72 hours if stored under refrigeration (5°C). As with all parenteral drug products, intravenous admixtures should be inspected visually for clarity, particulate matter, precipitate, discoloration, and leakage prior to administration, whenever solution and container permit. Solutions showing haziness, particulate matter, precipitate, discoloration, or leakage should be discarded.

Only limited data are available on the compatibility of **ZITHROMAX** for injection with other intravenous substances, therefore additives or other medications should not be added to **ZITHROMAX** for injection or infused simultaneously through the same intravenous line. If the same intravenous line is used for sequential infusion of several different drugs, the line should be flushed before and after infusion of **ZITHROMAX** for injection with an infusion solution compatible with **ZITHROMAX** for injection and with any other drug(s) administered via the common line. If **ZITHROMAX** for injection is to be given concomitantly with another drug, each drug should be given separately in accordance with tie recommended dosage and route of administration for each drug.

Reconstitute with 4.8 mL diluent for a concentration of 100 mg/mL.

Withdraw: 5 mL of reconstituted azithromycin dihydrate and further dilute to appropriate volume with appropriate diluent (see package insert).

How many full doses are available in this vial? ________ dose(s).

Does this reconstituted medication require a reconstitution label? ________

Explain: One dose

Note: The reconstituted solution must be further diluted prior to administration.

0.5g = 500mg/100 = 5

500mg/500 = 1

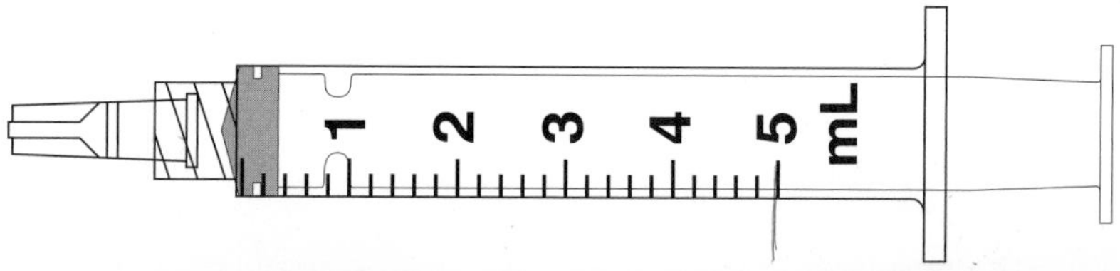

5. Order: *ceftriaxone 750 mg IM daily*

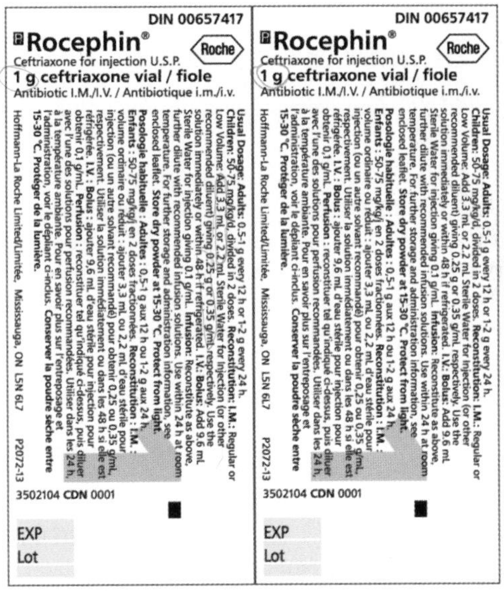

Label submitted by manufacturer for general information and may change; please always refer to the latest product monograph/label. ©Copyright 2007, Hoffman-LaRoche Limited.

Reconstitute with ________ mL diluent for an initial concentration of ________ mg/mL.
Give: ________ mL

How many full doses are available in this vial? ________ dose(s)

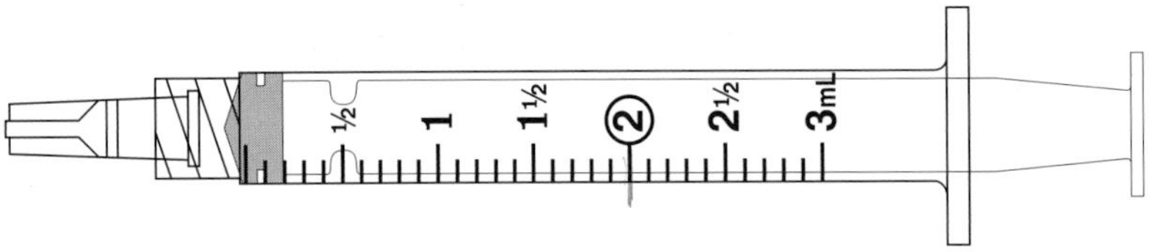

6. Order: *penicillin G sodium 1 000 000 units IM q6h*

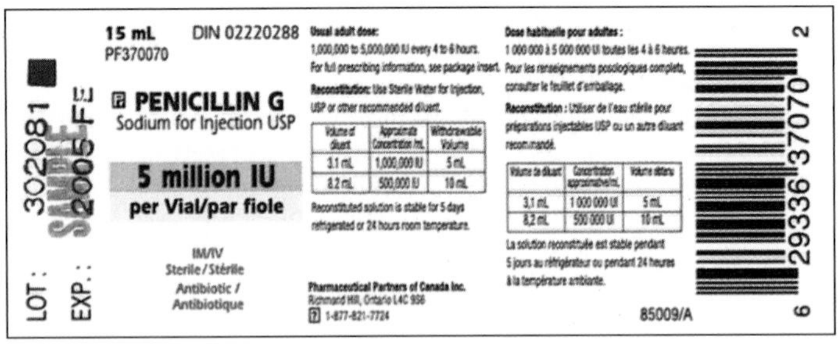

Pharmaceutical Partners of Canada Inc., Richmond Hill, ON

Describe the two concentrations and calculate the amount to give for each of the supply dosage concentrations.

Reconstitute with ________ mL diluent for a concentration of ________ units/mL, and give ________ mL.

Reconstitute with ________ mL diluent for a concentration of ________ units/mL, and give ________ mL.

Indicate the concentration you would choose and explain the rationale for your selection.

Select ________ units/mL and give ________ mL. Rationale: ____________________

____

How many full doses are available in this vial? ________ dose(s)

Prepare a reconstitution label for the remaining solution.

Reconstitution Label

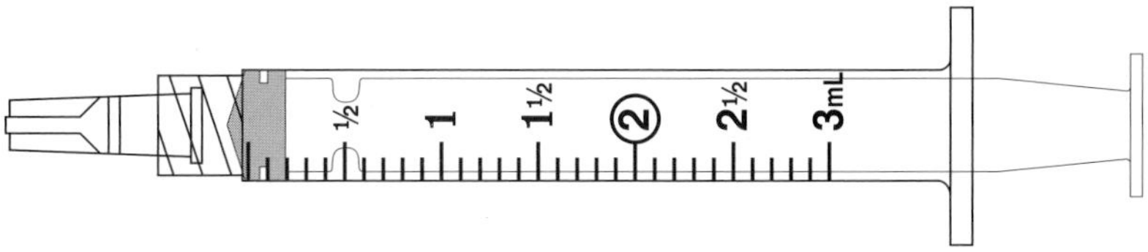

7. Order: *methylprednisolone sodium succinate 175 mg IM daily*

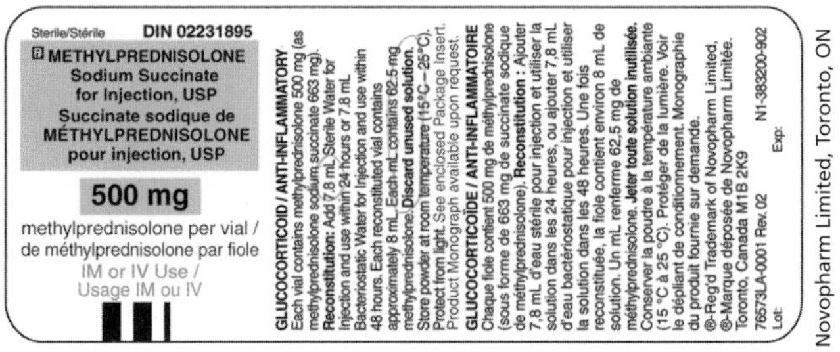

Reconstitute with __7.8__ mL diluent for a concentration of __62.5__ mg/mL.

Give: __2.8__ mL

How many full doses are available in this vial? __2__ dose(s).

Prepare a reconstitution label for the remaining solution.

Reconstitution Label

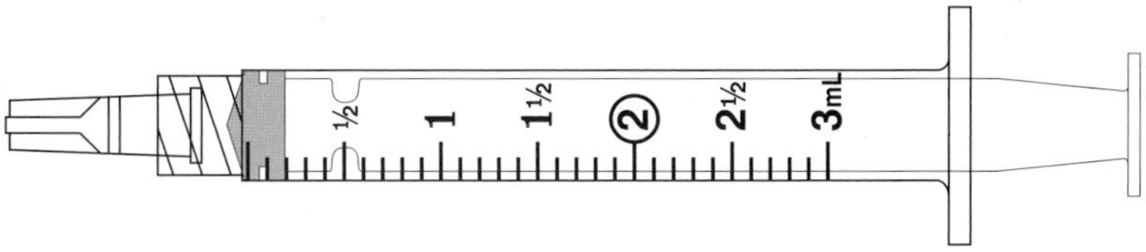

8. Order: *pipercillin 200 mg IM q6h*

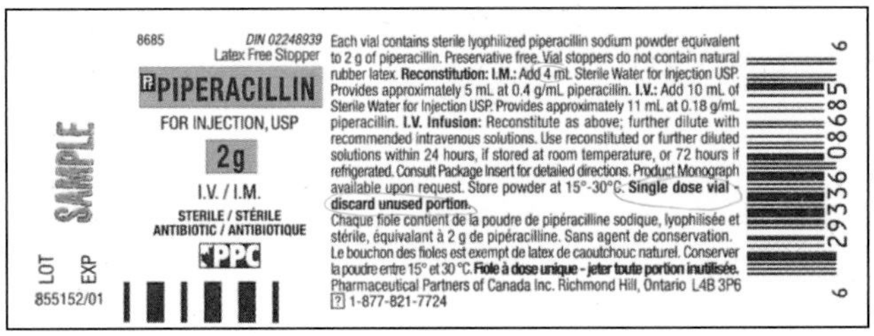

Pharmaceutical Partners of Canada Inc., Richmond Hill, ON

Reconstitute with __4__ mL diluent for a concentration of __0.4__ g/__5__ mL or __400__ mg/__0.4__ mL.

Give: __0.5__ mL

How many full doses are available in this vial? __Single use__ dose(s).

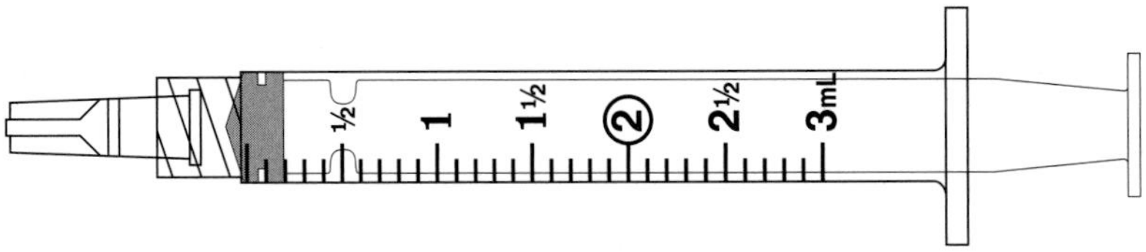

9. Order: *penicillin G sodium 500 000 units IM q6h*

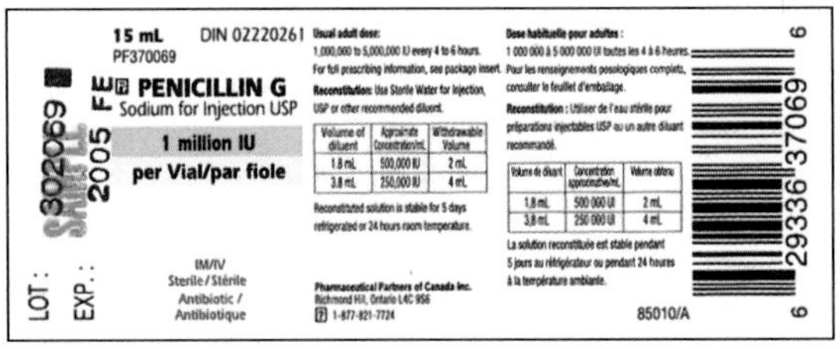

Pharmaceutical Partners of Canada Inc., Richmond Hill, ON

Describe the two concentrations and calculate the amount to give for each of the supply dosage concentrations.

Reconstitute with __1.8__ mL diluent for a concentration of ________ units/mL, and give ________ mL.

Reconstitute with ________ mL diluent for a concentration of ________ units/mL, and give ________ mL.

Indicate the concentration you would choose and explain the rationale for your selection.

Select ________ units/mL and give ________ mL. Rationale: ________________________

____

How many full doses are available in this vial? ________ dose(s)

Prepare a reconstitution label for the remaining solution.

Reconstitution Label

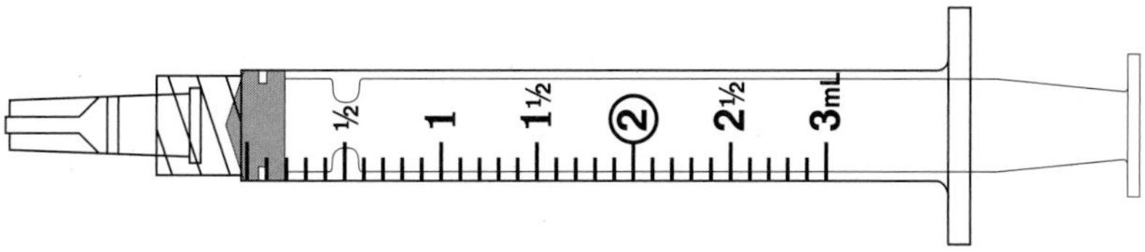

10. Order: *ampicillin sodium 500 mg IV q6h*

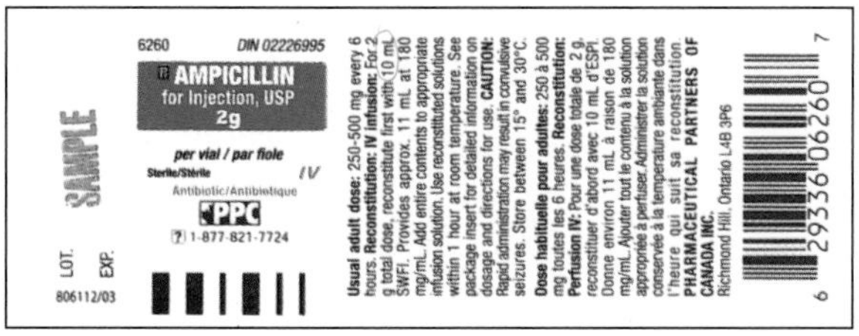

Pharmaceutical Partners of Canada Inc., Richmond Hill, ON

Reconstitute with __10__ mL diluent for a concentration of __1.8__ g/__11__ mL or __180__ mg/mL.

Give: __2.8__ mL

How many full doses are in this vial? __4__ dose(s)

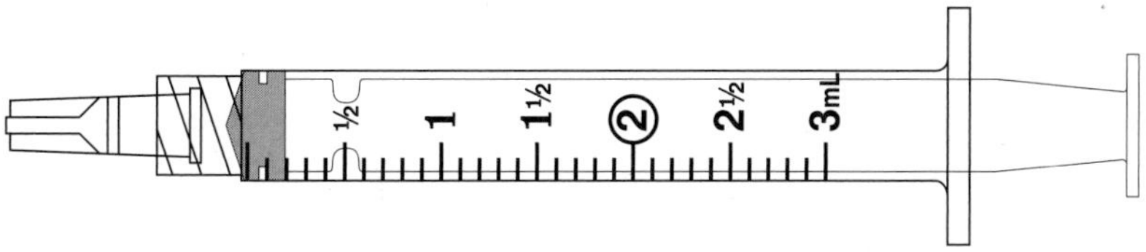

11. Order: *methylprednisolone sodium succinate 24 mg IM daily*

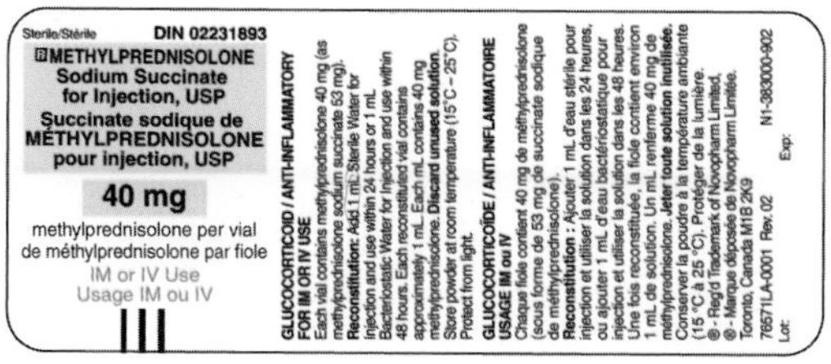

Novopharm Limited, Toronto, ON

Reconstitute with __1__ mL diluent for a concentration of __40__ mg/mL.

Give __0.6__ mL

How many full doses are available in this vial? __1__ dose(s)

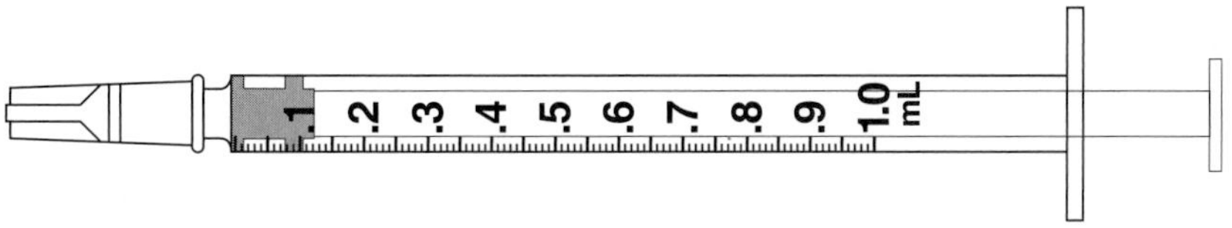

12. Order: *ceftazidime 250 mg IV q12h*

Reconstitute with __10__ mL diluent for a concentration of __0.18__ g/______ mL or __180__ mg/mL.

Give: __1.4__ mL

How many full doses are available in this vial? __4__ dose(s).

Will the drug remain potent to use all available doses? ________ Explain: ________

Prepare a reconstitution label for the remaining solution.

Reconstitution Label

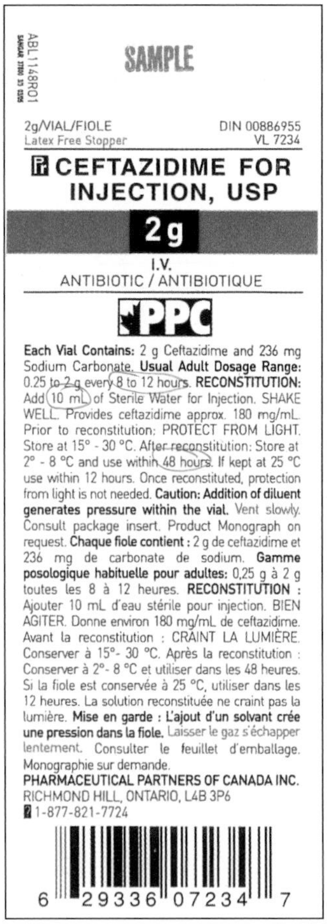

Pharmaceutical Partners of Canada Inc., Richmond Hill, ON

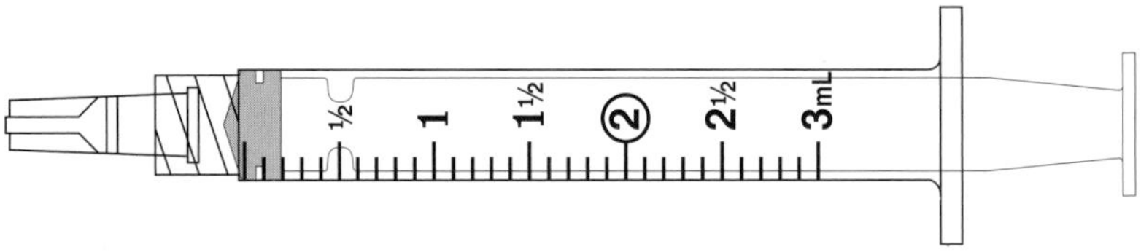

13. Order: *ceftriaxone 750 mg IV q6h in 50 mL D_5W (5% Dextrose & Water minibag administration solution)*

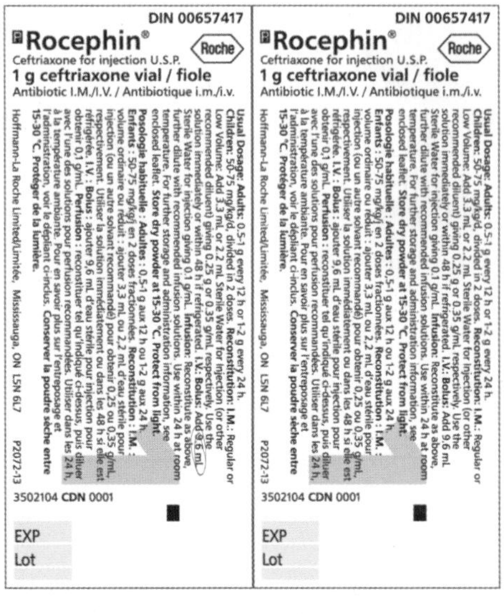

Label submitted by manufacturer for general information and may change; please always refer to the latest product monograph/label. ©Copyright 2007, Hoffman-LaRoche Limited.

Reconstitute vial with __9.6__ mL diluent for an initial concentration of __100__ mg/mL.
Withdraw: __7.5__ mL and inject in 50 mL minibag of D5W

How many full doses are available in this vial? __1__ dose(s)

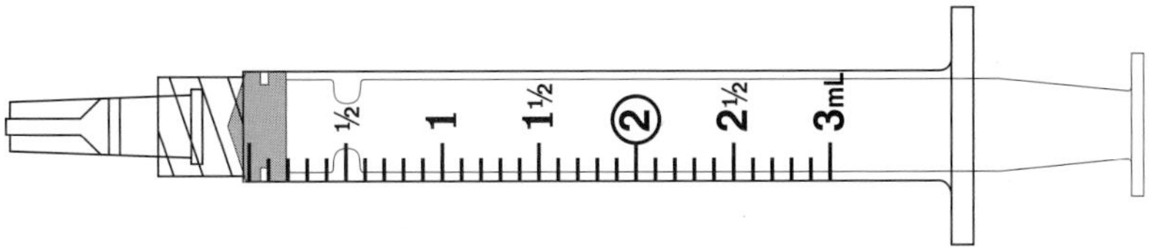

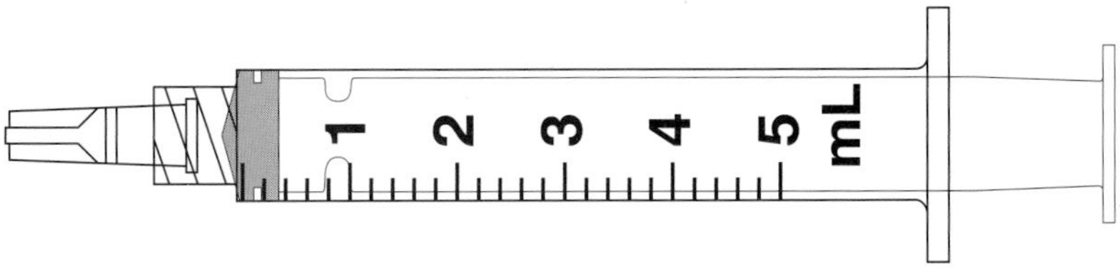

14. Order: *tobramycin sulfate 80 mg IV q8h*

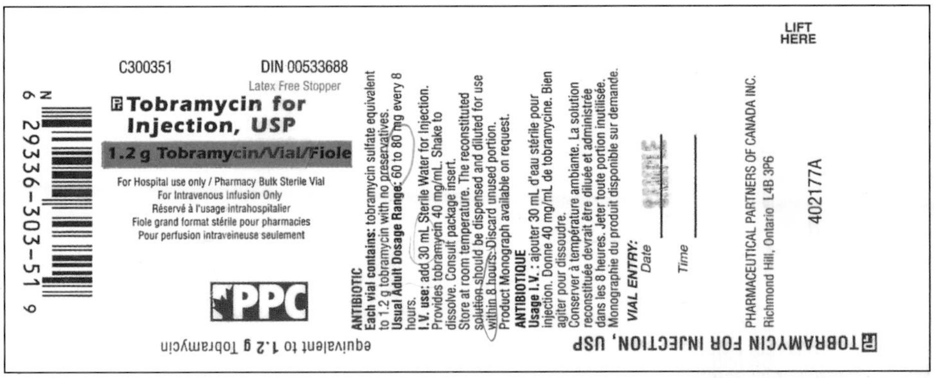

Pharmaceutical Partners of Canada Inc., Richmond Hill, ON

Reconstitute with __30__ mL diluent for a concentration of __40__ mg/mL.

Give: __2__ mL

How many full doses are available in this vial? __1__ dose(s).

Prepare a reconstitution label for the remaining solution.

Reconstitution Label

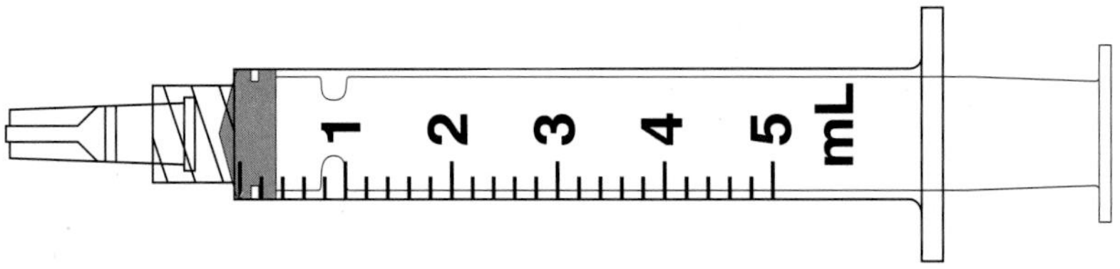

15. Order: *cefazolin 250 mg IM q6h*

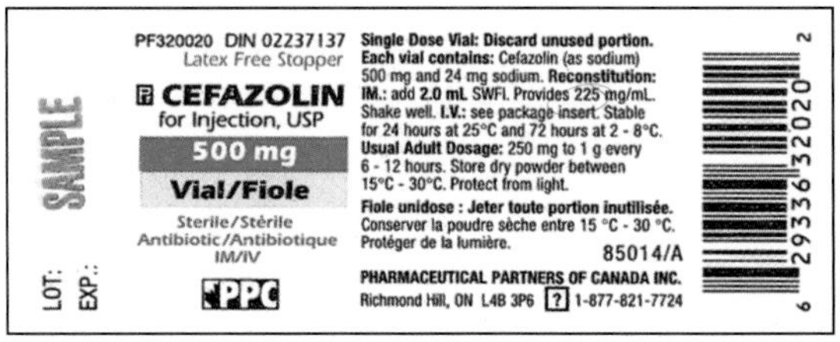

Pharmaceutical Partners of Canada Inc., Richmond Hill, ON

Reconstitute with ___2.0___ mL diluent for a concentration of ___225___ mg/mL.

Give: ___1.1___ mL

How many full doses are available in this vial? ___2___ dose(s).

Prepare a reconstitution label for the remaining solution.

Reconstitution Label

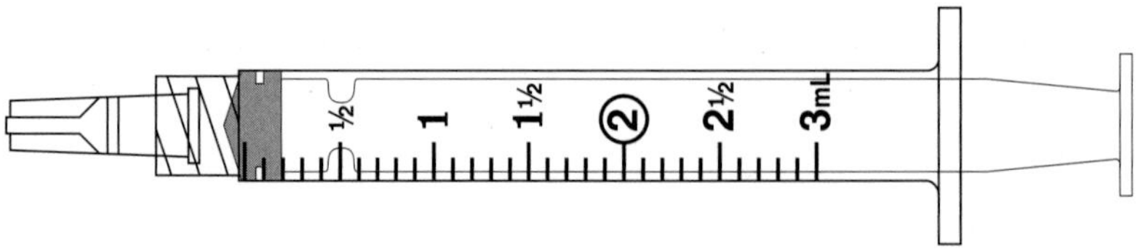

After completing these problems, see pages 478–482 to check your answers.

RECONSTITUTION OF NONINJECTABLE SOLUTIONS

The principles of reconstitution can also be applied to nutritional formulas. Although many solutions are specifically formulated to be used in full strength, in some cases the nurse or healthcare professional will find it necessary to dilute a liquid concentrate (*solute*) with water or saline (*solvent*) to make a weaker *solution.*

Solution Concentration

An important concept for understanding solution concentration or strength is that the amount of solvent used to decrease the total concentration is determined by the desired final strength of the solution. The *less* solvent added, the more concentrated the final solution strength; the *more* solvent added, the less concentrated the final solution strength. Think of orange juice concentrate as a way to illustrate this concept. The directions are for 3 cans of water to be added to 1 can of orange juice concentrate. The result is "reconstituted juice," a ready-to-drink beverage. If you like a stronger orange taste, you could add only 2 cans of water, making it a *more* concentrated juice, but you get *less total volume* to drink. If you have several people wanting to drink orange juice, you might choose to add 4 cans of water to the final total volume. You get *more* volume, but the orange juice is *less* concentrated; therefore, it is more dilute, because you have increased the water (solvent) content. Note that in either case, the amount of orange juice concentrate in the final solution is the same.

Medical written communication to express the strength of a solution uses either a ratio, percent, or fraction. The fraction is the preferred form because it is easily applied in calculation and helps explain the ratio of solute to total solution. Recall that a ratio or percent can also be expressed as a fraction.

RATIONALE FOR PRACTICE

When a fraction expresses the strength of a solution, made from a liquid concentrate:

- **The *numerator* of the fraction is the number of parts of *solute.***
- **The *denominator* of the fraction is the total number of parts of total *solution.***
- **The *difference* between the denominator (final solution) and the numerator (parts of solute) is the number of parts of *solvent.***

Let us describe some solutions made from liquid concentrates.

Example 1:

$\frac{1}{4}$ *strength reconstituted orange juice* made from canned frozen concentrate

$$\frac{1}{4}\text{ strength} = \frac{1\text{ part (can) of frozen orange juice concentrate}}{4\text{ parts (cans) of total reconstituted orange juice}}$$

- 1 part (can) frozen orange juice concentrate (*solute*, numerator)
- 4 parts (cans) of total reconstituted orange juice (*solution*, denominator)
- $4 - 1 = 3$ parts (cans) of water (*solvent*)

Three cans of water added to 1 can frozen orange juice concentrate makes 4 cans of a final reconstituted orange juice solution. The resulting $\frac{1}{4}$ strength reconstituted orange juice is comparable to the strength of fresh juice.

Example 2:

$\frac{1}{3}$ *strength nutritional formula*

- 1 part concentrate formula as the solute
- 3 parts of total solution
- 3 − 1 = 2 parts solvent (water)

Calculating Solutions

To prepare a prescribed solution of a certain strength from a solute, you can apply a similar formula to the one you learned for calculating dosages: $\frac{D}{H} \times Q = X$.

RATIONALE FOR PRACTICE

To prepare solutions,

1. **D (Desired solution strength) × Q (Quantity of desired solution) = X (Amount of solute) or you can apply ratio-proportion to find the amount of solute:**

   Ratio for desired solution strength $= \frac{\text{Amount of solute}}{\text{Quantity of desired solution}}$

2. **Quantity of desired solution − Amount of solute = Amount of solvent**

In this application, "D" is the strength of the desired solution, which is written as a fraction. "Q" is the amount of solution you desire to prepare, usually expressed as millilitres or ounces. The unknown "X" you are solving for is the quantity or amount of solute you will need to add to the solvent to prepare the desired solution. Let us now examine how this rule and formula are applied in healthcare.

TOPICAL SOLUTIONS/IRRIGANTS

Topical or irrigating solutions may be mixed from powders, salts, or liquid concentrates. Asepsis in all stages of preparing, using, and storing the solution is essential. Liquids can quickly harbour microorganisms. Our focus here is to review the essentials of reconstitution, but nurses and other healthcare professionals need to be alert at all times to the possibility of infection by contamination.

Most often nurses and other healthcare professionals will further dilute ready-to-use solutions, which are called *full-strength* or stock solutions, to create a less concentrated liquid. Consider the desired solution strength as well as the final volume needed for the task.

Example:

Hydrogen peroxide, which is usually available full strength as a 3% solution, can be drying to the skin and should not be directly applied undiluted. For use as a topical antiseptic, the therapeutic protocol is to reconstitute hydrogen peroxide to $\frac{1}{2}$ strength with normal saline used as the solvent. You decide to make 120 mL that can be kept in a sterile container at the patient's bedside for traction pin care.

Step 1 Convert No conversion is necessary.

Step 2 Think The fraction represents the desired solution strength: $\frac{1}{2}$ strength means 1 part solute (hydrogen peroxide) to 2 total parts solution. The amount of solvent is 2 − 1 = 1 part saline. Because you need 120 mL of solution, you estimate that you will need $\frac{1}{2}$ of it as solute and $\frac{1}{2}$ of it as solvent, or 60 mL hydrogen peroxide and 60 mL saline to make a total of 120 mL of $\frac{1}{2}$ strength hydrogen peroxide.

Step 3 Calculate $D \times Q = X$

$\frac{1}{2}$ (Strength of desired solution) $\times$ 120 mL (Quantity desired) $=$ X (Amount of solute)

$$\frac{1}{2} \times 120\,\text{mL} = 60\,\text{mL}$$

You could also use ratio-proportion, if you prefer.

Remember that $\frac{1}{2}$ strength $= \frac{1\text{ part solute}}{2\text{ parts total solution}}$. Here, the desired solution strength is $\frac{1}{2}$. The quantity of solution desired is 120 mL. You want to know how much solute (X mL) you will need.

$$\frac{1}{2} \times \frac{X\text{ mL (solute)}}{120\text{ mL (solution)}}$$

$60X = 120$

$$\frac{2X}{2} = \frac{120}{60}$$

$X = 60$ mL of solute

X (60 mL) is the quantity of solute (full-strength hydrogen peroxide) you will need to prepare the desired solution (120 mL of $\frac{1}{2}$ strength hydrogen peroxide). The amount of solvent is 120 mL $-$ 60 mL $=$ 60 mL. If you add 60 mL of full-strength hydrogen peroxide (solute) to 60 mL of normal saline (solvent), you will prepare 120 mL of a $\frac{1}{2}$ strength hydrogen peroxide topical antiseptic.

ORAL AND ENTERAL FEEDINGS

The principles of reconstitution are frequently applied to nutritional liquids for children and adults with special needs. Premature infants require increased calories for growth yet cannot take large volumes of fluid. Children who suffer from intestinal malabsorption require incremental changes as their bodies adjust to more concentrated formulas. Adults, especially older adults, also experience nutritional problems that can be remedied with liquid nutrition. Prepared solutions that are taken orally or through nasogastric, jejunal, or gastric (often a percutaneous endoscopic gastrostomy) feeding tubes are usually available and ready to use from manufacturers. Nutritional solutions may also be mixed from powders or liquid concentrates. Figure 10-13 shows examples of the three forms of one nutritional formula. Directions on the label detail how much water should be added to the powdered form or liquid concentrate. Nutritionists provide further expertise in creating complex solutions for special patient needs.

Asepsis in the preparation, use, and storage of nutritional liquids is essential. Because they contain sugars, such liquids have an increased risk of contamination during preparation and spoilage during storage and use. These are important concepts to teach a patient's family members.

Diluting Ready-to-Use Nutritional Liquids

Ready-to-use nutritional liquid products are those solutions that are normally administered directly from the container without any further dilution. Many ready-to-use products contain 68 calories per 100 mL and are used of children and adults. The manufacturer balances the solute (nutrition) and solvent (water) to create a balanced, full-strength solution. However, some children and adults require less than full-strength product for a short period to normalize intestinal absorption. Nutritional products are diluted with sterile water or tap water for oral use. Consult the institution policy regarding the use of tap water to reconstitute nutritional products. A few typical examples follow.

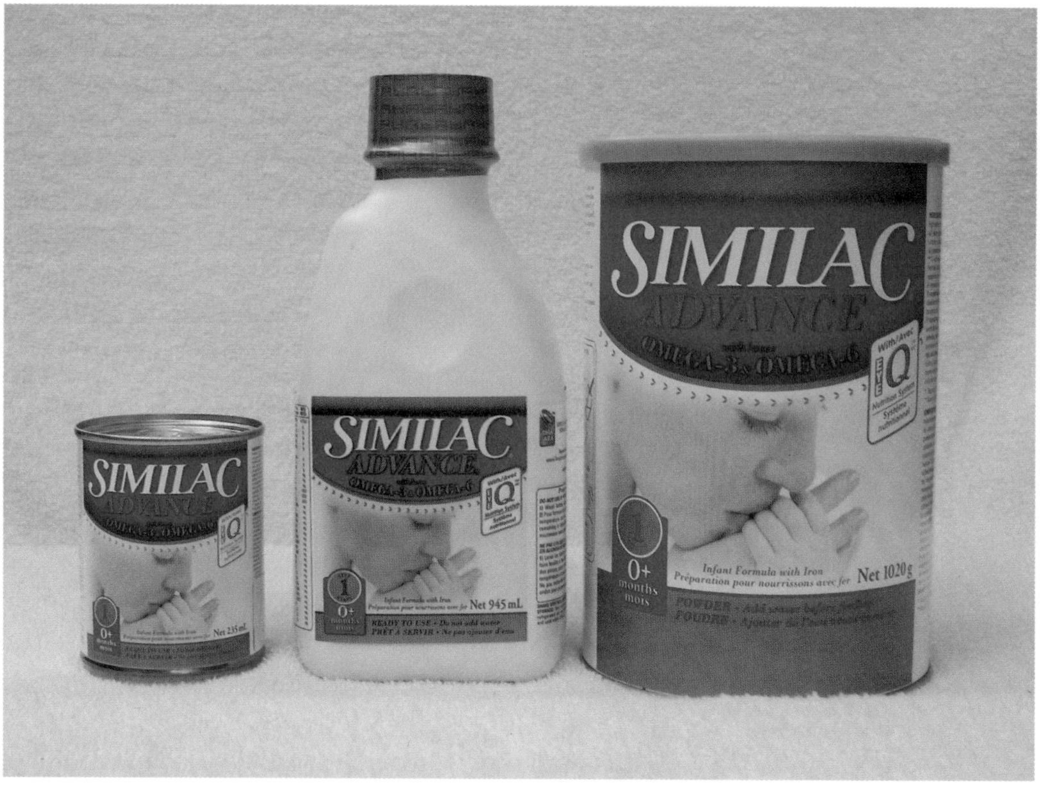

Lynn McLeod

FIGURE 10-13 Similac Advance LF Nutritional Formulas Can Labels

Example 1:

A physician orders *Ensure $\frac{1}{4}$ strength 120 mL q2h via NG tube × 3 feedings* for a patient who is recovering from gastric surgery. Available is a 235-mL can of Ensure ready-to-use product.

Step 1 Convert No conversion necessary.

Step 2 Think You need 120 mL total reconstituted meal replacement product for each of 3 feedings. This is a total of $120 \times 3 = 360$ mL. But you must dilute the full-strength Ensure to $\frac{1}{4}$ strength. You know that $\frac{1}{4}$ strength means 1 part Ensure to 4 parts solution. The solvent needed is $4 - 1 = 3$ parts water. You will need $\frac{1}{4}$ of the solution as solute ($\frac{1}{4} \times 360\,\text{mL} = 90\,\text{mL}$) and $\frac{3}{4}$ of the solution as solvent ($\frac{3}{4} \times 360\,\text{mL} = 270\,\text{mL}$). Therefore, if you mix 90 mL of full-strength Ensure with 270 mL of water, you will have 360 mL of $\frac{1}{4}$ strength Ensure.

Step 3 Calculate $D \times Q = \frac{1}{4} \times 360\text{ mL} = 90\text{ mL}$ full-strength Ensure

Or, use ratio-proportion.

$$\frac{1}{4} \quad \frac{X\text{ mL}}{360\text{ mL}}$$

$$4X = 360$$

$$\frac{4X}{4} = \frac{360}{4}$$

$X = 90$ mL of full-strength Ensure

You need 90 mL of Ensure (solute). Use 90 mL from the 235-mL can. The amount of solvent needed is 360 − 90 = 270 mL water. Add 270 mL water to 90 mL of full-strength Ensure to make a total of 360 mL of $\frac{1}{4}$ strength Ensure. There is now enough for 3 full feedings. Administer 120 mL to the patient for each feeding.

Example 2:

The physician orders *800 mL of $\frac{3}{4}$ strength Boost Plus through a gastrostomy tube over 8 h* to supplement a patient while he sleeps. Boost Plus ready-to-use product is available in 237-mL bottles.

Step 1 Convert No conversion necessary.

Step 2 Think The ordered solution strength is $\frac{3}{4}$. This means "3 parts solute to 4 total parts in solution." You know that $\frac{3}{4}$ of the 800 mL will be solute or full-strength Boost Plus ($\frac{3}{4} \times 800 = 600\,\text{mL}$) and $\frac{1}{4}$ of the solution will be solvent or water ($\frac{1}{4} \times 800 = 200\,\text{mL}$). This proportion of solute to solvent will reconstitute the Boost Plus to the required $\frac{3}{4}$ strength and total volume of 800 mL.

Step 3 Calculate $D \times Q = \frac{3}{4} \times 800\,\text{mL} = 600\,\text{mL}$ of full-strength Boost Plus

Or, use ratio-proportion.

$$\frac{3}{4} = \frac{X\text{ mL}}{800\text{ mL}}$$

$$4X = 2400$$

$$\frac{4X}{4} = \frac{2400}{4}$$

$X = 600$ mL of full-strength Boost Plus

You need 600 mL of the nutritional drink Boost Plus (solute). Because the bottle contains 237 mL, you will need 2.6 bottles (600 mL) to prepare the $\frac{3}{4}$ strength Boost Plus as ordered. The amount of solvent needed is 800 mL − 600 mL = 200 mL water. Add 200 mL water to 600 mL (2.6 bottles) of full-strength Boost Plus to make a total of 800 mL of $\frac{3}{4}$ strength Boost Plus for the full feeding.

QUICK REVIEW

- *Solute*—a concentrated or solid substance to be dissolved or diluted.
- *Solvent*—or diluent, a liquid substance that dissolves another substance to prepare a solution.
- *Solution*—the resulting mixture of a solute plus a solvent.
- When a fraction expresses the strength of a desired solution to be made from a liquid concentrate:
  - The *numerator* of the fraction is the number of parts of *solute*.
  - The *denominator* of the fraction is the total number of parts of *solution*.
  - The *difference between the denominator and the numerator* is the number of parts of *solvent*.
- To prepare solutions:

  1. D (Desired solution strength) × Q (Quantity of desired solution) = X (Amount of solute)

     or, Ratio for desired solution strength $= \frac{\text{Amount of solute}}{\text{Quantity of desired solution}}$

  2. Quantity of desired solution − Amount of solute = Amount of solvent.

REVIEW SET 25

Explain how you would prepare each of the following from ready-to-use nutritional formulas for the specified time period. Note which supply would require the least discard of unused product.

1. $\frac{1}{3}$ *strength Ensure 900 mL via NG tube over 9 h.* Supply: Ensure 235-mL can. ____________

2. $\frac{1}{4}$ *strength Isomil 120 mL PO q4h for 24 h.* Supply: Isomil 235-mL can. ____________

3. $\frac{2}{3}$ *strength Boost Plus 300 mL PO QID.* Supply: Boost Plus 237-mL bottle. ____________

4. $\frac{1}{2}$ *strength Ensure 780 mL via gastrostomy tube over 5 h.* Supply: Ensure 235-mL can. ____________

5. $\frac{1}{2}$ *strength Boost Plus 250 mL PO QID.* Supply: Boost Plus 237-mL bottle. ____________

6. $\frac{3}{4}$ *strength Isomil 240 mL PO q4h for 24 h.* Supply: Isomil 235-mL can. ____________

7. $\frac{2}{3}$ *strength Ensure 180 mL via gastrostomy tube over 2 h.* Supply: Ensure 235-mL can. ____________

8. $\frac{1}{4}$ *strength Ensure 480 mL via NG tube over 6 h.* Supply: Ensure 235-mL can. ____________

Prepare the following solutions using the same principles as used for preparing enteral feeding solutions with water as the diluent.

9. 70% solution from 50 mL of mouthwash. ____________

10. 20% solution from 80 mL of skin cleanser. ______________________

11. 2% solution from 5 mL of sodium bicarbonate. ______________________

12. 50% solution from 240 mL of hydrogen peroxide. ______________________

After completing these problems, see page 482 to check your answers.

CRITICAL THINKING SKILLS

Errors in formula dilution occur when the nurse fails to correctly calculate the amount of solute and solvent needed for the required solution strength.

error

Incorrect calculation of solute and solvent.

possible scenario

Suppose the physician ordered $\frac{1}{3}$ *strength Isomil 90 mL PO q3h for four feedings* for an infant recovering from gastroenteritis. The concentration will be increased after these feedings. The nurse knows she will give all four feedings during her 12-hour shift, so she requires 360 mL of product. She takes a 235-mL can of ready-to-use Isomil, removes 120 mL, and adds 360 mL of water for oral use. She thinks, "One-third means 120 mL of formula and 360 mL of water. This is easy!"

potential outcome

What the nurse has actually mixed is a $\frac{1}{4}$ strength solution. Because the infant is getting a more dilute solution than intended, the amount of water to solute is increased and the incremental tolerance of more concentrated product could be jeopardized. Thinking the child is tolerating $\frac{1}{3}$ strength, the physician might increase it to $\frac{2}{3}$ strength, and the infant may have problems digesting this more concentrated product. His progress could be jeopardized.

prevention

The nurse should have thought through the meaning of the terms of a solution. If so, she would have recognized that $\frac{1}{3}$ strength meant 1 part solute (formula) to 3 total parts of solution with 2 parts water, not 1 part formula to 3 parts water. She should have applied the calculation formula to determine the amount of solute (full-strength Isomil) needed and the amount of solvent (water) to add. If she did not know how to prepare the product, she should have conferred with another nurse or called the pharmacy or dietary services for assistance. Never guess. Think and calculate with accuracy.

PRACTICE PROBLEMS—CHAPTER 10

Calculate the amount you will prepare for one dose. Indicate the syringe you will select to measure the medication.

1. Order: *piperacillin sodium/tazobactam sodium 2.5 g IV q8h*

   Supply: 3.375-g vial of powdered piperacillin sodium/tazobactam sodium

   Directions: 1. Reconstitute piperacillin sodium/tazobactam sodium with 15 mL of a diluent from the list for a total solution volume of 17.36 mL at 0.194 g/mL.

   The concentration is ________ g/ ________ mL

   Give: ________ mL

   Select: ________ syringe

2. Order: *ampicillin sodium 500 mg IM q4h*

   Supply: ampicillin sodium 500 mg

   Directions: Reconstitute with 1.8 mL diluent for a concentration of 250 mg/mL

   Give: ________ mL

   Select: ________ syringe

3. Order: *cefazolin sodium 500 mg IV q6h*

   Supply: cefazolin sodium 1 g

   Directions: Reconstitute with 2.5 mL diluent to yield 3 mL with concentration of 330 mg/mL

   Give: ________ mL

   Select: ________ syringe

4. Order: *ceftriaxone sodium 750 mg IV q6h in 50 mL 5% Dextrose & Water IV solution*

   Supply: See label and package insert for ceftriaxone sodium IV vial.

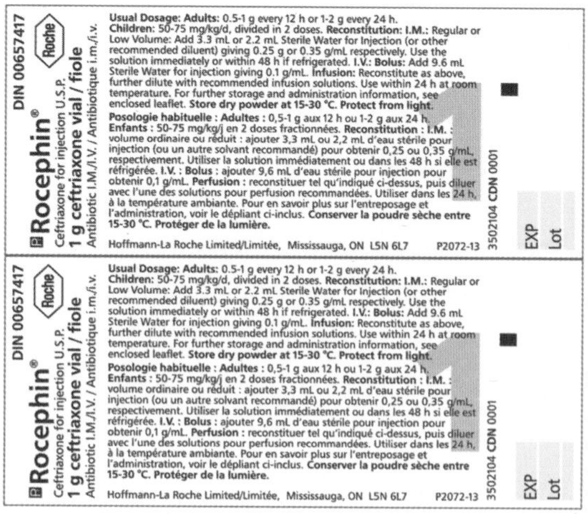

Label submitted by manufacturer for general information and may change; please always refer to the latest product monograph/label. ©Copyright 2007, Hoffman-LaRoche Limited.

Label submitted by manufacturer for general information and may change; please always refer to the latest product monograph/label. ©Copyright 2007, Hoffman-LaRoche Limited.

3599043 CDN
0504.1075

Rocephin®
Ceftriaxone for injection

Roche

Please refer to product monograph for full product information

Dosage and administration
ROCEPHIN (ceftriaxone sodium) may be administered intravenously or intramuscularly after reconstitution.
Dosage and route of administration should be determined by the severity of infection, susceptibility of the causative organisms, and condition of the patient. The intravenous route is preferable for patients with septicemia or other severe or life threatening infections.

Dosage
Adults

Type of infection	Route	Dose	Frequency	Total daily dose
Moderate and severe infections	I.V. or I.M.	1 or 2 g	q24 h	1 or 2 g
		0.5 or 1 g	q12 h	1 or 2 g

There is limited experience with daily doses of 3–4 g administered as single dose or two equally divided doses. The total daily dose should not exceed 4 g.

Uncomplicated gonorrhea	I.M.	0.25 g	Single dose	–

Infants and children (one month to 12 years of age)

Type of infection	Route	Dose	Frequency	Total daily dose
Serious miscellaneous infections	I.V. or I.M.	25 or 37.5 mg per kg	q12 h	50 or 75 mg per kg

The total daily dose should not exceed 2 g. If body weight is 50 kg or more the adult dose should be used.

Meningitis	I.V. or I.M.	50 mg/kg*	q12 h	100 mg/kg

* With or without a loading dose of 75 mg/kg.
The total daily dose should not exceed 4 g.

With the exception of gonorrhea, which is treated with a single dose, the administration of ROCEPHIN should be continued for a minimum of 48–72 hours after the patient defervesces or after evidence of bacterial eradication has been obtained, usually 4–14 days. In bone and joint infections the average duration of treatment during clinical trials was 6 weeks, with a range of 1–13 weeks, depending on the severity of the infection.
When treating infections caused by beta hemolytic streptococcus, it is recommended that therapy be continued for at least 10 days. The average duration of therapy for infections associated with beta hemolytic streptococcus during clinical trials was 2 weeks, with a range of 1–5 weeks, depending on the site and severity of the infection.

Prophylaxis
(vaginal or abdominal hysterectomy, coronary artery bypass surgery, biliary tract surgery)
For preoperative use as prophylaxis before vaginal or abdominal hysterectomy or coronary artery bypass surgery or biliary tract surgery in patients at risk of infection, a single dose of 1 g administered ½–2 hours before surgery is recommended.

Impairment of renal and/or hepatic function
In patients with mild to moderate renal impairment, changes in the dosage regimen are not required, provided liver function is intact. In cases of preterminal renal failure (creatinine clearance less than 10 mL per min), periodic monitoring of serum ceftriaxone concentrations is recommended. The daily dosage should be limited to 2 g or less. In patients with liver damage, there is no need for the dosage to be reduced provided renal function is intact. In cases of coexistent renal and clinically significant hepatic insufficiency, close monitoring of serum ceftriaxone concentrations, at regular intervals, is recommended. If there is evidence of accumulation, dosage should be decreased accordingly.

Administration
Intramuscular
The reconstituted solution of ROCEPHIN should be administered by deep intragluteal injection. It is recommended that not more than 1 g be injected at a single site. Pain on intramuscular injection is usually mild and less frequent when ROCEPHIN is administered in sterile 1% lidocaine solution.

Intravenous (bolus) injection
The reconstituted solution should be administered over approximately 5 minutes. If the distal port of an intravenous administration set is used, stop the primary flow, inject the reconstituted ROCEPHIN solution and then restart the primary flow. This will prevent mixing with the primary fluid and possible incompatibilities.

Short intravenous infusion
The further diluted intravenous solution should be given over a period of 10–15 minutes in infants and children and 20–30 minutes in adults.
Note: ROCEPHIN solution should not be physically mixed with aminoglycoside antibiotics nor administered at the same site because of possible chemical incompatibility. There have also been literature reports of physical incompatibilities between ceftriaxone and vancomycin, amsacrine, or fluconazole.

Reconstitution
For intramuscular use
Reconstitute ROCEPHIN powder with the appropriate diluent:
- Sterile Water for Injection
- 0.9% Sodium Chloride Injection
- 5% Dextrose Injection
- Bacteriostatic Water for Injection
- 1% Lidocaine Solution

Reconstitute as follows:
Regular volume reconstitution table (I.M.)*

Vial size	Volume to be added to vial mL	Approximate available volume mL	Approximate average concentration g/mL
0.25 g	0.9	1.0	0.25
1.0 g	3.3	4.0	0.25
2.0 g	6.6	8.0	0.25

*Shake well until dissolved.

Low volume reconstitution table (I.M.)*

Vial size	Volume to be added to vial mL	Approximate available volume mL	Approximate average concentration g/mL
0.25 g	Not recommended for this vial size		
1.0 g	2.2	2.8	0.35
2.0 g	4.4	5.6	0.35

*Shake well until dissolved.

Note: solutions prepared for intramuscular use or any solution containing lidocaine or bacteriostatic water for injection should never be administered intravenously.

For intravenous use
Reconstitute only with Sterile Water for Injection.

Reconstitute as follows:
Reconstitution table (I.V.)**

Vial size	Volume to be added to vial mL	Approximate available volume mL	Approximate average concentration g/mL
0.25 g	2.4	2.5	0.1
1.0 g	9.6	10.1	0.1
2.0 g	19.2	20.5	0.1

**Shake well until dissolved. The prepared solution may be further diluted to the desired volume with any of the "Solutions for I.V. Infusion" listed below.

Solutions for I.V. infusion
- 0.9% Sodium Chloride Injection
- 5% Dextrose Injection
- Dextrose and Sodium Chloride Injection

Pharmacy bulk vial reconstitution for preparation of intravenous infusion solutions
The closure of the pharmacy bulk vial shall be penetrated only one time after reconstitution, using a suitable sterile transfer device or dispensing set which allows measured dispensing for the contents.
Reconstitution table for bulk pharmacy vial***

Vial size	Volume to be added to vial mL	Approximate available volume mL	Approximate average concentration g/mL
10 g	95	101	0.1

***Shake well until dissolved. Withdraw the required amount and dilute with one of the "Solutions for I.V. infusion". Any unused solution remaining within a period of 8 hours should be discarded.

Stability and storage recommendations
ROCEPHIN sterile powder should be stored at a controlled room temperature (between 15 and 30°C) and protected from light.

Reconstituted solutions – Stability and storage recommendations
1. *For intramuscular use:* Solutions should be reconstituted immediately before use. If storage is required, these solutions may be stored under refrigeration and should be used within 48 hours.
2. *For I.V. bolus injection (without further dilution):* Reconstituted solutions should be administered within 24 hours when stored at room temperature and within 72 hours when refrigerated (2–8°C).
3. *For I.V. infusion:* Further diluted reconstituted solutions should be administered within 24 hours when stored at room temperature.
   a) Solutions further diluted with 0.9% Sodium Chloride Injection, or with 5% Dextrose Injection should be administered within 72 hours when stored under refrigeration (2–8°C).
   b) Solutions further diluted with Dextrose and Sodium Chloride Injection as diluent should not be refrigerated. These solutions are not physically compatible when refrigerated.
4. *Extended use of intravenous admixtures:* Although intravenous admixtures may often be physically and chemically stable for longer periods, **due to microbiological considerations, they are usually recommended for use within a maximum of 24 hours at room temperature or 72 hours when refrigerated (2–8°C).** Hospitals and institutions that have recognized admixture programs and use validated aseptic techniques for preparation of intravenous solutions may extend the storage times for ROCEPHIN admixtures with 0.9% Sodium Chloride Injection or 5% Dextrose Injection in glass or polyvinyl chloride infusion containers, in concentrations of 3 mg/mL to 40 mg per mL, to 7 days when stored under refrigeration (2–8°C).

   Warning
   As with all parenteral drug products, intravenous admixtures should be visually inspected prior to administration, whenever solution and container permit. Solutions showing any evidence of haziness or cloudiness, particulate matter, precipitation, discolouration or leakage should not be used.
5. *Frozen I.V. infusion solutions:* Hospitals and institutions that have recognized admixture programs and use validated aseptic techniques for preparation of intravenous solutions may freeze and store ROCEPHIN I.V. infusion solutions when prepared in accordance with the following instructions.
   I.V. infusion solutions prepared from reconstituted ROCEPHIN (ceftriaxone sodium) further diluted with 5% Dextrose Injection or 0.9% Sodium Chloride Injection, in flexible polyvinyl chloride infusion containers, in concentrations up to 40 mg ceftriaxone per mL, may be stored at –10 to –20°C for periods up to three months.
   The frozen solutions should be thawed in a refrigerator (2–8°C) overnight and should subsequently be used within 24 hours when stored at room temperature or seven days when stored under refrigeration (2–8°C).
   After thawing, check for leaks by squeezing the bag firmly. If leaks are found, discard the container as sterility may be impaired. Do not use unless the solution is clear and seals/outlet ports are intact. Ceftriaxone solutions range from light yellow to amber in colour. Parenteral drug products should be inspected visually for particulate matter and discolouration prior to administration whenever the solution and container permit.
   DO NOT REFREEZE the previously frozen ceftriaxone I.V. infusion solutions.

Incompatibility
ROCEPHIN should not be physically mixed with other antimicrobial agents, vancomycin, amsacrine, or fluconazole.
ROCEPHIN should not be added to blood products, protein hydrolysates or amino acids.
ROCEPHIN should not be added to solutions containing calcium.

Availability of dosage forms
1. ROCEPHIN vials containing sterile ceftriaxone sodium powder equivalent to 0.25 g, 1 g and 2 g of ceftriaxone.
2. ROCEPHIN Pharmacy Bulk vials containing sterile ceftriaxone sodium powder equivalent to 10 g ceftriaxone (not for direct administration). The availability of the pharmacy bulk vial is restricted to hospitals with a recognized intravenous admixture programme.

Product monograph dated March 5, 2004
This leaflet issued May 2005
© Copyright 1997–2004, Hoffmann-La Roche Limited
® Registered Trade-Mark of Hoffmann-La Roche Limited
Registered Trade-Mark
Hoffmann-La Roche Limited
Mississauga, ON L5N 6L7

P3367-07

Add ________ mL diluent to the vial.

The concentration is ________ mg/mL

Give: ________ mL

How many full doses are available in this vial? ________

Select: ________ syringe

5. Order: *cefepime hydrochloride 500 mg IM q12h*

   Supply: cefepime hydrochloride 1 g

   Directions: Reconstitute with 2.4 mL diluent for an approximate available volume of 3.6 mL and a concentration of 280 mg/mL.

   Give: ________ mL

   Select: ________ syringe

   How many full doses are available in this vial? ________ dose(s).

   Prepare a reconstitution label for the remaining solution. The drug is stable for up to 72 hours refrigerated.

Reconstitution Label

6. Order: *dalfopristin/quinupristin 375 mg IV q8h*

   Supply: dalfopristin/quinupristin 500 mg

   Directions: Reconstitute with 5 mL sterile water for a concentration of 100 mg/mL.

   Give: ________ mL

   Select: ________ syringe

   How many full doses are available in this vial? ________

Calculate one dose of each of the drug orders numbered 7 through 15. The labels show the medications you have available. Indicate which syringe you would select to measure the dose to be administered. Specify if a reconstitution label is required for multiple-dose vials.

7. Order: *cefazolin sodium 300 mg IM q8h*

   Reconstitute with ________ mL diluent for a concentration of ________ mg/mL and give ________ mL.

   Select: ________ syringe

   How many full doses are available in this vial? ________ dose(s)

   Is a reconstitution label required? ________

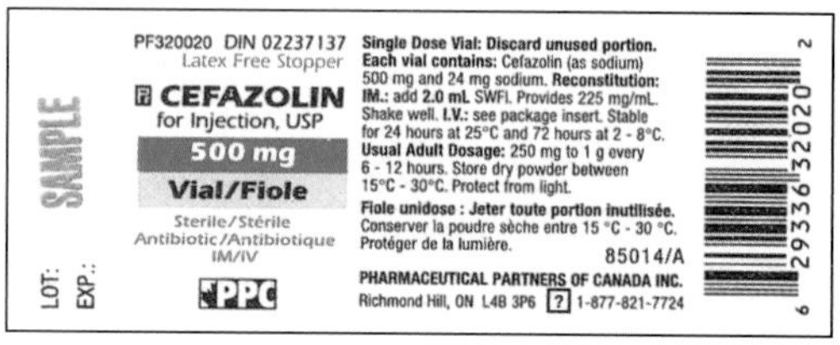

Pharmaceutical Partners of Canada Inc., Richmond Hill, ON

8. Order: *methylprednisolone sodium succinate 200 mg IV q6h*

   Reconstitute with ________ mL diluent for a concentration of ________ mg/mL and give ________ mL.

   Select: ________ syringe

   How many full doses are available in this vial? ________ dose(s)

   Is a reconstitution label required? ________

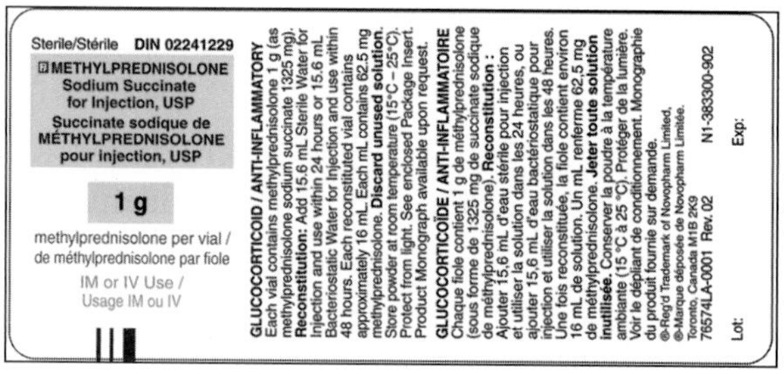

Novopharm Limited, Toronto, ON

9. Order: *cefazolin sodium 350 mg IM q12h*

   Reconstitute with ________ mL diluent for a concentration of ________ mg/mL and give ________ mL.

   Select: ________ syringe

   How many full doses are available in this vial? ________ dose(s)

   Is a reconstitution label required? ________

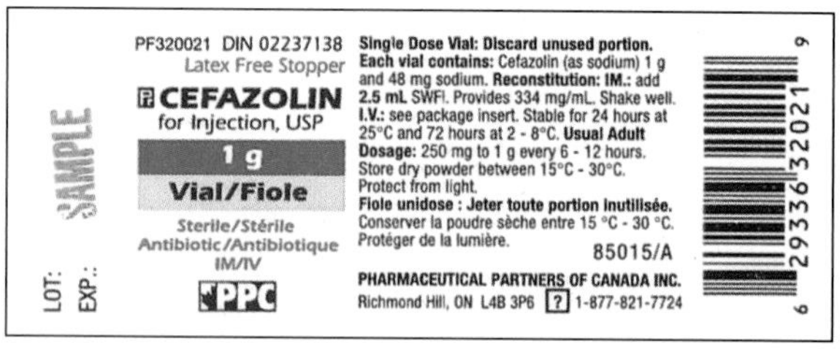

Pharmaceutical Partners of Canada Inc., Richmond Hill, ON

10. Order: *bacitracin 7500 units IM q12h*

Reconstitution of the 50,000 unit vial with 9.8 mL of diluent will result in a concentration of 5,000 units per mL. Solutions are stable for 1 week when refrigerated.

   Reconstitute with ________ mL diluent for a concentration of ________ units/mL and give ________ mL.

   Select: ________ syringe

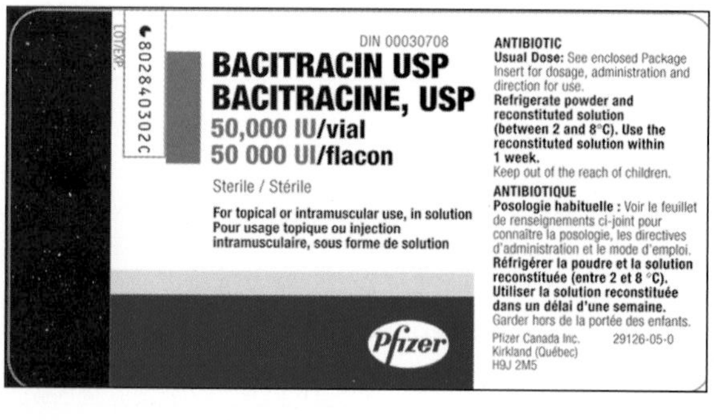

©Pfizer Canada Inc., Kirkland, Que

How many full doses are available in this vial?
________ dose(s)

Is a reconstitution label required? ________

11. Order: *ceftazidime 1.25 g IV q12h*

Reconstitute with ________ mL diluent for a concentration of ________ mg/ ________ mL make it mg and give ________ mL.

Select: ________ syringe

How many full doses are available in this vial?
________ dose(s)

Is a reconstitution label required? ________

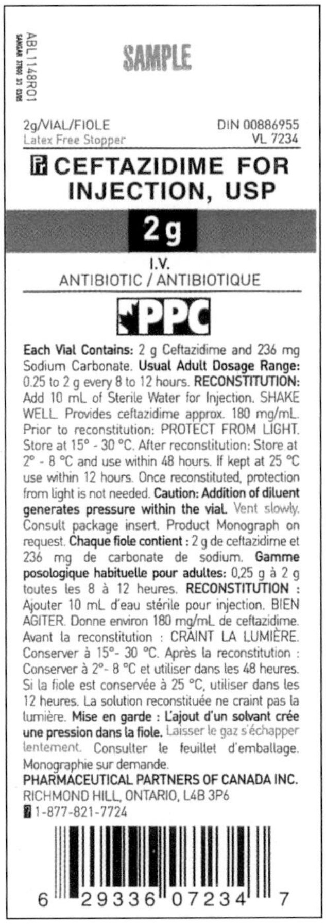

Pharmaceutical Partners of Canada Inc., Richmond Hill, ON

12. Order: *tobramycin sulfate 60 mg IV q8h*

Reconstitute with ________ mL diluent for a concentration of ________ mg/mL and give ________ mL.

Select: ________ syringe

How many full doses are available in this vial? ________ dose(s)

Is a reconstitution label required? ________

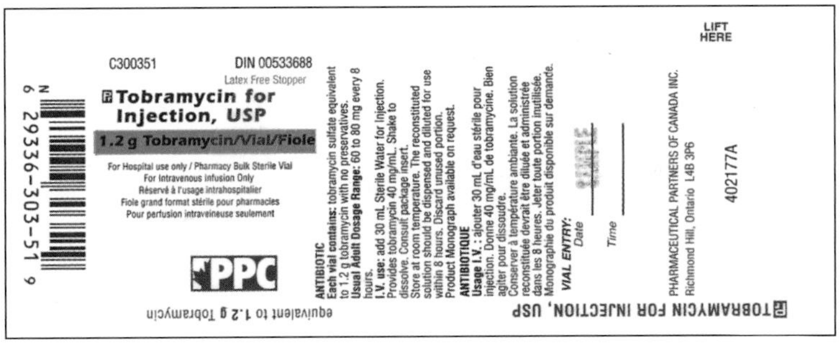

Pharmaceutical Partners of Canada Inc., Richmond Hill, ON

13. Order: *penicillin G sodium 2 000 000 units IM q8h*

Reconstitute with ________ mL diluent for a concentration of ________ units/mL and give ________ mL.

Select: ________ syringe

How many full doses are available in this vial? ________ dose(s)

Is a reconstitution label required? ________

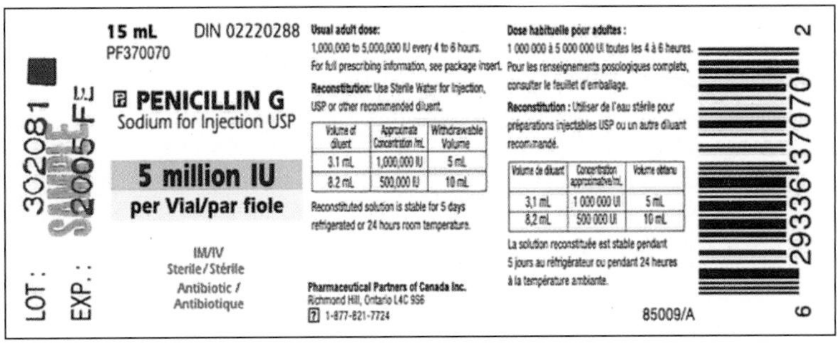

Pharmaceutical Partners of Canada Inc., Richmond Hill, ON

14. Order: *penicillin G sodium 1 000 000 units IM q8h*

    Reconstitute with ________ mL diluent for a concentration of ________ units/mL and give ________ mL.

    Select: ________ syringe

    How many full doses are available in this vial? ________ dose(s)

    Is a reconstitution label required? ________

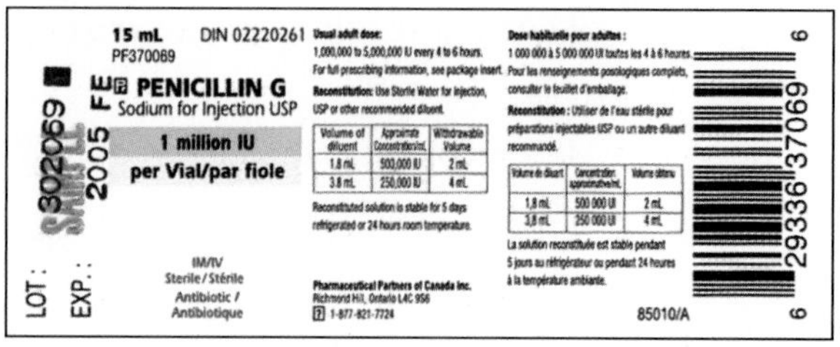

Pharmaceutical Partners of Canada Inc., Richmond Hill, ON

15. Order: *cefazolin sodium 400mg IM q8h*

    Reconstitute with ________ mL diluent for a concentration of ________ mg/mL and give ______ mL.

    Select: ________ syringe

    How many full doses are available in this vial? ________ dose(s)

    Is a reconstitution label required? ________

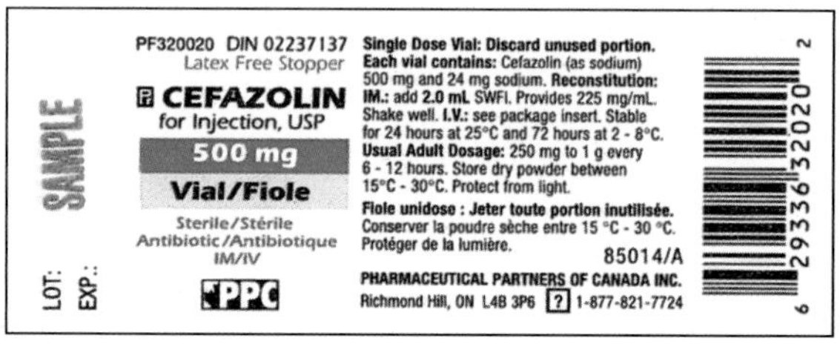

Pharmaceutical Partners of Canada Inc., Richmond Hill, ON

Explain how you would prepare each of the following hydrogen peroxide (solute) and normal saline (solvent) irrigation orders:

16. 480 mL of $\frac{1}{8}$ strength solution ________________

17. 320 mL of $\frac{3}{8}$ strength solution ________________

18. 80 mL of $\frac{5}{8}$ strength solution ________________

19. 540 mL of $\frac{2}{3}$ strength solution ________________

20. 500 mL of $\frac{7}{8}$ strength solution ________________

21. 1 L of $\frac{1}{4}$ strength solution ________________

Explain how you would prepare each of the following from ready-to-use nutritional formulas for the specified time period. Note how many cans or bottles of supply are needed and how much unused formula would remain from the used supply.

22. Order: *$\frac{1}{4}$ strength Enfamil 12 mL via NG tube hourly for 10 h*

    Supply: Enfamil 235-mL can

    ____

23. Order: *$\frac{3}{4}$ strength Boost Plus 360 mL over 4 h via gastrostomy*

    Supply: Sustacal 237-mL bottles

    ____

24. Order: *$\frac{2}{3}$ strength Ensure. Give 90 mL hourly for 5 h via NG tube.*

    Supply: Ensure 235-mL can

    ____

25. Order: $\frac{3}{8}$ *strength Enfamil.* Three patients need 960 mL of the $\frac{3}{8}$ strength Enfamil for one feeding each.

    Supply: Enfamil 235-mL can

    ____

26. Order: $\frac{1}{8}$ *strength Ensure. Give 160 mL stat via NG tube.*

    Supply: Ensure 235-mL can

    ____

27. Order: $\frac{1}{2}$ *strength Ensure 55 mL hourly for 10 h via gastrostomy tube*

    Supply: Ensure 235-mL can

    ____

The nurse is making up $\frac{1}{4}$ strength Enfamil formula for several infants in the nursery.

28. If 235-mL cans of ready-to-use Enfamil are available, how many cans of formula will be needed to make 1.4 L of reconstituted $\frac{1}{4}$ strength Enfamil? ________ can(s)

29. How many mL of water will be added to the Enfamil in question 28 to correctly reconstitute the $\frac{1}{4}$ strength Enfamil? ________ mL

30. Critical Thinking Skill: Describe the error that took place and the strategy that you would implement to prevent the medication error.

    possible scenario

    The order for your patient is *ceftazidime 250 mg IM stat and q8h.*

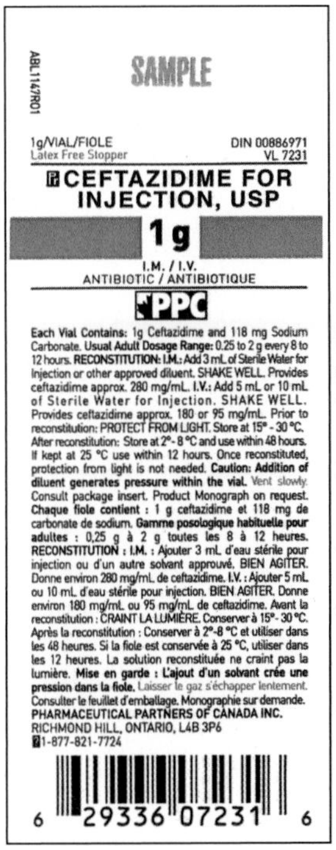

Pharmaceutical Partners of Canada Inc., Richmond Hill, ON

The nurse reconstituted the vial with 10.6 mL of sterile water for injection as diluent. Next the nurse calculated the dosage using the $\frac{D}{H} \times Q = X$ formula.

$$\frac{D}{H} \times Q = \frac{250\,\text{mg}}{95\,\text{mg}} \times 1 = 2.62 \text{ or } 2.6\text{ mL}$$

The nurse administered 2.6 mL of ceftazidime IM.

potential outcome

The nurse has administered a solution that is indicated for IV injection not IM. As the total solution would not be used, the vial would also be labelled incorrectly, resulting in the dosage strength for any further doses taken from this vial being incorrect.

prevention

____

____

After completing these problems, see pages 483–484 to check your answers.

CHAPTER 11

Pediatric and Adult Dosages Based on Body Weight

LEARNING OBJECTIVES

1. Calculate drug dosages based on body weight.
2. Verify the safety of medication orders.
3. Convert pounds to kilograms.
4. Consult a reputable drug resource to calculate the recommended safe dosage per kilogram of body weight.
5. Compare the ordered dosage with the recommended safe dosage.
6. Determine whether the ordered dosage is safe to administer.
7. Apply body weight dosage calculations to patients across the life span.

Body weight is an important consideration when calculating drug dosages for both adults and children. The prescriber is responsible for ordering the dosage of medications; however, before administering a drug, the nurse must know if the ordered dosage is accurate and safe. This is important for adults and critical for infants, children, frail older adults, and critically ill adults.

> **CAUTION**
>
> Those who administer drugs to patients are legally responsible for recognizing incorrect and unsafe dosages and for alerting the prescribing practitioner.

Safe drug administration remains the responsibility of the nurse who must verify the dosage to make sure that it is accurate. The nurse who is administering the drug is responsible for any errors in calculating the dosage. Therefore, it is important that the nurse check the drug label or the package insert for the recommended dosage of drugs. A reputable drug reference, the Hospital Formulary, and the hospital pharmacist are additional sources for detailed information.

A standard adult dosage is determined by the drug manufacturer. The dosage is usually recommended based on the requirements of an average-weight adult. Frequently an adult range is given, listing a minimum and maximum safe dosage, allowing the nurse to simply compare what is ordered to what is recommended.

Dosages for infants and children are based on their unique and changing body differences. The prescribing practitioner must consider the weight, height, body surface, age, and condition of the child as contributing factors to safe and effective medication dosages. The two methods currently used for calculating safe pediatric dosages are *body weight* (such as mg/kg) and *body surface area* (BSA, measured in square metres, m^2). The body weight method is more common in pediatric situations and is emphasized in this chapter. The BSA method is based on both weight and height. It is used primarily in oncology and critical care situations. BSA is discussed in Chapter 13. Although used most frequently in pediatrics, both the body weight and BSA methods are also used for adults, especially in critical care situations. The calculations are the same.

ADMINISTERING MEDICATIONS TO CHILDREN

Numerically, the infant's or child's dosage appears smaller, but *proportionally* pediatric dosages are frequently much larger per kilogram of body weight than the usual adult dosage. Infants—birth to 1 year—have a greater percentage of body water and diminished ability to absorb water-soluble drugs, necessitating dosages of oral and some parenteral drugs that are higher than those given to persons of larger size. Children—age 1 to 12 years—metabolize drugs more readily than adults, which necessitates higher dosages. Both infants and children, however, are growing, and their organ systems are still maturing. Immature physiological processes related to drug pharmacokinetics (absorption, distribution, metabolism, and excretion) place them at risk of overdose, toxic reactions, and even death. Adolescents—age 13 to 18 years—are often erroneously thought of as adults because of their body weight (greater than 50 kilograms) and mature physical appearance. In fact, they should still be regarded as physiologically immature, with unpredictable growth spurts and hormonal surges. Drug therapy for the pediatric population is further complicated because limited detailed pharmacological research has been carried out on children and adolescents. The infant or child, therefore, must be frequently evaluated for desired clinical responses to medications, and serum drug levels may be needed to help adjust some drug dosages. It is important to remember that administration of an incorrect dosage to adult patients is dangerous, but with a child, the risk is even greater. Therefore, using a reputable drug reference to verify safe pediatric dosages is a critical healthcare skill.

CONVERTING POUNDS TO KILOGRAMS

The body weight method uses calculations based on the patient's weight in kilograms. Recall that the pounds to kilograms conversion was introduced in Chapter 4.

REMEMBER

1 kg = 2.2 lb and 1 lb = 16 oz

Simply stated, weight in pounds is approximately twice the metric weight in kilograms; or weight in kilograms is approximately $\frac{1}{2}$ of weight in pounds. You can estimate kilograms by halving the weight in pounds.

MATH TIP

When converting pounds to kilograms, round kilogram weight to one decimal place (tenths).

Example 1:

Convert 45 lb to kg

Approximate equivalent: 1 kg = 2.2 lb

Think: $\frac{1}{2}$ of 45 = approximately 23

Smaller → Larger: (÷)

45 lb = 45 ÷ 2.2 = 20.45 kg = 20.5 kg

Example 2:

Convert 10 lb 12 oz to kg

Approximate equivalents: 1 kg = 2.2 lb

1 lb = 16 oz

Smaller → Larger: (÷)

$12 \text{ oz} = 12 \div 16 = \frac{\overset{3}{\cancel{12}}}{\underset{4}{\cancel{16}}} = \frac{3}{4} \text{ lb; so } 10 \text{ lb } 12 \text{ oz} = 10\frac{3}{4} \text{ lb}$

Think: $\frac{1}{2}$ of $10\frac{3}{4}$ = approximately 5

Smaller → Larger: (÷)

$10\frac{3}{4} \text{ lb} = 10.75 \div 2.2 = 4.88 \text{ kg} = 4.9 \text{ kg}$

BODY WEIGHT METHOD FOR CALCULATING SAFE PEDIATRIC DOSAGE

The most common method of prescribing and administering the therapeutic amount of medication for a child is to calculate the amount of drug according to the child's body weight in **kilograms.** The nurse then compares the child's *ordered dosage* to the recommended *safe dosage* from a reputable drug resource before administering the medication. The intent is to ensure that the ordered dosage is safe and effective *before* calculating the amount to give and administering the dose to the patient.

RATIONALE FOR PRACTICE

To verify safe pediatric dosage:

1. Convert the child's weight from pounds to kilograms (rounded to tenths).
2. Calculate the safe dosage in mg/kg or mcg/kg (rounded to tenths) for a child of this weight, as recommended by a reputable drug reference: **multiply mg/kg by child's weight in kg.**
3. Compare the *ordered dosage* to the *recommended dosage*, and decide if the dosage is safe.
4. If safe, calculate the amount to give and administer the dose; if the dosage seems unsafe, consult with the ordering practitioner before administering the drug.

NOTE: The *dosage per kg* may be mg/kg, mcg/kg, g/kg, mEq/kg, units/kg, etc.

For each pediatric medication order, it is important to question whether the dosage is safe. Let us work through some examples.

Single-Dosage Drugs

Example:

Single-dosage drugs are intended to be given once or prn. Dosage ordered by the body weight method is based on **mg/kg/dose, calculated by multiplying the recommended mg by the patient's kg weight for each dose.**

The physician orders *morphine sulfate 1.8 mg IM stat*. The child weighs 79 lb. Is this dosage safe?

1. **Convert lb to kg.** Approximate equivalent: 1 kg = 2.2 lb

   Think: $\frac{1}{2}$ of 79 = approximately 40

   Smaller → Larger: (÷)

   79 lb = 79 ÷ 2.2 = 35.90 kg = 35.9 kg

2. **Calculate mg/kg as recommended by a reputable drug resource.** A reputable drug resource indicates that the usual intramuscular (IM)/subcutaneous dosage may be initiated at 0.05 mg/kg/dose.

> **MATH TIP**
>
> Notice that the kg unit of measurement cancels out, leaving the unit as mg/dose.
>
> $$\frac{\text{mg}}{\cancel{\text{kg}}/\text{dose}} \times \cancel{\text{kg}} = \text{mg/dose}$$
>
> Or,
>
> $\text{mg}/\cancel{\text{kg}}/\text{dose} \times \cancel{\text{kg}} = \text{mg/dose}$

$0.005\ \text{mg}/\cancel{\text{kg}}/\text{does} \times 35.9\ \cancel{\text{kg}} = 1.79\text{mg/does} = 1.8\ \text{mg/dose}$

3. **Decide if the dosage is safe by comparing ordered and recommended dosages.** For this child's weight, 1.8 mg is the recommended dosage and 1.8 mg is the ordered dosage. Yes, the dosage is safe.
4. **Calculate 1 dose.** Apply the three steps of dosage calculation.

Order: *morphine sulfate 1.8 mg IM stat*

Supply: morphine sulfate 5 mg/mL (Figure 11-1)

Step 1 Convert No conversion is necessary.

Step 2 Think You want to give less than 1 mL. Estimate that you want to give less than 0.5 mL.

Step 3 Calculate

$$\frac{D}{H} \times Q = \frac{1.8\ \cancel{\text{mg}}}{5\ \cancel{\text{mg}}} \times 1\ \text{mL} = 0.36\ \text{mL}$$

Or, apply the ratio-proportion method.

$$\frac{5\ \text{mg}}{1\ \text{mL}} \times \frac{1.8\ \text{mg}}{X\ \text{mL}}$$

$5X = 1.8$

$$\frac{5X}{5} = \frac{1.8}{5}$$

$X = 0.36\ \text{mL}$

This is a small, child's dose. Measure 0.36 mL in a 1-mL syringe. Route is IM. Select the appropriate injection needle.

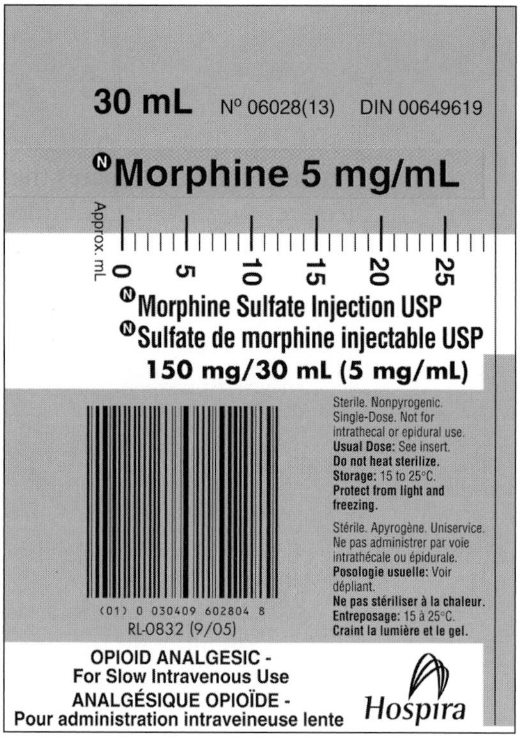
30 mL Nº 06028(13) DIN 00649619
Morphine 5 mg/mL
Approx. mL
0 5 10 15 20 25
Morphine Sulfate Injection USP
Sulfate de morphine injectable USP
150 mg/30 mL (5 mg/mL)
Sterile. Nonpyrogenic. Single-Dose. Not for intrathecal or epidural use. Usual Dose: See insert. Do not heat sterilize. Storage: 15 to 25°C. Protect from light and freezing.
Stérile. Apyrogène. Uniservice. Ne pas administrer par voie intrathécale ou épidurale. Posologie usuelle: Voir dépliant. Ne pas stériliser à la chaleur. Entreposage: 15 à 25°C. Craint la lumière et le gel.
(01) 0 030409 602804 8
RL-0832 (9/05)
OPIOID ANALGESIC - For Slow Intravenous Use
ANALGÉSIQUE OPIOÏDE - Pour administration intraveineuse lente
Hospira

Hospira Healthcare Corporation, Saint-Laurent, QUE

FIGURE 11-1 Morphine Label

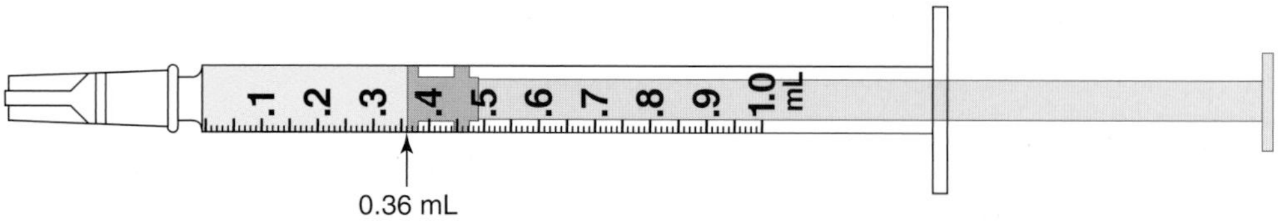
.1 .2 .3 .4 .5 .6 .7 .8 .9 1.0 mL
0.36 mL

Single-Dosage Range

Example:

Some single-dosage medications indicate a minimum and maximum range, or a safe dosage range.

The practitioner orders *hydroxyzine hydrochloride 20 mg IM q4h, prn for nausea*. The child weighs 44 lb. Is this a safe dosage?

1. **Convert lb to kg.** Approximate equivalent: 1 kg = 2.2 lb

   Think: $\frac{1}{2}$ of 44 = 22

   44 lb = 44 ÷ 2.2 = 20 kg

2. **Calculate recommended dosage.** A reputable drug resource indicates that the usual IM dosage is 0.5 mg to 1 mg/kg/dose every 4 to 6 hours as needed. Notice that the recommended dosage is represented as a range of "0.5–1 mg/kg/dose" for dosing flexibility. Calculate the minimum and maximum safe dosage range.

   Minimum per dose: $0.5 \text{ mg/}\cancel{\text{kg}}\text{/dose} \times 20 \cancel{\text{kg}} = 10 \text{ mg/dose}$

   Maximum per dose: $1 \text{ mg/}\cancel{\text{kg}}\text{/dose} \times 20 \cancel{\text{kg}} = 20 \text{ mg/dose}$

3. **Decide if the ordered dosage is safe.** The recommended dosage range is 10 mg to 20 mg, and the ordered dosage of 20 mg is within this range. Yes, the ordered dosage is safe.

4. **Calculate 1 dose.** Apply the three steps of dosage calculation.

   Order: *hydroxyzine hydrochloride 20 mg IM q4h, prn for nausea*

   Supply: hydroxyzine hydrochloride 50 mg/mL (Figure 11-2)

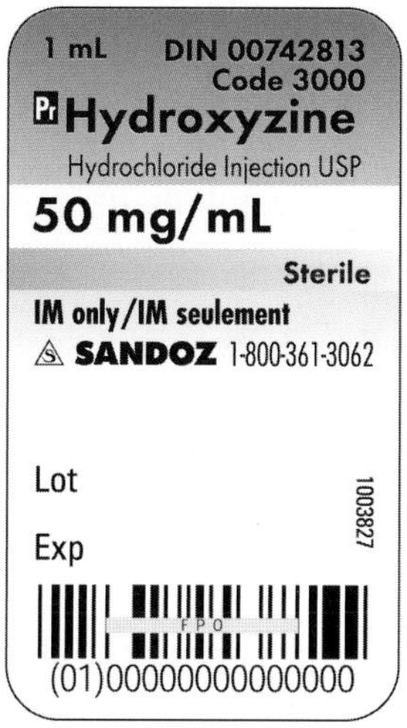

FIGURE 11-2 Hydroxyzine Hydrochloride Label

Step 1	**Convert**	No conversion is necessary.
Step 2	**Think**	Estimate that you want to give less than 1 mL; in fact, you want to give less than 0.5 mL.

Step 3 Calculate $\frac{D}{H} \times Q = \frac{2\cancel{0}\text{ mg}}{5\cancel{0}\text{ mg}} \times 1\text{ mL} = \frac{2}{5}\text{ mL} = 0.4\text{ mL}$

Or, apply the ratio-proportion method.

$$\frac{50\text{ mg}}{1\text{ mL}} \times \frac{20\text{ mg}}{X\text{ mL}}$$

$50X = 20$

$$\frac{50X}{50} = \frac{20}{50}$$

$X = 0.4\text{ mL}$

This is a small, child's dose. Measure it in a 1-mL syringe. Route is IM. Select the appropriate injection needle.

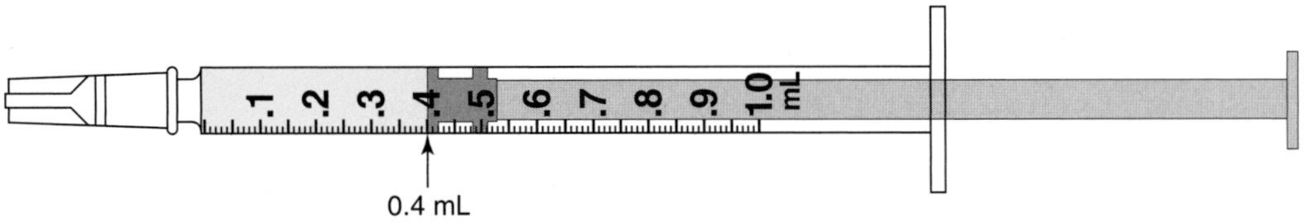

Routine or Round-the-Clock Drugs

Example:

Routine or round-the-clock drugs are intended to produce a continuous therapeutic effect over 24 hours. They are recommended as a *total daily dosage:* **mg/kg/day to be divided into some number of individual doses,** such as "three divided doses," "four divided doses," "divided doses every 8 hours," and so on. "Three divided doses" means the drug total daily dosage is divided equally and is administered three times per day, either TID or q8h. Likewise, "four divided doses" means the total daily drug dosage is divided equally and administered four times per day either QID or q6h. Recommendations like "divided doses every 8 hours" specify that the total daily drug dosage should be divided equally and administered q8h.

The practitioner orders *cefaclor 100 mg PO TID*. The child weighs $33\frac{1}{2}$ lb. Is this dosage safe?

1. **Convert lb to kg.** Approximate equivalent: 1 kg = 2.2 lb

   Think: $\frac{1}{2}$ of 33 = approximately 17

   $33\frac{1}{2}\text{ lb} = 33.5\text{ lb} = 33.5 \div 2.2 = 15.22\text{ kg} = 15.2\text{ kg}$

2. **Calculate recommended dosage.** The recommended dosage on the drug label (Figure 11-3) is, "Usual dose—Children, 20 mg per kg a day . . .in three divided doses." First, calculate the total daily dosage: $20\text{ mg/}\cancel{\text{kg}}\text{/day} \times 15.2\ \cancel{\text{kg}} = 304\text{ mg/day}$. Then, divide this total daily dosage into 3 doses: $304\text{ mg} \div 3\text{ doses} = 101.3\text{ mg/dose}$.

3. **Decide if the ordered dosage is safe.** Yes, the ordered dosage is safe, because this is an *oral* dose and 100 mg is a *reasonably safe* dosage for a 101.3 mg recommended single dosage. Think: To give 101.3 mg you would calculate $\frac{D}{H} \times Q = \frac{101.3\ \cancel{\text{mg}}}{125\ \cancel{\text{mg}}} \times 5\text{ mL} = 4.05\text{ mL}$, which would be rounded to 4 mL. Notice in step 4 that to administer 100 mg, the dose is also 4 mL because of rounding.

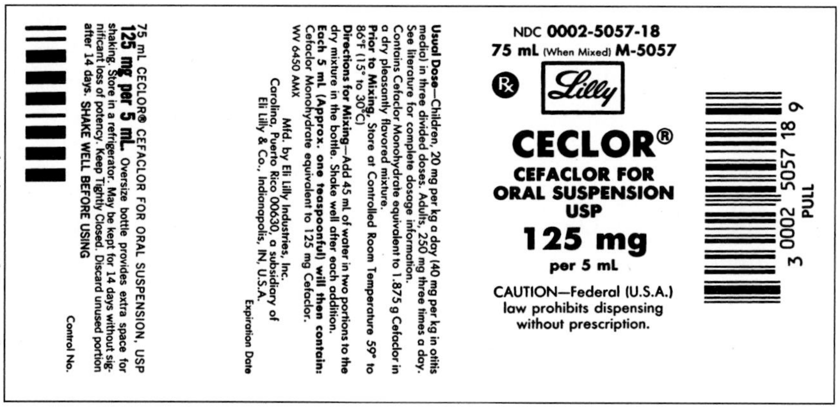

Courtesy of Eli Lilly and Company

FIGURE 11-3 Cefaclor Label

4. **Calculate 1 dose.** Apply the three steps of dosage calculation.

   Order: *cefaclor 100 mg PO TID*

   Supply: *cefaclor 125 mg/5 mL*

Step 1 Convert No conversion is necessary.

Step 2 Think You want to give less than 5 mL. Estimate that you want to give between 2.5 mL and 5 mL.

Step 3 Calculate

$$\frac{D}{H} \times Q = \frac{\overset{4}{\cancel{100}}\text{ mg}}{\underset{5}{\cancel{125}}\text{ mg}} \times 5\text{ mL} = \frac{4}{\cancel{5}}\text{ mL} \times \cancel{5}\text{ mL} = 4\text{ mL}$$

Or, apply the ratio-proportion method.

$$\frac{125\text{ mg}}{5\text{ mL}} \times \frac{100\text{ mg}}{X\text{ mL}}$$

$$125X = 500$$

$$\frac{125X}{125} = \frac{500}{125}$$

$$X = 4\text{ mL}$$

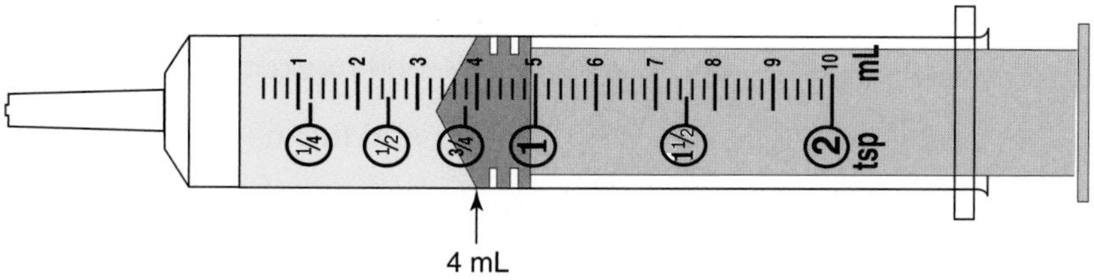

Total Daily Dosage Range per Kilogram

Example:

Many medications are recommended by a minimum and maximum mg/kg range per day to be divided into some number of doses. Amoxicillin is an antibiotic that is used to treat a variety of infections in adults and children. It is often given in divided doses round the clock for a total daily dosage.

The physician orders *amoxicillin 200 mg PO q8h* for a child who weighs 22 lb. Is this dosage safe?

1. **Convert lb to kg.** Approximate equivalent: 1 kg = 2.2 lb

   Think: $\frac{1}{2}$ of 22 = 11

   22 lb = 22 ÷ 2.2 = 10 kg

2. **Calculate recommended dosage.** Look at the label for amoxicillin (Figure 11-4). The label describes the recommended dosage as "20 to 40 mg/kg/day in divided doses every 8 hours. . . ."

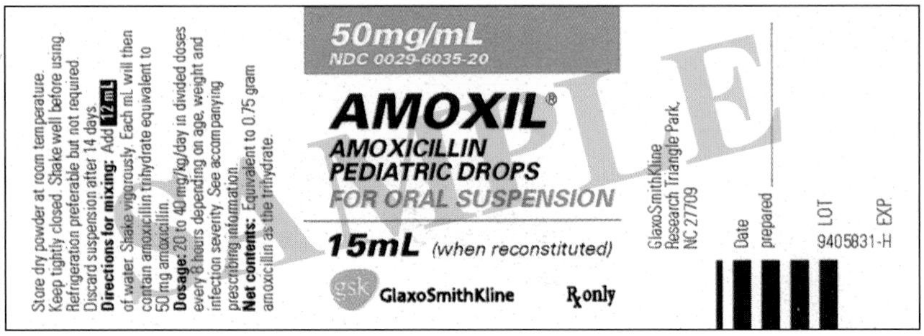

FIGURE 11-4 Amoxicillin Label

   Calculate the minimum and maximum dosage for each single dose. On the label, the recommendations are for the total daily dosage be divided and administered every 8 hours, resulting in 3 doses in 24 hours.

   Minimum total daily dosage: 20 mg/ ~~kg~~/day × 10 ~~kg~~ = 200 mg/day

   Minimum dosage for each single dose: 200 mg ÷ 3 doses = 66.7 mg/dose

   Maximum total daily dosage: 40 mg/~~kg~~/day × 10 ~~kg~~ = 400 mg/day

   Maximum dosage for each single dose: 400 mg ÷ 3 doses = 133.3 mg/dose

   The single dosage range is 66.7 to 133.3 mg/dose.

3. **Decide if the ordered dosage is safe.** The ordered dosage is 200 mg, and the allowable, safe dosage is 66.7 to 133.3 mg/dose. No, this dosage is too high and is not safe.

4. **Contact the prescriber to discuss the order.** You can save yourself a calculation step with the following shortcut, based on the total daily dosage.

   Calculate recommended minimum and maximum daily dosage range for *this* child.

   You know the total daily dosage is divided into 3 doses in 24 hours.

   Minimum total daily dosage: 20 mg/ ~~kg~~/day × 10 ~~kg~~ = 200 mg/day

   Maximum total daily dosage: 40 mg/ ~~kg~~/day × 10 ~~kg~~ = 400 mg/day

   Daily dosage per this order: 200 mg/ ~~dose~~ × 3 ~~doses~~/day = 600 mg/day

   Decide if the ordered daily dosage is safe. The ordered daily dosage is 600 mg, and the allowable safe daily dosage is 200 to 400 mg/day. No, the dosage ordered is too high and is not safe.

Total Daily Dosage Range per Kilogram with Maximum Daily Allowance

Example:

Some medications have a range of mg/kg/day recommended, with a maximum allowable total amount per day also specified.

The physician orders *cefazolin sodium 2.1 g IV q8h* for a child with a serious joint infection. The child weighs 95 lb. According to the usual IM or intravenous (IV) dosage of cefazolin sodium for infants older than 1 month and children is 25 to 50 mg/kg/day divided every 6–8 hours; for severe infections the dosage may be increased to 100 mg/kg/day. This means that regardless of how much the child weighs, the maximum safe allowance of this drug is 100 mg/kg per 24 hours.

1. **Convert lb to kg.** Approximate equivalent: 1 kg = 2.2 lb

   Think: $\frac{1}{2}$ of 95 = approximately 48

   95 lb = 95 ÷ 2.2 = 43.18 kg = 43.2 kg

2. **Calculate recommended dosage.**

   Minimum mg/kg/day: $25\,\text{mg/}\cancel{\text{kg}}\text{/day} \times 43.2\,\cancel{\text{kg}} = 1080\,\text{mg/day}$

   Minimum mg/dose: 1080 mg ÷ 3 doses = 360 mg/dose or 0.36 g/dose (360 mg/dose = 360 ÷ 1000 = 0.36 g/dose)

   Maximum mg/kg/day: $100\,\text{mg/}\cancel{\text{kg}}\text{/day} \times 43.2\,\cancel{\text{kg}} = 4320\,\text{mg/day}$

   Maximum mg/dose: 4320 mg ÷ 3 doses = 1440 mg/dose or 1.44 g/dose (1440 mg/dose = 1440 ÷ 1000 = 1.44 g/dose)

3. **Decide if the dosage is safe.** No, the dosage is too high. It exceeds both the highest mg/kg/dose extreme of the range (1440 mg/dose) and the maximum allowable dosage. At 4.32 g/day, no more than 1.44 g/dose would be allowed. The ordered dosage of 2.1 g is not safe, because 3 doses/day would deliver 6.3 g of the drug (2.1 g × 3 = 6.3 g). This example points out the importance of carefully reading all dosage recommendations.

4. **Contact the prescriber to discuss the order.**

Underdosage

Example:

Underdosage, as well as overdosage, can be unsafe. If the medication is necessary for the treatment or comfort of the patient, then giving too little can be just as dangerous as giving too much. Dosage that is less than the recommended therapeutic amount is also considered unsafe, because it may be ineffective.

The nurse notices a baby's fever has not decreased to less than 39.2°C in spite of several doses of ibuprofen that the physician ordered as an antipyretic. The order is *ibuprofen 40 mg PO q6h prn, temp more than 38.7°C*. The 7-month-old weighs $17\frac{1}{2}$ lb.

1. **Convert lb to kg.** Approximate equivalent: 1 kg = 2.2 lb

   Think: $\frac{1}{2}$ of $17\frac{1}{2}$ = approximately 9

   $17\frac{1}{2}$ lb = 17.5 lb = 17.5 ÷ 2.2 = 7.95 kg = 8 kg

2. **Calculate safe dosage.** According to the drug reference "Usual dosage . . .oral: Children: . . . Antipyretic: 6 months–12 years: Temperature less than 39.1°C: 5 mg/kg/dose; temperature more than or equal to 39.1°C: 10 mg/kg/dose; given every 6–8 hr; Maximum daily dose: 40 mg/kg/day."

   The recommended safe mg/kg dosage to treat this child's fever of 39.2°C is based on 10 mg/kg/dose. For the 8-kg child, per dose, $10\,\text{mg/kg/dose} \times 8\,\text{kg} = 80\,\text{mg/dose}$.

3. **Decide if the dosage is safe.** The nurse realizes that the dosage as ordered is insufficient to lower the child's fever. Because it is below the recommended therapeutic dosage, it is unsafe.

4. **Contact the physician.** Upon discussion with the physician, the physician agrees and revises the order to *ibuprofen 80 mg PO q6h prn, Temp more than 39.1°C* and *ibuprofen 40 mg PO q6h prn, Temp less than 39.1°C*. Underdosage with an antipyretic may result in serious complications of hyperthermia. Likewise, consider how underdosage with an antibiotic may lead to a superinfection and underdosage of a pain reliever may be inadequate to effectively treat the patient's pain, delaying recovery. Remember, the information in the drug reference provides important details related to specific use of medications and appropriate dosages for certain age groups to provide safe, therapeutic dosing. Both the physician and nurse must work together to ensure accurate and safe dosages that are within the recommended parameters as stated by the manufacturer on the label, in a drug insert, or in a reputable drug reference.

> **CAUTION**
>
> Once an adolescent attains a weight of 50 kg (110 lb) or greater, the standard adult dosage is frequently prescribed instead of a calculated dosage by weight. The healthcare professional must carefully verify that the order for a child's dosage *does not exceed* the maximum adult dosage recommended by the manufacturer.

COMBINATION DRUGS

Some medications contain two drugs combined into one solution or suspension. To calculate the safe dosage of these medications, you should consult a pediatric drug reference. Often you will need to calculate the *safe* dosage for each of the medications combined in the solution or suspension. Combination drugs are usually ordered by the amount to give or dose volume.

Example 1:

The physician orders *erythromycin ethylsuccinate/sulfisoxazole acetyl 6 mL PO q6h* for a child weighing 44 lb. According to the pediatric drug reference, this combination drug contains 200 mg of erythromycin ethylsuccinate with 600 mg of sulfisoxazole acetyl in every 5 mL oral suspension. The usual dosage for this drug is 50 mg erythromycin ethylsuccinate and 150 mg sulfisoxazole acetyl/kg/day in equally divided doses administered every 6 hours. Is the dose volume ordered safe?

Because this is a combination drug, notice that the order is for the dose volume (6 mL). To verify that the dose is safe, you must calculate the recommended dosage and the recommended quantity to give to supply that dosage for each drug component.

1. **Convert lb to kg.** Approximate equivalent: 1 kg = 2.2 lb

   Think: $\frac{1}{2}$ of 44 = 22

   44 lb = 44 ÷ 2.2 = 20 kg

2. **Calculate the safe dosage for each drug component.**

   erythromycin ethylsuccinate per day: $50\,\text{mg}/\cancel{\text{kg}}/\text{day} \times 20\,\cancel{\text{kg}} = 1000\,\text{mg}/\text{day}$; divided into 4 doses/day 1000 mg ÷ 4 doses = 250 mg/dose

   sulfisoxazole acetyl per day: $150\,\text{mg}/\cancel{\text{kg}}/\text{day} \times 20\,\cancel{\text{kg}} = 3000\,\text{mg}/\text{day}$; divided into 4 doses/day 3000 mg ÷ 4 doses = 750 mg/dose

3. **Calculate the volume of medication recommended for 1 dose for each drug component.**

   erythromycin ethylsuccinate: 250 mg is the recommended dosage; the supply has 200 mg/5 mL.

$$\frac{D}{H} \times Q = \frac{\overset{5}{\cancel{250\,mg}}}{\underset{4}{\cancel{200\,mg}}} \times 5\,mL = \frac{25}{4}\,mL = 6.25\,mL = 6\,mL \text{ recommended to deliver 250 mg}$$

erythromycin ethylsuccinate

As this is an oral dosage, it is safely and reasonably rounded to 6 mL.

Or, use ratio-proportion.

$$\frac{200\text{ mg}}{5\text{ mL}} = \frac{250\text{ mg}}{X\text{ mL}}$$

$200X = 1250$

$$\frac{200X}{200} = \frac{1250}{200}$$

X = 6.25 mL = 6 mL recommended to deliver 250 mg erythromycin ethylsuccinate

sulfisoxazole acetyl: 750 mg is the recommended dosage; 600 mg/5 mL is the supply.

$$\frac{D}{H} \times Q = \frac{\overset{5}{\cancel{750\,mg}}}{\underset{4}{\cancel{600\,mg}}} \times 5\,mL = \frac{25}{4}\,mL = 6.25\,mL = 6\,mL \text{ recommended to deliver 750 mg}$$

sulfisoxazole acetyl

Or, use ratio-proportion.

$$\frac{600\text{ mg}}{5\text{ mL}} = \frac{750\text{ mg}}{X\text{ mL}}$$

$600X = 3750$

$$\frac{600X}{600} = \frac{3750}{600}$$

X = 6.25 mL = 6 mL recommended to deliver 750 mg sulfisoxazole acetyl

4. **Decide if the dose ordered is safe.** The ordered dose is 6 mL, and the appropriate dose based on the recommended dosage for each component is 6 mL. The dose is safe. **Realize that because this is a combination product; 6 mL contains *both* medications delivered in this suspension.** Therefore, 6 mL is given, not 6 mL plus 6 mL.

Example 2:

The physician orders *sulfamethoxazole/trimethoprim suspension 7.5 mL PO q12h* for a child who weighs 22 lb. According to the drug reference, this combination drug contains trimethoprim 40 mg and sulfamethoxazole 200 mg in 5 mL oral suspension. Furthermore, the usual dose is based on the trimethoprim component, which is 6 to 12 mg/kg/day PO in divided doses q12h for a mild to moderate infection. Is this dose volume safe?

1. **Convert lb to kg.** Approximate equivalent: 1 kg = 2.2 lb

   Think: $\frac{1}{2}$ of 22 = 11

   22 lb = 22 ÷ 2.2 = 10 kg

2. **Calculate the safe dose for the trimethoprim range.**

   Trimethoprim minimum daily dosage: $6\,mg/\cancel{kg}/day \times 10\,\cancel{kg} = 60\,mg/day$

   Divided into 2 doses/day: 60 mg ÷ 2 doses = 30 mg/dose

   Trimethoprim maximum daily dosage: $12\,mg/\cancel{kg}/day \times 10\,\cancel{kg} = 120\,mg/day$

   Divided into 2 doses/day: 120 mg ÷ 2 doses = 60 mg/dose

3. **Calculate the volume of medication for the dosage range.**

Minimum dose volume: $\frac{D}{H} \times Q = \frac{\overset{3}{\cancel{30\,mg}}}{\underset{4}{\cancel{40\,mg}}} \times 5\,mL = \frac{15}{4}\,mL = 3.75\,mL$, minimum per dose

Or, use ratio-proportion.

$$\frac{40\,mg}{5\,mL} \times \frac{30\,mg}{X\,mL}$$

$$40X = 150$$

$$\frac{40X}{40} = \frac{150}{40}$$

$X = 3.75$ mL, minimum per dose

Maximum dose volume: $\frac{D}{H} \times Q = \frac{\overset{3}{\cancel{60\,mg}}}{\underset{2}{\cancel{40\,mg}}} \times 5\,mL = \frac{15}{2}\,mL = 7.5\,mL$, maximum per dose

Or, use ratio-proportion.

$$\frac{40\,mg}{5\,mL} = \frac{60\,mg}{X\,mL}$$

$$40X = 300$$

$$\frac{40X}{40} = \frac{300}{40}$$

$X = 7.5$ mL, maximum per dose

4. **Decide if the dose volume is safe.** Because the physician ordered 7.5 mL, the dosage is within the safe range and is a safe dose.

What dosage of trimethoprim did the physician actually order per dose for this child?

Using the formula, $\frac{D}{H} \times Q = X$, write in the quantities you already know.

$\frac{D\,mg}{40\,mg} \times 5\,mL = 7.5\,mL$ Solve for the unknown "D," desired dosage.

$\frac{5D}{40} \times \frac{7.5}{1}$ Notice you now have a ratio-proportion.

$$5D = 300$$

$$\frac{5D}{5} = \frac{300}{5}$$

$D = 60$ mg This is the dosage of trimethoprim you would give in one 7.5-mL dose, which matches the upper limit of the safe dosage range.

Or, you could have started with a ratio-proportion: ratio for dosage on hand equals ratio for desired dosage.

$\frac{40\,mg}{5\,mL} \times \frac{D\,mg}{7.5\,mL}$ The unknown "D" is the desired dosage.

$$5D = 300$$

$$\frac{5D}{5} = \frac{300}{5}$$

$$D = 60\,mg$$

Example 3:

The pediatric oral surgeon orders *acetaminophen and codeine phosphate suspension 10 mL PO q4h prn for pain* for a child weighing 42 lb, who had two teeth repaired. According to the drug reference, acetaminophen plus codeine phosphate is a combination drug containing 160 mg of acetaminophen and 8 mg of codeine phosphate per 5 mL. Safe dosage is based on the codeine component, which is 0.5 mg/kg/dose every 4 hours as needed. Is this dose volume safe?

1. **Convert lb to kg.** Approximate equivalent: 1 kg = 2.2 lb

   Think: $\frac{1}{2}$ of 42 = 21

   42 lb = 42 ÷ 2.2 = 19.09 kg = 19.1 kg

2. **Calculate the safe dosage range for the codeine phosphate.**

   codeine phosphate per dose: $0.5\,\text{mg}/\cancel{\text{kg}}/\text{dose} \times 19.1\,\cancel{\text{kg}} = 9.55\,\text{mg}/\text{dose} = 9.6\,\text{mg}/\text{dose}$

3. **Calculate the volume of medication for the recommended dose range.**

   Dose volume: $\frac{D}{H} \times Q = \frac{9.6\,\text{mg}}{8\,\text{mg}} \times 5\,\text{mL} = 6\,\text{mL}$, per dose

   Or, use ratio-proportion.

   $$\frac{8\,\text{mg}}{5\,\text{mL}} = \frac{9.6\,\text{mg}}{X\,\text{mL}}$$

   $$8X = 48$$

   $$\frac{18X}{18} = \frac{48}{8}$$

   X = 6 mL per dose

4. **Decide if the dose volume is safe.** The ordered dose of 10 mL exceeds the recommended safe dose range; the dose is not safe. Contact the physician to discuss the order.

Be sure to take the time to double-check pediatric dosage. The healthcare provider who administers the medication has the last opportunity to ensure safe drug administration.

ADULT DOSAGES BASED ON BODY WEIGHT

Some adult dosage recommendations are also based on body weight, although less frequently than for children. The information you learned about calculating and verifying children's body weight dosages can be applied to adults. It is important that you become familiar and comfortable with reading labels, drug inserts, and drug reference books to check any order that appears questionable.

See Figure 11-5 for the information found in a drug insert about the adult dosage recommendations for the drug potassium clavulanate/ticarcillin disodium. Notice that the adult dosage is recommended by body weight.

BODY WEIGHT DOSAGE CALCULATION WORKSHEET

Some students find the following worksheet helpful when calculating dosage ranges based on body weight for either adults or children. First convert the weight in lb to kg.

Example:

Order: *ticarcillin disodium/potassium clavulanate 4 gm IV q6h* for a patient with bacterial septicemia

Supply: ticarcillin disodium/potassium clavulanate 200 mg/mL

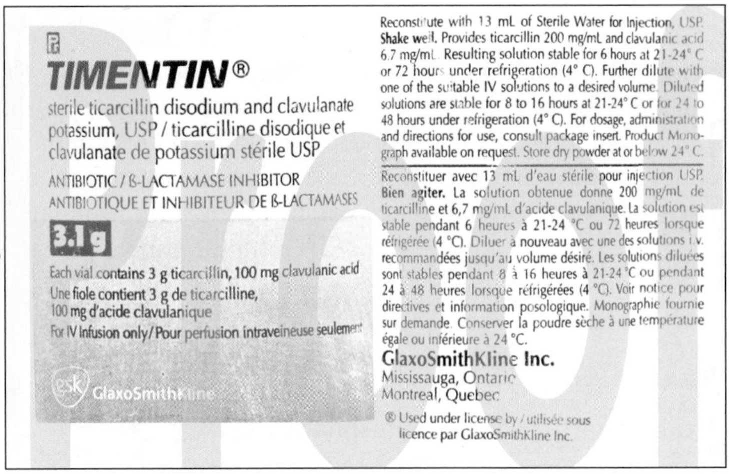

FIGURE 11-5 Section of Ticarcillin Disodium/Clavulanate Potassium Package Insert

Recommended adult dosage from the package insert: 200–300 mg/kg/day q4–6h for patients weighing less than 60 kg based on ticarcillin disodium content; 3.1 g q4–6h for patients weighing 60 kg or more

Patient's weight: 150 lb

Convert lb to kg.

Think: $\frac{1}{2}$ of 150 = 75

150 lb = 150 ÷ 2.2 = 68.2 kg

	Minimum Dosage	Maximum Dosage
Body Weight (kg)	68.2 kg	68.2 kg
× Recommended Dosage	× 200 mg/kg/day	× 300 mg/kg/day
Total Daily Dosage	13 640 mg/kg/day	20 460 mg/kg/day
÷ Number of Doses/Day	÷ 4 Doses/Day	÷ 4 Doses/Day
Dosage Range/Dose	3410 mg/dose q6h to	5115 mg/dose q6h

The ordered dosage of ticarcillin disodium/potassium clavulanate 4 g (or 4000 mg) is between the minimum (3.4 g or 3400 mg) and maximum (5.1 g or 5100 mg) recommended dose. Therefore, it is safe.

QUICK REVIEW

To use the body weight method to verify the safety of pediatric and adult dosages:

- Convert body weight from pounds and ounces to kilograms: 1 kg = 2.2 lb; 1 lb = 16 oz.
- Calculate the recommended safe dosage in mg/kg.
- Compare the ordered dosage with the recommended dosage to decide if the dosage is safe.
- If the dosage is safe, calculate the amount to give for one dose; if not, notify the prescriber.
- Combination drugs are ordered by dose volume. Check a reputable drug reference to be sure the dose ordered contains the safe amount of each drug as recommended.

REVIEW SET 26

Calculate 1 dose of safe pediatric dosages.

1. Order: *cloxacillin sodium 125 mg PO q6h* for a child who weighs 36 lb. The recommended dosage of cloxacillin sodium for children weighing less than 20 kg is 50–100 mg/kg/day PO in equally divided doses q6h for moderate to severe infections to a maximum of 4 g/day.

Child's weight: ________ kg

Recommended minimum daily dosage for this child: ________ mg/day

Recommended minimum single dosage for this child: ________ mg/dose

Recommended maximum daily dosage for this child: ________ mg/day

Recommended maximum single dosage for this child: ________ mg/dose

Is the dosage ordered safe? ________

2. Cloxacillin sodium is available as an oral suspension of 125 mg per 5 mL. If the dosage ordered in question 1 is safe, give ________ mL. If not safe, explain why not and describe what the nurse should do. ____

____

3. Order: *chloramphenicol sodium succinate 55 mg IV q12h* for an 8-day-old infant who weighs 2200 g. The recommended dosage of chloramphenicol sodium succinate for neonates under 2 weeks of age is 25 mg/kg/day divided q6h; and for neonates over 14 days to 4 weeks of age is 50 mg/kg/day divided q6h.

Infant's weight: ________ kg

Recommended daily dosage for this infant: ________ mg/day

Recommended single dosage for this infant: ________ mg/dose

Is the dosage ordered safe? ________

4. Chloramphenicol sodium succinate is available as a solution for injection of 1 g per 10 mL. If the dosage ordered in question 3 is safe, give ________ mL. If not safe, explain why not and describe what the nurse should do. ____

____

5. Order: *cefixime 120 mg PO daily* for a child who weighs 33 lb. The recommended dosage of cefixime for children under 50 kg is 8 mg/kg PO once daily or 4 mg/kg PO q12h.

Child's weight: ________ kg

Recommended single dosage for this child: ________ mg/dose

Is the dosage ordered safe? ________

6. Cefixime is available as a suspension of 100 mg per 5 mL in a 50-mL bottle. If the dosage ordered in question 5 is safe, give ________ mL. If not safe, explain why not and describe what the nurse should do. ____

____

How many doses are available in the bottle of cefixime? ________ dose(s)

7. Order: *acetaminophen 480 mg PO q4h prn for temperature more than or equal to 38.3°C.* The child's weight is 32 kg. The recommended child's dosage of acetaminophen is 10–15 mg/kg/dose PO q4–6h for fever. No more than 65 mg/kg/day for a maximum of 5 days is recommended.

Child's weight: ________ kg

Recommended minimum single dosage for this child: ________ mg/dose

Recommended maximum single dosage for this child: ________ mg/dose

Is the dosage ordered safe? ________

8. Acetaminophen is available as a suspension of 160 mg per 5 mL. If the dosage ordered in question 7 is safe, give ________ mL. If not safe, explain why not and describe what the

nurse should do. ______________________________

____

9. Order: *cephalexin 125 mg PO q6h* for a child who weighs 44 lb. The recommended pediatric dosage of cephalexin is 25–50 mg/kg/day in 2–4 equally divided doses to a maximum of 1 g daily.

   Child's weight: ________ kg

   Recommended minimum daily dosage for this child: ________ mg/day

   Recommended minimum single dosage for this child: ________ mg/dose

   Recommended maximum daily dosage for this child: ________ mg/day

   Recommended maximum single dosage for this child: ________ mg/dose

   Is the dosage ordered safe? ________

10. Cephalexin is available in an oral suspension of 125 mg per 5 mL. If the dosage ordered in question 9 is safe, give ________ mL. If not safe, explain why not and describe what the nurse should do. ______________________________

____

The labels provided represent the drugs available to answer questions 11 through 25. Verify safe dosages, indicate the amount to give, and draw an arrow on the accompanying measuring device. Explain unsafe dosages and describe the appropriate action to take.

11. Order: *tobramycin sulfate 8 mg IV q12h* for an infant who weighs 5000 g and is 1 week old. The recommended pediatric dosage of tobramycin sulfate is up to 4 mg/kg/day administered q12h.

   Infant's weight: ________ kg

   Recommended daily single dosage for this infant: ________ mg/dose

   Recommended total daily dosage for this infant: ________ mg/day

   Is the dosage ordered safe? ________

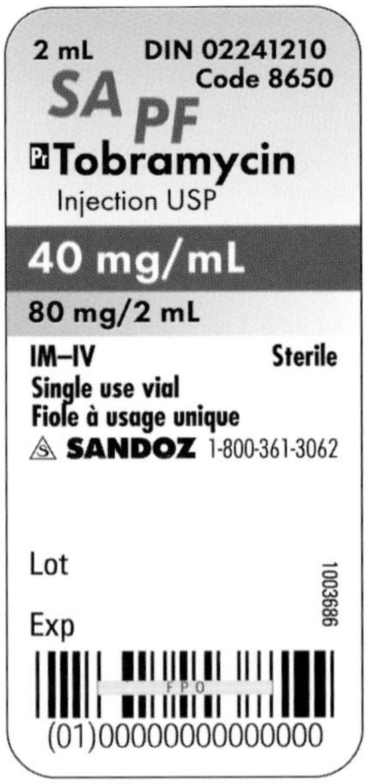

12. If the dosage ordered in question 11 is safe, give ________ mL. If not safe, explain why not and describe what the nurse should do.

____

____

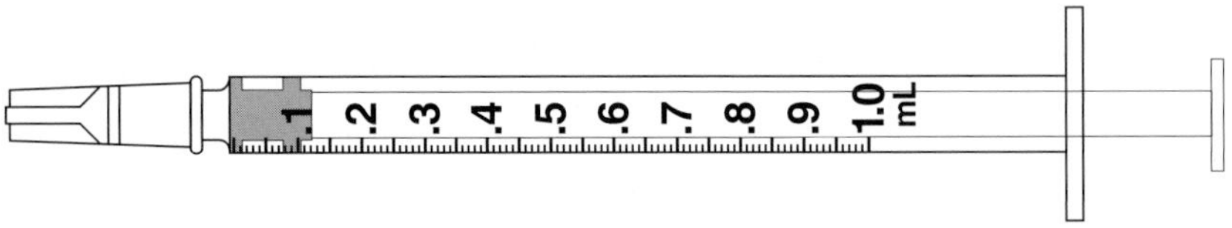

13. Order: *ceftazidime 34 mg IV q12h* for an infant who is 1 month old and weighs 7 lb 8 oz. The recommended daily dosage of ceftazidime for infants and children is as follows: 1–2 months is 12.5–25 mg/kg administered q12h (maximum 6 g/day); 2 months–12 years is 10–33 mg/kg administered q8h (maximum 6 g/day).

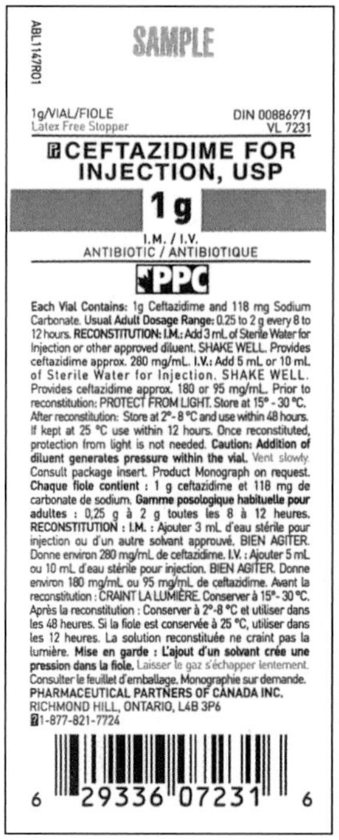

Pharmaceutical Partners of Canada Inc., Richmond Hill, ON

Child's weight: ________ kg

Recommended minimum single dosage for this child: ________ mg

Recommended maximum single dosage for this child: ________ mg

Is the dosage ordered safe? ________

14. If the dosage ordered in question 13 is safe, give ________ mL. If not safe, explain why not and describe what the nurse should do. ____

____

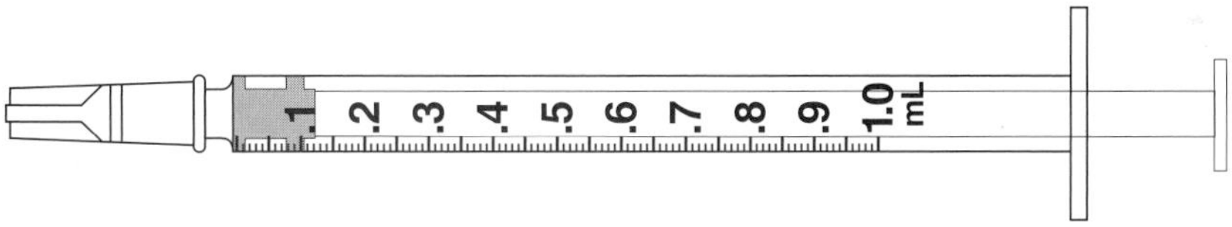

15. Order: *trimethoprim/sulfamethoxazole pediatric suspension 2.5 mL PO q12h* for a child who weighs 15 kg and has an urinary tract infection. The recommended dosage of trimethoprim and sulfamethoxazole for such infections in children is based on the trimethoprim at 8 mg/kg/day administered in 2 equal doses.

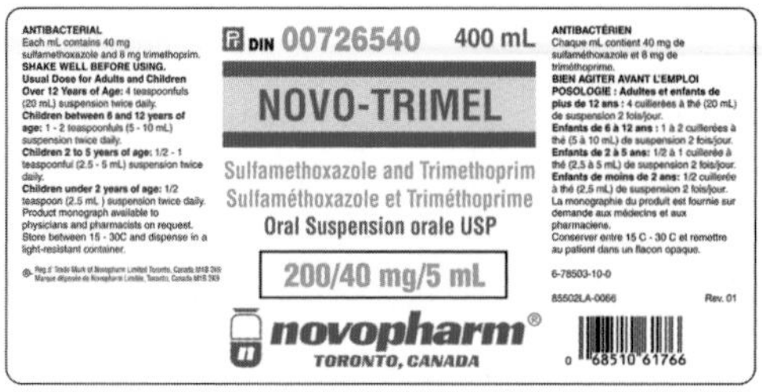

Novopharm Limited, Toronto, ON

Recommended daily trimethoprim dosage for this child: ________ mg/day

Recommended single trimethoprim dosage for this child: ________ mg/dose

Recommended single dose for this child: ________ mL/dose

Is the dose ordered safe? ________

16. If the dose ordered in question 15 is safe, give ________ mL. If not safe, explain why not and describe what the nurse should do. ____

____

The dose ordered is equivalent to ________ teaspoons.

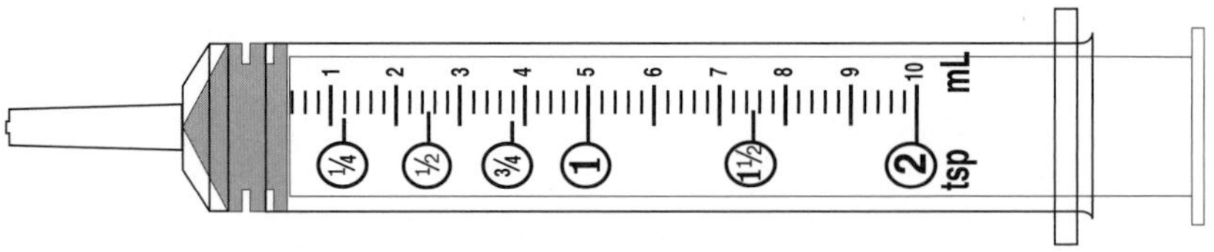

17. Order: *gentamicin sulfate 40 mg IV q8h* for a premature neonate who is 5 days old and weighs 1800 g. The recommended dosage of gentamicin sulfate for premature and full-term neonates 1 week of age or less is 6mg/kg/day administered q12h; and for infants older than 1 week 6 mg/kg/day administered q8h.

    Neonate's weight: ________ kg

    Recommended single dosage for this neonate: ________ mg/dose

    Is the ordered dosage safe? ________

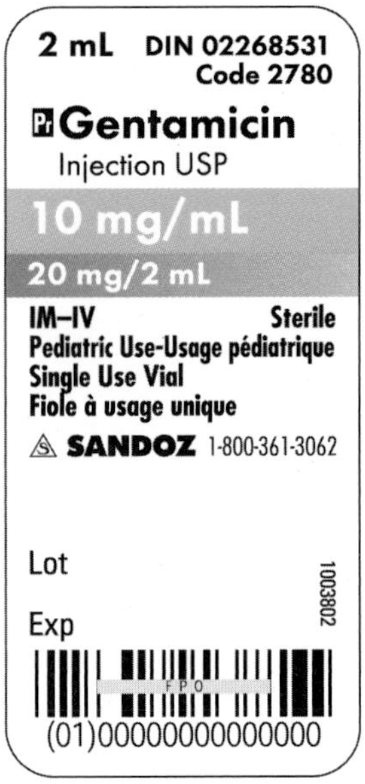

18. If the dosage ordered in question 17 is safe, give ________ mL. If not safe, explain why not and describe what the nurse should do. ____

    ____

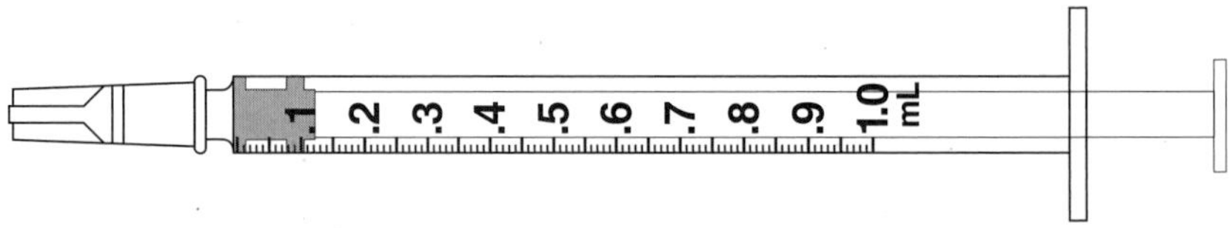

19. Order: *digoxin 0.15 mg PO q12h* for a maintenance dose for a 9-year-old child who weighs 70 lb. The recommended maintenance pediatric dosage of digoxin tablets and elixir is 7–10 mcg/kg/day divided and given in 2 equal doses per day.

    Child's weight: ________ kg

    Recommended minimum daily dosage for this child: ________ mg/day

    Recommended minimum single dosage for this child: ________ mg/dose

    Recommended maximum daily dosage for this child: ________ mg/day

    Recommended maximum single dosage for this child: ________ mg/dose

    Is the dosage ordered safe? ________

20. If the dosage ordered in question 19 is safe, give ________ mL. If not safe, explain why not and describe what the nurse should do. ______________________________

____

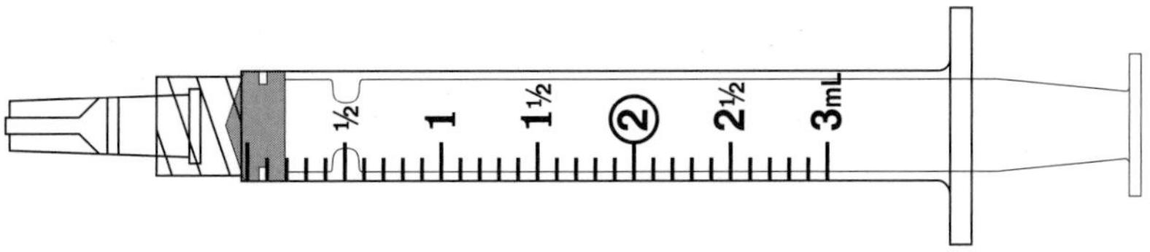

21. Order: *amoxicillin oral suspension 100 mg PO q8h* for a child who weighs 39 lb.
Recommended dosage: See label.

Child's weight: 17.7 kg

Recommended minimum daily dosage for this child: 354 mg/day

Recommended minimum single dosage for this child: 118 mg/dose

Recommended maximum daily dosage for this child: 708 mg/day

Recommended maximum single dosage for this child: 236 mg/dose

Is the dosage ordered safe? no underdose

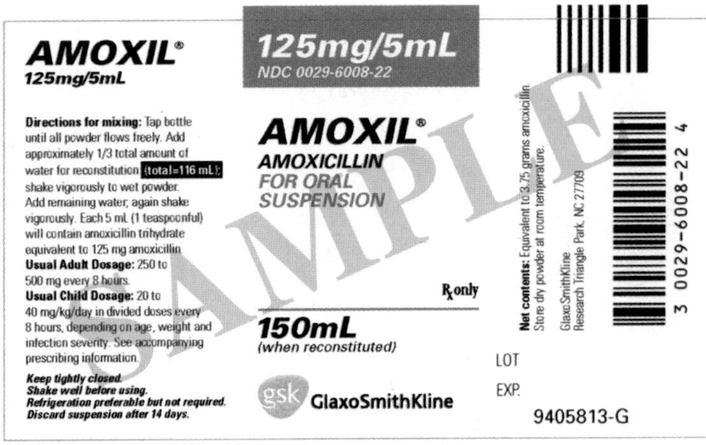

22. If the dosage ordered in question 21 is safe, give ________ mL. If not safe, explain why not and describe what the nurse should do. ______________________________

____

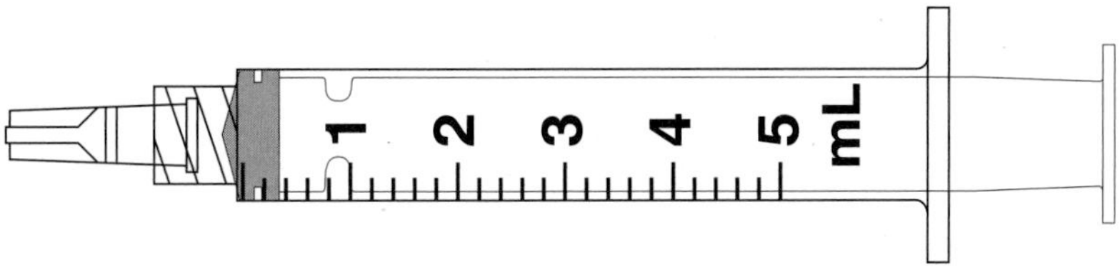

23. Order: *meropenem 325 mg IV q8h* for a 9-year-old child who weighs 55 lb. Recommended dosage for infants and children over 3 months of age and weighing up to 50 kg: 10–40 mg/kg q8h.

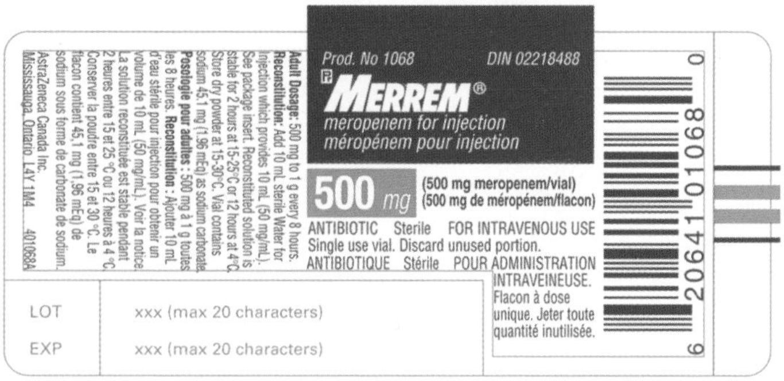
Prod. No 1068
DIN 02218488
MERREM®
meropenem for injection
méropénem pour injection
500 mg
(500 mg meropenem/vial)
(500 mg de méropénem/flacon)
ANTIBIOTIC Sterile FOR INTRAVENOUS USE
Single use vial. Discard unused portion.
ANTIBIOTIQUE Stérile POUR ADMINISTRATION INTRAVEINEUSE.
Flacon à dose unique. Jeter toute quantité inutilisée.
LOT
xxx (max 20 characters)
EXP
xxx (max 20 characters)

AstraZeneca Canada Inc., Mississauga, ON

Child's weight: ________ kg

Recommended minimum daily dosage for this child: ________ mg/day

Recommended minimum single dosage for this child: ________ mg/dose

Recommended maximum daily dosage for this child: ________ mg/day

Recommended maximum single dosage for this child: ________ mg/dose

Is the dosage ordered safe? ________

24. If the dosage ordered in question 23 is safe, give ________ mL. If not safe, explain why not and describe what the nurse should do. ____

____

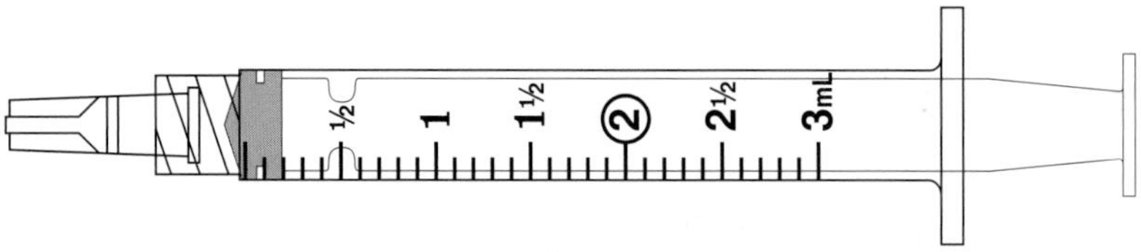
½
1
1½
2
2½
3mL

25. Order: *meropenem 275 mg IV daily* for a 7-year-old child who weighs 21 kg. Recommended dosage: See question 23.

Is the ordered dosage safe? ________ Explain: ________________________________

____

Refer to the following information from the label for ticarcillin disodium and clavulanate potassium to answer questions 26 through 30.

The package insert contains information regarding adult and child dosages. The recommended dosage for adults (60 kg or greater) is 3.1 g every 4 to 6 hours. For patients weighing less than 60 kg, the recommended dosage is 200 to 300 mg/kg/day, based on ticarcillin disodium content, given in divided doses every 4 to 6 hours.

Dosage in Infants and Children: Infections Dosage Schedule is calculated according to Total Daily Dosage (mg/kg/day) based on ticarcillin disodium.

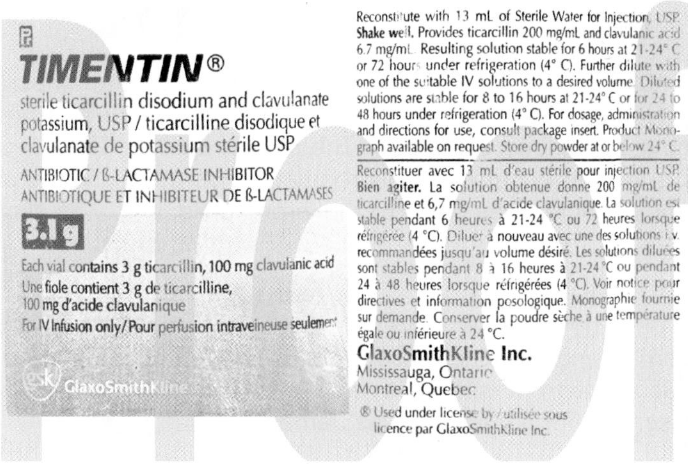

26. What is the recommended adult dosage of ticarcillin disodium and clavulanate potassium for patients weighing less than 60 kg?

____

27. What is the recommended adult dosage of ticarcillin disodium and clavulanate potassium for adults weighing more than 60 kg?

____

28. What daily dosage range of ticarcillin disodium and clavulanate potassium should you expect for an adult who weighs 130 lb? ________ g to ________ g/day

29. What single dosage range of ticarcillin disodium and clavulanate potassium administered q4h should you expect for the adult described in question 28? ________ g to ________ g/dose

30. What single dosage range of ticarcillin disodium and clavulanate potassium administered q6h should you expect for the adult described in question 28? ________ g to ________ g/dose

After completing these problems, see pages 484–486 to check your answers.

CRITICAL THINKING SKILLS

Medication errors in pediatrics often occur when the nurse fails to properly identify the child before administering the dose.

error

Failing to identify the child before administering a medication.

possible scenario

Suppose the physician ordered *ampicillin 500 mg IV q6h* for a child diagnosed with pneumonia. The nurse calculated the dosage to be safe, checked that the child had no allergies, and prepared the medication. The child had been assigned to a semiprivate room. The nurse entered the room and noted only one child in the room and administered the IV ampicillin to that child, without

(continues)

(continued)

checking the identification of the child. Within an hour of the administered ampicillin the child began to break out in hives and had signs of respiratory distress. The nurse asked the child's mother, "Does Johnny have any known allergies?" The mother replied, "This is James, not Johnny, and yes, James is allergic to penicillin. His roommate, Johnny, is in the playroom." At this point the nurse realized the ampicillin was given to the wrong child, who was allergic to penicillin.

potential outcome

James's physician would have been notified and he would likely have ordered epinephrine subcutaneously stat (given for anaphylactic reactions), followed by close monitoring of the child. Anaphylactic reactions can range from mild to severe. Ampicillin is a derivative of penicillin and would not have been prescribed for a child such as James.

prevention

This error could easily have been avoided had the nurse remembered the cardinal rule of *identifying the child* before administering *any* medication. Children are mobile, and the identity of a child should not be assumed simply because the child is in a particular room. The correct method of identifying the child is to check the wrist or ankle band and compare it to the medication administration record with the child's name, room number, physician, and patient's identification number. Finally, remember that the first of the *ten rights* of medication administration is the *right patient*.

PRACTICE PROBLEMS—CHAPTER 11

Convert the following weights to kilograms. Round to one decimal place.

1. 12 lb = ________ kg
2. 8 lb 4 oz = ________ kg
3. 1570 g = ________ kg
4. 2300 g = ________ kg
5. 34 lb = ________ kg
6. 6 lb 10 oz = ________ kg
7. 52 lb = ________ kg
8. 890 g = ________ kg
9. The recommended dosage of tobramycin sulfate for adults with serious, non–life-threatening infections is 3 mg/kg/day in 3 equally divided doses q8h. What should you expect the total daily dosage of tobramycin sulfate to be for an adult with a serious infection who weighs 80 kg? ________ mg/day
10. What should you expect the single dosage of tobramycin sulfate to be for the adult described in question 9? ________ mg/dose

The labels provided represent the drugs available to answer questions 11 through 42. Verify safe dosages and indicate the amount to give and draw an arrow on the accompanying measuring device. Explain unsafe dosages and describe the appropriate action to take.

11. Order: *gentamicin sulfate 40 mg IV q8h* for a child who weighs 43 lb. The recommended dosage for children is 3–6 mg/kg/day administered q8h.

    Child's weight: ________ kg

    Recommended minimum single dosage for this child: ________ mg/dose

    Recommended maximum single dosage for this child: ________ mg/dose

    Is the ordered dosage safe? ________

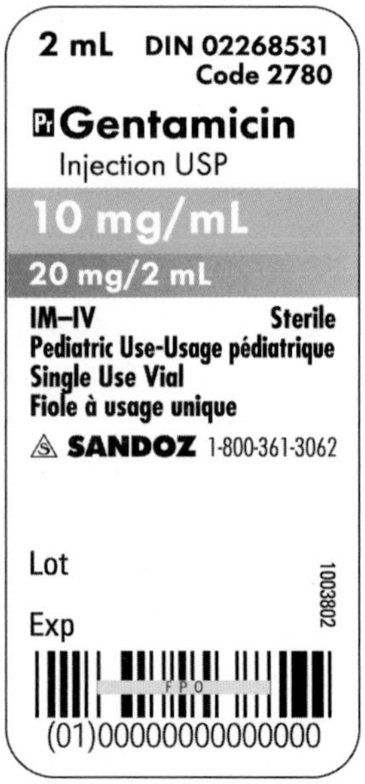
2 mL DIN 02268531
Code 2780
Gentamicin
Injection USP
10 mg/mL
20 mg/2 mL
IM–IV Sterile
Pediatric Use-Usage pédiatrique
Single Use Vial
Fiole à usage unique
SANDOZ 1-800-361-3062
Lot
Exp
10038802
(01)00000000000000

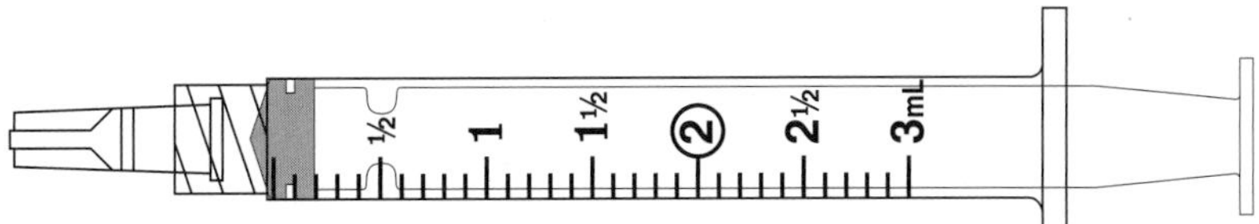

12. If the dosage ordered in question 11 is safe, give ________ mL. If not safe, explain why not and describe what the nurse should do. ____

____

13. Order: *furosemide oral solution 10 mg PO BID* (maximum 2 mg/kg/day) for a child who weighs 16 lb. The recommended pediatric dosage is 0.5–2 mg/kg/day BID.

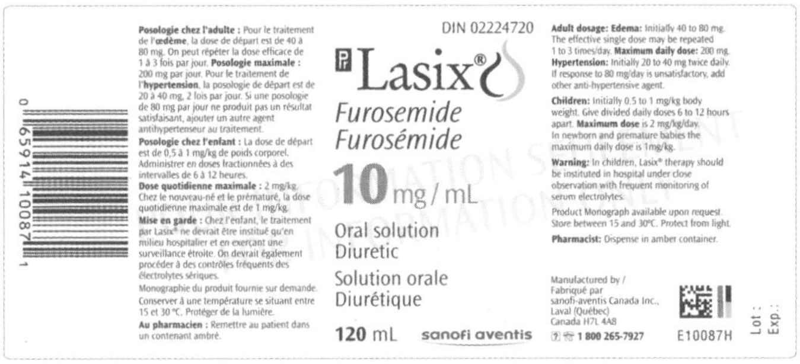

Sanofi-aventis Canada, Laval, QUE

Child's weight: ________ kg

Recommended minimum single dosage for this child: ________ mg/dose

Recommended maximum single dosage for this child: ________ mg/dose

Is the ordered dosage safe? ________

14. If the dosage ordered in question 13 is safe, give ________ mL. If not safe, explain why not and describe what the nurse should do. ____

____

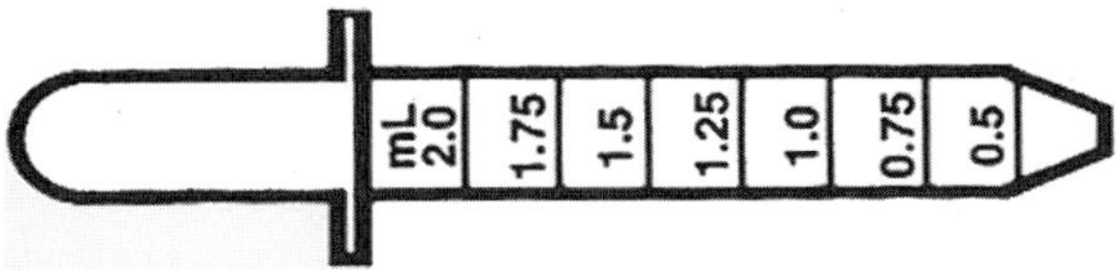

15. Order: *phenytoin oral suspension 250 mg PO BID* for a child who is 7 years old and weighs 50 lb. The recommended daily maintenance dosage for children is 4–8 mg/kg/day in 2 divided doses per day, not to exceed 300 mg/day.

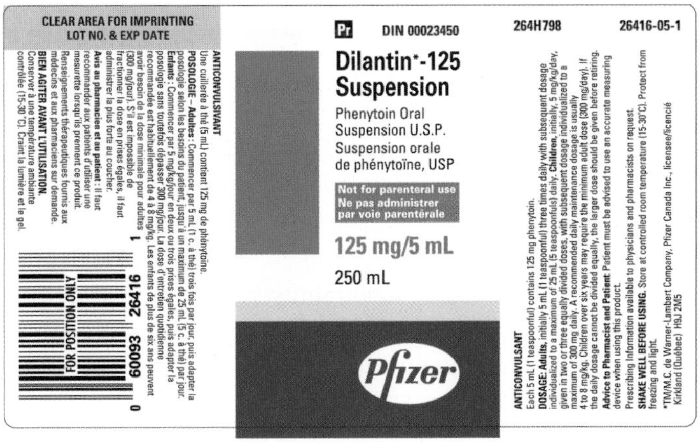

©Pfizer Canada Inc., Kirkland, Que

Child's weight: ________ kg

Recommended mimimum daily dosage for this child: ________ mg/day

Recommended mimimum single dosage for this child: ________ mg/dose

Recommended maximum daily dosage for this child: ________ mg/day

Recommended maximum single dosage for this child: ________ mg/day

Is the dosage ordered safe? ________

16. If the dosage ordered in question 15 is safe, give ________ mL. If not safe, explain why not and describe what the nurse should do. ____

____

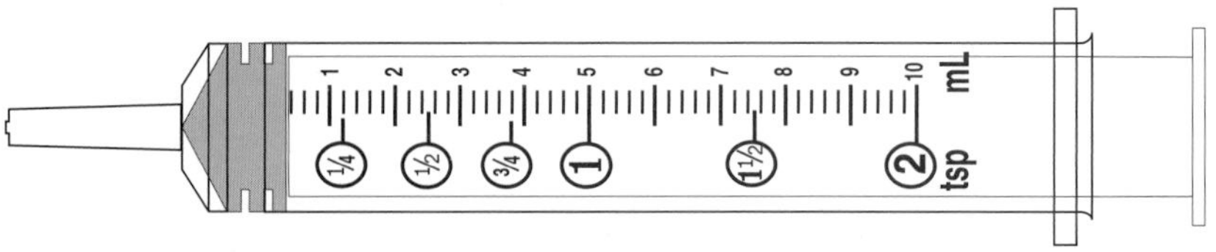

17. Order: *valproic acid 150 mg PO BID* for a child who is 10 years old and weighs 64 lb. The recommended dosage for adults and children 10 years and older is 10–15 mg/kg/day up to a maximum of 60 mg/kg/day. If the total daily dosage exceeds 250 mg, divide the dose.

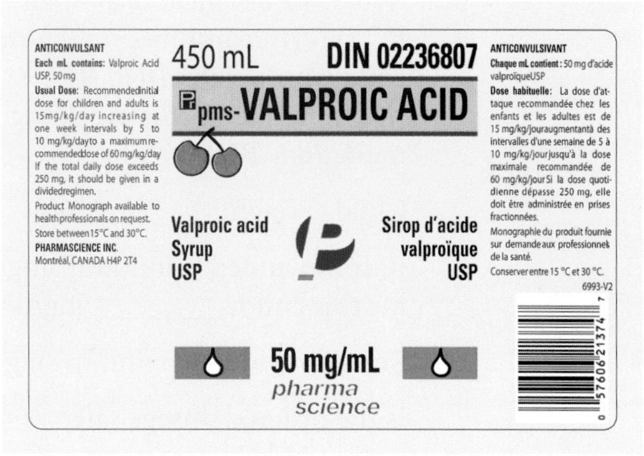

Pharmascience Inc., Montreal, Que

Child's weight: ________ kg

Recommended minimum daily dosage for this child: ________ mg/day

Recommended minimum single dosage for this child: ________ mg/dose

Recommended maximum daily dosage for this child: ________ mg/day

Recommended maximum single dosage for this child: ________ mg/dose

Is the dosage ordered safe? ________

18. If the dosage ordered in question 17 is safe, give ________ mL. If not safe, explain why not and describe what the nurse should do. ____

____

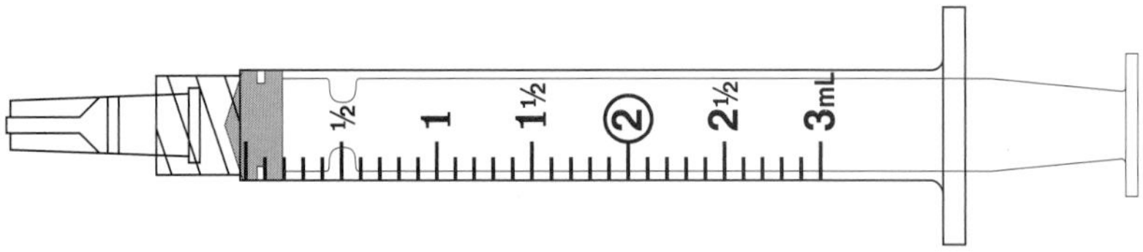

19. Order: *bacitracin 750 units IM q8h* for an infant who weighs 2500 g. The recommended dosage for infants 2.5 kg and below: 900 units/kg/day in 2–3 divided doses; infants over 2.5 kg: 1000 units/kg/day in 2–3 divided doses. Reconstitute the 50 000 unit vial with 9.8 mL of diluent for a concentration of 5000 units/mL.

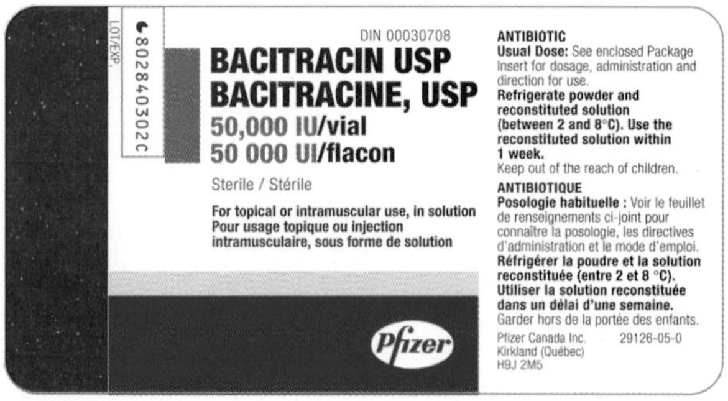

©Pfizer Canada Inc., Kirkland, Que

Child's weight: ________ kg

Recommended daily dosage for this child: ________ units/day

Recommended single dosage for this child: ________ units/dose

Is the ordered dosage safe? ________

20. If the dosage ordered in question 19 is safe, reconstitute with ________ mL diluent for a total solution volume of ________ mL with a concentration of ________ units/mL. Give ________ mL. If not safe, explain why not and describe what the nurse should do.

____

____

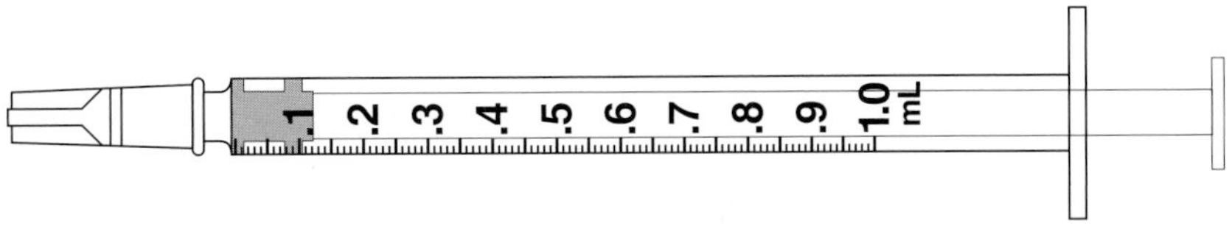

21. Order: *amoxicillin oral suspension 150 mg PO q8h* for a child who weighs 41 lb. Recommended dosage: See label below.

Child's weight: ________ kg

Recommended minimum daily dosage for this child: ________ mg/day

Recommended minimum single dosage for this child: ________ mg/dose

Recommended maximum daily dosage for this child: ________ mg/day

Recommended maximum single dosage for this child: ________ mg/dose

Is the dosage ordered safe? ________

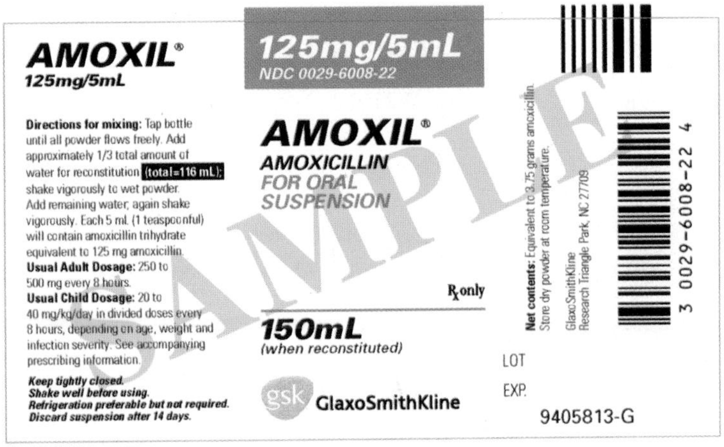

GlaxoSmithKline, Research Triangle Park, NC (Labels reproduced with permission of GlaxoSmithKline)

22. If the dosage ordered in question 21 is safe, give ________ mL. If not safe, explain why not and describe what the nurse should do. ____

____

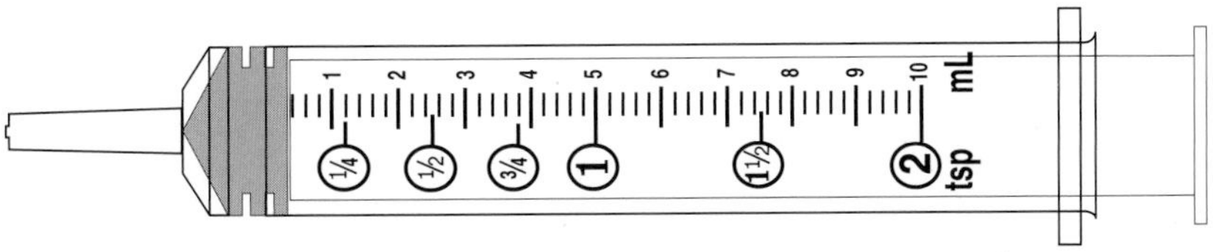

23. Order: *cefaclor oral suspension 187 mg PO BID* for a child with otitis media and who weighs $20\frac{1}{2}$ lb. Recommended dosage: See label.

    Child's weight: ________ kg

    Recommended daily dosage for this child: ________ mg/day

    Recommended single dosage for this child: ________ mg/dose

    Is the dosage ordered safe? ________

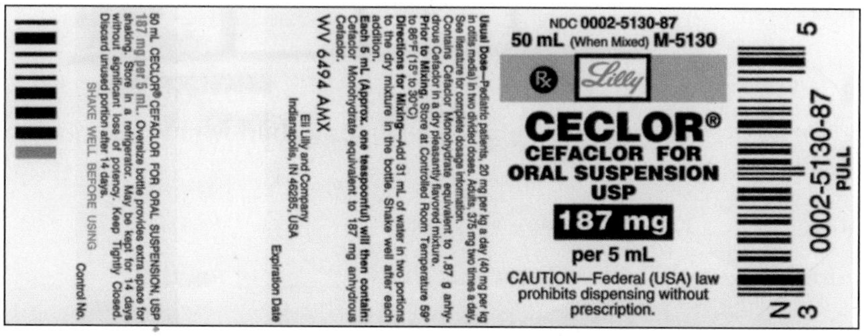

Courtesy of Eli Lilly and Company

24. If the dosage ordered in question 23 is safe, give ________ mL. If not safe, explain why not and describe what the nurse should do. ____

    ____

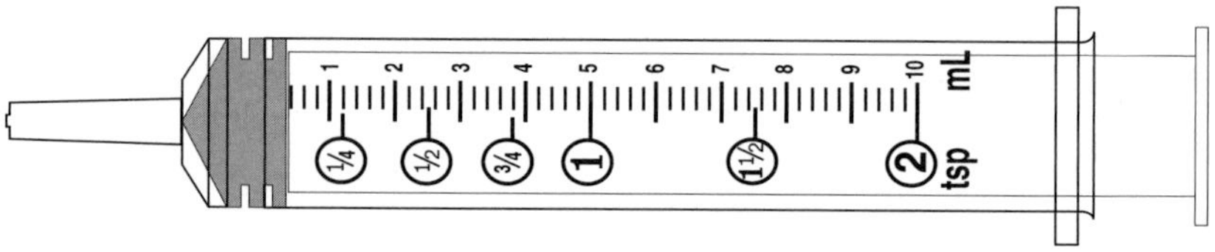

25. Order: *naloxone hydrochloride 100 mcg subcutaneous stat* for a child who weighs 22 lb. Recommended pediatric dosage: 0.01 mg/kg/dose.

    Child's weight: ________ kg

    Recommended single dosage for this child: ________ mg/dose

    Is the dosage ordered safe? ________

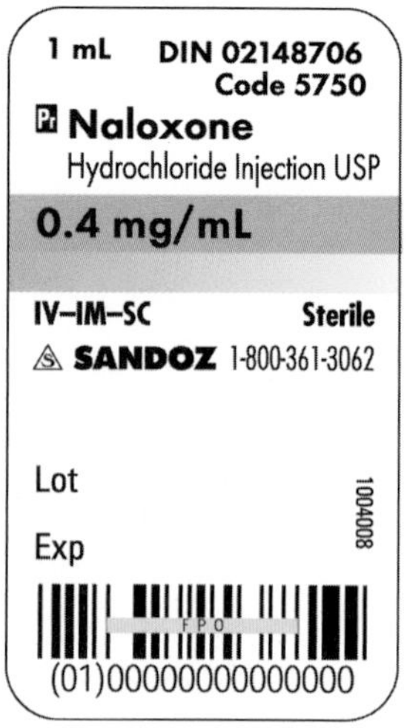

26. If the dosage ordered in question 25 is safe, give ________ mL. If not safe, explain why not and describe what the nurse should do.

    ____

    ____

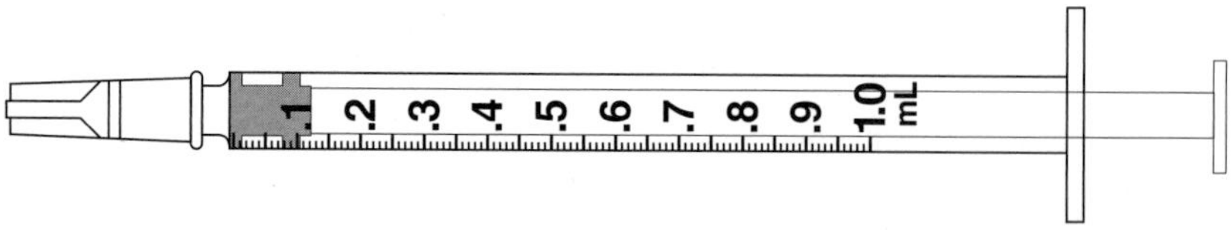

27. Order: *tobramycin sulfate 40 mg IV q8h* for a child who weighs 14 kg. The recommended pediatric dosage of tobramycin sulfate is 6 to 7.5 mg/kg/day in 3 or 4 equally divided doses.

    Recommended minimum single dosage for this child: ________ mg/dose

    Recommended maximum single dosage for this child: ________ mg/dose

    Is the dosage ordered safe? ________

28. If the dosage ordered in question 27 is safe, give ________ mL. If not safe, explain why not and describe what the nurse should do.

    ____

    ____

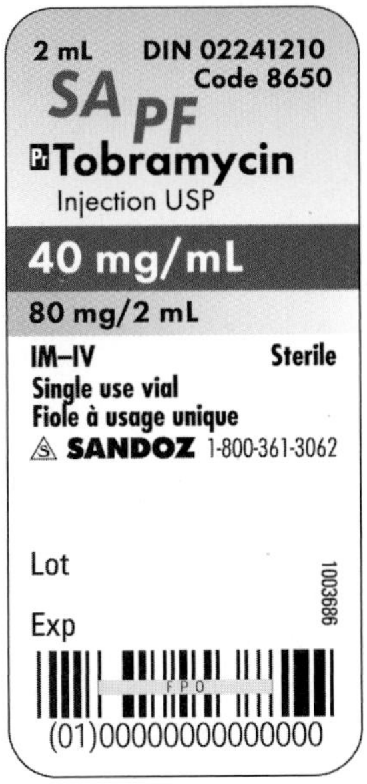

29. Order: *ceftriaxone sodium 1 g IV q12h* for a child who weights 20 lb and has a serious infection. The recommended pediatric dosage of ceftriaxone sodium is a total daily dosage of 25–37.5 mg/kg, given in equally divided doses twice a day, not to exceed 50–75 mg/kg (2 g/day).

    Child's weight: ________ kg

    Recommended minimum daily dosage for this child: ________ mg/day

    Recommended maximum single dosage for this child: ________ mg/dose

    Is the dosage ordered safe? ________

30. If the dosage ordered in question 29 is safe, give ________ mL. If not safe, explain why not and describe what the nurse should do.

    ____

    ____

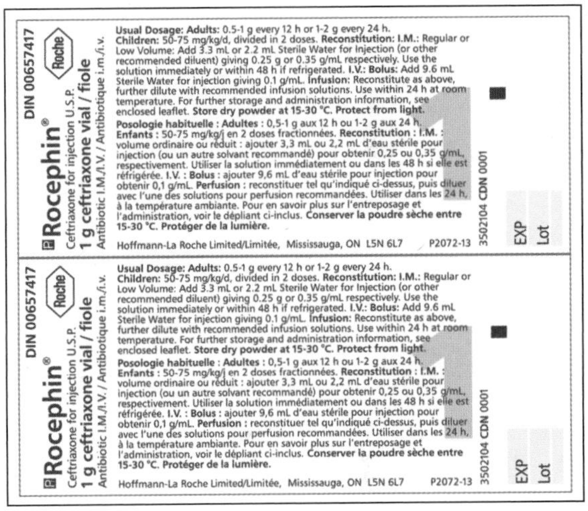

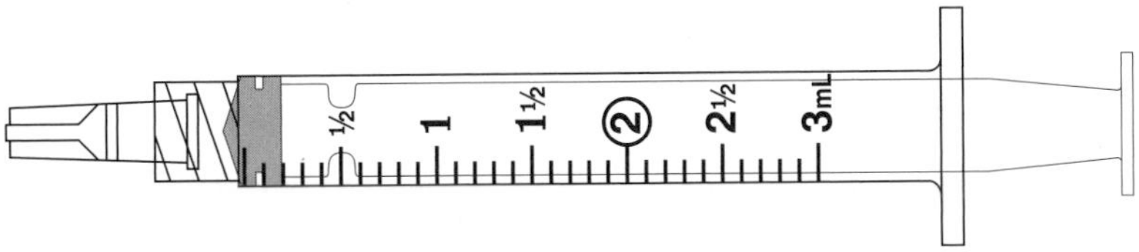

31. Order: *glycopyrrolate 50 mcg IM 60 min pre-op* for a child who weighs 11.4 kg. The recommended pre-anesthesia dosage of glycopyrrolate for a child is 0.005 mg/kg of body weight given intramuscularly.

    Recommended single dosage for this child: ________ mg/dose

    Is the dosage ordered safe? ________

32. If the dosage ordered in question 31 is safe, give ________ mL. If not safe, explain why not and describe what the nurse should do.

    ____

    ____

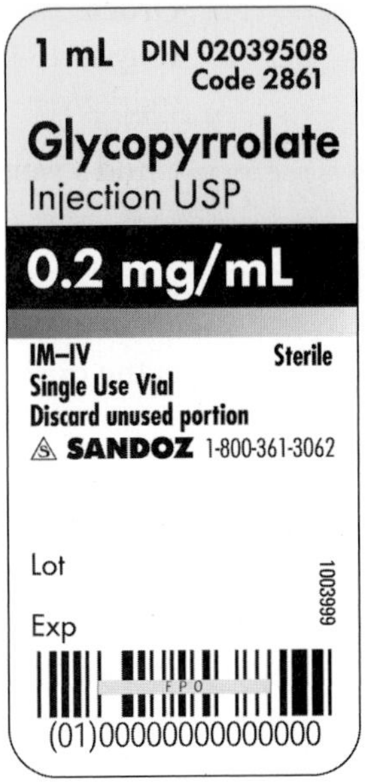

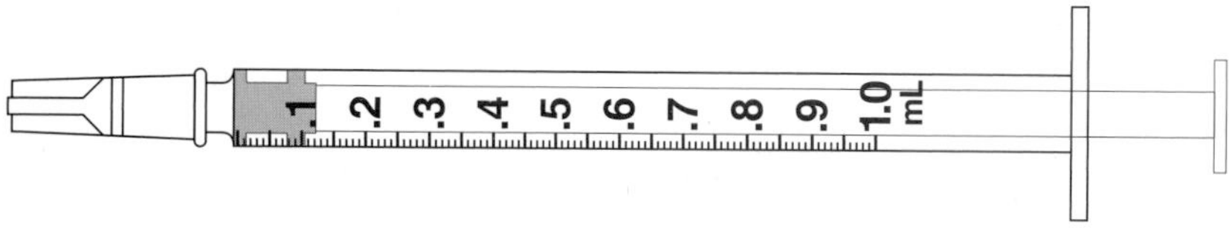

33. Order: *ceftazidime 400 mg IV q8h* for a 6-month-old infant who weighs 18 lb and has a serious infection. The recommended dosage of ceftazidime for infants and children 2 months–12 years is 10–33 mg/kg q8h.

    Child's weight: _________ kg

    Recommended minimum single dosage for this child: _________ mg/dose

    Recommended maximum single dosage for this child: _________ mg/dose

    Is the dosage ordered safe? _________

34. If the dosage ordered in question 33 is safe, reconstitute with _________ mL diluent for a total solution volume of _________ mL with a concentration of _________ mg/mL. Give _________ mL. If not safe, explain why not and describe what the nurse should do.

    ____

    ____

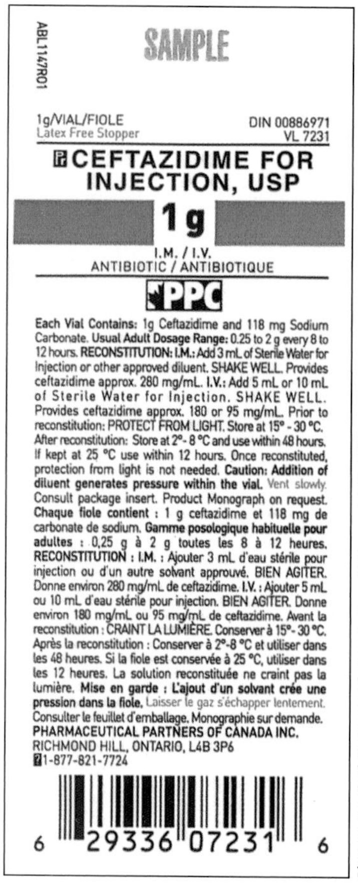

Pharmaceutical Partners of Canada Inc., Richmond Hill, ON

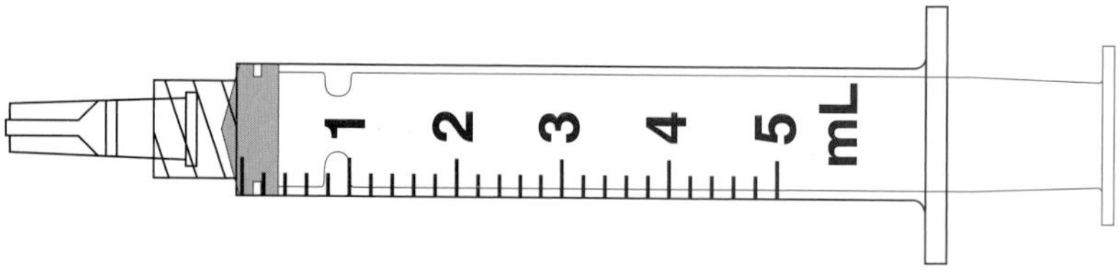

35. Order: *amoxicillin trihydrate/clavulanate potassium 200 mg PO q12h* for a 5-year-old child who weighs 45 lb. The recommended dosage of this combination drug is based on the amoxicillin at 25 mg/kg/day in divided doses q12h or 20 mg/kg/day in divided doses q8h.

    Child's weight: _________ kg

    Recommended daily dosage for this child: _________ mg/day

    Recommended single dosage for this child: _________ mg/dose

    Is the dosage ordered safe? _________

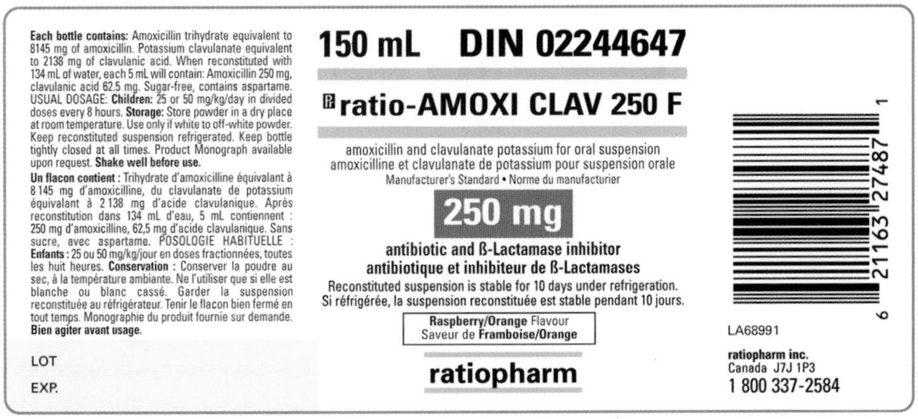

Ratiopharm Inc., Mississauga, ON

36. If the dosage ordered in question 35 is safe, give ________ mL. If not safe, explain why not and describe what the nurse should do. ____

____

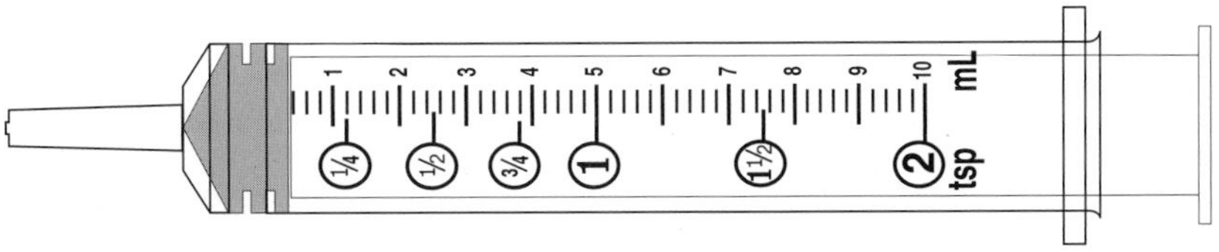

37. Order: *cefaclor oral suspension 75 mg PO TID* for a child with an upper respiratory infection who weighs 18 lb. Recommended dosage: See label.

Child's weight: ________ kg

Recommended daily dosage for this child: ________ mg/day

Recommended single dosage for this child: ________ mg/dose

Is the dosage ordered safe? ________

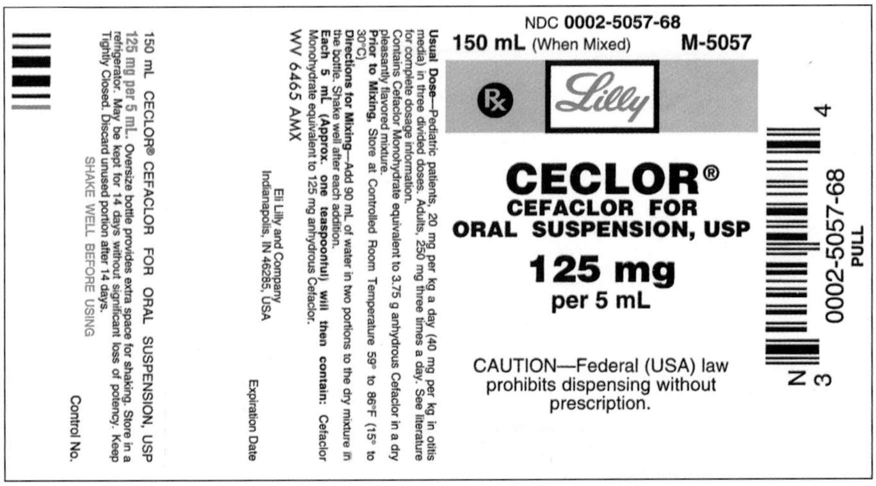

Courtesy of Eli Lilly and Company

38. If the dosage ordered in question 37 is safe, give ________ mL. If not safe, explain why not and describe what the nurse should do. ____

____

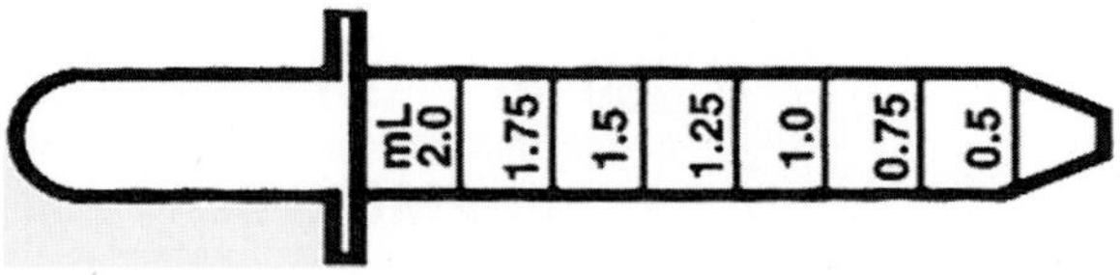

mL
2.0
1.75
1.5
1.25
1.0
0.75
0.5

39. Order: *cephalexin oral suspension 125 mg PO QID × 10 days* for a 4-year-old child who weighs 45 lb and has tonsillitis. Recommended dosage for children 25–50 mg/kg/day in 4 divided doses.

Child's weight: ________ kg

Recommended minimum daily dosage for this child: ________

Recommended single minimum dose: ________

Recommended maximum daily dosage for this child: ________

Recommended single maximum dose:________

Is the dosage ordered safe? ________

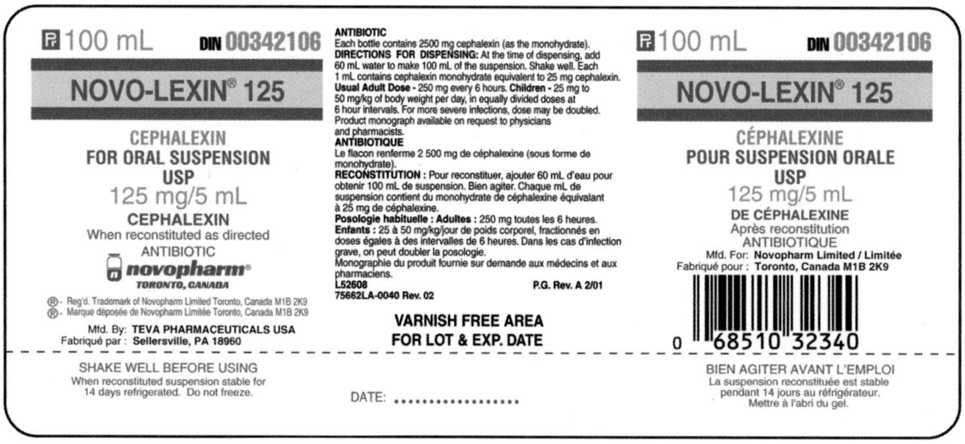

Pr 100 mL DIN 00342106
NOVO-LEXIN® 125
CEPHALEXIN
FOR ORAL SUSPENSION
USP
125 mg/5 mL
CEPHALEXIN
When reconstituted as directed
ANTIBIOTIC
novopharm®
TORONTO, CANADA
®- Reg'd. Trademark of Novopharm Limited Toronto, Canada M1B 2K9
®- Marque déposée de Novopharm Limitée Toronto, Canada M1B 2K9
Mfd. By: TEVA PHARMACEUTICALS USA
Fabriqué par : Sellersville, PA 18960
SHAKE WELL BEFORE USING
When reconstituted suspension stable for 14 days refrigerated. Do not freeze.
ANTIBIOTIC
Each bottle contains 2500 mg cephalexin (as the monohydrate).
DIRECTIONS FOR DISPENSING: At the time of dispensing, add 60 mL water to make 100 mL of the suspension. Shake well. Each 1 mL contains cephalexin monohydrate equivalent to 25 mg cephalexin.
Usual Adult Dose - 250 mg every 6 hours. Children - 25 mg to 50 mg/kg of body weight per day, in equally divided doses at 6 hour intervals. For more severe infections, dose may be doubled.
Product monograph available on request to physicians and pharmacists.
ANTIBIOTIQUE
Le flacon renferme 2 500 mg de céphalexine (sous forme de monohydrate).
RECONSTITUTION : Pour reconstituer, ajouter 60 mL d'eau pour obtenir 100 mL de suspension. Bien agiter. Chaque mL de suspension contient du monohydrate de céphalexine équivalant à 25 mg de céphalexine.
Posologie habituelle : Adultes : 250 mg toutes les 6 heures.
Enfants : 25 à 50 mg/kg/jour de poids corporel, fractionnés en doses égales à des intervalles de 6 heures. Dans les cas d'infection grave, on peut doubler la posologie.
Monographie du produit fournie sur demande aux médecins et aux pharmaciens.
L52608 P.G. Rev. A 2/01
75662LA-0040 Rev. 02
VARNISH FREE AREA
FOR LOT & EXP. DATE
DATE: ....
Pr 100 mL DIN 00342106
NOVO-LEXIN® 125
CÉPHALEXINE
POUR SUSPENSION ORALE
USP
125 mg/5 mL
DE CÉPHALEXINE
Après reconstitution
ANTIBIOTIQUE
Mfd. For: Novopharm Limited / Limitée
Fabriqué pour : Toronto, Canada M1B 2K9
0 68510 32340
BIEN AGITER AVANT L'EMPLOI
La suspension reconstituée est stable pendant 14 jours au réfrigérateur.
Mettre à l'abri du gel.

Novopharm Limited, Toronto, ON

40. If the dosage ordered in question 39 is safe, give ________ mL. If not safe, explain why not and describe what the nurse should do. ____

____

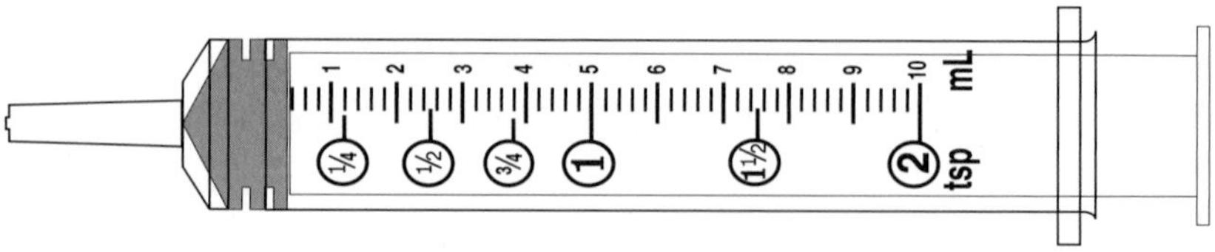

1
2
3
4
5
6
7
8
9
10
mL
¼
½
¾
1
1½
2
tsp

41. Order: *clarithromycin 175 mg PO q12h* for a child who weighs 51 lb. Recommended dosage for children: See label.

Child's weight: ________ kg

Recommended daily dosage for this child: ________ mg/day

Recommended single dosage for this child: ________ mg/dose

Is the dosage ordered safe? ________

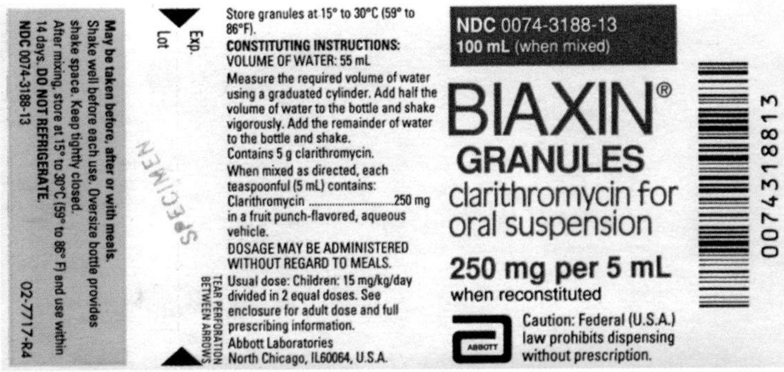

Courtesy of Abbott Laboratories, Inc.

42. If the dosage ordered in question 41 is safe, give ________ mL. If not safe, explain why not and describe what the nurse should do. ______________________________

____

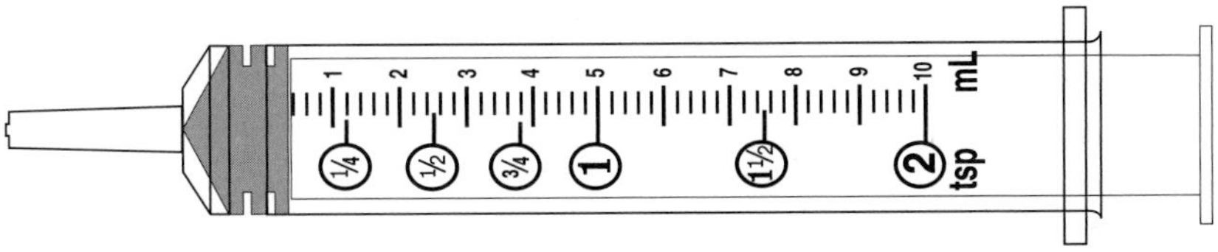

Questions 43 through 48 ask you to apply the steps on your own to determine safe dosages, just as you would do in the clinical setting. Calculate the amount to give and mark an arrow on the measuring device, or explain unsafe dosages and describe the appropriate action.

43. Order: *methylprednisolone 10 mg IM q6h* for a child who weighs 95 lb. Recommended pediatric dosage: Not less than 0.5 mg/kg/day

    If the dosage ordered is safe, give ________ mL. If not safe, explain why not and describe what the nurse should do. ______________________________

    ____

    ____

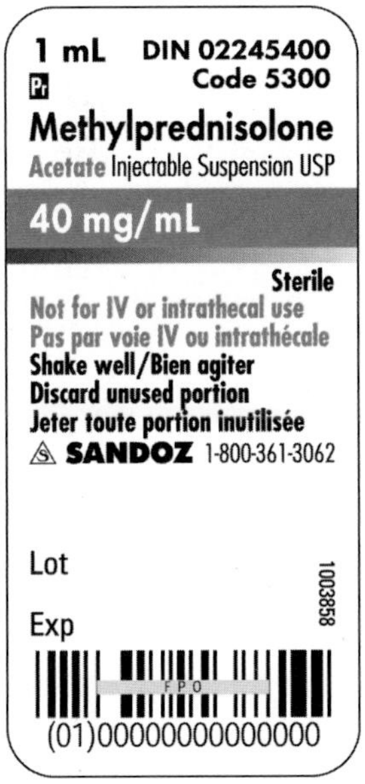

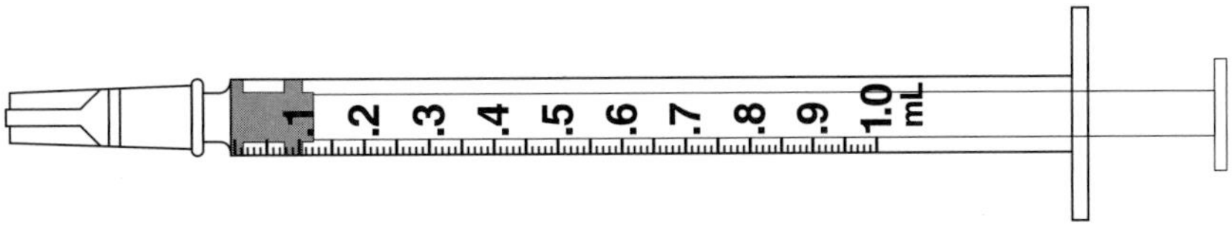

44. Order: *salbutamol 1.4 mg PO TID* for a 2-year-old child who weighs 31 lb. Recommended dosage: 0.1 mg/kg, not to exceed 2 mg TID.

If the dosage ordered is safe, give ________ mL. If not safe, explain why not and describe what the nurse should do. ____

____

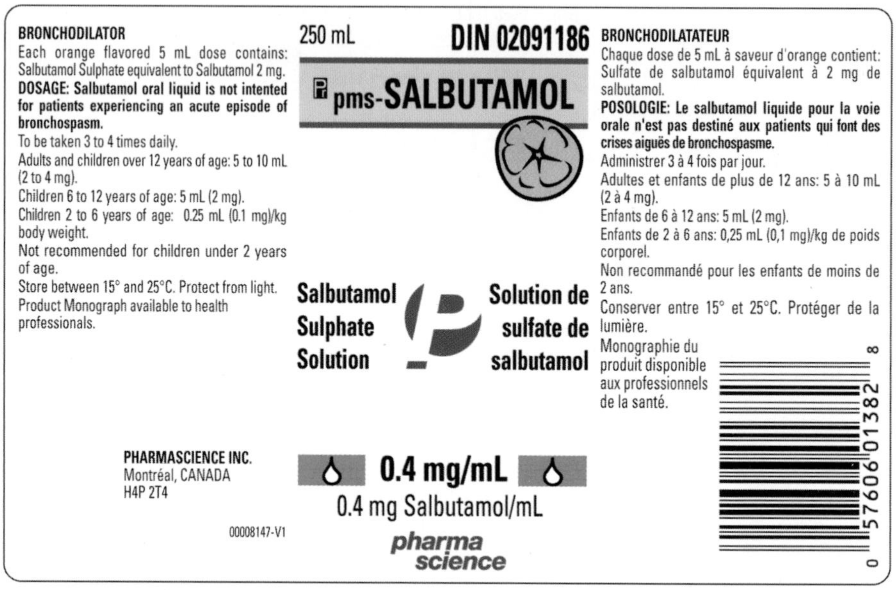

Pharmascience Inc., Montreal, Que

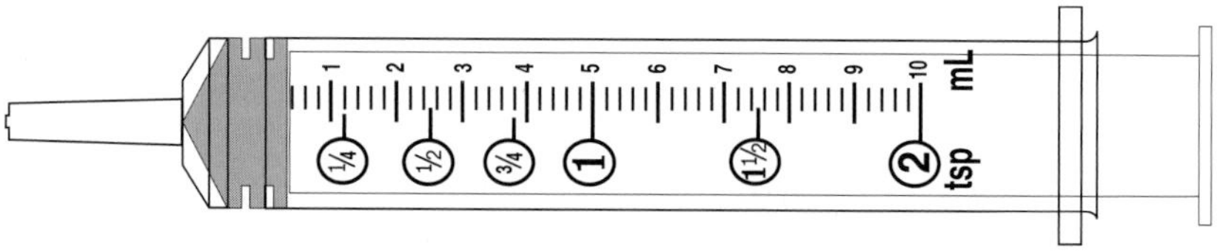

45. Order: *penicillin G sodium 450 000 units IM q6h* for a child who weighs 12 kg and has a streptococcal infection. Recommended pediatric dosage for streptococcal infections is 150 000 units/kg/day given in equal doses divided q4–6h.

If the dosage ordered is safe, reconstitute to a dosage supply of ________ units/mL and give ________ mL. If not safe, explain why not and describe what the nurse should do.

____

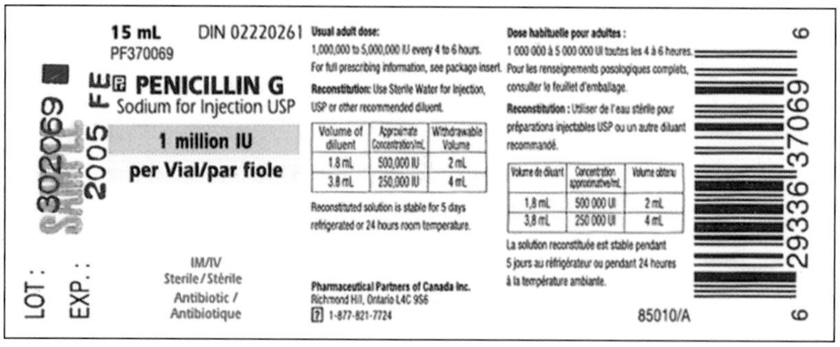

Pharmaceutical Partners of Canada Inc., Richmond Hill, ON

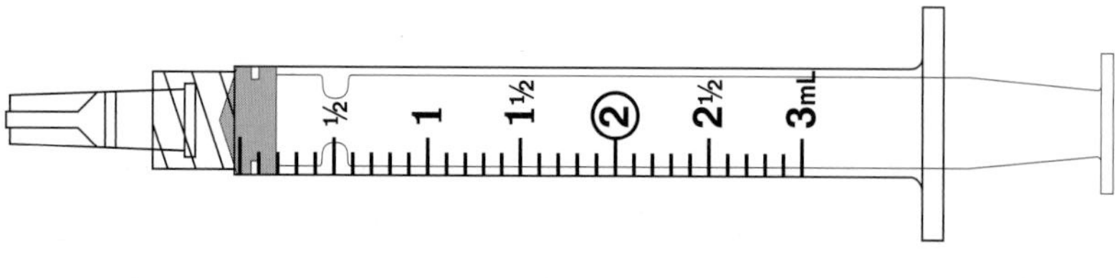

46. Order: *clonazepam 1 mg PO BID* for a 9-year-old child on initial therapy who weighs 56 lb. The recommended initial pediatric dosage of clonazepam for children up to 10 years or 30 kg is 0.01–0.03 mg/kg/day in 2–3 divided doses up to a maximum of 0.05 mg/kg/day.

    If the dosage ordered is safe, give ________ tablet(s). If not safe, explain why not and describe what the nurse should do. ____

    ____

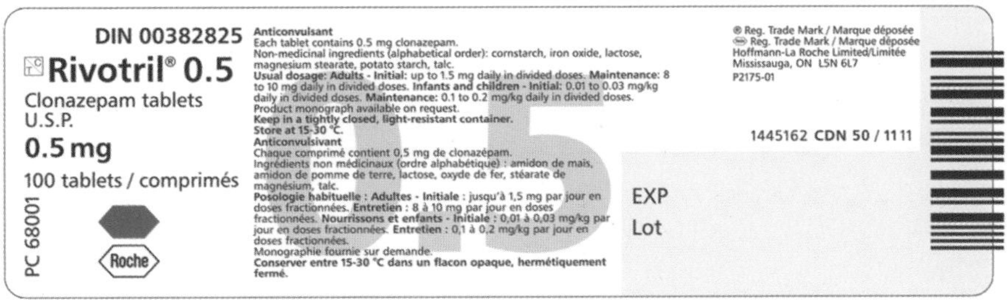

47. Order: *meperidine hydrochloride 20 mg subcutaneously q3–4h prn for pain* for a child who weighs 18 lb. Recommended pediatric dosage: 1.1–1.8 mg/kg q3–4h prn; do not exceed adult dosage of 50–100 mg/dose.

    If the dosage ordered is safe, give ________ mL. If not safe, explain why not and describe what the nurse should do. ____

    ____

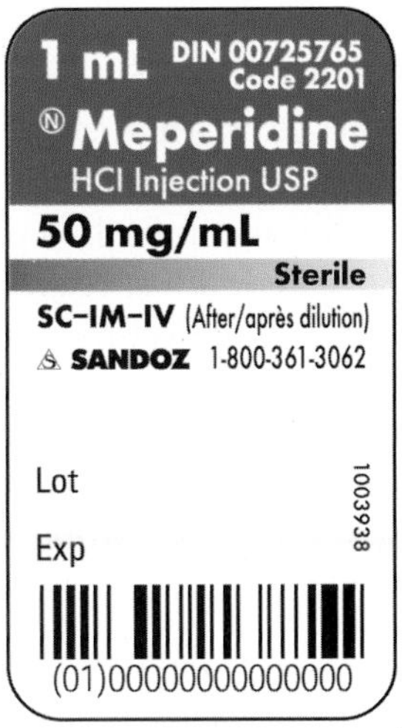

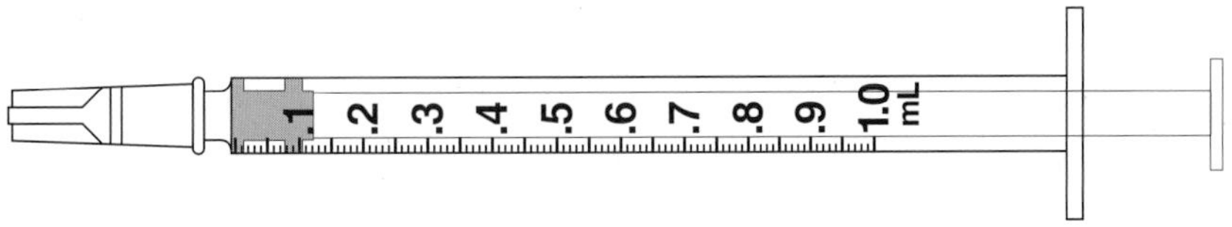

48. Order: *cefazolin sodium 250 mg IM q8h* for a 3-year-old child who weighs 35 lb. The recommended pediatric dosage of cefazolin sodium for children over 1 month: 25–50 mg/kg/day in 3–4 divided doses.

    If the dosage ordered is safe, give ________ mL. If not safe, explain why not and describe what the nurse should do. ____

    ____

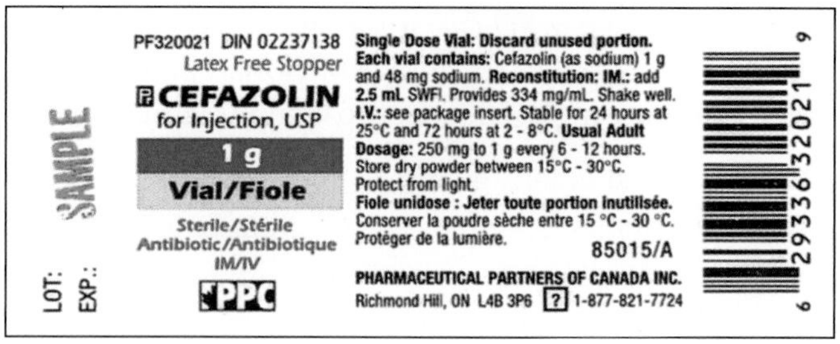

Pharmaceutical Partners of Canada Inc., Richmond Hill, ON

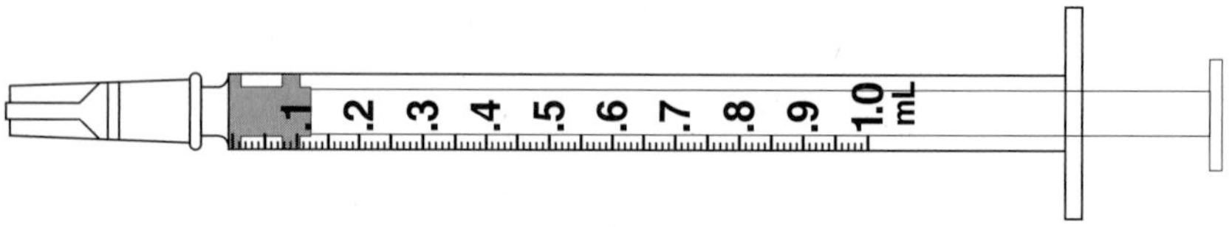

49. Refer back to questions 43 through 48. Identify which drugs require a reconstitution label.

____

____

50. Critical Thinking Skill: Describe the strategy or strategies you would implement to prevent this medication error.

possible scenario

Suppose the family practice resident ordered *tobramycin sulfate 110 mg IV q8h* for a child with cystic fibrosis who weighs 10 kg. The pediatric reference guide states that the safe dosage of tobramycin sulfate for a child with severe infections is 7.5 mg/kg/day in 3 equally divided doses. The nurse received five admissions the evening of this order and thought, "I'm too busy to calculate the safe dosage this time." The pharmacist prepared and labelled the medication in a syringe and the nurse administered the first dose of the medication. An hour later, the resident arrived on the pediatric unit and inquired if the nurse had given the first dose. When the nurse replied "yes," the resident became pale and stated, "I just realized that I ordered an adult dose of tobramycin sulfate. I hoped that the medication had not yet been given."

potential outcome

The resident's next step would likely have been to discontinue the tobramycin sulfate and order a stat tobramycin sulfate level. The level would most likely have been elevated, and the child would have required close monitoring for renal damage and hearing loss.

prevention

____

____

After completing these problems, see pages 486–490 to check your answers.

SECTION 3 SELF-EVALUATION

Chapter 8: Oral Dosage of Drugs

The following labels (A–N) represent the drugs you have available on your medication cart for the patient care orders in questions 1 through 10. Select the correct label and identify the letter that corresponds to fill these medication orders. Calculate the amount to give.

1. Order: *allopurinol 0.2 g PO daily*

   Select label ________ and give ________ tab

2. Order: *clonazepam 1 mg daily*

   Select label ________ and give ________ tab

3. Order: *lorazepam 1 mg*

   Select label ________ and give ________ tab

4. Order: *cephalexin 187.5 mg PO q6h × 5 days*

   Select label ________ and give ________ mL

5. Order: *potassium chloride 16 mEq PO daily*

   Select label ________ and give ________ mL

6. Order: *procainamide hydrochloride 1 g q6h*

   Select label ________ and give ________ cap/tab

7. Order: *spironolactone 75 mg PO daily*

   Select label ________ and give ________ tab

8. Order: *lisinopril 7.5 mg PO daily*

   Select label ________ and give ________ tab

9. Order: *furosemide 12.5 mg PO BID*

   Select label ________ and give ________ mL

10. Order: *cefixime 70 mg BID*

    Select label ________ and give ________ mL

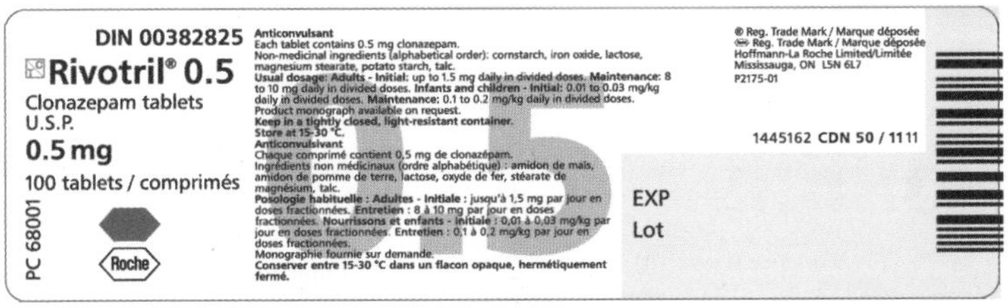

Label submitted by manufacturer for general information and may change; please always refer to the latest product monograph/label. ©Copyright 2007, Hoffman-LaRoche Limited.

A

Novopharm Limited, Toronto, ON

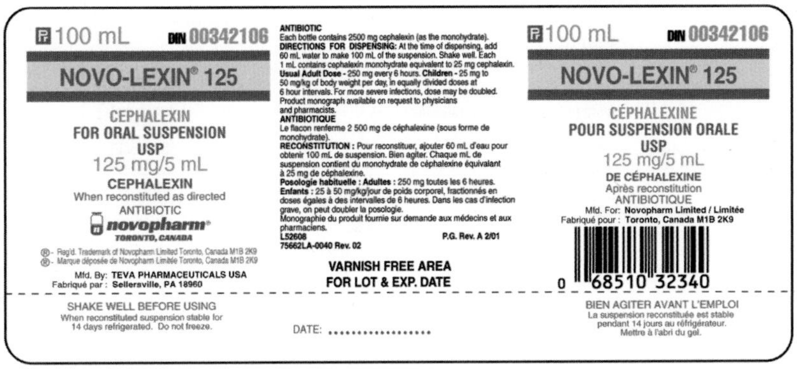

B

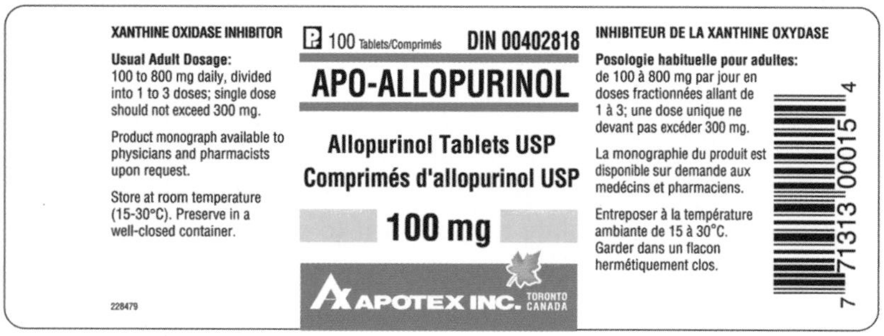

C

Apotex Inc., Weston, ON

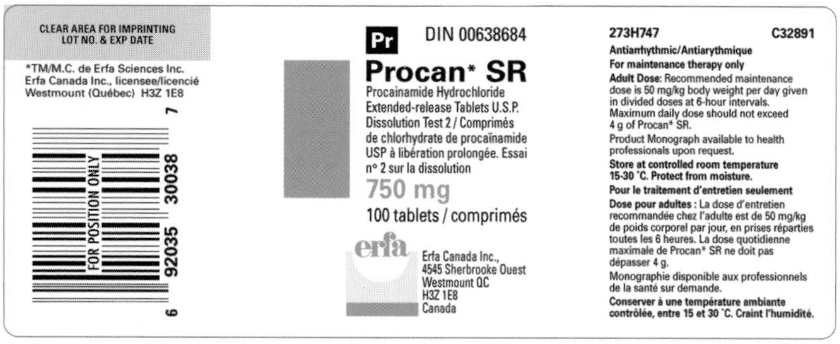

D

Erfa Canada Inc., Westmount, QUE

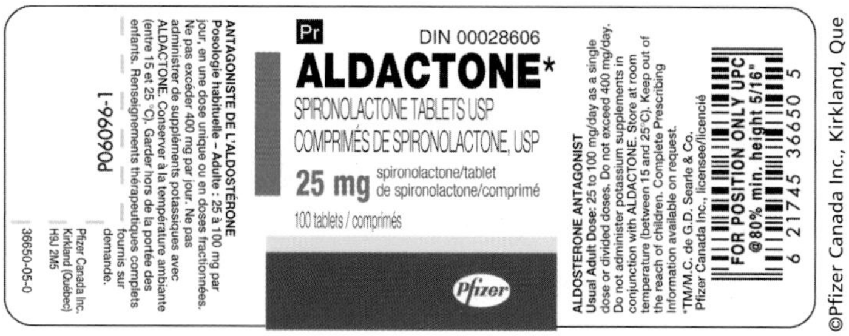

E

©Pfizer Canada Inc., Kirkland, Que

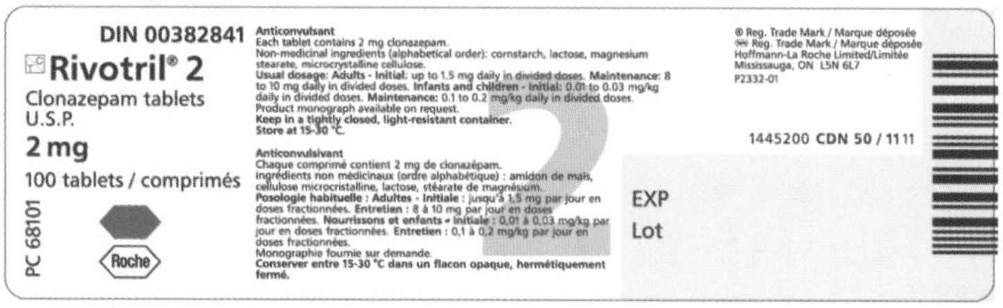

F

Label submitted by manufacturer for general information and may change; please always refer to the latest product monograph/label. ©Copyright 2007, Hoffman-LaRoche Limited.

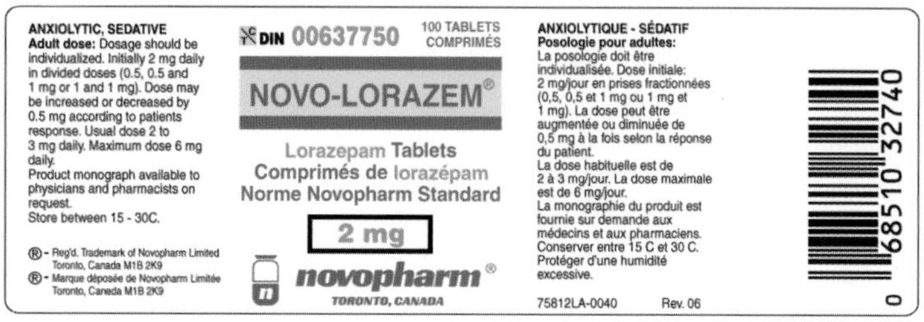

G

Novopharm Limited, Toronto, ON

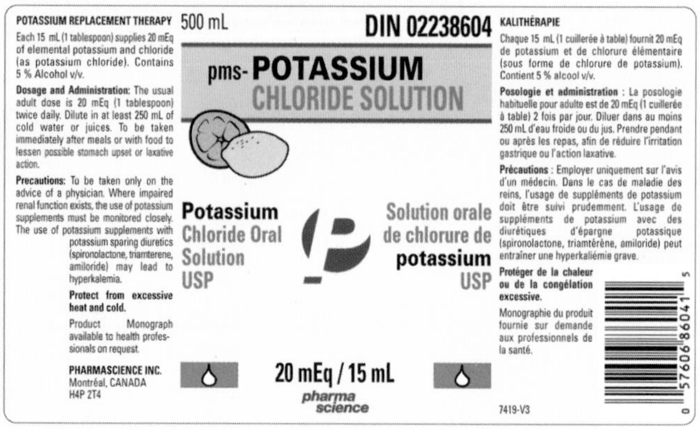

Pharmascience Inc., Montreal, Que

H

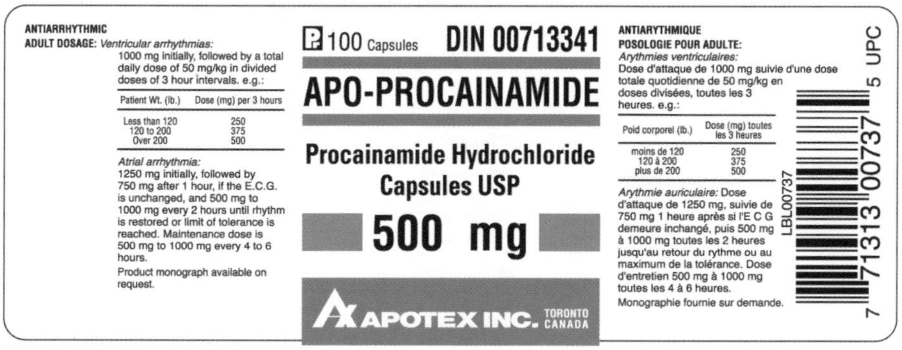
ANTIARRHYTHMIC
ADULT DOSAGE: Ventricular arrhythmias: 1000 mg initially, followed by a total daily dose of 50 mg/kg in divided doses of 3 hour intervals. e.g.:
Patient Wt. (lb.) | Dose (mg) per 3 hours
Less than 120 250
120 to 200 375
Over 200 500
Atrial arrhythmia: 1250 mg initially, followed by 750 mg after 1 hour, if the E.C.G. is unchanged, and 500 mg to 1000 mg every 2 hours until rhythm is restored or limit of tolerance is reached. Maintenance dose is 500 mg to 1000 mg every 4 to 6 hours.
Product monograph available on request.
Pr 100 Capsules DIN 00713341
APO-PROCAINAMIDE
Procainamide Hydrochloride Capsules USP
500 mg
APOTEX INC. TORONTO CANADA
ANTIARYTHMIQUE
POSOLOGIE POUR ADULTE:
Arythmies ventriculaires: Dose d'attaque de 1000 mg suivie d'une dose totale quotidienne de 50 mg/kg en doses divisées, toutes les 3 heures. e.g.:
Poids corporel (lb.) | Dose (mg) toutes les 3 heures
moins de 120 250
120 à 200 375
plus de 200 500
Arythmie auriculaire: Dose d'attaque de 1250 mg, suivie de 750 mg 1 heure après si l'E C G demeure inchangé, puis 500 mg à 1000 mg toutes les 2 heures jusqu'au retour du rythme ou au maximum de la tolérance. Dose d'entretien 500 mg à 1000 mg toutes les 4 à 6 heures.
Monographie fournie sur demande.
LBL00737
7 71313 00737 5 UPC

Apotex Inc., Weston, ON

I

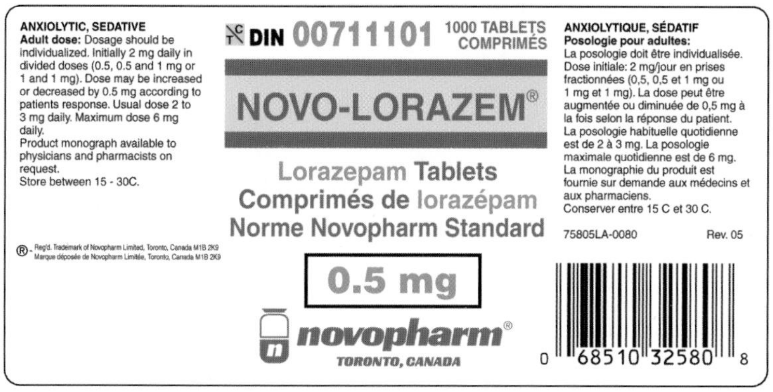
ANXIOLYTIC, SEDATIVE
Adult dose: Dosage should be individualized. Initially 2 mg daily in divided doses (0.5, 0.5 and 1 mg or 1 and 1 mg). Dose may be increased or decreased by 0.5 mg according to patients response. Usual dose 2 to 3 mg daily. Maximum dose 6 mg daily.
Product monograph available to physicians and pharmacists on request.
Store between 15 - 30C.
® - Reg'd. Trademark of Novopharm Limited, Toronto, Canada M1B 2K9 / Marque déposée de Novopharm Limitée, Toronto, Canada M1B 2K9
DIN 00711101 1000 TABLETS COMPRIMÉS
NOVO-LORAZEM®
Lorazepam Tablets
Comprimés de lorazépam
Norme Novopharm Standard
0.5 mg
novopharm®
TORONTO, CANADA
ANXIOLYTIQUE, SÉDATIF
Posologie pour adultes: La posologie doit être individualisée. Dose initiale: 2 mg/jour en prises fractionnées (0,5, 0,5 et 1 mg ou 1 mg et 1 mg). La dose peut être augmentée ou diminuée de 0,5 mg à la fois selon la réponse du patient. La posologie habituelle quotidienne est de 2 à 3 mg. La posologie maximale quotidienne est de 6 mg. La monographie du produit est fournie sur demande aux médecins et aux pharmaciens.
Conserver entre 15 C et 30 C.
75805LA-0080 Rev. 05
0 68510 32580 8

Novopharm Limited, Toronto, ON

J

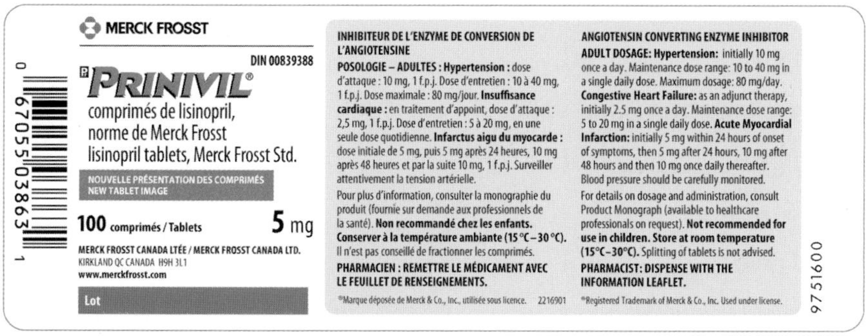
0 67055 03863 1
MERCK FROSST
DIN 00839388
Pr PRINIVIL®
comprimés de lisinopril, norme de Merck Frosst
lisinopril tablets, Merck Frosst Std.
NOUVELLE PRÉSENTATION DES COMPRIMÉS
NEW TABLET IMAGE
100 comprimés / Tablets 5 mg
MERCK FROSST CANADA LTÉE / MERCK FROSST CANADA LTD.
KIRKLAND QC CANADA H9H 3L1
www.merckfrosst.com
Lot
INHIBITEUR DE L'ENZYME DE CONVERSION DE L'ANGIOTENSINE
POSOLOGIE – ADULTES : Hypertension : dose d'attaque : 10 mg, 1 f.p.j. Dose d'entretien : 10 à 40 mg, 1 f.p.j. Dose maximale : 80 mg/jour. Insuffisance cardiaque : en traitement d'appoint, dose d'attaque : 2,5 mg, 1 f.p.j. Dose d'entretien : 5 à 20 mg, en une seule dose quotidienne. Infarctus aigu du myocarde : dose initiale de 5 mg, puis 5 mg après 24 heures, 10 mg après 48 heures et par la suite 10 mg, 1 f.p.j. Surveiller attentivement la tension artérielle.
Pour plus d'information, consulter la monographie du produit (fournie sur demande aux professionnels de la santé). Non recommandé chez les enfants. Conserver à la température ambiante (15 °C – 30 °C). Il n'est pas conseillé de fractionner les comprimés.
PHARMACIEN : REMETTRE LE MÉDICAMENT AVEC LE FEUILLET DE RENSEIGNEMENTS.
®Marque déposée de Merck & Co., Inc., utilisée sous licence. 2216901
ANGIOTENSIN CONVERTING ENZYME INHIBITOR
ADULT DOSAGE: Hypertension: initially 10 mg once a day. Maintenance dose range: 10 to 40 mg in a single daily dose. Maximum dosage: 80 mg/day. Congestive Heart Failure: as an adjunct therapy, initially 2.5 mg once a day. Maintenance dose range: 5 to 20 mg in a single daily dose. Acute Myocardial Infarction: initially 5 mg within 24 hours of onset of symptoms, then 5 mg after 24 hours, 10 mg after 48 hours and then 10 mg once daily thereafter. Blood pressure should be carefully monitored.
For details on dosage and administration, consult Product Monograph (available to healthcare professionals on request). Not recommended for use in children. Store at room temperature (15°C–30°C). Splitting of tablets is not advised.
PHARMACIST: DISPENSE WITH THE INFORMATION LEAFLET.
®Registered Trademark of Merck & Co., Inc. Used under license.
9751600

Merck Frosst Canada Ltd., Kirkland, QUE

K

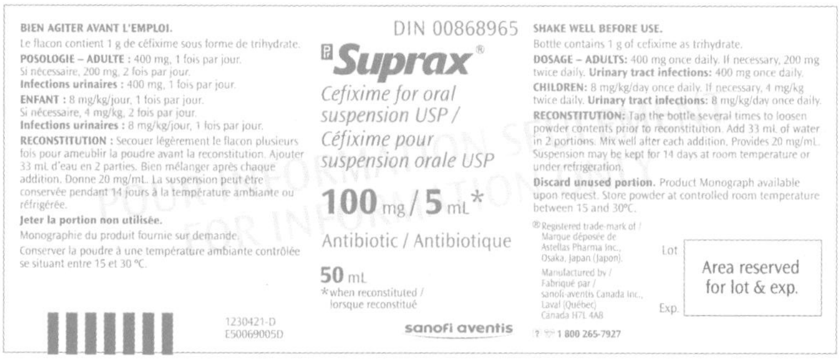
BIEN AGITER AVANT L'EMPLOI.
Le flacon contient 1 g de céfixime sous forme de trihydrate.
POSOLOGIE – ADULTE : 400 mg, 1 fois par jour. Si nécessaire, 200 mg, 2 fois par jour. Infections urinaires : 400 mg, 1 fois par jour.
ENFANT : 8 mg/kg/jour, 1 fois par jour. Si nécessaire, 4 mg/kg, 2 fois par jour. Infections urinaires : 8 mg/kg/jour, 1 fois par jour.
RECONSTITUTION : Secouer légèrement le flacon plusieurs fois pour ameublir la poudre avant la reconstitution. Ajouter 33 mL d'eau en 2 parties. Bien mélanger après chaque addition. Donne 20 mg/mL. La suspension peut être conservée pendant 14 jours à la température ambiante ou réfrigérée.
Jeter la portion non utilisée.
Monographie du produit fournie sur demande.
Conserver la poudre à une température ambiante contrôlée se situant entre 15 et 30 °C.
1230421-D
E50069005D
DIN 00868965
Pr Suprax®
Cefixime for oral suspension USP /
Céfixime pour suspension orale USP
100 mg / 5 mL*
Antibiotic / Antibiotique
50 mL
*when reconstituted / lorsque reconstitué
sanofi aventis
SHAKE WELL BEFORE USE.
Bottle contains 1 g of cefixime as trihydrate.
DOSAGE – ADULTS: 400 mg once daily. If necessary, 200 mg twice daily. Urinary tract infections: 400 mg once daily.
CHILDREN: 8 mg/kg/day once daily. If necessary, 4 mg/kg twice daily. Urinary tract infections: 8 mg/kg/day once daily.
RECONSTITUTION: Tap the bottle several times to loosen powder contents prior to reconstitution. Add 33 mL of water in 2 portions. Mix well after each addition. Provides 20 mg/mL. Suspension may be kept for 14 days at room temperature or under refrigeration.
Discard unused portion. Product Monograph available upon request. Store powder at controlled room temperature between 15 and 30°C.
® Registered trade-mark of / Marque déposée de Astellas Pharma Inc., Osaka, Japan (Japon).
Manufactured by / Fabriqué par / sanofi-aventis Canada Inc., Laval (Québec) Canada H7L 4A8
1 800 265-7927
Lot
Exp.
Area reserved for lot & exp.

Sanofi-aventis Canada, Laval, QUE

L

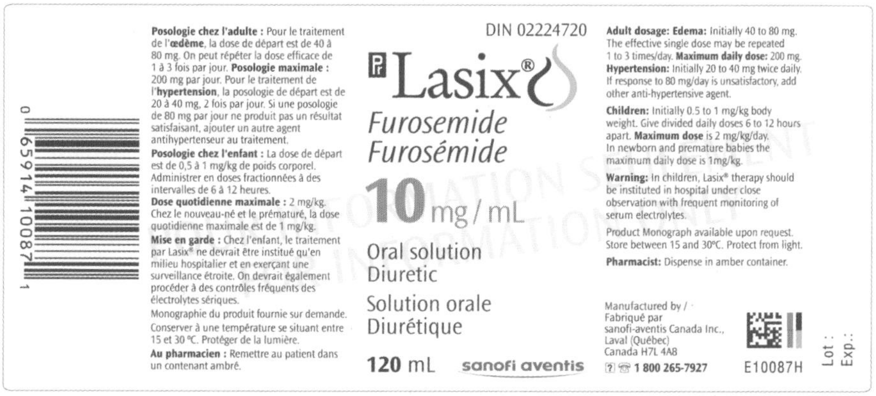
0 65914 10087 1
Posologie chez l'adulte : Pour le traitement de l'œdème, la dose de départ est de 40 à 80 mg. On peut répéter la dose efficace de 1 à 3 fois par jour. Posologie maximale : 200 mg par jour. Pour le traitement de l'hypertension, la posologie de départ est de 20 à 40 mg, 2 fois par jour. Si une posologie de 80 mg par jour ne produit pas un résultat satisfaisant, ajouter un autre agent antihypertenseur au traitement.
Posologie chez l'enfant : La dose de départ est de 0,5 à 1 mg/kg de poids corporel. Administrer en doses fractionnées à des intervalles de 6 à 12 heures.
Dose quotidienne maximale : 2 mg/kg. Chez le nouveau-né et le prématuré, la dose quotidienne maximale est de 1 mg/kg.
Mise en garde : Chez l'enfant, le traitement par Lasix® ne devrait être institué qu'en milieu hospitalier et en exerçant une surveillance étroite. On devrait également procéder à des contrôles fréquents des électrolytes sériques.
Monographie du produit fournie sur demande.
Conserver à une température se situant entre 15 et 30 °C. Protéger de la lumière.
Au pharmacien : Remettre au patient dans un contenant ambré.
DIN 02224720
Pr Lasix®
Furosemide
Furosémide
10 mg / mL
Oral solution
Diuretic
Solution orale
Diurétique
120 mL
sanofi aventis
Adult dosage: Edema: Initially 40 to 80 mg. The effective single dose may be repeated 1 to 3 times/day. Maximum daily dose: 200 mg. Hypertension: Initially 20 to 40 mg twice daily. If response to 80 mg/day is unsatisfactory, add other anti-hypertensive agent.
Children: Initially 0.5 to 1 mg/kg body weight. Give divided daily doses 6 to 12 hours apart. Maximum dose is 2 mg/kg/day. In newborn and premature babies the maximum daily dose is 1mg/kg.
Warning: In children, Lasix® therapy should be instituted in hospital under close observation with frequent monitoring of serum electrolytes.
Product Monograph available upon request. Store between 15 and 30°C. Protect from light.
Pharmacist: Dispense in amber container.
Manufactured by / Fabriqué par sanofi-aventis Canada Inc., Laval (Québec) Canada H7L 4A8
1 800 265-7927
E10087H
Lot :
Exp.:

Sanofi-aventis Canada, Laval, QUE

M

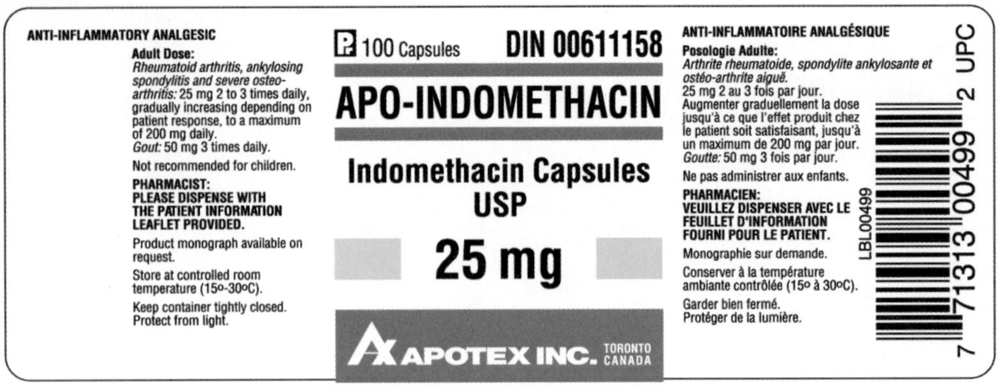
ANTI-INFLAMMATORY ANALGESIC
Adult Dose:
Rheumatoid arthritis, ankylosing spondylitis and severe osteo-arthritis: 25 mg 2 to 3 times daily, gradually increasing depending on patient response, to a maximum of 200 mg daily.
Gout: 50 mg 3 times daily.
Not recommended for children.
PHARMACIST: PLEASE DISPENSE WITH THE PATIENT INFORMATION LEAFLET PROVIDED.
Product monograph available on request.
Store at controlled room temperature (15o-30oC).
Keep container tightly closed. Protect from light.
100 Capsules
DIN 00611158
APO-INDOMETHACIN
Indomethacin Capsules USP
25 mg
APOTEX INC. TORONTO CANADA
ANTI-INFLAMMATOIRE ANALGÉSIQUE
Posologie Adulte:
Arthrite rheumatoïde, spondylite ankylosante et ostéo-arthrite aiguë.
25 mg 2 au 3 fois par jour. Augmenter graduellement la dose jusqu'à ce que l'effet produit chez le patient soit satisfaisant, jusqu'à un maximum de 200 mg par jour.
Goutte: 50 mg 3 fois par jour.
Ne pas administrer aux enfants.
PHARMACIEN: VEUILLEZ DISPENSER AVEC LE FEUILLET D'INFORMATION FOURNI POUR LE PATIENT.
Monographie sur demande.
Conserver à la température ambiante contrôlée (15o à 30oC).
Garder bien fermé.
Protéger de la lumière.
LBL00499
7 71313 00499 2 UPC

Apotex Inc., Weston, ON

N

Chapter 9: Parenteral Dosage of Drugs

The following labels (A–H) represent the drugs that are available on your medication cart for the patient care orders in questions 11 through 18. Select the correct label and identify the letter that corresponds to fill these parenteral medication orders. Calculate the amount to give.

11. Order: *vitamin B_{12} 0.2 mg subcutaneous daily × 10 days*

    Select label ________ and give ________ mL

12. Order: *diazepam 2.5 mg IV stat*

    Select label ________ and give ________ mL

13. Order: *epinephrine 200 mcg subcutaneous stat*

    Select label ________ and give ________ mL

14. Order: *furosemide 8 mg IM daily*

    Select label ________ and give ________ mL

15. Order: *gentamicin sodium 60 mg IV q8h*

    Select label ________ and give ________ mL

16. Order: *heparin sodium 7500 units subcutaneous stat*

    Select label ________ and give ________ mL

17. Order: *morphine sulfate 7.5 mg subcutaneous q4h, prn for pain*

    Select label ________ and give ________ mL

18. Order: *naloxone hydrochloride 0.3 mg IM stat*

    Select label ________ and give ________ mL

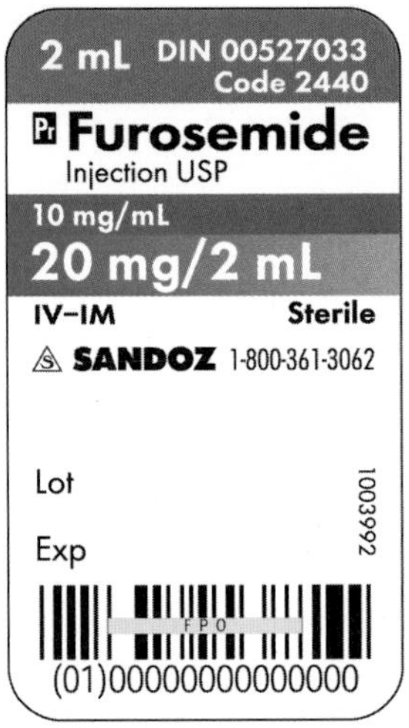
2 mL DIN 00527033
Code 2440
Furosemide
Injection USP
10 mg/mL
20 mg/2 mL
IV–IM Sterile
SANDOZ 1-800-361-3062
Lot
Exp
1003992
(01)00000000000000

A

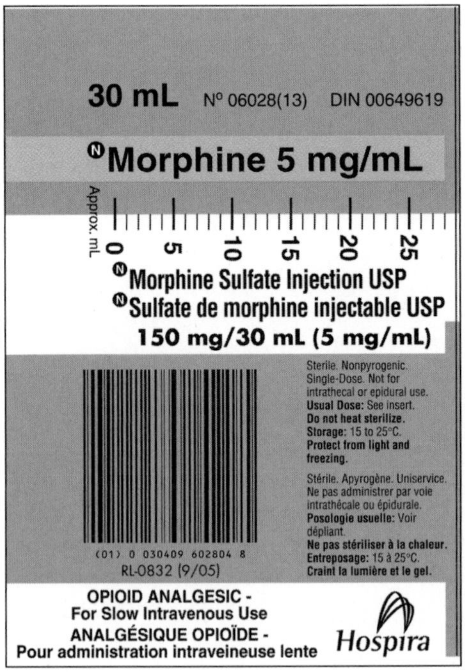
30 mL Nº 06028(13) DIN 00649619
Morphine 5 mg/mL
Approx. mL
0 5 10 15 20 25
Morphine Sulfate Injection USP
Sulfate de morphine injectable USP
150 mg/30 mL (5 mg/mL)
Sterile. Nonpyrogenic. Single-Dose. Not for intrathecal or epidural use. Usual Dose: See insert. Do not heat sterilize. Storage: 15 to 25°C. Protect from light and freezing.
Stérile. Apyrogène. Uniservice. Ne pas administrer par voie intrathécale ou épidurale. Posologie usuelle: Voir dépliant. Ne pas stériliser à la chaleur. Entreposage: 15 à 25°C. Craint la lumière et le gel.
(01) 0 030409 602804 8
RL-0832 (9/05)
OPIOID ANALGESIC - For Slow Intravenous Use
ANALGÉSIQUE OPIOÏDE - Pour administration intraveineuse lente
Hospira

B

Hospira Healthcare corporation, Saint-Laurent, QUE

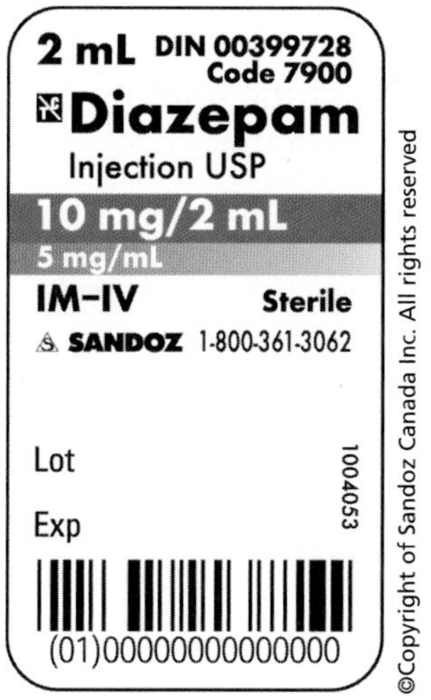

C

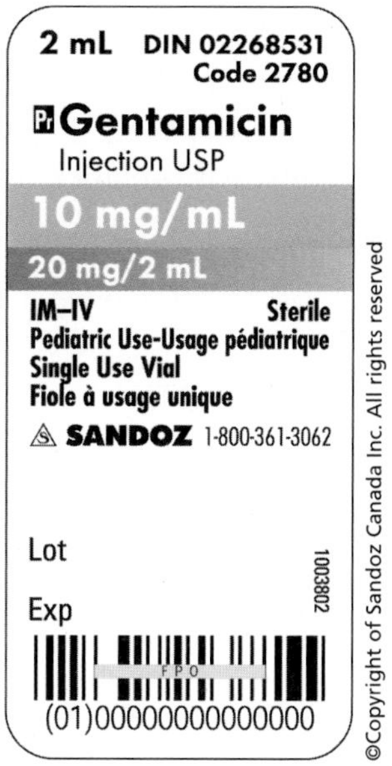

D

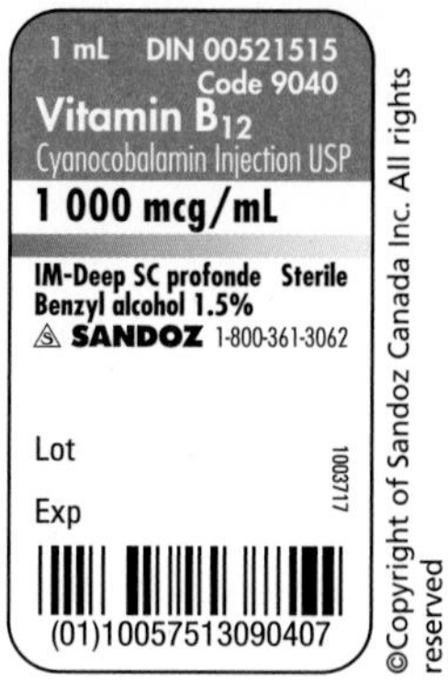

E

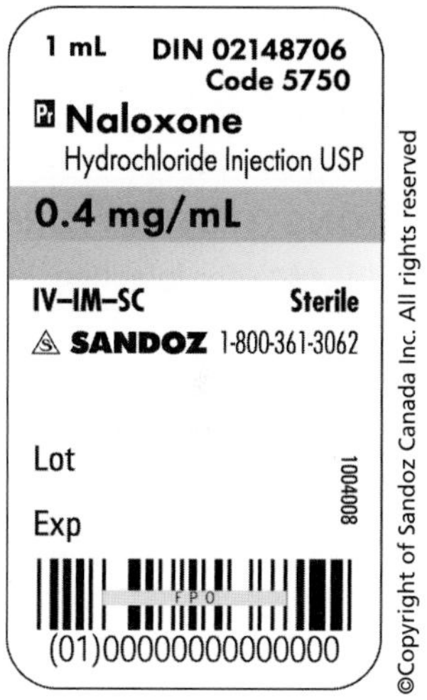

H

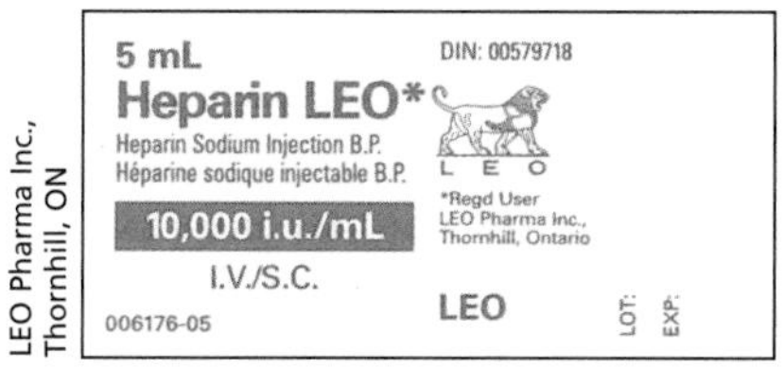

F

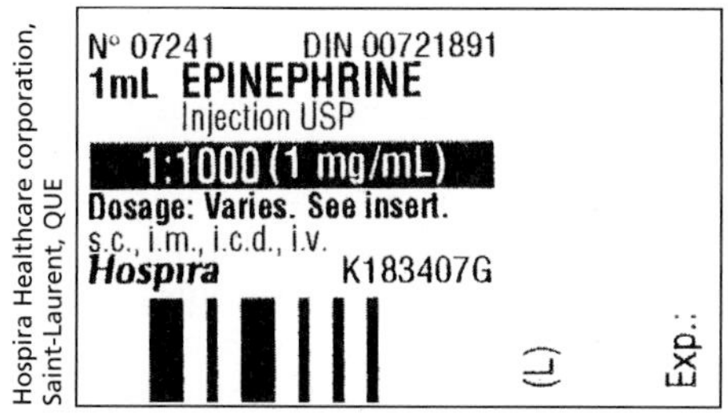

G

For questions 19 and 20, mark the amount to give on the correct syringe.

19. Order: *Humulin N 100-unit insulin 48 units subcutaneous 15 min before breakfast*

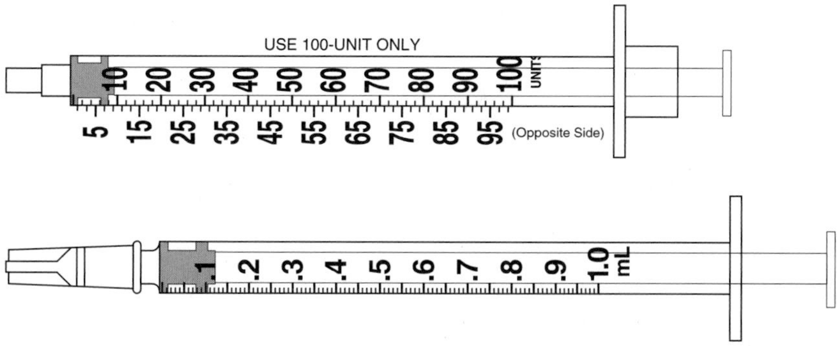

20. Order: *Humulin R 100-unit insulin 12 units with Humulin N 100-unit insulin 28 units subcutaneous 15 min before dinner*

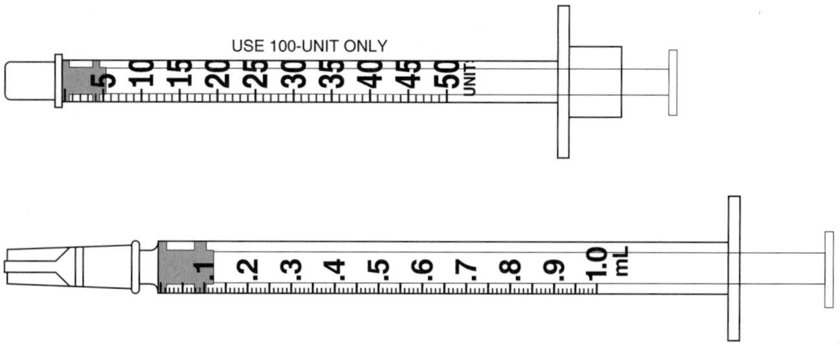

Chapter 10: Reconstitution of Solutions

For questions 21 through 26, specify the amount of diluent to add and the resulting solution concentration. Calculate the amount to give and indicate the dose with an arrow on the accompanying syringe. Finally, make a reconstitution label, if required.

21. Order: *azithromycin dihydrate 400 mg IV daily. See package insert for instructions on dilution.*

    Reconstitute with ________ mL diluent for a total solution volume of ________ mL with a concentration of ________ mg/mL.

    Withdraw: ________ mL and further dilute prior to administration

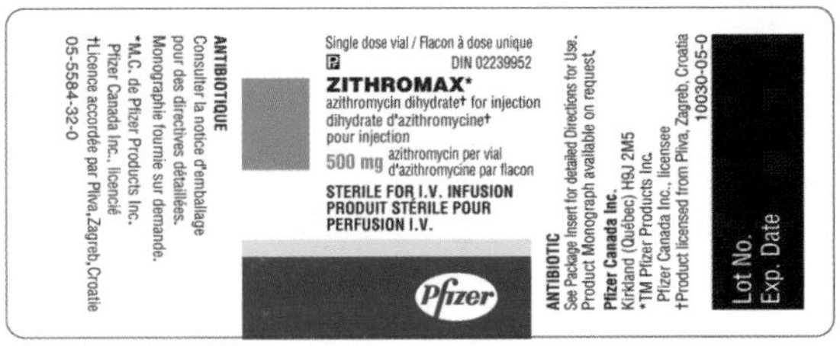

RECONSTITUTION DIRECTIONS

ZITHROMAX for Injection:

RECONSTITUTION OF ZITHROMAX FOR INJECTION

Strength	Reconstitution Solution	Volume to be Added	Approximate Volume Available	Nominal Concentration
500 mg	Sterile Water for Injection	4.8 mL	5 mL	100 mg/mL

Prepare the initial solution of ZITHROMAX for Injection by adding 4.8 mL of Sterile Water for Injection to the 500 mg vial. Shake the vial until all of the drug is dissolved. Since the vial is evacuated, it is recommended that a standard 5 mL (non-automated) syringe be used to ensure that the exact volume of 4.8 mL is dispensed. Each mL of reconstituted solution contains azithromycin dihydrate equivalent to 100 mg azithromycin. Reconstituted solution is stable for 24 hours when stored below 30°C. **The reconstituted solution must be further diluted prior to administration.**

Dilution of reconstituted solution: To provide azithromycin over a concentration range of 1.0–2.0 mg/mL, transfer 5 mL of the 100 mg/mL azithromycin solution into the appropriate amount of the following diluents:

Final Infusion Concentration (mg/mL)	Amount of Diluent (mL)
1.0 mg/mL	500 mL
2.0 mg/mL	250 mL

Appropriate Diluents

0.9% Sodium Chloride Injection
5% Dextrose in Water for Injection
0.45% Sodium Chloride Injection
Lactated Ringer's Injection
5% Dextrose in 0.45% Sodium Chloride Injection with 20 mEq Potassium Chloride
5% Dextrose in Lactated Ringer's Injection
5% Dextrose in 0.3% Sodium Chloride Injection
5% Dextrose in 0.45% Sodium Chloride Injection
Normosol-M in 5% Dextrose

Diluted solutions prepared in this manner are stable for 24 hours at or below room temperature (30°C), or for 72 hours if stored under refrigeration (5°C). As with all parenteral drug products, intravenous admixtures should be inspected visually for clarity, particulate matter, precipitate, discoloration and leakage prior to administration, whenever solution and container permit. Solutions showing haziness, particulate matter, precipitate, discoloration or leakage should be discarded.

Only limited data are available on the compatibility of ZITHROMAX for Injection with other intravenous substances, therefore additives or other medications should not be added to ZITHROMAX for Injection or infused simultaneously through the same intravenous line. If the same intravenous line is used for sequential infusion of several different drugs, the line should be flushed before and after infusion of ZITHROMAX for Injection with an infusion solution compatible with ZITHROMAX for Injection and with any other drug(s) administered via the common line. If ZITHROMAX for Injection is to be given concomitantly with another drug, each drug should be given separately in accordance with the recommended dosage and route of administration for each drug.

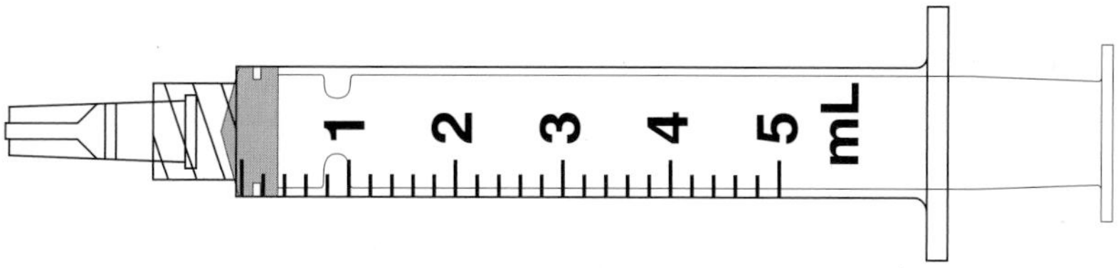

22. Order: *vancomycin hydrochloride 500 mg IV q6h*

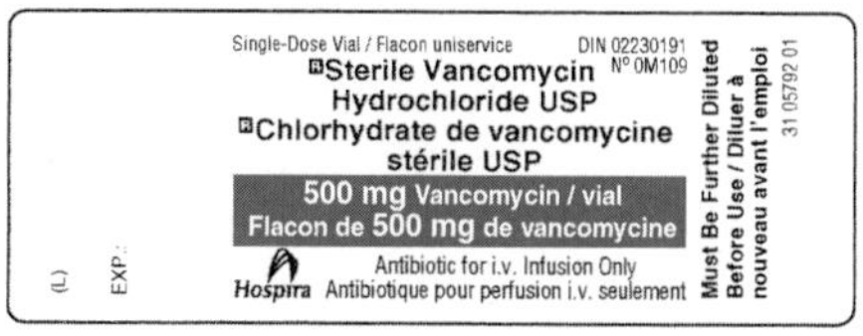

Hospira Healthcare corporation, Saint-Laurent, QUE

See package instructions for dilution.

Reconstitute with ________ mL diluent with a concentration of ________ mg/mL.

Withdraw: ________ mL and further dilute prior to administration

Reconstitution
Flip-Top Vial

Solution for Reconstitution: Sterile Water for Injection USP
Reconstitute as follows:

Reconstitution Table			
Flip-Top Vial Size	Volume to Be Added to Vial	Approx. Available Volume	Vancomycin in Concentration
500 mg	10 mL	10.3 mL	50 mg/mL
1 g	20 mL	20.6 mL	50 mg/mL

NOTE: FURTHER DILUTION IS REQUIRED
For Intermittent Intravenous Infusion

500 mg viat Re constituted solutions must be diluted with at least 100 mL of 0.9% Sodium Chloride Injection or 5% Dextrose in Sterile Water for Injection U.S.P.

1 g vial: Re constituted solutions must be diluted with at least 200 mL of 0.9% Sodium Chloride Injection or 5% Dextrose in Sterile Water for Injection U.S.P.

For Continuous Intravenous Infusion

The vials reconstituted according to the above table should be further diluted to the desired volume with one of the following intravenous solutions:
- 5% Dextrose Injection
- 3.3% Dextrose Injection and 0.3% Sodium Chloride Injection Lootated Ringer's Injection
- 0.9% Sodium Chloride Injection

A concentration of no greater than 5 mg/mL is recommended.

Stability and Storage Recommendations
Dry Powder

Vancomycin hydrochloride powder should be stored between 20 and 25°C (see "Controlled Room Temperature" in USP). Protect from freezing.

Solutions

Reconstituted solutions and further diluted infusion mixtures should be used within 24 hours if kept at room temperature or within 72 hours if stored under refrigeration (2 to 8°C). If prepared in a facility with a recognized parenteral intravenous admixture program, such mixtures may be kept up to 96 hours if stored under refrigeration (2 to 8°C).

NOTE: As with all parenteral drug products, intravenous admixtures should be inspected visually for clarity, particulate matter, precipitation, discolouration and leakage prior to administration whenever solution and container permit. Solutions showing haziness, particulate matter, precipitate, discolouration or leakage should not be used. Discard unused portion.

Hospira Healthcare corporation, Saint-Laurent, QUE

23. Order: *ceftazidime 200 mg IM q6h*

Reconstitute with ________ mL diluent for a concentration of ________ mg/mL.

Give: ________ mL

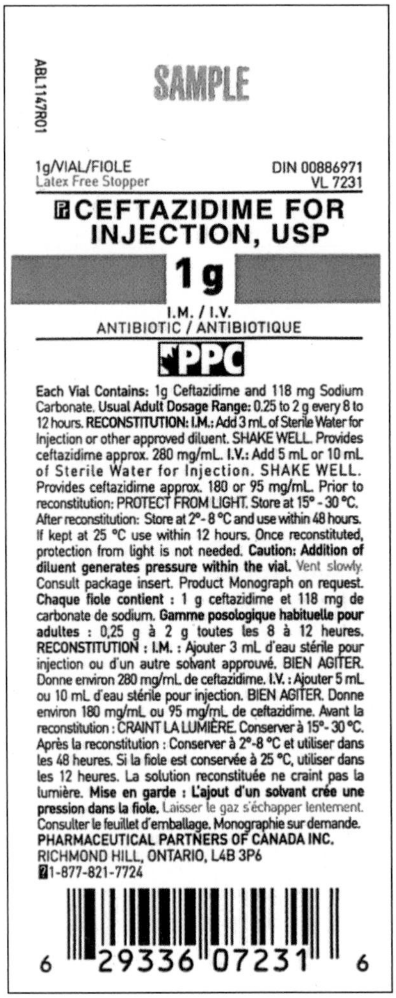

Pharmaceutical Partners of Canada Inc., Richmond Hill, ON

24. Order: *cefazolin sodium 750 mg IM q8h*

Reconstitute with ________ mL diluent for a concentration of ________ mg/mL.

Give: ________ mL

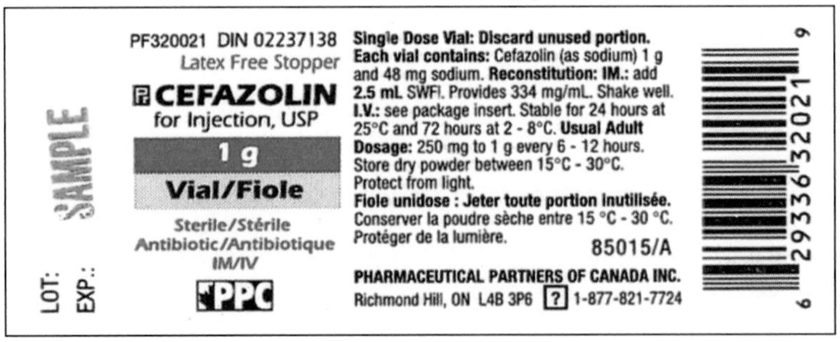

Pharmaceutical Partners of Canada Inc., Richmond Hill, ON

25. Order: *methylprednisolone sodium succinate 250 mg IV q6h*

Reconstitute with ________ mL diluent for a total solution volume of ________ mL with a concentration of ________ mg/mL.

Give: ________ mL

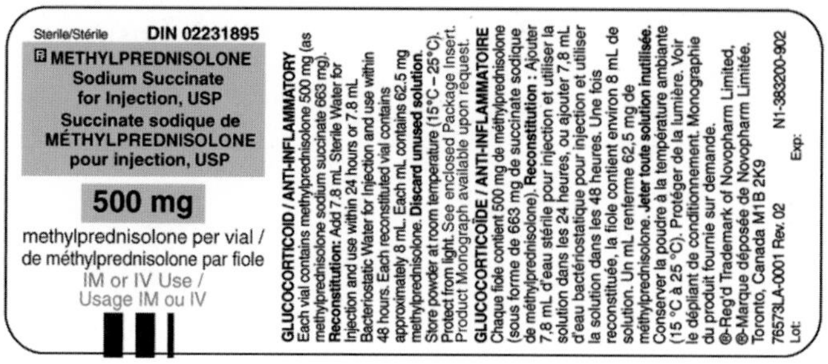
Sterile/Stérile DIN 02231895
METHYLPREDNISOLONE Sodium Succinate for Injection, USP
Succinate sodique de MÉTHYLPREDNISOLONE pour injection, USP
500 mg
methylprednisolone per vial / de méthylprednisolone par fiole
IM or IV Use / Usage IM ou IV
GLUCOCORTICOID / ANTI-INFLAMMATORY
Reconstitution: Add 7.8 mL Sterile Water for Injection and use within 24 hours or 7.8 mL Bacteriostatic Water for Injection and use within 48 hours. Each reconstituted vial contains approximately 8 mL. Each mL contains 62.5 mg methylprednisolone. Discard unused solution.
GLUCOCORTICOÏDE / ANTI-INFLAMMATOIRE
N1-383200-902

Novopharm Limited, Toronto, ON

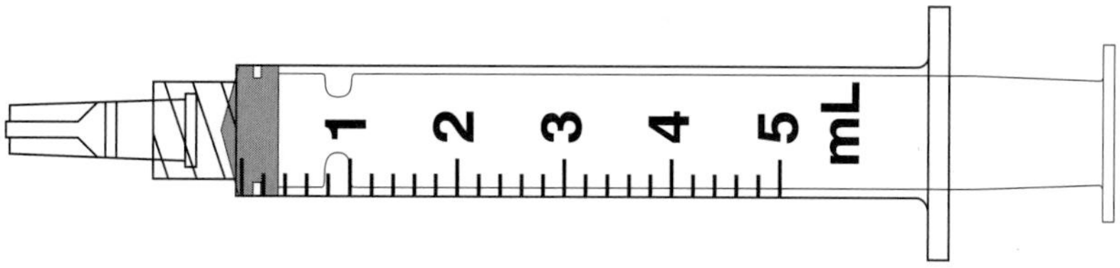
1
2
3
4
5
mL

26. Order: *tobramycin sulfate 100 mg IV q8h*

Reconstitute with ________ mL diluent for a total solution volume of ________ mL with a concentration of ________ mg/mL.

Withdraw: ________ mL and further dilute before administration

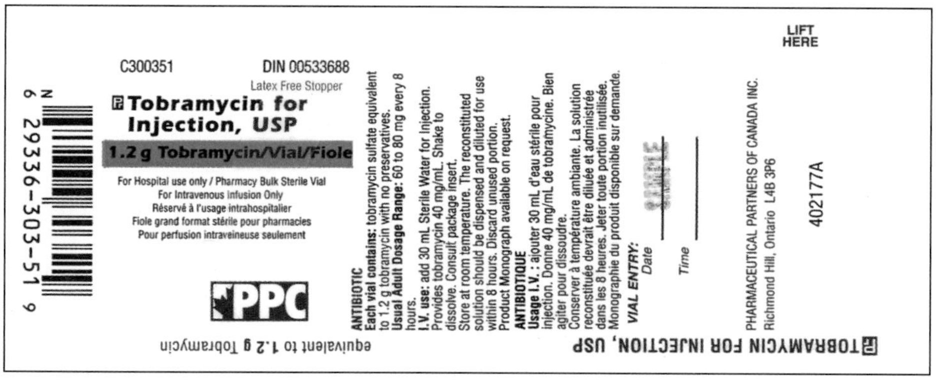
LIFT HERE
C300351
DIN 00533688
Latex Free Stopper
Tobramycin for Injection, USP
1.2 g Tobramycin/Vial/Fiole
For Hospital use only / Pharmacy Bulk Sterile Vial
For Intravenous Infusion Only
Réservé à l'usage intrahospitalier
Fiole grand format stérile pour pharmacies
Pour perfusion intraveineuse seulement
PPC
equivalent to 1.2 g Tobramycin
ANTIBIOTIC
Each vial contains: tobramycin sulfate equivalent to 1.2 g tobramycin with no preservatives.
Usual Adult Dosage Range: 60 to 80 mg every 8 hours.
I.V. use: add 30 mL Sterile Water for Injection. Provides tobramycin 40 mg/mL. Shake to dissolve. Consult package insert.
Store at room temperature. The reconstituted solution should be dispensed and diluted for use within 8 hours. Discard unused portion.
Product Monograph available on request.
VIAL ENTRY: Date Time
PHARMACEUTICAL PARTNERS OF CANADA INC.
Richmond Hill, Ontario L4B 3P6
402177A
TOBRAMYCIN FOR INJECTION, USP

Pharmaceutical Partners of Canada Inc., Richmond Hill, ON

27. How many full doses are available of the medication supplied for question 26? ________ dose(s)

28. Will the medication supplied expire before it is used up for the order in question 26? ________ Explain: ____________________

Prepare the following therapeutic solutions.

29. 360 mL of $\frac{1}{3}$-strength hydrogen peroxide diluted with normal saline

Supply: 60 mL stock hydrogen peroxide solution

Add ________ mL solute and ________ mL solvent

30. 240 mL $\frac{3}{4}$-strength Ensure

    Supply: 240-mL can of Ensure

    Add ________ mL Ensure and ________ mL water

Refer to the following order for questions 31 and 32.

Order: *Give $\frac{2}{3}$-strength Ensure 240 mL via NG tube q3h.*

Supply: Ready-to-use Ensure 240-mL can and sterile water.

31. How much Ensure and water is needed for 24-hour supply for this patient? ________ ml Ensure and ____________mL water

32. How many cans of Ensure are needed to prepare this order for 1 day and how much would be discarded? ________ cans and discard ________ mL

Use the following information to answer questions 33 and 34.

You will prepare formula to feed nine infants in the nursery. Each infant has an order for *120 mL of $\frac{1}{2}$-strength Isomil formula q3h.* You have 240-mL cans of ready-to-use Isomil and sterile water.

33. How many cans of formula will you need to open to prepare the reconstituted formula for all nine infants for one feeding each? ________ can(s)

34. How many millilitres of sterile water will you add to the Isomil to reconstitute the formula for one feeding for all nine infants? ________ mL

Chapter 11—Pediatric and Adult Dosages Based on Body Weight

Calculate and assess the safety of the following dosages. Mark safe dosages on the measuring device supplied.

35. Order: *morphine sulfate 6 mg IV q4h prn severe pain* for a child who weighs 30.5 kg. Recommended pediatric dosage: 100–200 mcg/kg q4h, up to a maximum of 15 mg/dose.

    If the dosage ordered is safe, give ________ mL. If not safe, explain why not and describe what you should do. ____________

    ____

    ____

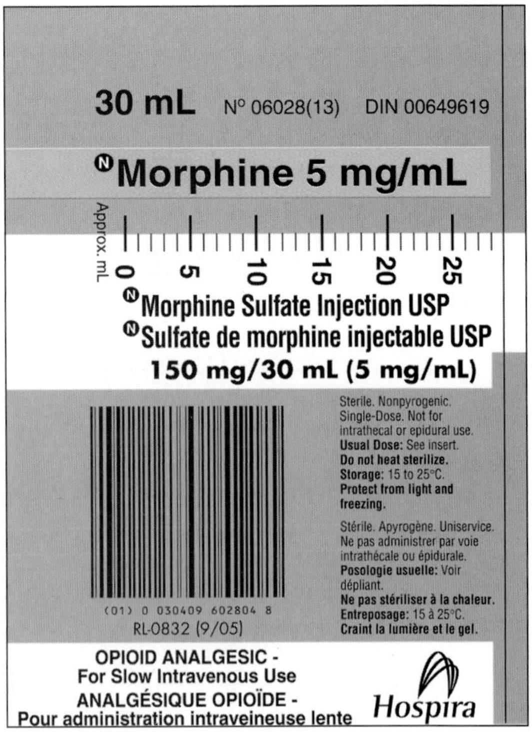

Hospira Healthcare corporation, Saint-Laurent, QUE

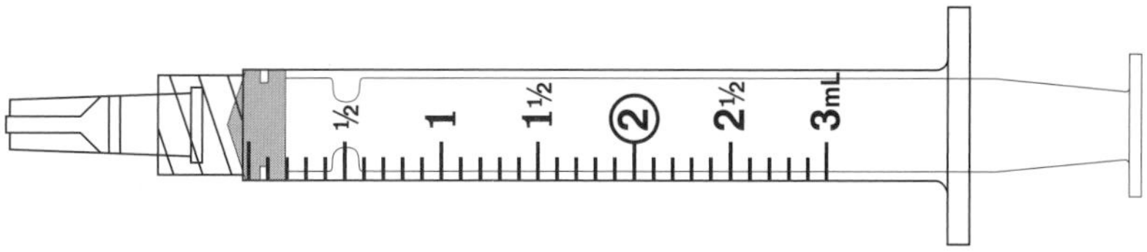

36. Order: *amoxicillin trihydrate suspension 75 mg PO q8h* for a 6.8 kg baby. Recommended dosage: See label.

If the dosage ordered is safe, reconstitute with ________ mL diluent for a total solution volume of ________ mL and a concentration of ________ mg/mL and give ___________ mL. If not safe, explain why not and describe what you should do. ____________________

____

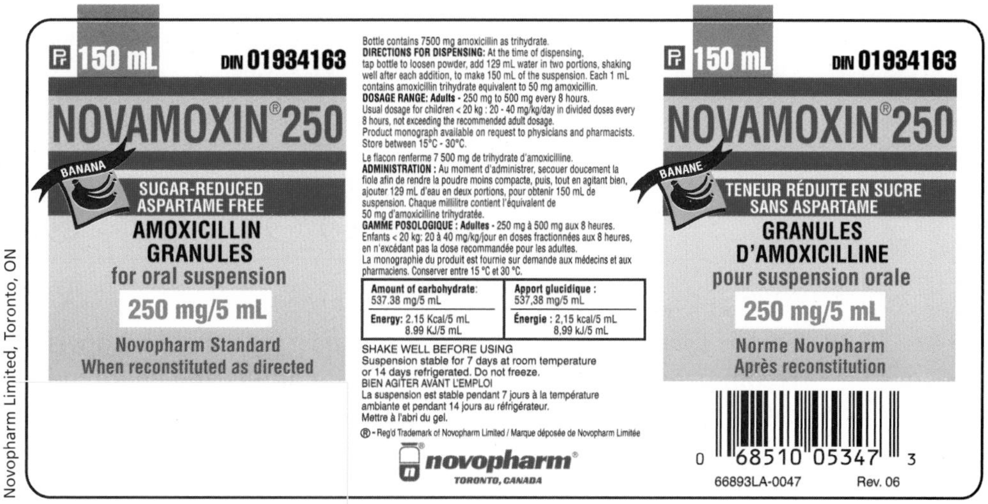

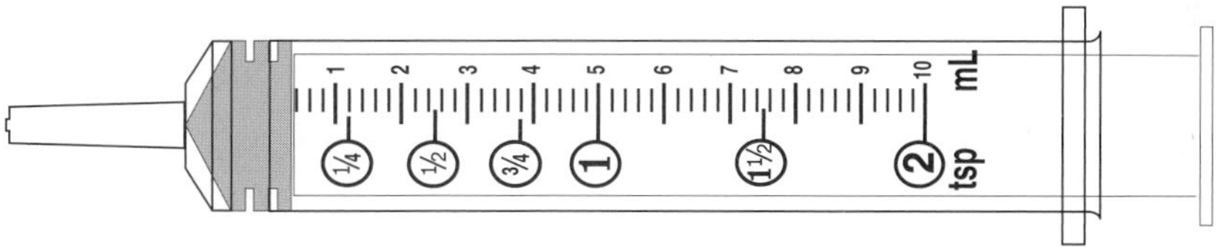

37. Order: *phenytoin sodium 200 mg IV* for a child who weighs 20 kg who is experiencing a generalized convulsive status epilepticus. Recommended pediatric IV dosage for short-term management of an acute seizure is 15–20 mg/kg. If the dosage ordered is safe and within effective range, give ________ mL. If not safe, explain why not and describe what you should do. ____

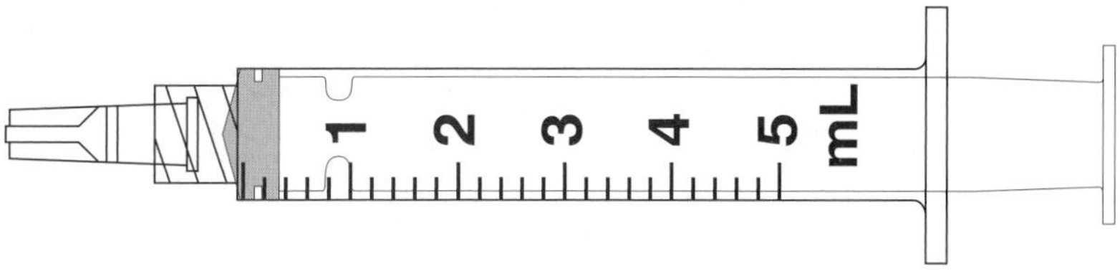

38. Order: *cefaclor 187 mg PO QID* for a child with otitis media and who weighs 7.3 kg. Recommended dosage: See label.

If the dosage ordered is safe, reconstitute with ________ mL diluent for a total solution volume of ________ mL and a concentration of ________ mg/mL. Give ________ mL. If not safe, explain why not and describe what you should do. ________________________

____

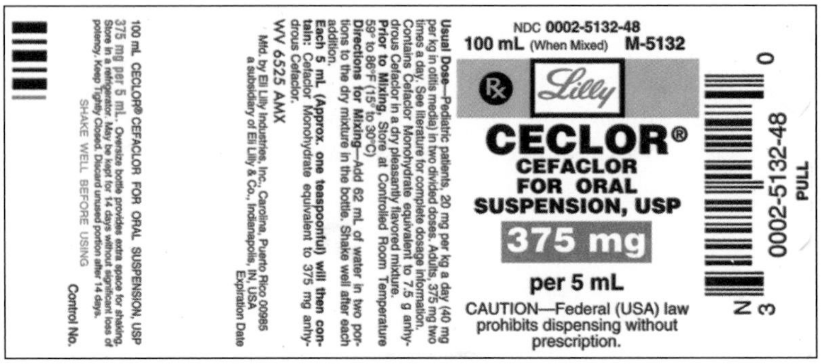

Courtesy of Eli Lilly and Company

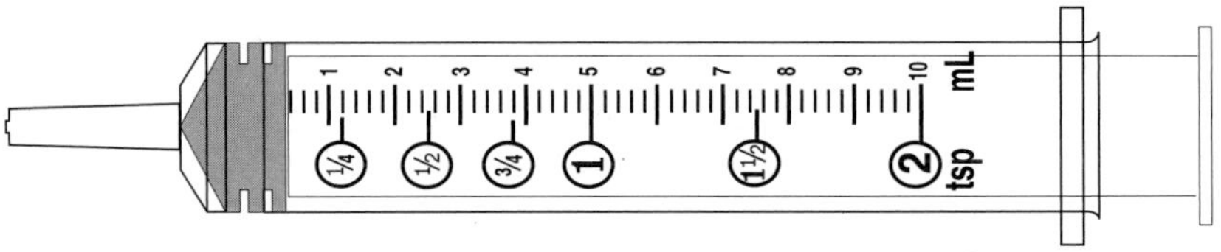

39. Order: *tobramycin sulfate 30 mg IM q8h* for a child who weighs 7.3 kg. The recommended dosage of tobramycin for adults and children is 6–7.5 mg/kg/day in 3 divided doses, not to exceed 1.5 g/day.

If the ordered dosage is safe, give ________ mL. If not safe, explain why not and describe what you should do. ________________________

____

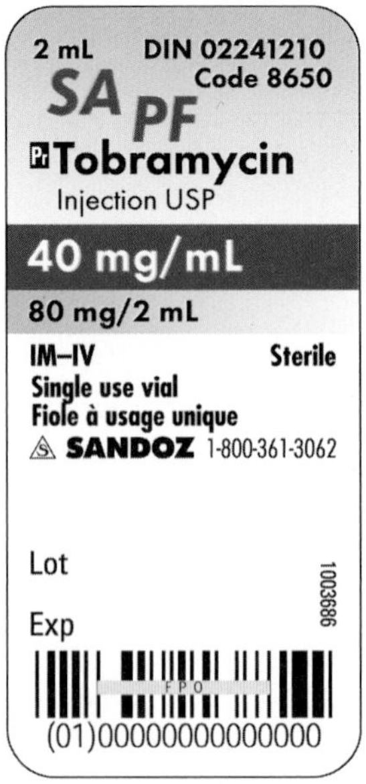

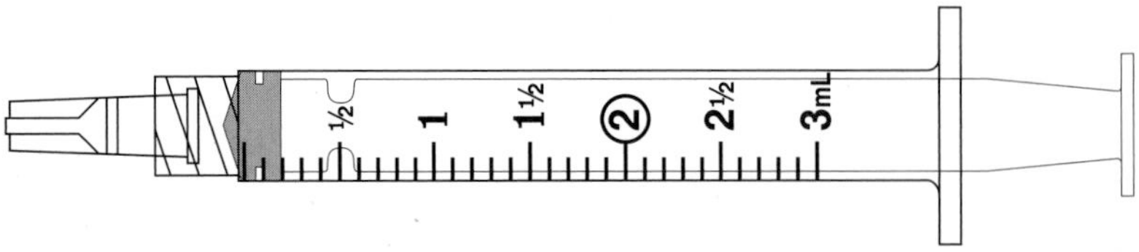

40. Refer to the recommended dosage of tobramycin in question 39. What dosage range would you expect the single q8h dosage of tobramycin sulfate to be for an adult who weighs 125 kg?

    Minimum ________ mg/dose Maximum ________ mg/dose

After completing these problems, see pages 490–493 to check your answers. Give yourself 2 points for each correct answer.

Perfect score = 100 My score = ________

Mastery score = 86 or higher (35 correct)

SECTION

4

Advanced Calculations

CHAPTER

12

Intravenous Solutions, Equipment, and Calculations

LEARNING OBJECTIVES

1. Identify common intravenous (IV) solutions and equipment.
2. Calculate the amount of specific components in common IV fluids.
3. Define the following terms: IV, peripheral line, central line, primary IV, secondary IV, saline locks, intravenous piggyback (IVPB), and IV push.
4. Calculate millilitres per hour: mL/h.
5. Recognize the calibration or drop factor in drops (gtt) per mL (gtt/mL) from information on the IV tubing package.
6. Apply the formula method to calculate IV flow rate in gtt/min.
7. Apply the shortcut method to calculate IV flow rate in gtt/min.
8. Calculate small-volume piggyback IVs (IVPB).
9. Calculate rate for IV push medications.
10. Calculate IV infusion time.
11. Calculate IV infusion volume.
12. Recalculate IV flow rates and determine the amount of increase or decrease.

Intravenous (IV) is the administration of fluids or medication through a vein. IV fluids are ordered for a variety of reasons: to replace lost fluids, to maintain fluid and electrolyte balance, or to administer IV medications. The type of fluid ordered is individualized according to the patient and the rationale for its use. *Replacement fluids* are often ordered due to losses that may occur from hemorrhage, vomiting, or diarrhea. *Maintenance fluids* sustain normal fluid and electrolyte balance. They may be used for the patient who is not yet depleted but is beginning to show symptoms of depletion. They may also be ordered for the patient who has the potential to become depleted, such as the patient who is allowed nothing by mouth (NPO) for surgery.

IV fluids and drugs may be administered by two methods: *continuous* and *intermittent* infusion. Continuous IV infusions replace or maintain fluid and electrolytes and serve as a vehicle for drug administration. Intermittent, such as IV piggyback (IVPB) and IV push, infusions are used for IV administration of drugs and supplemental fluids. Intermittent peripheral infusion devices, also known as saline or heparin locks, are used to maintain venous access without continuous fluid infusion.

IV therapy is an important and challenging nursing role. This chapter covers the essential information and presents step-by-step calculations to help you gain a thorough understanding and mastery of this subject. To begin we will analyze IV solutions.

IV SOLUTIONS

IV solutions are ordered by a physician or prescribing practitioner; however, they are administered and monitored by the nurse. It is the responsibility of the nurse to ensure that the correct IV fluid is administered to the correct patient at the prescribed rate. IV fluids can be supplied in plastic solution bags (which is more common) or glass bottles, with the volume of the IV fluid container typically varying from 50 mL to 1000 mL. Some IV bags may contain more than 1000 mL. Solutions used for total parenteral nutrition often contain 2000 mL or more in a single bag. The IV solution bag or bottle will be labelled with the exact components and amount of the IV solution. Healthcare practitioners frequently use abbreviations when communicating about the IV solution. Therefore, it is important to know the common IV solution components and the solution concentration strengths represented by such abbreviations.

Solution Components

Glucose (dextrose), water, saline (sodium chloride or NaCl), and selected electrolytes and salts are found in IV fluids. Dextrose and sodium chloride are the two most common solute components. Learn these common IV component abbreviations.

REMEMBER

Common IV Component Abbreviations

Abbreviation	Solution Component
D	Dextrose
W	Water
S	Saline
NS	Normal Saline
NaCl	Sodium Chloride
RL	Ringer's Lactate
LR	Lactated Ringer's

Solution Strength

The abbreviation letters indicate the solution components, and the numbers indicate the solution strength or concentration of the components. The numbers may be written as subscripts in the patient care order.

Example 1:

Suppose an order includes D_5W. This abbreviation means "dextrose 5% in water" and is supplied as 5% dextrose injection (see Figure 12-1). This means that the solution strength of the solute (dextrose) is 5%. The solvent is water. Recall from Chapter 7 that parenteral solutions expressed in a percent indicate X g per 100 mL. Read the IV bag label and notice that "each 100 mL contains 5 g dextrose. . . ." For every 100 mL of solution, there is 5 g of dextrose.

Example 2:

Suppose a nurse writes D_5LR in the nurse's notes. This abbreviation means "dextrose 5% in Lactated Ringer's" and is supplied as Lactated Ringer's and 5% dextrose injection (see Figure 12-2).

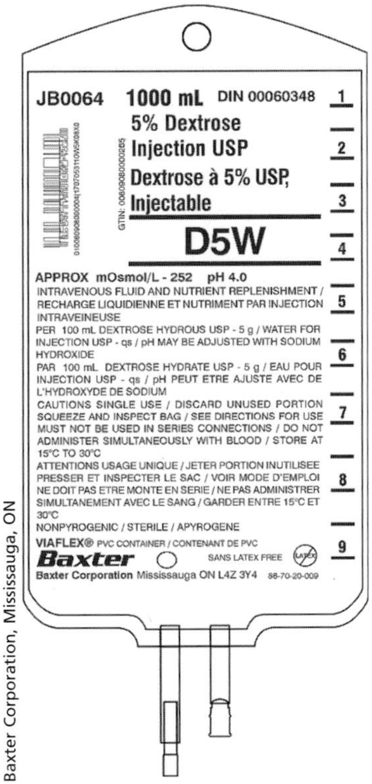

Baxter Corporation, Mississauga, ON

FIGURE 12-1 IV Solution Label: D_5W

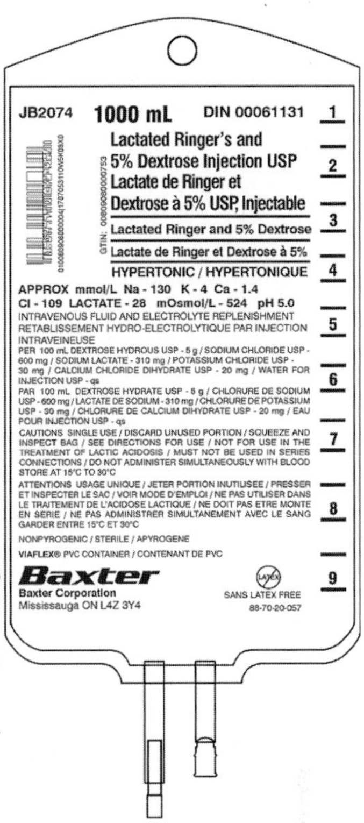

Baxter Corporation, Mississauga, ON

FIGURE 12-2 IV Solution Label: D_5LR

Example 3:

A written order is for, *D_5NS 1000 mL IV q8h.* This order means "administer 1000 mL 5% dextrose in normal saline intravenously every 8 hours" and is supplied as 5% dextrose and 0.9% sodium chloride (see Figure 12-3). *Normal saline is the common term for 0.9% sodium chloride.* Another name is *physiologic saline.* The concentration of sodium chloride in normal saline is 0.9 g (or 900 mg) per 100 mL of solution.

Another common saline IV concentration is 0.45% sodium chloride (NaCl) (see Figure 12-4). Notice that 0.45% NaCl is $\frac{1}{2}$ the strength of 0.9% NaCl, which is normal saline. Thus, it is typically written as "$\frac{1}{2}$ NS" for $\frac{1}{2}$ normal saline. Other saline solution strengths include 0.33% NaCl (also abbreviated as $\frac{1}{3}$ NS) and 0.225% NaCl (also abbreviated as $\frac{1}{4}$ NS). In Canada, 0.33% NaCl and 0.225% NaCl are available only with 5% dextrose.

The goal of IV therapy, achieved through fluid infusion, is to maintain or regain fluid and electrolyte balance. When dextrose or saline (*solute*) is diluted in water for injection (*solvent*), the result is a *solution* that can be administered to maintain or approximate the normal blood plasma. Blood or serum concentration is called *tonicity* or *osmolarity* and is measured in milliOsmoles per litre or mOsm/L. IV fluids are concentrated and classified as *isotonic* (the same tonicity or osmolarity as blood and other body serums), *hypotonic* (lower tonicity or osmolarity than blood and other body serums), or *hypertonic* (higher tonicity or osmolarity than blood and other body serums). Normal saline (0.9% NaCl or physiologic saline) is an isotonic solution. The osmolarity of a manufactured solution is detailed on the printed label. Look for the mOsm/L in the fine print under the solution name in Figures 12-1 through 12-4.

Figure 12-5 compares the three solution concentrations to normal serum osmolarity. Parenteral therapy is determined by unique patient needs, and these basic factors must be considered when ordering and infusing IV solutions.

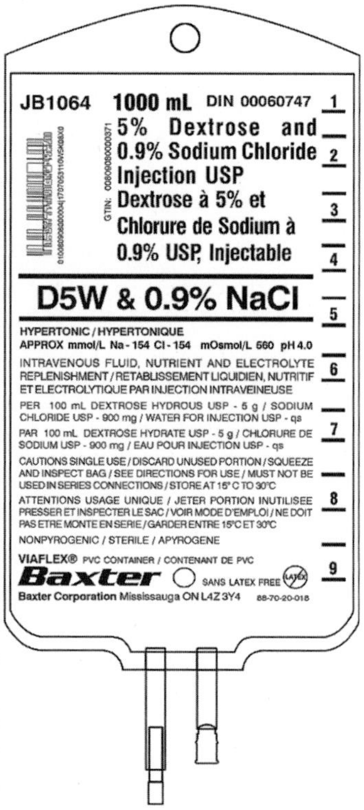

FIGURE 12-3 IV Solution Label: D_5NS

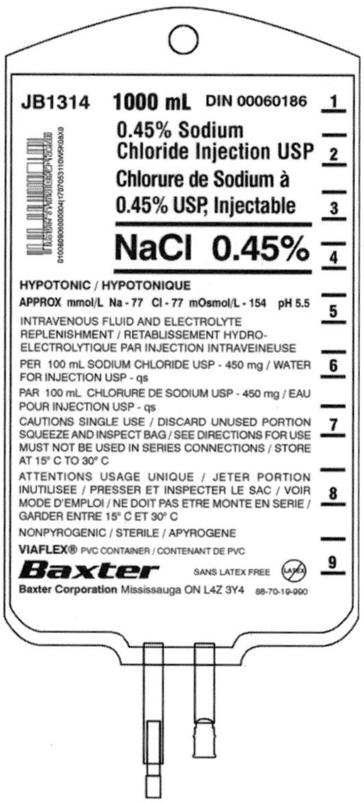

FIGURE 12-4 IV Solution Label: 0.45% NaCl

See page 221 for a review of *solute, solvent,* and *solution. Osmolality* refers to the concentration of particles in a solution. *Osmolarity* is the number of solutes in a solution. *Osmotic concentration* determinations are usually expressed as either milliosmoles/kilogram (mOsm/kg) of solvent (osmolality) or milliosmoles/litre (mOsm/L) of solution (osmolarity).

Normal Serum Osmolarity
(Normal Average Tonicity—All Ages)
280–320 mOsm/L

Hypotonic (less than 250 mOsm/L) *Solvent exceeds solute—* used to dilute excess serum electrolytes, as in hyperglycemia	**Isotonic** (250–375 mOsm/L) *Solvent and solutes are* balanced—used to expand volume and maintain normal tonicity	**Hypertonic** (more than 375 mOsm/L) *Solutes exceed solvent—* used to correct electrolyte imbalances, as in loss from excess vomiting and diarrhea
Example of IV solution: *0.45% saline* (154 mOsm/L)	Examples of IV solution: *0.9% saline* (308 mOsm/L) *Lactated Ringer's* (273 mOsm/L) *5% dextrose in water* (252 mOsm/L)	Example of IV solution: *5% dextrose and 0.9% NaCl* (560 mOsm/L) *5% dextrose and Lactated Ringer's* (525 mOsm/L)

FIGURE 12-5 Comparison of IV Solution Concentrations by Osmolarity

Solution Additives

Electrolytes also may be added to the basic IV fluid. Potassium chloride (KCl) is a common IV additive and is measured in *milliequivalents* (mEq). The order is usually written to indicate the amount of milliequivalents *per litre* (1000 mL) to be added to the IV fluid. As potassium chloride is a high-risk medication in Canada, solutions are available pre-prepared.

Example:

The physician orders *D_5NS with 20 mEq KCl/L*. This means to add 20 milliequivalents potassium chloride per litre of 5% dextrose and 0.9% sodium chloride IV solution.

QUICK REVIEW

- Pay close attention to IV abbreviations: *letters* indicate the solution components and *numbers* indicate the concentration or solution strength.
- Dextrose and sodium chloride (NaCl) are common IV solutes.
- Solution strength expressed as a percent (%) indicates X g per 100 mL.
- Normal saline is 0.9% sodium chloride: 0.9 g NaCl/100 mL solution.
- IV solution tonicity or osmolarity is measured in mOsm/L.
- D_5W and normal saline are common isotonic solutions.

REVIEW SET 27

For each of the following IV solutions labelled A through H:

a. Specify the *letter* of the illustration corresponding to the fluid abbreviation.

b. List the *solute(s)* of each solution, and identify the *strength (g/mL)* of each solute.

c. Identify the *osmolarity (mOsm/L)* of each solution.

d. Identify the *tonicity (isotonic, hypotonic, or hypertonic)* of each solution.

	a. Letter of Matching Illustration	b. Components and Strength	c. Osmolarity (mOsm/L)	d. Tonicity
1. NS	______	______	______	______
2. D_5W	______	______	______	______
3. D_5NS	______	______	______	______
4. $D_5\frac{1}{2}NS$	______	______	______	______
5. $D_5\frac{1}{4}NS$	______	______	______	______
6. D_5LR	______	______	______	______
7. NS with 20 mEq KCl/L	______	______	______	______
8. $\frac{1}{2}NS$	______	______	______	______

After completing these problems, see page 494 to check your answers.

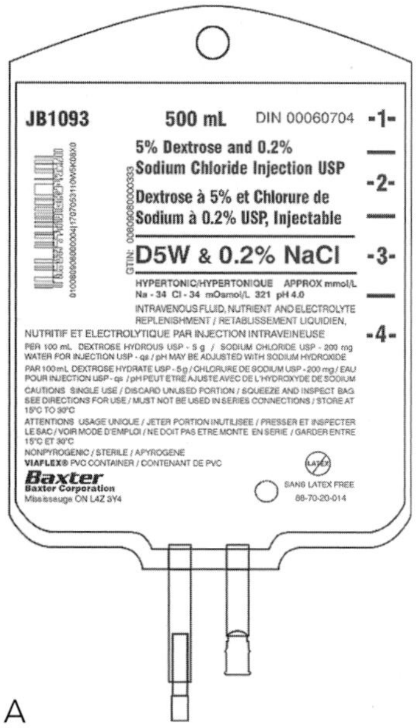
JB1093 500 mL DIN 00060704
5% Dextrose and 0.2% Sodium Chloride Injection USP
Dextrose à 5% et Chlorure de Sodium à 0.2% USP, Injectable
D5W & 0.2% NaCl
Baxter
-1- -2- -3- -4-

Baxter Corporation, Mississauga, ON

A

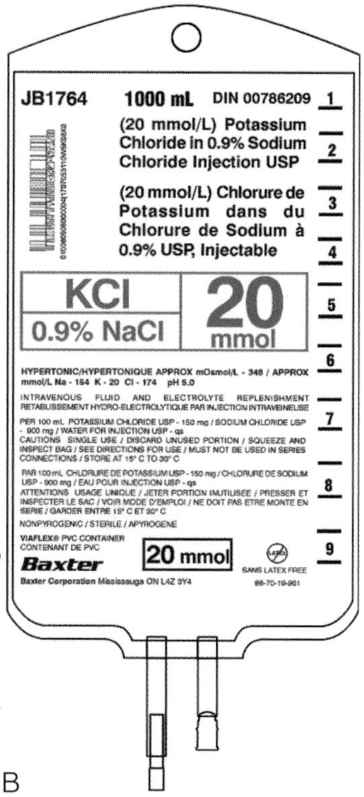
JB1764 1000 mL DIN 00786209
(20 mmol/L) Potassium Chloride in 0.9% Sodium Chloride Injection USP
(20 mmol/L) Chlorure de Potassium dans du Chlorure de Sodium à 0.9% USP, Injectable
KCl 20
0.9% NaCl mmol
20 mmol
Baxter
1 2 3 4 5 6 7 8 9

Baxter Corporation, Mississauga, ON

B

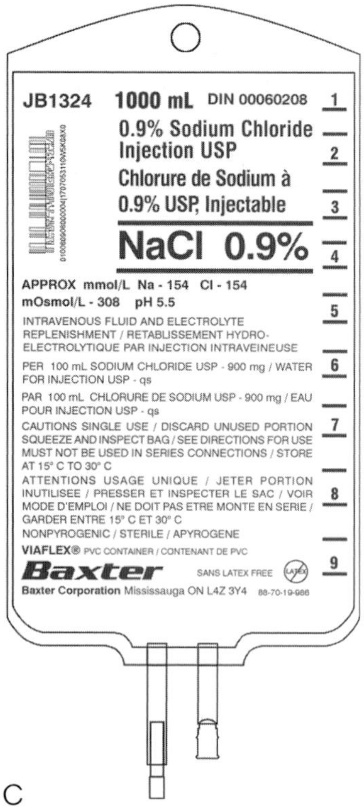
JB1324 1000 mL DIN 00060208
0.9% Sodium Chloride Injection USP
Chlorure de Sodium à 0.9% USP, Injectable
NaCl 0.9%
APPROX mmol/L Na - 154 Cl - 154
mOsmol/L - 308 pH 5.5
INTRAVENOUS FLUID AND ELECTROLYTE REPLENISHMENT / RETABLISSEMENT HYDRO-ELECTROLYTIQUE PAR INJECTION INTRAVEINEUSE
PER 100 mL SODIUM CHLORIDE USP - 900 mg / WATER FOR INJECTION USP - qs
PAR 100 mL CHLORURE DE SODIUM USP - 900 mg / EAU POUR INJECTION USP - qs
CAUTIONS SINGLE USE / DISCARD UNUSED PORTION SQUEEZE AND INSPECT BAG / SEE DIRECTIONS FOR USE MUST NOT BE USED IN SERIES CONNECTIONS / STORE AT 15° C TO 30° C
ATTENTIONS USAGE UNIQUE / JETER PORTION INUTILISEE / PRESSER ET INSPECTER LE SAC / VOIR MODE D'EMPLOI / NE DOIT PAS ETRE MONTE EN SERIE / GARDER ENTRE 15° C ET 30° C
NONPYROGENIC / STERILE / APYROGENE
VIAFLEX® PVC CONTAINER / CONTENANT DE PVC
Baxter SANS LATEX FREE
Baxter Corporation Mississauga ON L4Z 3Y4
1 2 3 4 5 6 7 8 9

Baxter Corporation, Mississauga, ON

C

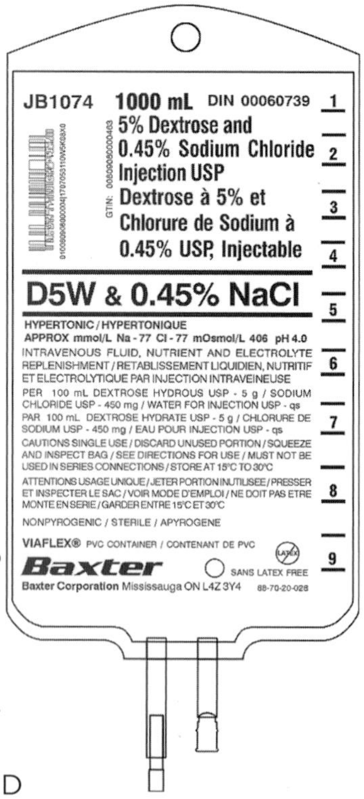
JB1074 1000 mL DIN 00060739
5% Dextrose and 0.45% Sodium Chloride Injection USP
Dextrose à 5% et Chlorure de Sodium à 0.45% USP, Injectable
D5W & 0.45% NaCl
HYPERTONIC / HYPERTONIQUE
APPROX mmol/L Na - 77 Cl - 77 mOsmol/L 406 pH 4.0
INTRAVENOUS FLUID, NUTRIENT AND ELECTROLYTE REPLENISHMENT / RETABLISSEMENT LIQUIDIEN, NUTRITIF ET ELECTROLYTIQUE PAR INJECTION INTRAVEINEUSE
NONPYROGENIC / STERILE / APYROGENE
VIAFLEX® PVC CONTAINER / CONTENANT DE PVC
Baxter SANS LATEX FREE
Baxter Corporation Mississauga ON L4Z 3Y4
1 2 3 4 5 6 7 8 9

Baxter Corporation, Mississauga, ON

D

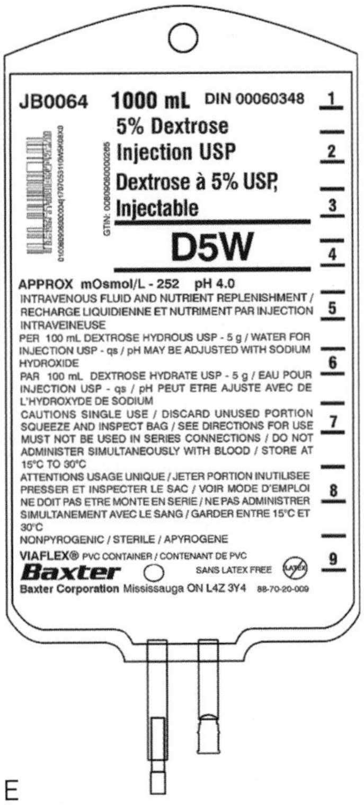
JB0064 1000 mL DIN 00060348
5% Dextrose Injection USP
Dextrose à 5% USP, Injectable
D5W
APPROX mOsmol/L - 252 pH 4.0
INTRAVENOUS FLUID AND NUTRIENT REPLENISHMENT / RECHARGE LIQUIDIENNE ET NUTRIMENT PAR INJECTION INTRAVEINEUSE
PER 100 mL DEXTROSE HYDROUS USP - 5 g / WATER FOR INJECTION USP - qs / pH MAY BE ADJUSTED WITH SODIUM HYDROXIDE
PAR 100 mL DEXTROSE HYDRATE USP - 5 g / EAU POUR INJECTION USP - qs / pH PEUT ETRE AJUSTE AVEC DE L'HYDROXYDE DE SODIUM
CAUTIONS SINGLE USE / DISCARD UNUSED PORTION SQUEEZE AND INSPECT BAG / SEE DIRECTIONS FOR USE MUST NOT BE USED IN SERIES CONNECTIONS / DO NOT ADMINISTER SIMULTANEOUSLY WITH BLOOD / STORE AT 15°C TO 30°C
ATTENTIONS USAGE UNIQUE / JETER PORTION INUTILISEE PRESSER ET INSPECTER LE SAC / VOIR MODE D'EMPLOI NE DOIT PAS ETRE MONTE EN SERIE / NE PAS ADMINISTRER SIMULTANEMENT AVEC LE SANG / GARDER ENTRE 15°C ET 30°C
NONPYROGENIC / STERILE / APYROGENE
VIAFLEX® PVC CONTAINER / CONTENANT DE PVC
Baxter
SANS LATEX FREE
Baxter Corporation Mississauga ON L4Z 3Y4 88-70-20-009
1
2
3
4
5
6
7
8
9

Baxter Corporation, Mississauga, ON

E

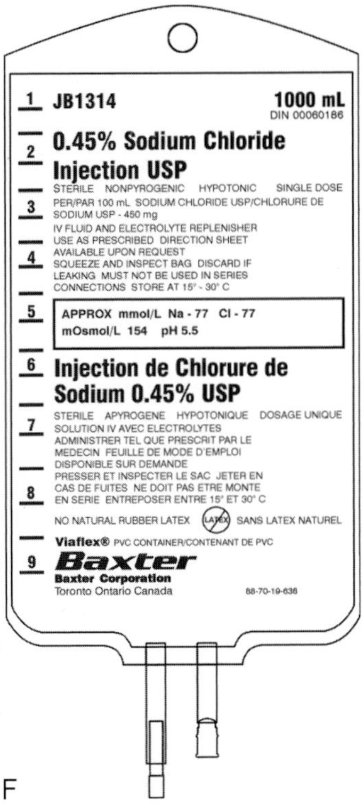
JB1314 1000 mL
DIN 00060186
0.45% Sodium Chloride Injection USP
STERILE NONPYROGENIC HYPOTONIC SINGLE DOSE
PER/PAR 100 mL SODIUM CHLORIDE USP/CHLORURE DE SODIUM USP - 450 mg
IV FLUID AND ELECTROLYTE REPLENISHER
USE AS PRESCRIBED DIRECTION SHEET AVAILABLE UPON REQUEST
SQUEEZE AND INSPECT BAG DISCARD IF LEAKING MUST NOT BE USED IN SERIES CONNECTIONS STORE AT 15° - 30° C
APPROX mmol/L Na - 77 Cl - 77
mOsmol/L 154 pH 5.5
Injection de Chlorure de Sodium 0.45% USP
STERILE APYROGENE HYPOTONIQUE DOSAGE UNIQUE
SOLUTION IV AVEC ELECTROLYTES
ADMINISTRER TEL QUE PRESCRIT PAR LE MEDECIN FEUILLE DE MODE D'EMPLOI DISPONIBLE SUR DEMANDE
PRESSER ET INSPECTER LE SAC JETER EN CAS DE FUITES NE DOIT PAS ETRE MONTE EN SERIE ENTREPOSER ENTRE 15° ET 30° C
NO NATURAL RUBBER LATEX SANS LATEX NATUREL
Viaflex® PVC CONTAINER/CONTENANT DE PVC
Baxter
Baxter Corporation
Toronto Ontario Canada
88-70-19-636
1
2
3
4
5
6
7
8
9

Baxter Corporation, Mississauga, ON

F

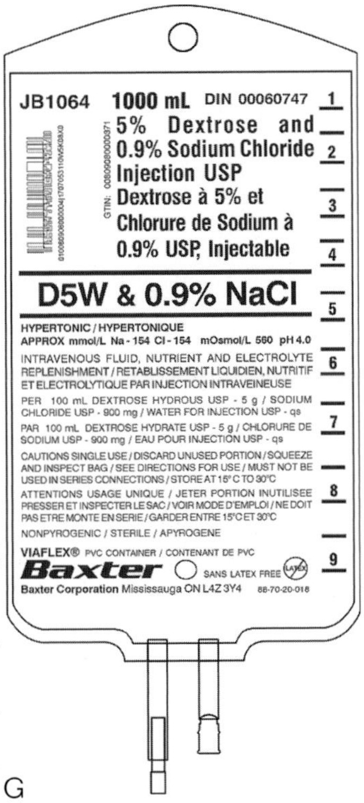
JB1064 1000 mL DIN 00060747
5% Dextrose and 0.9% Sodium Chloride Injection USP
Dextrose à 5% et Chlorure de Sodium à 0.9% USP, Injectable
D5W & 0.9% NaCl
HYPERTONIC / HYPERTONIQUE
APPROX mmol/L Na - 154 Cl - 154 mOsmol/L 560 pH 4.0
INTRAVENOUS FLUID, NUTRIENT AND ELECTROLYTE REPLENISHMENT / RETABLISSEMENT LIQUIDIEN, NUTRITIF ET ELECTROLYTIQUE PAR INJECTION INTRAVEINEUSE
PER 100 mL DEXTROSE HYDROUS USP - 5 g / SODIUM CHLORIDE USP - 900 mg / WATER FOR INJECTION USP - qs
PAR 100 mL DEXTROSE HYDRATE USP - 5 g / CHLORURE DE SODIUM USP - 900 mg / EAU POUR INJECTION USP - qs
CAUTIONS SINGLE USE / DISCARD UNUSED PORTION / SQUEEZE AND INSPECT BAG / SEE DIRECTIONS FOR USE / MUST NOT BE USED IN SERIES CONNECTIONS / STORE AT 15°C TO 30°C
ATTENTIONS USAGE UNIQUE / JETER PORTION INUTILISEE PRESSER ET INSPECTER LE SAC / VOIR MODE D'EMPLOI / NE DOIT PAS ETRE MONTE EN SERIE / GARDER ENTRE 15°C ET 30°C
NONPYROGENIC / STERILE / APYROGENE
VIAFLEX® PVC CONTAINER / CONTENANT DE PVC
Baxter
SANS LATEX FREE
Baxter Corporation Mississauga ON L4Z 3Y4 88-70-20-018
1
2
3
4
5
6
7
8
9

Baxter Corporation, Mississauga, ON

G

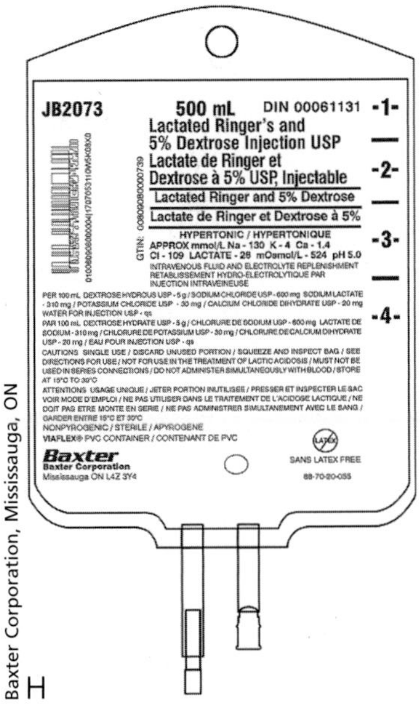
JB2073 500 mL DIN 00061131
Lactated Ringer's and 5% Dextrose Injection USP
Lactate de Ringer et Dextrose à 5% USP, Injectable
Lactated Ringer and 5% Dextrose
Lactate de Ringer et Dextrose à 5%
HYPERTONIC / HYPERTONIQUE
APPROX mmol/L Na - 130 K - 4 Ca - 1.4 Cl - 109 LACTATE - 28 mOsmol/L - 524 pH 5.0
INTRAVENOUS FLUID AND ELECTROLYTE REPLENISHMENT
RETABLISSEMENT HYDRO-ELECTROLYTIQUE PAR INJECTION INTRAVEINEUSE
PER 100 mL DEXTROSE HYDROUS USP - 5 g / SODIUM CHLORIDE USP - 600 mg SODIUM LACTATE - 310 mg / POTASSIUM CHLORIDE USP - 30 mg / CALCIUM CHLORIDE DIHYDRATE USP - 20 mg WATER FOR INJECTION USP - qs
PAR 100 mL DEXTROSE HYDRATE USP - 5 g / CHLORURE DE SODIUM USP - 600 mg LACTATE DE SODIUM - 310 mg / CHLORURE DE POTASSIUM USP - 30 mg / CHLORURE DE CALCIUM DIHYDRATE USP - 20 mg / EAU POUR INJECTION USP - qs
CAUTIONS SINGLE USE / DISCARD UNUSED PORTION / SQUEEZE AND INSPECT BAG / SEE DIRECTIONS FOR USE / NOT FOR USE IN THE TREATMENT OF LACTIC ACIDOSIS / MUST NOT BE USED IN SERIES CONNECTIONS / DO NOT ADMINISTER SIMULTANEOUSLY WITH BLOOD / STORE AT 15°C TO 30°C
ATTENTIONS USAGE UNIQUE / JETER PORTION INUTILISEE / PRESSER ET INSPECTER LE SAC VOIR MODE D'EMPLOI / NE PAS UTILISER DANS LE TRAITEMENT DE L'ACIDOSE LACTIQUE / NE DOIT PAS ETRE MONTE EN SERIE / NE PAS ADMINISTRER SIMULTANEMENT AVEC LE SANG / GARDER ENTRE 15°C ET 30°C
NONPYROGENIC / STERILE / APYROGENE
VIAFLEX® PVC CONTAINER / CONTENANT DE PVC
Baxter
Baxter Corporation
Mississauga ON L4Z 3Y4
SANS LATEX FREE
88-70-20-055
-1-
-2-
-3-
-4-

Baxter Corporation, Mississauga, ON

H

CALCULATING COMPONENTS OF IV SOLUTIONS WHEN EXPRESSED AS A PERCENT

Recall from Chapter 7 that solution strength expressed as a percent (%) indicates X g per 100 mL. Understanding this concept allows you to calculate the total amount of solute per IV order.

Example 1:

Order: *D_5W 1000 mL*

Calculate the amount of dextrose in 1000 mL D_5W.

This can be calculated using ratio-proportion.

Recall that % indicates g per 100 mL; therefore, 5% dextrose is 5 g dextrose per 100 mL of solution.

$$\frac{5\text{ g}}{100\text{ mL}} \times \frac{X\text{ g}}{1000\text{ mL}}$$

$$100X = 5000$$

$$\frac{100X}{100} = \frac{5000}{100}$$

$$X = 50\text{ g}$$

1000 mL of D_5W contains 50 g of dextrose.

Example 2:

Order: *$D_5\frac{1}{4}NS$ 500 mL*

Calculate the amount of dextrose and sodium chloride in 500 mL.

D_5 = dextrose 5% = 5 g dextrose per 100 mL

$$\frac{5\text{ g}}{100\text{ mL}} \times \frac{X\text{ g}}{500\text{ mL}}$$

$$100X = 2500$$

$$\frac{100X}{100} = \frac{2500}{100}$$

$$X = 25\text{ g dextrose}$$

$\frac{1}{4}$NS = 0.225% NaCl = 0.225 g NaCl per 100 mL

(Recall that NS or normal saline is 0.9% NaCl; therefore, $\frac{1}{4}$ NS is $\frac{1}{4} \times 0.9\% = 0.225\%$ NaCl.)

$$\frac{0.225\text{ g}}{100\text{ mL}} \times \frac{X\text{ g}}{500\text{ mL}}$$

$$100X = 112.5$$

$$\frac{100X}{100} = \frac{112.5}{100}$$

$$X = 1.125\text{ g NaCl}$$

500 mL $D_5\frac{1}{4}$ NS contains 25 g dextrose and 1.125 g sodium chloride.

This concept is important because it helps you to understand that IV solutions provide much more than fluid. They also provide other components. For example, now you know what you are administering to your patient when the IV order prescribes D_5W. Think, "I am hanging D_5W IV solution. Do I know what this fluid contains? Yes, it contains dextrose as the solute and water as the solvent in the concentration of 5 g of dextrose in every 100 mL of solution." Regular monitoring and careful understanding of IV infusions cannot be stressed enough.

QUICK REVIEW

- Solution concentration expressed as a percent is X g of solute per 100 mL solution.

REVIEW SET 28

Calculate the amount of dextrose and/or sodium chloride in each of the following IV solutions.

1. 1000 mL of D_5NS

   dextrose ________ g

   sodium chloride ________ g

2. 500 mL of $D_5 \frac{1}{2}NS$

   dextrose ________ g

   sodium chloride ________ g

3. 250 mL of $D_{10}W$

   dextrose ________ g

4. 750 mL of NS

   sodium chloride ________ g

5. 500 mL of D_5 0.33% NaCl

   dextrose ________ g

   sodium chloride ________ g

6. 3 L of D_5NS

   dextrose ________ g

   sodium chloride ________ g

7. 0.5 L of $D_{10} \frac{1}{4}NS$

   dextrose ________ g

   sodium chloride ________ g

8. 300 mL of D_{12} 0.9% NaCl

   dextrose ________ g

   sodium chloride ________ g

9. 2 L of D_5 0.225% NaCl

   dextrose ________ g

   sodium chloride ________ g

10. 0.75 L of 0.45% NaCl

    sodium chloride ________ g

After completing these problems, see page 494 to check your answers.

IV SITES

IV fluids are administered via a *peripheral line,* such as a vein in the arm, leg, or sometimes a scalp vein for infants, if other sites are inaccessible. Blood flowing through these veins can usually sufficiently dilute the components in IV fluids. Glucose or dextrose is usually concentrated between 5% and 10% for short-term IV therapy. Because glucose is a hypertonic (higher osmolality) solution and has a higher osmotic pressure than the cells in the body, peripheral veins can only accommodate a maximum glucose concentration of 12%. As well, the rate of infusion in peripheral veins should not exceed 200 mL in 1 hour.

IV fluids that are transparent flow smoothly into relatively small peripheral veins. When blood transfusion or replacement is needed, a larger vein is preferred to facilitate ease of blood flow. Whole blood or its components, especially packed cells, can be viscous and must be infused within a short period of time.

IV fluids may also be administered via a *central line,* in which a special catheter is inserted to access a large vein in the chest. The subclavian vein, for example, may be used for a central line. Central lines may be accessed either directly through the chest wall or indirectly via a neck vein or peripheral vein in the arm. If a peripheral vein is used to access a central vein, you may see the term *peripherally inserted central catheter* or *PICC line.* Larger veins can accommodate higher concentrations of glucose (up to 35%) and other nutrients, and faster rates of IV fluids (more than 200 mL in 1 hour). They are often utilized if the patient is expected to need IV therapy for an extended period of time.

MONITORING IVs

The nurse is responsible for monitoring the patient regularly during an IV infusion.

> **CAUTION**
>
> Generally the IV site and infusion should be checked *at least every 30 minutes to 1 hour* (according to institution policy) for volume of remaining fluids, correct infusion rate, and signs of complications.

The major complications associated with IV therapy are phlebitis and infiltration. *Phlebitis* occurs when the vein becomes irritated, red, or painful. *Infiltration* occurs when the IV catheter becomes dislodged from the vein and IV fluid escapes into the subcutaneous tissue. Should phlebitis or infiltration occur, the IV is discontinued and another IV site is chosen to restart the IV. The patient should be instructed to notify the nurse of any pain or swelling.

PRIMARY AND SECONDARY IVs

Primary IV tubing packaging and set are shown in Figures 12-6 and 12-7. This IV set is used to set up a typical or *primary IV.* Primary IV tubing includes a drip chamber, one or more injection ports, and a roller clamp, and is long enough to be attached to the hub of the IV catheter positioned in the patient's vein. The drip chamber is squeezed until it is approximately one half full of IV fluid, and IV fluid is run through the tubing prior to attaching it to the IV catheter to ensure that no air is in the tubing. The nurse can either regulate the rate manually using the roller clamp (see Figure 12-7 a) or place the tubing in an electronic infusion pump (see Figures 12-11 through 12-14).

An IV bag may be labelled with an infusion label (see Figure 12-7 b), often referred to as a *flow strip* or *time tape* that provides a visual check for the nurse to monitor if the IV solution is infusing on time as prescribed. The label is attached to the IV bag and identifies the time the solution was hung and how the IV should be progressing, such as at 25 gtt/min. Each hour from the start time to the stop time the nurse should mark the label using a pen (not a marker as the ink may penetrate the plastic and flow into the solution) at the level where the solution should be. Be sure to check the institution policy before using an infusion label. An infusion label may also be required for solutions infused through electronic infusion devices.

Secondary IV tubing is used when giving medications. Secondary tubing is "piggybacked" into the primary line (see Figure 12-8). This type of tubing generally is shorter and also contains a drip chamber and roller clamp. This gives access to the primary IV catheter without having to start another IV. You will notice that in this type of setup, the *secondary IV* set or *piggyback* (IVPB) is hung higher than

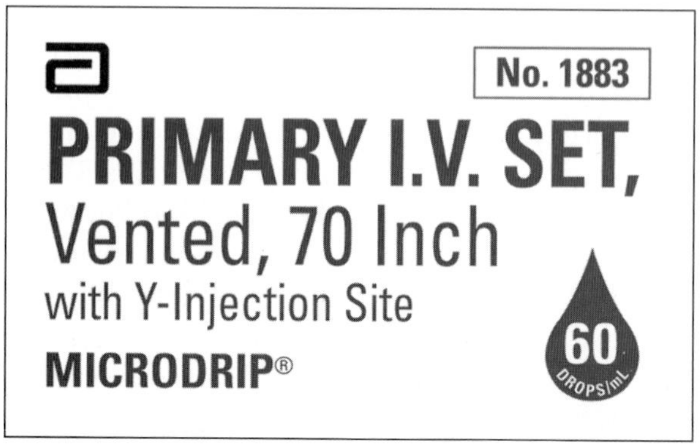
No. 1883
PRIMARY I.V. SET,
Vented, 70 Inch
with Y-Injection Site
MICRODRIP®
60
DROPS/mL

Courtesy of Abbott Laboratories, Inc.

FIGURE 12-6 Primary Intravenous Infusion Set

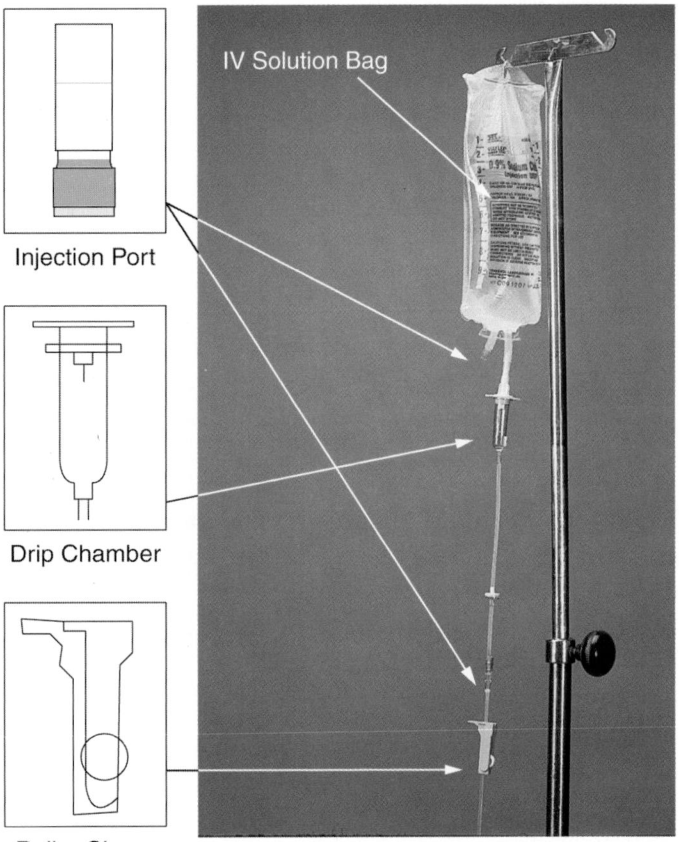
IV Solution Bag
Injection Port
Drip Chamber
Roller Clamp

Cengage Learning

FIGURE 12-7 (a) Standard Straight Gravity Flow IV System

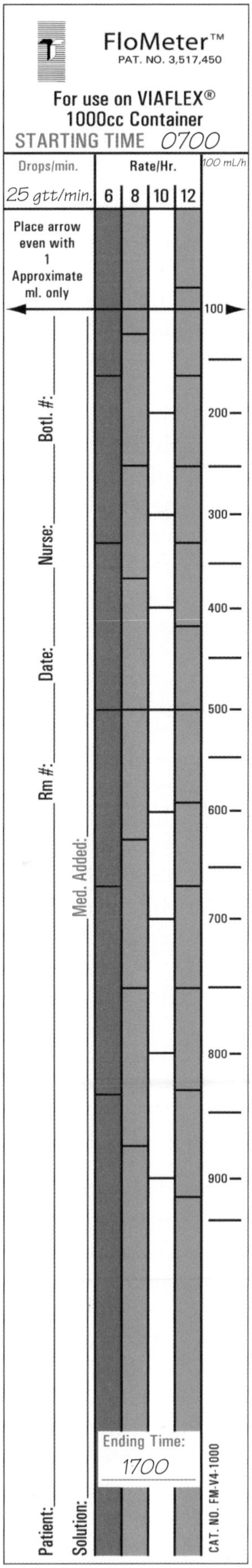
FloMeter™
PAT. NO. 3,517,450
For use on VIAFLEX®
1000cc Container
STARTING TIME 0700
Drops/min.
25 gtt/min.
Rate/Hr.
6 8 10 12
100 mL/h
Place arrow even with 1
Approximate ml. only
100 0800
200 0900
300 1000
400 1100
500 1200
600 1300
700 1400
800 1500
900 1600
Botl. #:
Nurse:
Date:
Rm #:
Med. Added:
Patient:
Solution:
Ending Time:
1700
CAT. NO. FM-V4-1000

Courtesy TimeMed

FIGURE 12-7 (b) Infusion Label

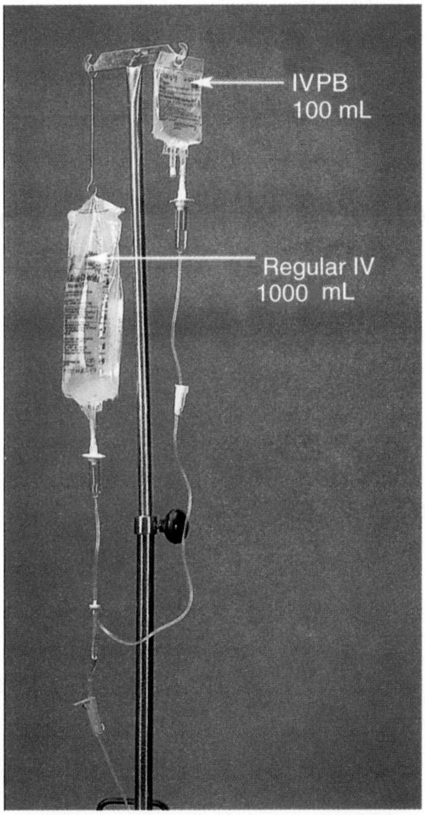
IVPB
100 mL
Regular IV
1000 mL

Cengage Learning

FIGURE 12-8 IV with Piggyback (IVPB)

the primary IV to allow the secondary set of medication to infuse first. When administering primary IV fluids, choose primary IV tubing; when hanging piggybacks, select secondary IV tubing. IVPBs are discussed further at the end of this chapter (see page 347).

BLOOD ADMINISTRATION TUBING

When blood is administered, a Y-type blood set (see Figure 12-9) is commonly used. The "Y" refers to the two spikes that are attached above the drip chamber. One spike is attached to the blood container, and the other spike is attached to normal saline. Normal saline is used to dilute packed cells and to flush the IV tubing at the beginning and at the end of the transfusion. Blood is usually infused manually by gravity, and the roller clamp on the line is used to adjust the rate. Some electronic pumps, such as the Alaris or Baxter pumps, may also be used for infusion of blood. In such cases, the nurse would program the pump in millilitres per hour and then the pump would regulate the blood infusion. Blood infusion is calculated the same as any other IV fluid. All blood components are transfused through a standard blood filter (170–260 micron) to ensure removal of particles such as fibrin and other microaggregates from stored human blood that may cause harm to the patient. Medications are never added to blood products as the effect of the medication on the blood is not known. As well, if a reaction did occur, it would be difficult to determine whether the reaction was as a result of the blood or the medication. If the transfusion had to be stopped for whatever reason, the entire dose of medication would not be administered. A separate IV line is used if medications are required during the transfusion period.

IV FLOW RATE

The *flow rate* of an IV infusion is ordered by the physician. It is the nurse's responsibility to regulate, monitor, and maintain the flow rate. Regulation of IV therapy is a critical skill in nursing. Because the fluids administered are infusing directly into the patient's circulatory system, careful monitoring is essential to be sure the patient does not receive too much or too little IV fluid and medication. It is also important for the nurse to accurately set and maintain the flow rate to administer the prescribed volume of the IV solution within the specified time period. The nurse records the IV fluids administered and IV flow rates on the IV administration record (see Figure 12-10).

IV solutions are usually ordered for a certain volume to run for a period of time, such as *125 mL/h* or *1000 mL/8 h*. The nurse will use electronic or manual regulating equipment to monitor the flow rate. The calculations you must perform to set the flow rate will depend on the equipment used to administer the IV solutions.

ELECTRONIC INFUSION DEVICES

Frequently, IV solutions are regulated electronically by an infusion device, such as a controller or pump. The use of an electronic infusion device will be determined by the need to strictly regulate the IV. Manufacturers supply special volumetric tubing that must be used with their infusion devices. This special tubing ensures accurate, consistent IV infusions. Each device can be set for a specific flow rate and will set off an alarm if this rate is interrupted. Electronic units today are powered by direct (wall) current as well as an internal rechargeable battery. The battery takes over when the unit is unplugged, to allow for portability and patient ambulation. Electronic infusion devices ensure the precise infusion of volumes of fluids or medications.

Controllers (see Figure 12-11) depend on gravity to maintain the desired flow rate by a compression/decompression mechanism that pinches the IV tubing, rather than forcing IV fluid into the system. They are often referred to as *electronic flow clamps* because they monitor the selected rate of infusion by either drop counting (drops per minute) or volumetric delivery (millilitres per hour).

Infusion pumps (see Figure 12-12) do not rely on gravity but maintain the flow by displacing fluid at the prescribed rate. Resistance to flow within the system causes positive pressure in relation to the

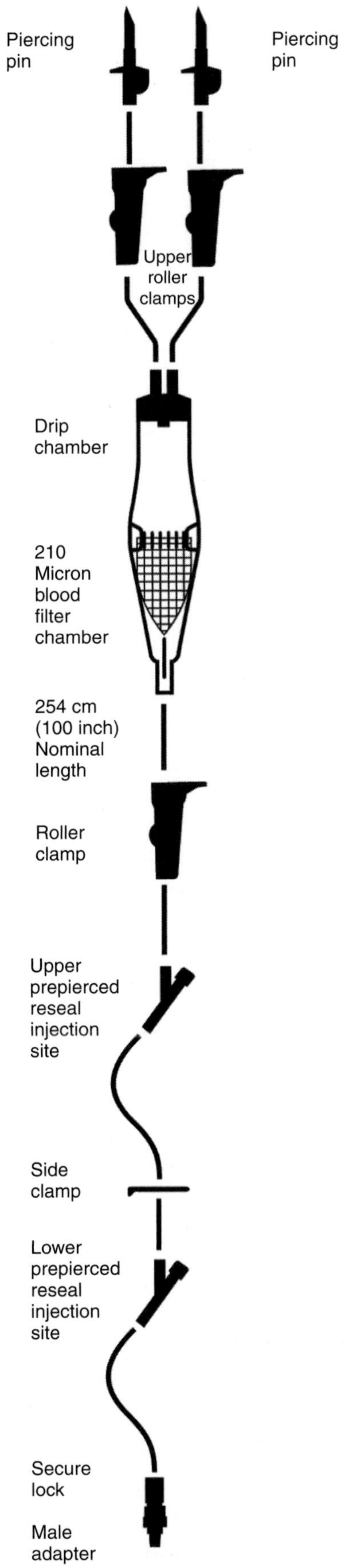
Piercing pin
Piercing pin
Upper roller clamps
Drip chamber
210 Micron blood filter chamber
254 cm (100 inch) Nominal length
Roller clamp
Upper prepierced reseal injection site
Side clamp
Lower prepierced reseal injection site
Secure lock
Male adapter

FIGURE 12-9 Y-Type Blood Set

Page: 1 of 1 DATE: 11/10/xx through

Correct	I.V. Order	Rate	Time	Initial	Site / Infusion Port	Pump / Other	Tubing Change
✓	D_5 ½ NS	100 mL/hr	0900	GP	LH / PIV	☐✓	✓

CIRCULATORY ACCESS SITE

Time	Gauge	Length	Type	Site	# Attempts	Dressing Change	Site Condition	IV Lock	Initial	Time Catheter D/C Intact	Site Condition	Reason Code	Initial
0800	22	1½"	I	LH	1	✓	0	☐	GP				

Type: I - Insyte; B - Butterfly; C - Cathlon; CVC - CVC; T - Tunnelled; IP - Implanted Port; PICC - PICC; A - Arterial Line; SG - Swan Ganz; DL - Dual Lumen Peripheral; UAC - UAC; UVC - UVC

Site: L - Left; R - Right; H - Hand; FA - Forearm; UA - Upper Arm; SC - Subclavian; C - Chest; A - Antecubital; F - Femoral; J - Jugular; FT - Foot; S - Scalp; U - Umbilical; RA - Radial

Dressing Change: T - Transparent; A - Air Occlusive; B - Bandaid; PR - Pressure Dressing

Reason Code: 1 - Infiltrate; 2 - Physician Order; 3 - Client Removed; 4 - Clotted; 5 - Phlebitis; 6 - Site Rotation; 7 - Leaking; 8 - Positional; 9 - Not Patent; 10 - Family Refused

Other: D - Dial-a-flow

Infusion Port: PIV - Peripheral IV; CVC - CVC; SG - Swan Ganz; D - Distal; M - Middle; P - Proximal; R - Red; BL - Blue; V - Venous; S - Sideport; AN - Access Needle; A - Arterial

Site Condition: 0; 1+; 2+; 3+; 4+; 5+

Tubing Change: P - Primary; S - Secondary; E - Extension; T - 3 Way Stopcock; H - Hemodynamic

ALLERGIES: NKA

Initial / Signature - Circulatory Access Site(s) checked hourly.

GP / G. Pickar, RN

Reconciled by:

Smith, James 43y M
Dr. Jones Medical Service
Admitted 01-01-xx Rm 237-1
Adm. # 6634297

IV ADMINISTRATION RECORD

602-0203 (2-94)dlg)MPC#32258)

FIGURE 12-10 IV Administration Record

flow rate. The nurse or other user may preset a pressure alarm threshold. When the pressure sensed by the device reaches this threshold, the device stops pumping and sets off an alarm. The amount of change in pressure that results from infiltration or phlebitis may be insufficient to reach the alarm threshold. Therefore, users should not expect the device to stop infusing in the presence of these conditions. Electronic infusion pumps are used for administering low fluid volumes (e.g., less than 20 mL/h) or in high-risk patients.

A *syringe pump* (see Figure 12-13) is a type of electronic infusion pump. Also called a *syringe infusion system,* it is used to infuse fluids or medications directly from a syringe. It is most often used for neonates and children when small volumes of medication are delivered at low rates. It is also used in anaesthesia, in labour and delivery, and in critical care when the drug cannot be mixed with other solutions or medications, or to reduce the volume of diluent fluid delivered to the patient. Syringe pumps can deliver in up to 16 different modes, including millilitres per hour, volume/time, dose or body weight modes, mass modes such as units per hour, and other specialty modes.

Electronic volumetric pumps are large-volume infusion pumps that infuse fluids into the vein under pressure and against resistance and do not rely on gravity. These pumps are programmed so that a uniform amount of fluid is delivered per hour. There is a wide range of electronic pumps available.

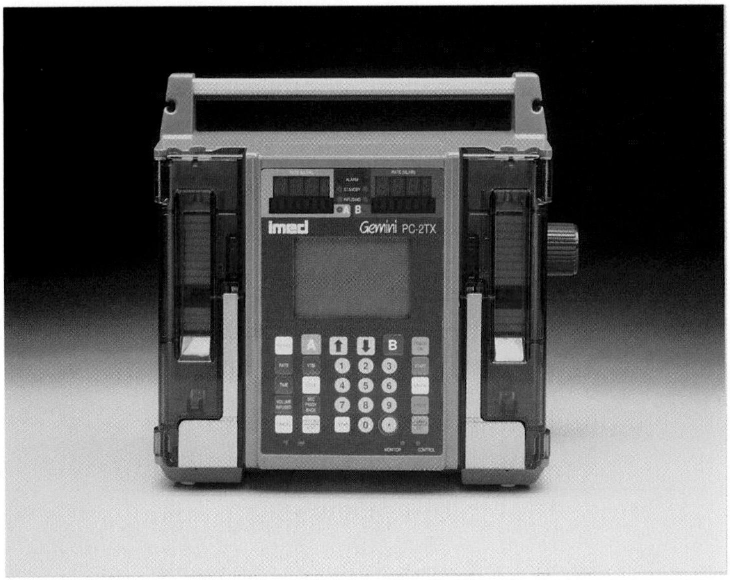

Photo courtesy of Alaris Medical Systems

FIGURE 12-11 Volumetric Infusion Controller/Pump

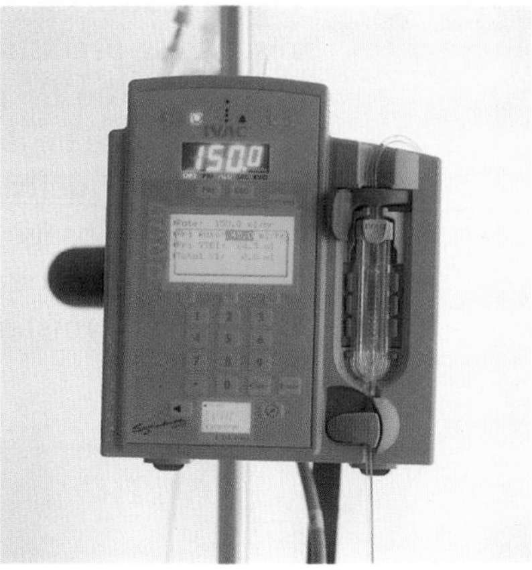

Photo courtesy of Alaris Medical Systems

FIGURE 12-12 Infusion Pump

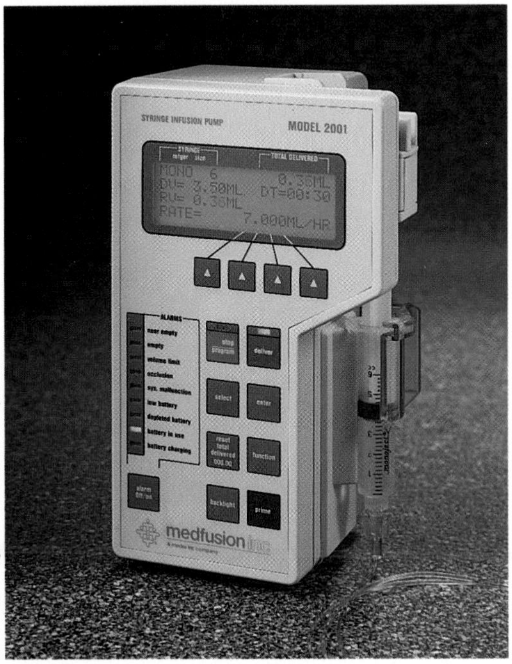

Photo courtesy of Alaris Medical Systems

FIGURE 12-13 Syringe Pump

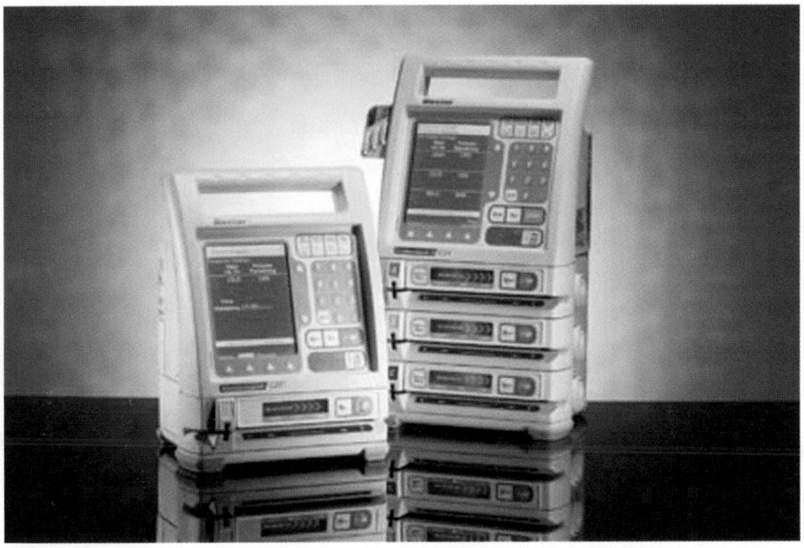

Baxter Corporation, Mississauga, ON

FIGURE 12-14 CC3 Volumetric Infusion Pump

Because these pumps deliver millilitres per hour (mL/h), any millilitre calculation that results in a decimal fraction must be rounded to a whole millilitre. Recently, the arrival of more sophisticated pumps called *smart pumps* allows infusions to be set by pump rate and the drug dosage to be administered. Other types of pumps allow decimal increments per millimetre. Such pumps are most often used in critical care units or to administer chemotherapeutic agents. Many hospitals in Canada are replacing volumetric pumps with smart pumps.

Smart pumps are infusion devices that improve precision in medication delivery. The smart pump consists of customized software that includes a reference of drugs. When medication levels are outside prescribed limits, the dose error reduction software is designed to alert the nurse. Smart pumps keep records of all alerts, including the time, date, drug, concentration, programmed rate, and volume infused, providing useful quality control information.

Add-on syringe pump systems for small-volume IV push or bolus infusions can also be added to some smart pumps while multiple infusions can be delivered through one pump. Others can figure in a patient's age or clinical condition. Smart pumps can be used to administer patient-controlled analgesia.

A *patient-controlled analgesia pump* (see Figure 12-15) is used to allow the patient to self-administer IV medication to control postoperative and other types of severe pain. The physician or other prescribing practitioner orders the pain medication, which is contained in a prefilled syringe locked securely in the IV pump. The patient presses the control button and receives the pain medication immediately. The dose, frequency, and a safety "lock out" time are ordered and programmed into the pump, which delivers an individual therapeutic dose. The pump stores information about the frequency and dosage of the drug requested by and delivered to the patient. The nurse can display this information to document and evaluate pain management effectiveness. The nurse can also use such a pump to administer other IV push medications.

CAUTION

All electronic infusion devices must be monitored frequently (at least every 30 minutes to 1 hour) to ensure proper and safe functioning. Check the policy in your facility.

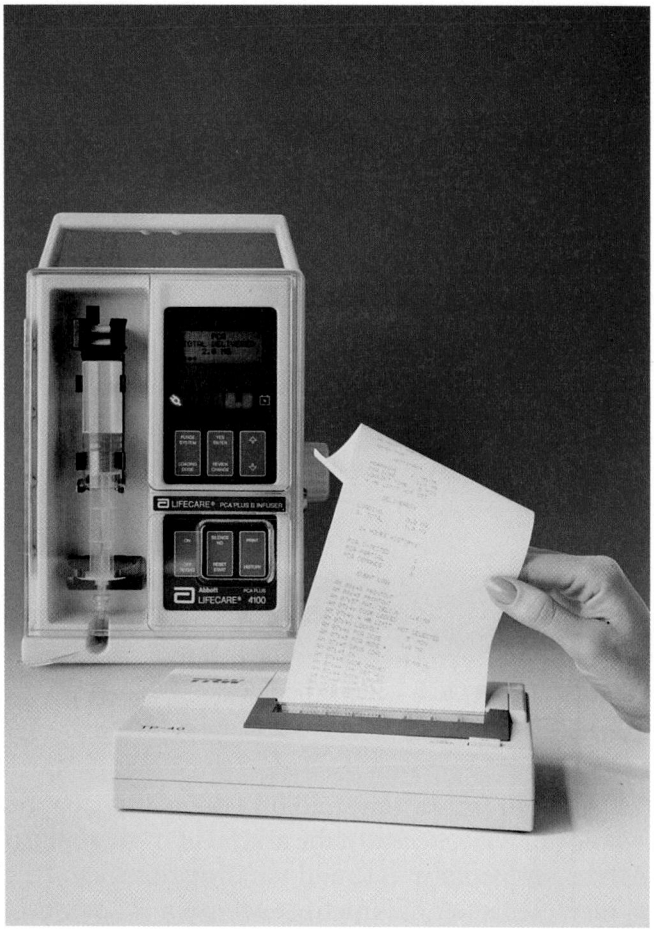

FIGURE 12-15 Abbott Lifecare Patient-Controlled Analgesia Plus II Infusion System

CALCULATING FLOW RATES FOR ELECTRONIC REGULATORS IN mL/h

When an electronic infusion regulator is used, the IV volume is ordered by the physician and programmed into the device by the nurse. These devices are regulated in millilitres per hour. Usually the physician orders the IV volume to be delivered in millilitres per hour. If not, the nurse must calculate it.

> **RULE**
>
> **To regulate an IV volume by electronic infusion pump or controller calibrated in millilitres per hour, calculate:**
>
> $$\frac{\textbf{Total mL ordered}}{\textbf{Total h ordered}} = \textbf{mL/h (rounded to a whole number)}$$

Example:

Order: *D_5W 250 mL IV over the next 2 h by infusion pump*

Step 1 Think. The pump is set by the rate of millilitres per hour. So, if 250 mL is to be infused in 2 hours, how much will be infused in 1 hour? Of course, 125 mL will be infused in 1 hour. You would set the pump at 125 mL per hour.

Step 2 Use the formula:

$$\frac{\text{Total mL ordered}}{\text{Total h ordered}} = \text{mL/h}$$

$$\frac{250 \text{ mL}}{2 \text{ h}} = \frac{125 \text{ mL}}{1 \text{ h}}$$

Therefore, set the pump at 125 mL per hour (125 mL/h).

In most cases it is easy to calculate mL/h by dividing total millilitres by total hour. However, an IV with medication added or an IVPB may be ordered to be administered in *less than 1 hour* by an electronic infusion device, but the pump or controller must still be set in mL/h.

> **RULE**
>
> $$\frac{\textbf{Total mL ordered}}{\textbf{Total min ordered}} \times \textbf{60 min/h} = \textbf{mL/h (rounded to a whole number)}$$

Example:

Order: *ampicillin 500 mg IV in 50 mL $D_5\frac{1}{2}NS$ in 30 min (to be infused by controller)*

Step 1 Think. If 50 mL is to be infused in 30 minutes, then 100 mL will be infused in 60 minutes, because 100 mL is twice as much as 50 mL and 60 minutes is twice as much as 30 minutes. Set the rate of the controller at 100 mL/h to infuse 50 mL/30 min (for the infusion of the drug, then re-assess rate).

Step 2 $$\frac{\text{Total mL ordered}}{\text{Total min ordered}} \times 60 \text{ min/h} = \text{mL/h}$$

$$\frac{50 \text{ mL}}{\cancel{30}_{1} \cancel{\text{min}}} \times \frac{\cancel{60}^{2} \cancel{\text{min}}}{1 \text{ h}} = 100 \text{ mL/h}$$

Or, you can use ratio-proportion.

$$\frac{50 \text{ mL}}{30 \text{ min}} \times \frac{X \text{ mL}}{60 \text{ min}}$$

$30X = 3000$

$$\frac{30X}{30} = \frac{3000}{30}$$

$X = 100 \text{ mL}/60 \text{ min}$ or 100 mL/h

QUICK REVIEW

- $\frac{\text{Total mL ordered}}{\text{Total h ordered}} = \text{mL/h}$
- If the infusion time is less than 1 hour, then $\frac{\text{Total mL ordered}}{\text{Total min ordered}} \times 60 \text{ min/h} = \text{mL/h}$
- Round mL/h to a whole number.

REVIEW SET 29

Calculate the flow rate at which you will program the electronic infusion regulator for the following IV orders.

1. *1 L D_5W IV to infuse in 10 h*

   Flow rate: ________ mL/h

2. *1800 mL normal saline IV to infuse in 15 h*

   Flow rate: ________ mL/h

3. *2000 mL D_5W IV in 24 h*

   Flow rate: ________ mL/h

4. *100 mL NS IVPB in 30 min*

   Flow rate: ________ mL/h

5. *30 mL antibiotic in D_5W IV in 15 min*

   Flow rate: ________ mL/h

6. *2.5 L NS IV in 20 h*

   Flow rate: ________ mL/h

7. *500 mL D_5LR IV in 4 h*

   Flow rate: ________ mL/h

8. *600 mL 0.45% NaCl IV in 3 h*

   Flow rate: ________ mL/h

9. *150 mL antibiotic in D_5W IV in 2 h*

   Flow rate: ________ mL/h

10. *3 L NS IV in 24 h*

    Flow rate: ________ mL/h

11. *1.5 L LR Injection IV in 24 h*

    Flow rate: ________ mL/h

12. *240 mL $D_{10}W$ IV in 10 h*

    Flow rate: ________ mL/h

13. *750 mL D_5W IV in 5 h*

    Flow rate: ________ mL/h

14. *1.5 L D_5NS IV in 12 h*

    Flow rate: ________ mL/h

15. *380 mL D_5 0.45% NaCl IV in 9 h*

    Flow rate: ________ mL/h

After completing these problems, see page 494 to check your answers.

MANUALLY REGULATED IVs

When an electronic infusion device is not used, the nurse manually regulates the IV rate. To do this, the nurse must calculate the ordered IV rate based on a certain *number of drops per minute (gtt/min)*. This actually represents the ordered millilitres per hour, as you will shortly see in the calculation.

The number of drops dripping per minute into the IV drip chamber (Figures 12-6 and 12-17) are counted and regulated by opening or closing the roller clamp. To count the drops, place your watch at the level of the drip chamber and count the drops as they fall during a 1-minute period (referred to as the *watch count*). This manual, gravity flow rate depends on the IV tubing calibration called the *drop factor*.

RULE

Drop factor = gtt/mL

The drop factor is the number of drops per millilitre (gtt/mL) a particular IV tubing set will deliver. It is stated on the IV tubing package (Figure 12-7) and varies according to the manufacturer of the IV equipment. Standard or *macrodrop* IV tubing sets have a drop factor of 10 or 15 gtt/mL. All microdrip (or minidrip) IV tubing has a drop factor of 60 gtt/mL. Hospitals typically stock 1 macrodrop tubing for routine adult IV administration and the microdrip tubing for situations requiring more exact measurement, such as patients on restricted fluid intake (e.g., patients in heart failure or kidney failure).

Figure 12-16 compares macro- and microdrops. See figure 12-17 for an illustration of the size and number of drops in 1 mL for each drop factor. Notice that the fewer the number of drops per millilitre, the larger the actual drop size.

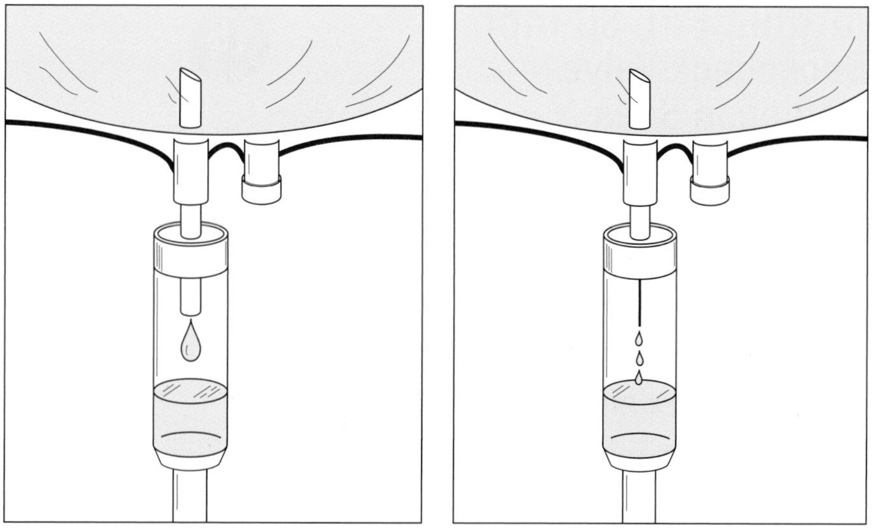

FIGURE 12-16 Intravenous Drip Chambers; Comparison of (a) Macrodrops and (b) Microdrops

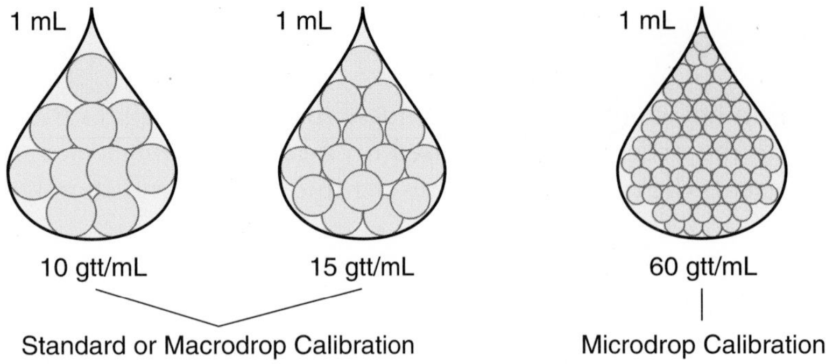

FIGURE 12-17 Comparison of Calibrated Drop Factors

QUICK REVIEW

- Drop factor = gtt/mL
- The drop factor is stated on the IV tubing package
- Macrodrop factors: 10 or 15 gtt/mL
- Microdrop factor: 60 gtt/mL

REVIEW SET 30

Identify the drop factor calibration of the IV tubing pictured.

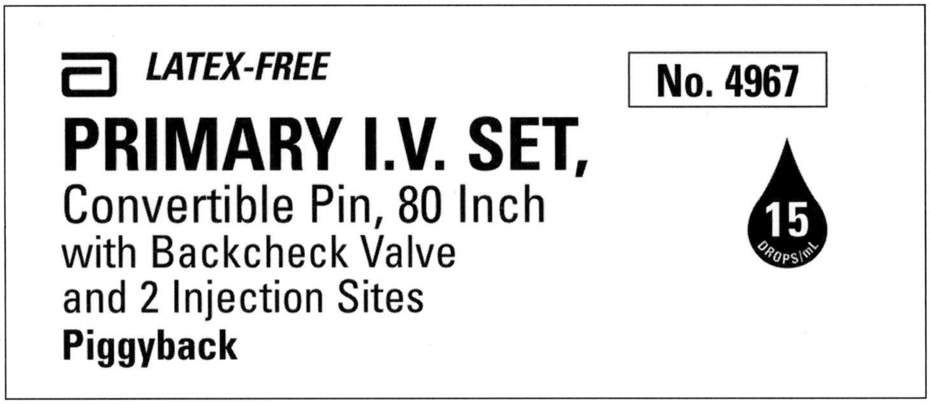

Courtesy of Abbott Laboratories, Inc.

1. ______ gtt/mL

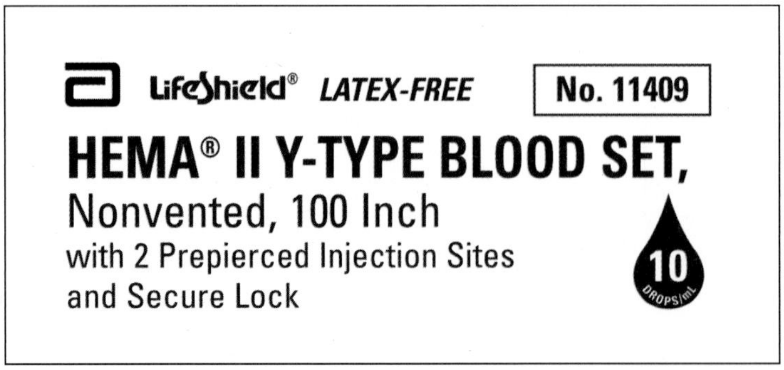

Courtesy of Abbott Laboratories, Inc.

2. ______ gtt/mL

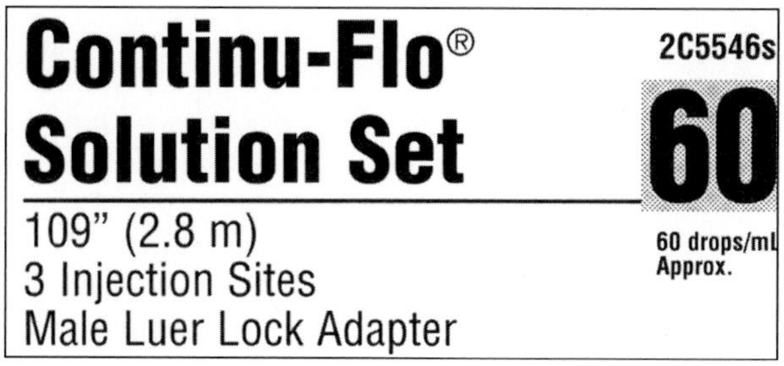

Courtesy of Abbott Laboratories, Inc.

3. ______ gtt/mL

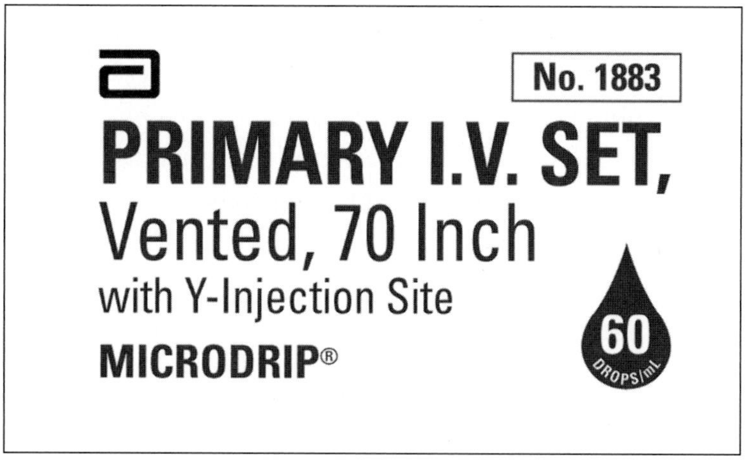

Courtesy of Abbott Laboratories, Inc.

4. ______ gtt/mL

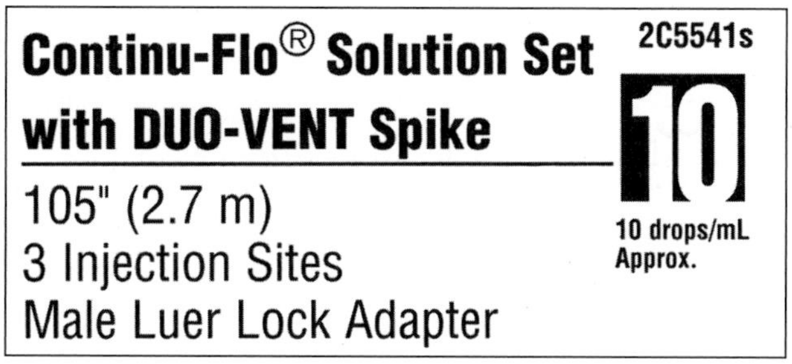

Courtesy of Abbott Laboratories, Inc.

5. ______ gtt/mL

After completing these problems, see page 495 to check your answers.

CALCULATING FLOW RATES FOR MANUALLY REGULATED IVs IN gtt/min

In this section you will learn two methods to calculate IV flow rate for manually regulated IVs: the formula method and the shortcut method.

Formula Method

The formula method can be used to determine the flow rate in drops per minute (*gtt/min*). IV fluid and medication orders are written as a specific volume to be infused in a certain time period. Most IV fluid orders are written as "X mL/h," which means X mL in 60 minutes. However, some IV medications are to be administered in less than 1 hour; for example, over 30 minutes.

RULE

The formula method to calculate IV flow rate for manually regulated IVs ordered in mL/h, or for a prescribed number of minutes, is:

$$\frac{V}{T} \times C = R$$

$$\frac{\text{Volume (mL)}}{\text{Time (min)}} \times \text{Calibration or drop factor (gtt/mL)} = \text{Rate (gtt/min)}$$

In this formula:

V = *volume* per hour to be infused in mL; ordered by the prescriber.
C = *calibration* of tubing (drop factor) in gtt/mL.
T = *time* ordered by the prescriber or pharmacy; converted to minutes.
R = *rate* of flow in gtt/min. Think: The unknown is the "watch count."

MATH TIP

Carry calculations to one decimal place. Round gtt/min to the nearest whole number, because you can watch-count only whole drops.

Some examples of how to calculate the flow rate or "watch count" in gtt/min follow.

Example 1:

Order: *D_5W IV @ 125 mL/h.* The infusion set is calibrated for a drop factor of 10 gtt/mL. Calculate the IV flow rate in gtt/min. Notice that the mL cancel out, leaving *gtt/min.*

$$\frac{V}{T} \times C = \frac{125\text{ mL}}{60\text{ min}} \times 10\text{ gtt/mL} = \frac{125\ \cancel{\text{mL}}}{\underset{6}{\cancel{60}}\text{ min}} \times \frac{\overset{1}{\cancel{10}}\text{ gtt}}{1\ \cancel{\text{mL}}} = \frac{125\text{ gtt}}{6\text{ min}} = 20.8\text{ gtt/min} = 21\text{ gtt/min}$$

Use your watch to count the drops and adjust the roller clamp to deliver 21 gtt/min.

Example 2:

Order: *Lactated Ringer's IV @ 150 mL/h.* The drop factor is 15 gtt/mL.

$$\frac{V}{T} \times C = \frac{150\ \cancel{\text{mL}}}{\underset{4}{\cancel{60}}\text{ min}} \times \overset{1}{\cancel{15}}\text{ gtt/}\cancel{\text{mL}} = \frac{150\text{ gtt}}{4\text{ min}} = 37.5\text{ gtt/min} = 38\text{ gtt/min}$$

Example 3:

Order: *ampicillin 500 mg IV in 100 mL of NS, infuse over 20 min*

The drop factor is 10 gtt/mL. Notice that the time is less than 1 hour.

$$\frac{V}{T} \times C = \frac{100\ \cancel{\text{mL}}}{20\text{ min}} \times 10\text{ gtt/}\cancel{\text{mL}} = \frac{1000\text{ gtt}}{20\text{ min}} = 50\text{ gtt/min}$$

MATH TIP

When the IV drop factor is 60 gtt/mL (microdrip sets), the flow rate in gtt/min is the same as the volume ordered in mL/h.

Example 4:

Order: *D_5W NS IV @ 50 mL/h.* The drop factor is 60 gtt/mL. Notice that the order, 50 mL/h, is *the same as the flow rate* of 50 gtt/min when the drop factor is 60 gtt/mL.

$$\frac{V}{T} \times C = \frac{50 \cancel{\text{mL}}}{\cancel{60} \text{ min}} \times \cancel{60} \text{ gtt}/\cancel{\text{mL}} = 50 \text{ gtt/min}$$

Sometimes the prescriber will order a total IV volume to be infused over a total number of hours. In such cases, first calculate the mL/h, then calculate gtt/min.

RULE

The formula method to calculate IV flow rate for manually regulated IVs ordered in total volume and total hours is:

STEP 1 $\frac{\text{Total mL}}{\text{Total hours}} = \text{mL/h}$

STEP 2 $\frac{V}{T} \times C = R$

Example:

Order: *NS IV 3000 mL/24 h.* Drop factor is 15 gtt/min.

Step 1 $\frac{\text{Total mL}}{\text{Total h}} = \frac{3000 \text{ mL}}{24 \text{ h}} = 125 \text{ mL/h}$

Step 2

$$\frac{V}{T} \times C = R: \frac{125 \text{ mL}}{60 \text{ min}} \times 15 \text{ gtt/mL} = \frac{125 \cancel{\text{mL}}}{\underset{4}{\cancel{60}} \text{ min}} \times \frac{\overset{1}{\cancel{15}} \text{ gtt}}{1 \cancel{\text{mL}}} = \frac{125 \text{ gtt}}{4 \text{ min}} = 31.3 \text{ gtt/min} = 31 \text{ gtt/min}$$

QUICK REVIEW

- The formula method to calculate the flow rate, or watch count, in gtt/min for manually regulated IV rates ordered in mL/h or mL/min is:

  $\frac{\text{Volume (mL)}}{\text{Time (min)}} \times \text{Calibration or drop factor (gtt/mL)} = \text{Rate (gtt/min)}$
- When total volume and total hours are ordered, first calculate mL/h.
- When the drop factor calibration is 60 (microdrop sets), then the flow rate in gtt/min is the same as the ordered volume in mL/h.
- Round gtt/min to a whole number.

REVIEW SET 31

1. State the rule for the formula method to calculate IV flow rate in gtt/min when mL/h is known. ________

Calculate the flow rate or watch count in gtt/min.

2. Order: *3000 mL D_5W IV @ 125 mL/h*

   Drop factor: 10 gtt/mL

   ________ gtt/min

3. Order: *250 mL LR IV @ 50 mL/h*

   Drop factor: 60 gtt/mL

   ________ gtt/min

4. Order: *100 mL NS bolus IV to infuse in 60 min*

   Drop factor: 10 gtt/mL

   ________ gtt/min

5. Order: *$D_5 \frac{1}{2}$ NS IV with 20 mEq KCl per litre to run at 25 mL/h*

   Drop factor: 60 gtt/mL

   ________ gtt/min

6. Order: *Two 500-mL units of whole blood IV to be infused in 4 h*

   Drop factor: 10 gtt/mL

   ________ gtt/min

7. Total parenteral nutrition is ordered for 1240 mL to infuse in 12 hours using an infusion set with tubing calibrated to 15 gtt/mL.

   ________ gtt/min

8. Order: *D_5NS IV @ 150 mL/h*

   Drop factor: 10 gtt/mL

   ________ gtt/min

9. Order: *150 mL NS bolus IV to infuse in 45 min*

   Drop factor: 15 gtt/mL

   ________ gtt/min

10. Order: *80 mL D_5W antibiotic solution IV to infuse in 60 min*

    Drop factor: 60 gtt/mL

    ________ gtt/min

11. Order: *480 mL packed red blood cells IV to infuse in 4 h*

    Drop factor: 10 gtt/mL

    ________ gtt/min

12. Order: *D_5W IV @ 120 mL/h*

    Drop factor: 15 gtt/mL

    ________ gtt/min

13. Order: *D_5 0.33% NaCl IV @ 50 mL/h*

    Drop factor: 10 gtt/mL

    ________ gtt/min

14. Order: *2500 mL LR IV @ 165 mL/h*

    Drop factor: 10 gtt/mL

    ________ gtt/min

15. Order: *3500 mL D_5LR IV to run at 160 mL/h*

    Drop factor: 15 gtt/mL

    ________ gtt/min

After completing these problems, see page 495 to check your answers.

Shortcut Method

By converting the volume and time in the formula method to mL/h (or mL/60 min), you can use a shortcut to calculate flow rate. This shortcut is derived from the drop factor (C), which cancels out each time and reduces the 60 minutes (T). You are left with the *drop factor constant.* Look at these examples.

Example 1:

Administer *normal saline 1000 mL IV at 125 mL/h* with a microdrop infusion set calibrated for *60 gtt/mL*. Use the formula $\frac{V}{T} \times C = R$.

$$\frac{V}{T} \times C = \frac{125 \not{mL}}{\underset{1}{\not{60}} \text{ min}} \times \overset{1}{\not{60}} \text{ gtt}/\not{mL} = \frac{125 \text{ gtt}}{(1) \text{ min}} = 125 \text{ gtt/min}$$

The drop factor constant for an infusion set with 60 gtt/mL is 1. Therefore, to administer 125 mL/h, set the flow rate at 125 gtt/min. Recall that when the drop factor is 60, then gtt/min = mL/h.

Example 2:

Administer *125 mL/h IV* with *10 gtt/mL* infusion set.

$$\frac{V}{T} \times C = \frac{125 \not{mL}}{\underset{6}{\not{60}} \text{ min}} \times \overset{1}{\not{10}} \text{ gtt}/\not{mL} = \frac{125 \text{ gtt}}{(1) \text{ min}} = 20.8 \text{ gtt/min} = 21 \text{ gtt/min}$$

Drop factor constant = 6

Each drop factor constant is obtained by dividing 60 by the drop factor calibration from the infusion set.

REMEMBER

Drop Factor	Drop Factor Constant
10 gtt/mL	$\frac{60}{10} = 6$
15 gtt/mL	$\frac{60}{15} = 4$
60 gtt/mL	$\frac{60}{60} = 1$

Most hospitals consistently use infusion equipment manufactured by one company. Each manufacturer typically supplies 1 macrodrop and 1 microdrop system. You will become familiar with the supplier used where you work; therefore, the shortcut method is practical, quick, and simple to use.

RULE

The shortcut method to calculate IV flow rate is:

$$\frac{\text{mL/h}}{\text{Drop factor constant}} = \text{gtt/min}$$

Let us examine three examples using the shortcut method.

Example 1:

The IV order reads: *D_5W IV @ 125 mL/h*. The infusion set is calibrated for a drop factor of 10 gtt/mL. Drop factor constant: 6

$$\frac{\text{mL/h}}{\text{Drop factor constant}} = \text{gtt/min}$$

$$\frac{125 \text{ mL/h}}{6} = 20.8 \text{ gtt/min} = 21 \text{ gtt/min}$$

Example 2:

Order reads *LR IV @ 150 mL/h*. The drop factor is 15 gtt/mL. Drop factor constant: 4

$$\frac{\text{mL/h}}{\text{Drop factor constant}} = \text{gtt/min}$$

$$\frac{150 \text{ mL/h}}{4} = 37.5 \text{ gtt/min} = 38 \text{ gtt/min}$$

Example 3:

Order reads: *D_5W NS IV @ 50 mL/h*. The drop factor is 60 gtt/mL. Drop factor constant: 1

$$\frac{\text{mL/h}}{\text{Drop factor constant}} = \text{gtt/min}$$

$$\frac{50 \text{ mL/h}}{1} = 50 \text{ gtt/min}$$

Remember, when the drop factor is 60 (microdrop), set the flow rate at the same gtt/min as the mL/h.

CAUTION

For the shortcut method to work, the rate has to be written in millilitres per hour. The shortcut method will not work if the time is less than 1 hour or is calculated in minutes, such as 15 or 75 minutes.

QUICK REVIEW

- The drop factor constant is 60 ÷ drop factor.

Drop Factor	Drop Factor Constant
10 gtt/mL	6
15 gtt/mL	4
60 gtt/mL	1 → Set the flow rate at the same gtt/min as the mL/h.

- $$\frac{\text{mL/h}}{\text{Drop factor constant}} = \text{gtt/min}$$

REVIEW SET 32

1. The drop factor constant is derived by dividing ________ by the drop factor calibration.

Determine the drop factor constant for each of the following infusion sets.

2. 60 gtt/mL ________
3. 15 gtt/mL ________
4. 10 gtt/mL ________
5. State the rule for the shortcut method to calculate the IV flow rate in gtt/min. ________

____

Calculate the IV flow rate in gtt/min using the shortcut method.

6. Order: *1000 mL D_5W IV to infuse @ 200 mL/h*

   Drop factor: 15 gtt/mL

   Flow rate: ________ gtt/min

7. Order: *750 mL D_5W IV to infuse @ 125 mL/h*

   Drop factor: 15 gtt/mL

   Flow rate: ________ gtt/min

8. Order: *500 mL D_5W 0.45% Saline IV to infuse @ 165 mL/h*

   Drop factor: 10 gtt/mL

   Flow rate: ________ gtt/min

9. Order: *2 L NS IV to infuse at 60 mL/h with microdrop infusion set of 60 gtt/mL*

   Flow rate: ________ gtt/min

10. Order: *400 mL D_5W IV to infuse @ 50 mL/h*

    Drop factor: 10 gtt/mL

    Flow rate: ________ gtt/min

11. Order: *3 L NS IV to infuse @ 125 mL/h*

    Drop factor: 15 gtt/mL

    Flow rate: ________ gtt/min

12. Order: *500 mL D_5LR IV to infuse in 6 h*

    Drop factor: 10 gtt/mL

    Flow rate: ________ gtt/min

13. Order: *0.5 L 0.45% NaCl IV to infuse in 20 h*

    Drop factor: 60 gtt/mL

    Flow rate: ________ gtt/min

14. Order: *650 mL D_5 0.33% NaCl IV to infuse in 10 h*

    Drop factor: 10 gtt/mL

    Flow rate: ________ gtt/min

15. Order: *250 mL $\frac{2}{3}$; $\frac{1}{3}$ IV to infuse in 5 h*

    Drop factor: 60 gtt/mL

    Flow rate: ________ gtt/min

After completing these problems, see page 495 to check your answers.

SUMMARY

Calculating mL/h to program infusion devices and calculating gtt/min to watch-count manually regulated IVs are two major IV calculations you need to know. Further, you have learned to calculate the supply dosage of certain IV solutes. These important topics warrant additional reinforcement and review.

QUICK REVIEW

- Solution strength expressed as a percent (%) indicates X g of solute per 100 mL of solution.
- When regulating IV flow rate for an electronic infusion device, calculate mL/h.
- When calculating IV flow rate to regulate an IV manually, calculate mL/h, find the drop factor, and calculate gtt/min by using the:

  Formula Method $\frac{V}{T} \times C = R$

  or Shortcut Method $\frac{\text{mL/h}}{\text{Drop factor constant}} = \text{gtt/min}$

- Carefully monitor patients receiving IV fluids every 30 minutes to 1 hour.
  - Check remaining IV fluids.
  - Check IV flow rate.
  - Observe IV site for complications.

REVIEW SET 33

Calculate the IV flow rate for these manually regulated IV administrations.

1. Order: *3000 mL 0.45% NaCl IV for 24 h*

   Drop factor: 15 gtt/mL

   Flow rate: ________ mL/h

   Flow rate: ________ gtt/min

2. Order: *200 mL D_5W IV to run @ 100 mL/h*

   Drop factor: Microdrop, 60 gtt/mL

   Flow rate: ________ gtt/min

3. Order: *800 mL $D_5 \frac{1}{3}$ NS IV for 8 h*

   Drop factor: 10 gtt/mL

   Flow rate: ________ mL/h

   Flow rate: ________ gtt/min

4. Order: *1000 mL NS IV @ 50 mL/h*

   Drop factor: 60 gtt/mL

   Flow rate: ________ gtt/min

5. Order: *1500 mL D_5W IV for 12 h*

   Drop factor: 15 gtt/mL

   Flow rate: ________ mL/h

   Flow rate: ________ gtt/min

6. Order: *theophylline 0.5 g IV in 250 mL D_5W to run over 2 h*

   Drop factor: 60 gtt/mL

   Flow rate: ________ mL/h

   Flow rate: ________ gtt/min

7. Order: *2500 mL D_5 0.45% NaCl IV @ 105 mL/h*

   Drop factor: 10 gtt/mL

   Flow rate: ________ gtt/min

8. Order: *500 mL D_5 0.45% NaCl IV @ 100 mL/h*

   Drop factor: 10 gtt/mL

   Flow rate: ________ gtt/min

9. Order: *1200 mL NS IV @ 150 mL/h*

   Drop factor: 10 gtt/mL

   Flow rate: ________ gtt/min

10. Order: *1000 mL D_5 0.45% NaCl to infuse over 8 h*

    Drop factor: On electronic infusion pump

    Flow rate: ________ mL/h

Calculate the IV flow rate for these electronically regulated IV administrations.

11. Order: *2000 mL D_5NS to infuse over 24 h*

    Drop factor: On electronic infusion controller

    Flow rate: ________ mL/h

12. Order: *500 mL LR to infuse over 4 h*

    Drop factor: On electronic infusion controller

    Flow rate: ________ mL/h

13. Order: *100 mL IV antibiotic to infuse in 30 min via electronic infusion pump*

    Flow rate: ________ mL/h

14. Order: *50 mL IV antibiotic to infuse in 20 min via electronic infusion pump*

    Flow rate: ________ mL/h

15. Order: *150 mL IV antibiotic to infuse in 45 min via electronic infusion pump*

    Flow rate: ________ mL/h

What is the total dosage of the solute(s) the patient will receive for each of the following orders?

16. *3000 mL $\frac{1}{2}$ NS IV*		NaCl: ________ g
17. *200 mL D_{10} NS IV*	D: ________ g	NaCl: ________ g
18. *2500 mL NS IV*		NaCl: ________ g
19. *650 mL D_5 0.33% NaCl IV*	D: ________ g	NaCl: ________ g
20. *1000 mL $D_5\frac{1}{4}$ NS IV*	D: ________ g	NaCl: ________ g

After completing these problems, see page 496 to check your answers.

ADJUSTING IV FLOW RATE

IV fluids, particularly those with medicines added (called *additives*), are viewed as medications with specific dosages (rates of infusion, in this case). It is the responsibility of the nurse to maintain this rate of flow through careful calculations and close observation at regular intervals. Various circumstances, such as gravity, condition, and movement of the patient, can alter the set flow rate of an IV, causing the IV to run ahead of or behind schedule.

CAUTION

It is not the discretion of the nurse to arbitrarily speed up or slow down the flow rate to catch up the IV. This practice can result in serious conditions of over- or underhydration and electrolyte imbalance. Avoid off-schedule IV flow rates by regularly monitoring IVs at least every 30 minutes to 1 hour. Check the institution policy.

During your regular monitoring of the IV, if you find that the rate is not progressing as scheduled or is significantly ahead of or behind schedule, the physician may need to be notified as warranted by the patient's condition, hospital policy, or good nursing judgment. Some hospital policies allow the flow rate per minute to be adjusted a certain percentage of variation. A rule of thumb is that the flow rate per minute may be adjusted by **up to 25% more or less** than the original rate depending on the condition of the patient. In such cases, assess the patient. If the patient is stable, recalculate the flow rate to administer the total millilitres remaining over the number of hours remaining of the original order.

RATIONAL FOR PRACTICE

- Check for institution policy regarding correcting off-schedule IV rates and the percentage of variation allowed. This variation generally should not exceed 25%.
- If adjustment is permitted, use the following formula to recalculate the mL/h and gtt/min for the time remaining and the percentage of variation.

Step 1 $\frac{\text{Remaining volume}}{\text{Remaining hours}} = \text{Recalculated mL/h}$

Step 2 $\frac{V}{T} \times C = \text{gtt/min}$

Step 3 $\frac{\text{Adjusted gtt/min} - \text{Ordered gtt/min}}{\text{Ordered gtt/min}} = \text{\% variation}$

The *% variation* will be positive (+) if the administration is slow and the rate has to be increased, and negative (−) if the administration is too fast and the rate has to be decreased.

Example 1:

The order reads *1000 mL D_5W IV @ 125 mL/h for 8 h.* The drop factor is 10 gtt/mL, and the IV is correctly set at 21 gtt/min. You would expect that after 4 hours, one-half of the total or 500 mL of the solution would be infused ($125 \text{ mL/}\cancel{h} \times 4 \cancel{h} = 500 \text{ mL}$). However, when you check the IV bag the fourth hour after starting the IV, you find 600 mL remaining. The rate of flow is *behind schedule*, and the hospital allows a 25% IV flow variation with careful patient assessment and if the patient's condition is stable. The patient is stable, so you decide to calculate a new flow rate for the remaining 600 mL to complete the IV fluid order in the remaining 4 hours.

Step 1 $\frac{\text{Remaining volume}}{\text{Remaining hours}} = \text{Recalculated mL/h}$

$$\frac{600 \text{ mL}}{4\text{h}} = 150 \text{ mL/h}$$

Step 2 $\frac{V}{T} \times C = \frac{150 \cancel{\text{mL}}}{\underset{6}{\cancel{60}} \text{ min}} \times \overset{1}{\cancel{10}} \text{ gtt/}\cancel{\text{mL}} = \frac{150 \text{ gtt}}{6 \text{ min}} = 25 \text{ gtt/min (adjusted flow rate)}$

You could also use the shortcut method.

$$\frac{\text{mL/h}}{\text{Drop factor constant}} = \text{gtt/min}$$

$$\frac{150 \text{ mL/h}}{6} = 25 \text{ gtt/min}$$

Step 3 $\frac{\text{Adjusted gtt/min} - \text{Ordered gtt/min}}{\text{Ordered gtt/min}} = \text{\% of variation}$

$\frac{25 - 21}{21} = \frac{4}{21} = 0.19 = 19\%$; within the acceptable 25% of variation depending on policy and patient's condition

Compare 25 gtt/min (in the last example) with the starting flow rate of 21 gtt/min. You can see that adjusting the total remaining volume over the total remaining hours changes the flow rate per minute little. Most patients can tolerate this small amount of increase per minute over several hours. However, trying to catch up the lost 100 mL in 1 hour can be dangerous. To infuse an extra 100 mL in

1 hour, with a drop factor of 10, you would need to speed up the IV to a much faster rate. Calculate what that rate would be.

$$\frac{V}{T} \times C = \frac{100 \cancel{mL}}{\underset{6}{\cancel{60}} \text{ min}} \times \overset{1}{\cancel{10}} \text{ gtt}/\cancel{mL} = \frac{100 \text{ gtt}}{6 \text{ min}} = 16.7 \text{ gtt/min} = 17 \text{ gtt/min more than the original rate}$$

To catch up the IV over the next hour, the flow rate would have to be 17 drops per minute faster than the original 21 drops per minute rate. The infusion would have to be set at $17 + 21 = 38$ gtt/min for 1 hour and then slowed to the original rate. Such an increase would be $\frac{38 - 21}{21} = \frac{17}{21} = 81\%$ greater than the ordered rate. This could present a serious problem. **Do not do it! If permitted by institution policy, the flow rate for the remainder of the order must be recalculated when the IV is off-schedule, and should never exceed a 25% adjustment.**

Example 2:

The order is for *500 mL LR to run over 10 h @ 50 mL/h.* The drop factor is 60 gtt/mL and the IV is correctly infusing at 50 gtt/min. After $2\frac{1}{2}$ hours, you find 300 mL remaining. Almost one-half of the total volume has already infused in about one-quarter the time. This IV infusion is *ahead of schedule.* You would compute a new flow rate of 300 mL to complete the IV fluid order in the remaining $7\frac{1}{2}$ hours. The patient would require close assessment for fluid overload.

Step 1 $\frac{\text{Remaining volume}}{\text{Remaining hours}} = \text{Recalculated mL/h}$

$$\frac{300 \text{ mL}}{7.5 \text{ h}} = 40 \text{ mL/h}$$

Step 2 $\frac{V}{T} \times C = \frac{40 \cancel{mL}}{\underset{1}{\cancel{60}} \text{ min}} \times \overset{1}{\cancel{60}} \text{ gtt/mL} = 40 \text{ gtt/min (adjusted flow rate)}$

Or, you know when drop factor is 60, then mL/h = gtt/min.

Step 3 $\frac{\text{Adjusted gtt/min} - \text{Ordered gtt/min}}{\text{Ordered gtt/min}} = \%\text{ of variation}$

$$\frac{40 - 50}{50} = \frac{-10}{50} = -0.2 = -20\% \text{ within the acceptable 25\% of variation}$$

Remember, the negative percent of variation (−20%) indicates that the adjusted flow rate will be decreased.

Recall that the recalculated flow rate should not vary from the original rate by more than 25%. If the recalculated rate does vary from the original by more than 25%, contact your supervisor or the prescriber for further instructions. The original order may have to be revised. Regular monitoring helps to prevent or minimize this problem.

Patients who require close monitoring for IV fluids will most likely have the IV regulated by an electronic infusion device. Because of the nature of their condition, "catching up" IVs, if off-schedule, is not recommended. If an IV regulated by an infusion pump or controller is off-schedule or inaccurate, suspect that the infusion pump may need recalibration. Consult with your supervisor, as appropriate.

QUICK REVIEW

- Regular IV monitoring and patient assessment at least every 30 minutes to 1 hour is important to maintain prescribed IV flow rate.
- Do not arbitrarily speed up or slow down IV flow rates that are off-schedule.
- Check hospital policy regarding adjustment of off-schedule IV flow rates and the percentage of variation allowed. If permitted, a rule of thumb is a maximum 25% variation for patients in stable condition.
- To recalculate off-schedule IV flow rate:

Step 1 $\frac{\text{Remaining volume}}{\text{Remaining hours}} = \text{Recalculated mL/h}$

Step 2 $\frac{V}{T} \times C = \text{gtt/min}$

Step 3 $\frac{\text{Adjusted gtt/min} - \text{Ordered gtt/min}}{\text{Ordered gtt/min}} = \text{\% variation}$

- Contact the prescriber for a new IV fluid order if the recalculated IV flow rate variation exceeds the allowed variation or if the patient's condition is unstable.

REVIEW SET 34

Compute the flow rate in drops per minute. Institution policy permits recalculation of IVs when off-schedule, with a maximum variation in rate of 25% for stable patients. Compute the percentage of variation.

1. Order: *1500 mL Lactated Ringer's IV for 12 h @ 125 mL/h*

   Drop factor: 10 gtt/mL

   Original flow rate: ________ gtt/min

   After 6 hours, there are 850 mL remaining; describe the appropriate nursing action now.

   Time remaining: ________ h

   Recalculated flow rate: ________ mL/h

   Recalculated flow rate: ________ gtt/min

   Variation: ________ %

   Action: ____

2. Order: *1000 mL Lactated Ringer's IV for 6 h @ 167 mL/h*

   Drop factor: 15 gtt/mL

   Original flow rate: ________ gtt/min

   After 4 hours, there are 360 mL remaining; describe the appropriate nursing action now.

   Time remaining: ________ h

   Recalculated flow rate: ________ mL/h

   Recalculated flow rate: ________ gtt/min

   Variation: ________ %

   Action: ____

3. Order: *1000 mL D_5W IV for 8 h @ 125 mL/h*

   Drop factor: 10 gtt/mL

   Original flow rate: ________ gtt/min

   After 4 hours, there are 800 mL remaining; describe the appropriate nursing action now.

   Time remaining: ________ h

   Recalculated flow rate: ________ mL/h

   Recalculated flow rate: ________ gtt/min

   Variation: ________ %

   Action: ____

4. Order: *2000 mL NS IV for 12 h @ 167 mL/h*

   Drop factor: 10 gtt/mL

   Original flow rate: ________ gtt/min

   After 8 hours, there are 750 mL remaining; describe the appropriate nursing action now.

   Time remaining: ________ h

   Recalculated flow rate: ________ mL/h

   Recalculated flow rate: ________ gtt/min

   Variation: ________ %

   Action: ____

5. Order: *1000 mL NS IV for 8 h @ 125 mL/h*

   Drop factor: 10 gtt/mL

   Original flow rate: ________ gtt/min

   After 4 hours, there are 750 mL remaining; describe the appropriate nursing action now.

   Time remaining: ________ h

   Recalculated flow rate: ________ mL/h

   Recalculated flow rate: ________ gtt/min

   Variation: ________ %

   Action: ____

6. Order: *2000 mL NS IV for 16 h @ 125 mL/h*

   Drop factor: 15 gtt/mL

   Original flow rate: ________ gtt/min

   After 6 hours, 650 mL of fluid have infused; describe the appropriate nursing action now.

   Solution remaining: ________ mL   Time remaining: ________ h

   Recalculated flow rate: ________ mL/h

   Recalculated flow rate: ________ gtt/min

   Variation: ________ %

   Action: ____

7. Order: *900 mL NS IV for 6 h @ 150 mL/h*

   Drop factor: 10 gtt/mL

   Original flow rate: ________ gtt/min

   After 3 hours, there are 700 mL remaining; describe the appropriate nursing action now.

   Time remaining: ________ h

   Recalculated flow rate: ________ mL/h

   Recalculated flow rate: ________ gtt/min

   Variation: ________ %

   Action: ____

8. Order: *500 mL D_5NS IV for 5 h @ 100 mL/h*

   Drop factor: 10 gtt/mL

   Original flow rate: ________ gtt/min

   After 2 hours, there are 250 mL remaining; describe the appropriate nursing action now.

   Time remaining: ________ h

   Recalculated flow rate: ________ mL/h

   Recalculated flow rate: ________ gtt/min

   Variation: ________ %

   Action: ____

9. Order: *1 L NS IV for 20 h @ 50 mL/h*

   Drop factor: 15 gtt/mL

   Original flow rate: ________ gtt/min

   After 10 hours, there are 600 mL remaining; describe the appropriate nursing action now.

   Time remaining: ________ h

   Recalculated flow rate: ________ mL/h

   Recalculated flow rate: ________ gtt/min

   Variation: ________ %

   Action: ____

10. Order: *1000 mL D_5W IV for 10 h @ 100 mL/h*

    Drop factor: 60 gtt/mL

    Original flow rate: ________ gtt/min

    After 5 hours, there are 500 mL remaining; describe the appropriate nursing action now.

    Time remaining: ________ h

    Recalculated flow rate: ________ mL/h

    Recalculated flow rate: ________ gtt/min

    Variation: ________ %

    Action: ____

After completing these problems, see pages 496–497 to check your answers.

INTERMITTENT IV INFUSIONS

Sometimes the patient requires supplemental fluid therapy or IV medications but does not need continuous replacement or maintenance IV fluids. Several intermittent IV infusion systems are available to administer IV drugs. These include IVPB, IV locks for IV push drugs, the ADD-Vantage system (see Figure 12-19), and volume control sets (such as a buretrol). Volume control sets are discussed in Chapter 13.

IV Piggybacks

A medication may be ordered to be dissolved in a small amount of IV fluid (usually 50 or 100 mL; however, piggyback bags are available in 25, 50, 100, and 250 mL) and run "piggyback" to the regular IV fluids (Figure 12-8). The amount of solution in the piggyback bag is determined by the medication being administered. The IV piggyback (IVPB) hangs higher than the primary line to provide increased pressure than the primary line, which allows the IVPB fluid to infuse first. Most IVPB sets have an extender so that the primary bag can be lowered.

The IVPB medication may come premixed by the manufacturer or pharmacy or the nurse may need to properly prepare it. Whichever the case, it is always the responsibility of the nurse to accurately and safely administer the medication. The infusion time may be less than 60 minutes, so it is important to carefully read the order and recommended infusion time.

Sometimes the patient care order for the IVPB medication will not include an infusion time or rate. When this is the case, it is understood that the nurse will follow the manufacturer's guidelines for infusion rates, keeping in mind the amount of fluid accompanying the medication and any standing orders that limit fluid amounts or rates. Appropriate infusion times are readily available in many drug reference books. Reference books are usually available on most nursing units, or you can consult with a hospital pharmacist.

Example 1:

Order: *cephazolin 0.5 g in 100 mL D_5W IVPB to run over 30 min*

Drop factor: 10 gtt/mL

What is the flow rate in gtt/min?

$$\frac{V}{T} \times C = \frac{100\ \cancel{mL}}{\underset{3}{\cancel{30}}\ \text{min}} \times \overset{1}{\cancel{10}}\ \text{gtt}/\cancel{mL} = \frac{100\ \text{gtt}}{3\ \text{min}} = 33.3\ \text{gtt/min} = 33\ \text{gtt/min}$$

Example 2:

If an infusion pump or controller is used to administer the same order as in Example 1, remember that you would need to program the device in *mL/h*.

Step 1 Think If 100 mL will be administered in 30 minutes or 1/2 hour, then 200 mL will be administered in 60 minutes or 1 hour.

Step 2 Calculate Use ratio-proportion to calculate mL/h.

$$\frac{100\ \text{mL}}{30\ \text{min}} \rightleftarrows \frac{X\ \text{mL}}{60\ \text{min}} \quad (1\ \text{h} = 60\ \text{min})$$

$$30X = 6000$$

$$\frac{30X}{30} = \frac{6000}{30}$$

$$X = 200\ \text{mL/h}$$

Set the electronic IVPB regulator to 200 mL/h.

Saline and Heparin IV Locks for IV Push Drugs

IV locks can be attached to the hub of the peripheral IV catheter that is positioned in the vein. The lock may be referred to as a *saline lock*, meaning that saline is used to flush or maintain the IV catheter patency, or a *heparin lock* if heparin is used to maintain the IV catheter patency. However, heparin is usually not required for the maintenance of peripheral IV locks. Sometimes a more general term, such as *intermittent peripheral infusion device*, may be used. Medications can be given *IV push*, meaning that a syringe is attached to the lock and medication is pushed in. An *IV bolus*, usually a quantity of IV fluid, can be run in over a specified period of time (such as 30 minutes to 1 hour) through an IV setup that is attached to the lock. Using an IV lock device allows for intermittent medication and fluid infusion. Many institutions are now recommending the use of 0.9% sodium chloride injection as a flush rather than heparin. The use of saline eliminates the risks associated with heparin use. Saline locks are also being used for outpatient and home care medication therapy. Refer to the policy at your hospital or healthcare agency regarding the frequency, volume, and concentration of saline or heparin to be used to maintain the IV lock.

> **CAUTION**
>
> Heparin lock flush solution is usually concentrated to 10 units/mL or 100 units/mL. Much higher concentrations of heparin are given IV or subcutaneously, so carefully check the concentration.

Dosage calculations for IV push injections are the same as calculations for intramuscular injections. The IV push route of administration is often preferred when immediate onset of action is desired for persons with small or wasted muscle mass, poor circulation, or for drugs that have limited absorption from body tissues.

Drug literature and institutional guidelines recommend an acceptable rate (per minute or per incremental amount of time) for IV push drug administration. Most timed IV push administration recommendations are for 1–5 minutes or more. For smooth manual administration of IV push drugs, calculate the incremental volume to administer over 15-second intervals. You should time the administration with a digital or sweep second-hand watch or clock.

> **CAUTION**
>
> IV drugs are potent and rapid acting. Never infuse IV push drugs more rapidly than recommended by institution policy or pharmacology literature. Some drugs require further dilution after reconstitution for IV push administration. Carefully read package inserts and reputable drug resources for minimum dilution and minimum time for IV administration. IV push drugs are usually administered by certified registered nurses in specialized and critical care units. Patients receiving IV push drugs often require additional monitoring.

Example 1:

Order: *lorazepam 3 mg IV push 20 min preoperatively*

Supply: lorazepam 4 mg/mL with drug literature guidelines of "IV infusion not to exceed 2 mg/min"

How much lorazepam should you prepare?

Step 1 **Convert** No conversion is necessary.

Step 2 **Think** You want to give less than 1 mL.

Step 3 **Calculate** $\frac{D}{H} \times Q = \frac{3 \not{mg}}{4 \not{mg}} \times 1 \text{ mL} = 0.75 \text{ mL}$

What is a safe infusion time?

Use $\frac{D}{H} \times Q$ to calculate the time required to administer the drug as ordered. In this problem, "Q" represents the quantity (or amount) of time for the supply rate: 1 min.

$$\frac{D}{H} \times Q = \frac{3\ \cancel{mg}}{4\ \cancel{mg}} \times 1\ min = \frac{3}{4}\ min = \frac{3}{4}\ min\ (45\ seconds)$$

Or use ratio-proportion to calculate the time required to administer the drug as ordered.

$$\frac{4\ mg}{1\ min} \nearrow\!\!\!\!\swarrow \frac{3\ mg}{X\ min}$$

$$4X = 3$$

$$\frac{4X}{2} = \frac{3}{2}$$

$$X = \frac{3}{4}\ min\ (45\ seconds)$$

Administer 0.75 mL over $\frac{3}{4}$ min. (45 seconds)

How much should you infuse every 15 seconds?

Convert: 1 min = 60 sec; $\frac{3}{4}$ min = 45 sec

$$\frac{0.75\ mL}{45\ sec} \nearrow\!\!\!\!\swarrow \frac{X\ mL}{15\ sec}$$

$$45X = 11.25$$

$$\frac{45X}{45} = \frac{11.25}{45}$$

$$X = 0.25\ mL$$

Administer 0.25 mL of lorazepam 4 mg/mL infused IV push every 15 seconds will deliver 3 mg of lorazepam.

This is a small amount. Use a 1-mL syringe to prepare 0.75 mL and slowly administer 0.13 mL every 15 seconds.

Example 2:

Order: *cefazolin 1500 mg IV push q8h*

Supply: cefazolin 1 g powder with directions, "For direct IV administration, reconstitute each 1 g in 10 mL sterile water and give slowly over 3–5 minutes."

How much cefazolin should you prepare?

Step 1 **Convert** 1 g = 1 × 1000 = 1000 mg

Step 2 **Think** If 1 g (or 1000 mg) requires 10 mL for dilution, then two 1 g vials will be required. Therefore, to administer 1500 mg, you will prepare more than 10 mL and less than 20 mL.

Step 3 **Calculate** $\frac{D}{H} \times Q = \frac{\overset{3}{\cancel{1500}}\ \cancel{mg}}{\underset{\underset{1}{\cancel{4}}}{\cancel{2000}}\ \cancel{mg}} \times \overset{5}{\cancel{20}}\ mL = 15\ mL$

What is a safe infusion time?

This amount is larger than the lorazepam dosage from Example 1, so you should use the longer infusion time recommendation (1 g per 5 min). Remember *Q* is the quantity of time to infuse the dosage you have on hand.

$$\frac{D}{H} \times Q = \frac{\overset{3}{\cancel{1500\ \text{mg}}}}{\underset{2}{\cancel{1000\ \text{mg}}}} \times 5\ \text{min} = \frac{15}{2}\ \text{min} = 7.5\ \text{min}$$

Administer 15 mL over 7.5 min.

How much should you infuse every 15 seconds?

Convert: 1 min = 60 sec

7.5 min = 7.5 × 60 = 450 sec

$$\frac{15\ \text{mL}}{450\ \text{sec}} \times \frac{X\ \text{mL}}{15\ \text{sec}}$$

450 X = 225

$$\frac{450\ X}{450} = \frac{225}{450}$$

Administer 0.5 mL of cefazolin 2 g/20 mL infused IV push every 15 seconds to deliver 1500 mg of cefazolin.

Reconstitute two vials of the medication as directed. *Use a 20-mL syringe to withdraw 15 mL and slowly infuse 0.5 mL every 15 seconds.*

ADD-Vantage System

Another type of IV medication setup commonly used in hospitals is the ADD-Vantage system by Abbott Laboratories (Figure 12-19). This system uses a specially designed IV bag with a medication vial port. The medication vial comes with the ordered dosage and medication prepared in a powder form. The medication vial is attached to the special IV bag, and together they become the IVPB container. The powder is dissolved by the IV fluid and used within a specified time. This system maintains asepsis and eliminates the extra time and equipment (syringe and diluent vials) associated with reconstitution of powdered medications. Several drug manufacturers currently market many common IV antibiotics using products similar to the ADD-Vantage system.

Premixed Intravenous Solutions

A large number of premixed IV solutions are available. There are some advantages to using prepared solutions. Usually such mixtures have a longer shelf life as they have been sterilized after the preparation process. The correct amount of medication has been added to the correct volume and type of IV solution, which decreases the time involved in preparing a medication. This is particularly important during an emergency situation when a patient requires fluids but also a medication to be administered quickly.

Premixed potassium chloride admixtures are available in several concentrations and various IV solutions. Examples of other medications premixed in IV solutions are heparin sodium, lidocaine hydrochloride, nitroglycerin, dobutamine hydrochloride, and dopamine hydrochloride. Medications such as levofloxacin and metoclopramide hydrochloride are also available premixed in minibags for single use. See Figure 12-18 for an example of the premixed medication levofloxacin, including preparation and administration instructions.

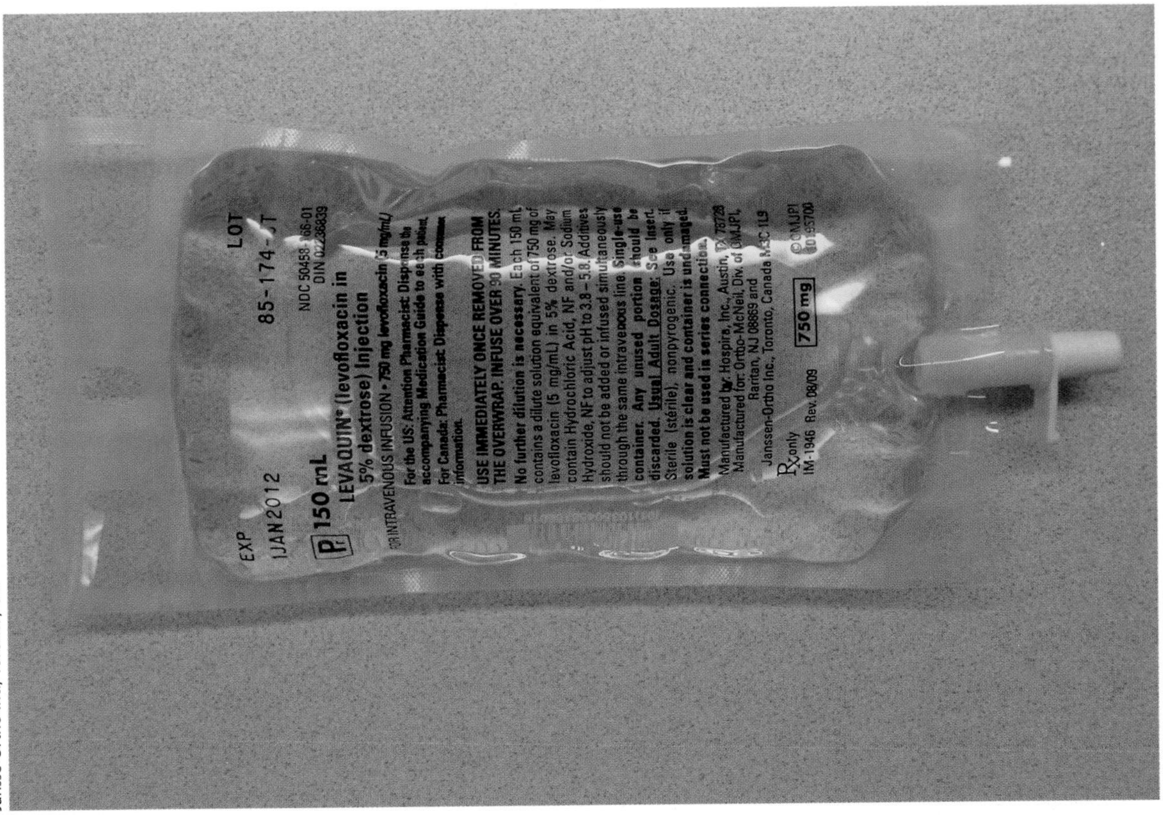

Jansse-Ortho Inc., Toronto, ON

Levofloxacin is an example of a premixed single-use flexible minibag, 5 mg/mL in 5% dextrose. It is available in 250 mg, 500 mg, and 750 mg of levofloxacin in 50 mL, 100 mL, and 150 mL, respectively. Instructions for use are as follows:

To open:

1. Tear outer wrap at the notch and remove solution container.
2. Check the container for minute leaks by squeezing the inner bag firmly. If leaks are found, or if the seal is not intact, discard the solution, as the sterility may be compromised.
3. Do not use if the solution is cloudy or a precipitate is present.
4. Use sterile equipment.
5. **WARNING: Do not use flexible containers in series connections.** Such use could result in air embolism due to residual air being drawn from the primary container before administration of the fluid from the secondary container is complete.

To administer:

1. Close flow control clamp of administration set.
2. Remove cover from port at bottom of container.
3. Insert piercing pin of administration set into port with a twisting motion until the pin is firmly seated.

NOTE: See full directions on administration set carton.

4. Suspend container from hanger.
5. Squeeze and release drip chamber to establish proper fluid level in chamber during infusion of levofloxacin injection in PREMIX flexible containers.
6. Open flow control clamp to expel air from set. Close clamp.
7. Regulate rate of administration with flow control clamp.

Jansse-Ortho Inc., Toronto, ON

FIGURE 12-18 Premixed Medication Solutions

QUICK REVIEW

- Intermittent IV infusions typically require more or less than 60 minutes of infusion time.
- Calculate IVPB flow rate in gtt/min: $\frac{V}{T} \times C = R$.
- Use a proportion to calculate IVPB flow rate in mL/h for an electronic infusion device.
- Use the three-step dosage calculation method to calculate the amount to give for IV push medications: convert, think, calculate ($\frac{D}{H} \times Q = X$).
- Use $\frac{D}{H} \times Q = X$ to calculate safe IV push time in minutes and seconds as recommended by reputable drug reference.

REVIEW SET 35

Calculate the IVPB or IV push flow rate.

1. Order: *cefazolin 1 g in 100 mL D_5W IVPB to be infused over 45 min*

   Drop factor: 60 gtt/mL

   Flow rate: ________ gtt/min

2. Order: *cefazolin 1 g in 100 mL D_5W IVPB to be administered by electronic infusion controller to infuse in 45 min*

   Flow rate: ________ mL/h

3. Order: *cefazolin 2 g IVPB diluted in 50 mL D_5W to infuse in 15 min*

   Drop factor: 15 gtt/mL

   Flow rate: ________ gtt/min

4. Order: *cefazolin 2 g IVPB diluted in 50 mL D_5W to infuse in 15 min by an electronic infusion pump*

   Flow rate: ________ mL/h

5. Order: *50 mL IVPB antibiotic solution to infuse in 30 min*

   Drop factor: 60 gtt/mL

   Flow rate: ________ gtt/min

6. Order: *piperacillin/tazobactam 3 g in 100 mL D_5W IVPB to be infused over 40 min*

   Drop factor: 10 gtt/mL

   Flow rate: ________ gtt/min

7. Order: *cefazolin 1.5 g in 50 mL D_5W IVPB to be infused over 15 min*

   Drop factor: 15 gtt/mL

   Flow rate: ________ gtt/min

8. Order: *meropenem 1 g in 100 mL D_5W IVPB to be infused over 30 min*

   Use infusion pump.

   Flow rate: ________ mL/h

9. Order: *cefazolin 750 mg in 50 mL NS IVPB to be infused over 20 min*

   Use infusion pump.

   Flow rate: ________ mL/h

10. Order: *oxacillin sodium 900 mg in 125 mL D_5W IVPB to be infused over 45 min*

    Use infusion pump.

    Flow rate: ________ mL/h

11. Order: *cefazolin 0.5 g in 100 mL D_5W IVPB to be infused over 15 min*

    Drop factor: 10 gtt/mL

    Flow rate: ________ gtt/min

12. Order: *cefazolin 500 mg in 50 mL NS IVPB to be infused over 20 min*

    Drop factor: 10 gtt/mL

    Flow rate: ________ gtt/min

13. Order: *meropenem 1 g in 100 mL D_5W IVPB to be infused over 50 min*

    Use infusion pump.

    Flow rate: ________ mL/h

14. Order: *ampicillin 900 mg in 125 mL D_5W IVPB to be infused over 20 min*

    Drop factor: 10 gtt/mL

    Flow rate: ________ gtt/min

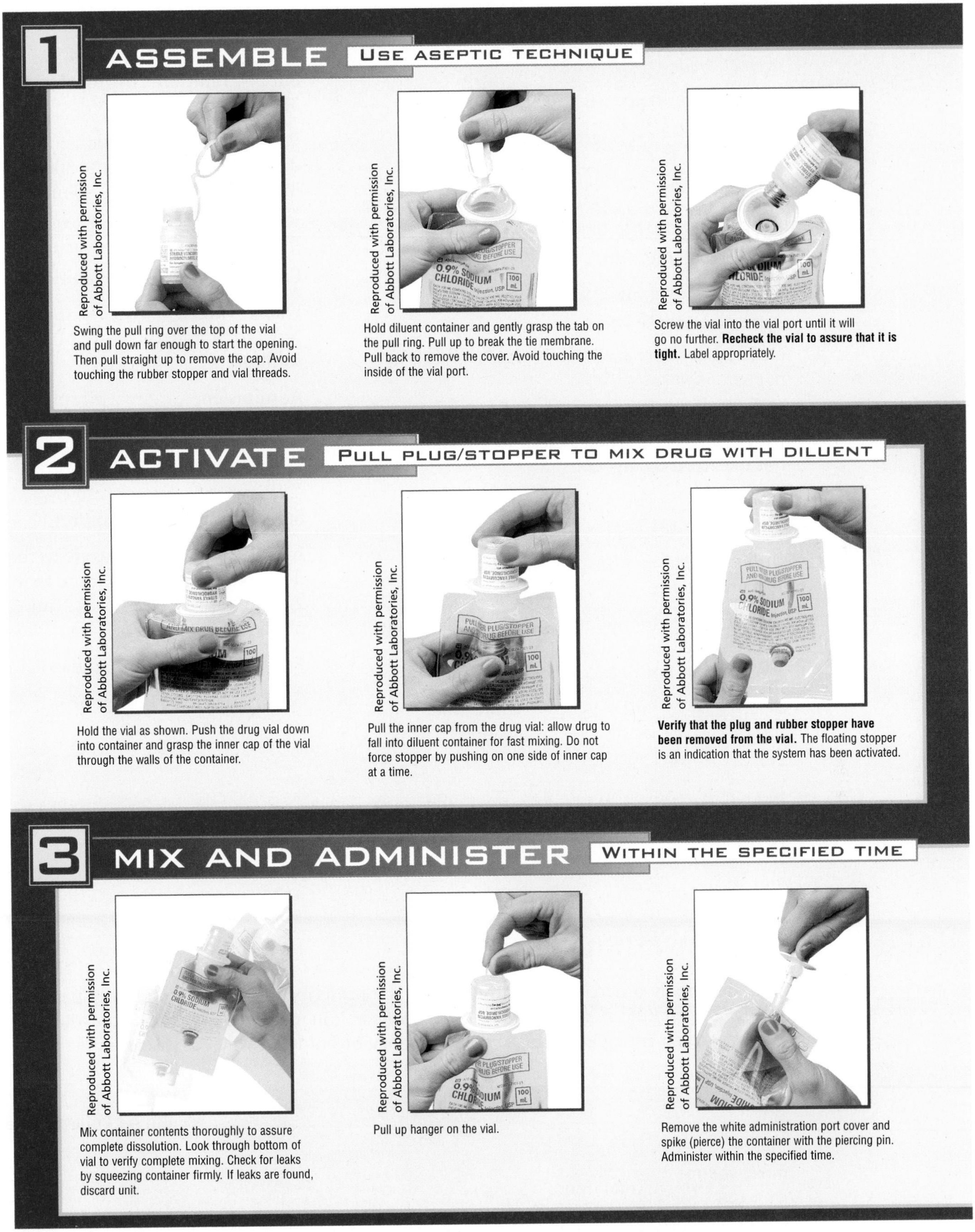
1 ASSEMBLE USE ASEPTIC TECHNIQUE
Reproduced with permission of Abbott Laboratories, Inc.
Swing the pull ring over the top of the vial and pull down far enough to start the opening. Then pull straight up to remove the cap. Avoid touching the rubber stopper and vial threads.
Reproduced with permission of Abbott Laboratories, Inc.
Hold diluent container and gently grasp the tab on the pull ring. Pull up to break the tie membrane. Pull back to remove the cover. Avoid touching the inside of the vial port.
Reproduced with permission of Abbott Laboratories, Inc.
Screw the vial into the vial port until it will go no further. Recheck the vial to assure that it is tight. Label appropriately.
2 ACTIVATE PULL PLUG/STOPPER TO MIX DRUG WITH DILUENT
Reproduced with permission of Abbott Laboratories, Inc.
Hold the vial as shown. Push the drug vial down into container and grasp the inner cap of the vial through the walls of the container.
Reproduced with permission of Abbott Laboratories, Inc.
Pull the inner cap from the drug vial: allow drug to fall into diluent container for fast mixing. Do not force stopper by pushing on one side of inner cap at a time.
Reproduced with permission of Abbott Laboratories, Inc.
Verify that the plug and rubber stopper have been removed from the vial. The floating stopper is an indication that the system has been activated.
3 MIX AND ADMINISTER WITHIN THE SPECIFIED TIME
Reproduced with permission of Abbott Laboratories, Inc.
Mix container contents thoroughly to assure complete dissolution. Look through bottom of vial to verify complete mixing. Check for leaks by squeezing container firmly. If leaks are found, discard unit.
Reproduced with permission of Abbott Laboratories, Inc.
Pull up hanger on the vial.
Reproduced with permission of Abbott Laboratories, Inc.
Remove the white administration port cover and spike (pierce) the container with the piercing pin. Administer within the specified time.

FIGURE 12-19 ADD-Vantage System: Medications Can Be Added to Another Solution Being Infused

15. Order: *piperacillin/tazobactam 1.3 g in 100 mL D_5W IVPB to be infused over 30 min*

    Drop factor: 60 gtt/mL

    Flow rate: _________ gtt/min

16. Order: *furosemide 120 mg IV push stat*

    Supply: furosemide 10 mg/mL with drug insert, which states, "IV injection not to exceed 40 mg/min."

    Give: _________ mL/ _________ min or _________ mL/15 sec

17. Order: *phenytoin sodium 150 mg IV push stat*

    Supply: phenytoin sodium 250 mg/5 mL with drug insert, which states, "IV infusion not to exceed 50 mg/min."

    Give: _________ mL/ _________ min or _________ mL/15 sec

18. Order: *morphine sulfate 6 mg IV push q3h prn, pain*

    Supply: morphine sulfate 10 mg/mL with drug reference recommendation, which states, "IV infusion not to exceed 2.5 mg/min."

    Give: _________ mL/ _________ min and _________ sec or _________ mL/15 sec

19. Order: *ranitidine hydrochloride 300 mg IV push stat*

    Supply: ranitidine hydrochloride 300 mg/2 mL

    Package insert instructions: "For direct IV injection, dilute 300 mg in 0.9% NaCl to a total volume of 20 mL. Inject over at least 2 minutes."

    Prepare _________ mL ranitidine.

    Dilute with _________ mL 0.9% NaCl for a total of 20 mL of solution.

    Administer _________ mL/min or _________ mL/15 sec.

20. Order: *midazolam 1.5 mg IV push stat*

    Supply: midazolam 1 mg/mL

    Instructions: "Slowly titrate to the desired effect using no more than 2.5 mg initially given over 2-min period."

    Prepare _________ mL midazolam.

    Give _________ mL/min or _________ mL/15 sec.

After completing these problems, see pages 497–498 to check your answers.

CALCULATING IV INFUSION TIME

IV solutions are usually ordered to be administered at a prescribed number of millilitres per hour, such as *1000 mL Lactated Ringer's IV to run at 125 mL per hour.* You may need to calculate the total infusion time so that you can anticipate when to add a new bag or bottle, or when to discontinue the IV.

RULE

To calculate IV infusion time:

- $\frac{\text{Total volume}}{\text{L/h}} = \text{Total hours}$

Or use ratio-proportion—ratio for prescribed flow rate in mL/h = ratio for total mL per X total hours:

- $\frac{\text{mL}}{\text{h}} = \frac{\text{Total mL}}{\text{X Total h}}$

Example 1:

1000 mL LR IV to run at 125 mL/h. How long will this IV last?

$$\frac{\overset{8}{\cancel{1000}}\ \cancel{\text{mL}}}{\underset{1}{\cancel{125}}\ \cancel{\text{mL}}/\text{h}} = 8\ \text{h}$$

Or, use ratio-proportion.

$$\frac{125\ \text{mL}}{1\ \text{h}} = \frac{1000\ \text{mL}}{\text{X h}}$$

$$125\text{X} = 1000$$

$$\frac{125\text{X}}{125} = \frac{1000}{125}$$

$$\text{X} = 8\ \text{h}$$

Example 2:

1000 mL D_5W IV to infuse at 60 mL/h to begin at 0600. At what time will this IV be complete?

$$\frac{1000\ \cancel{\text{mL}}}{60\ \cancel{\text{mL}}/\text{h}} = 16.67\ \text{h} = 16\frac{2}{3}\ \text{h} = \frac{2}{3}\ \text{h} = \frac{2}{3} \times 60 = 40\ \text{min; total time:16 h and 40 min}$$

Or, use ratio-proportion:

$$\frac{60\ \text{mL}}{1\ \text{h}} \times \frac{1000\ \text{mL}}{\text{X h}}$$

$$60\ \text{X} = 1000$$

$$\frac{60\text{X}}{60} = \frac{1000}{60}$$

$$\text{X} = 16.6\ \text{h} = 16\frac{2}{3}\ \text{h} = 16\ \text{h and 40 min}$$

The IV will be complete at 0600 + 1640 = 2240 (or 10:40 PM).

You can also determine the infusion time if you know the volume, flow rate in gtt/min, and drop factor. Calculate the infusion time by using the $\frac{V}{T} \times C = R$ formula; T, time in minutes, is unknown.

RULE

Use the formula method to calculate time (T):

$$\frac{V}{T} \times C = R$$

Example:

80 mL D_5W IV at 20 microdrops/min

The drop factor is 60 gtt/mL. Calculate the infusion time.

Step 1 $\frac{V}{T} \times C = R$: $\frac{80\ \text{mL}}{\text{T min}} \times 60\ \text{gtt/mL} = 20\ \text{gtt/min}$

$$\frac{80\ \cancel{\text{mL}}}{\text{T min}} \times \frac{60\ \text{gtt}}{1\ \cancel{\text{mL}}} = \frac{20\ \text{gtt}}{1\ \text{min}}$$

$$\frac{4800 \text{ gtt}}{\text{T min}} = \frac{20 \text{ gtt}}{1 \text{ min}}$$

Then you apply ratio-proportion.

$$\frac{4800}{\text{T}} \times \frac{20}{1}$$

$$20\text{T} = 4800$$

$$\frac{20\text{T}}{20} = \frac{4800}{20}$$

$$\text{T} = 240 \text{ min}$$

Step 2 Convert: minutes to hours

$$240 \text{ min} = \frac{240}{60} = 4 \text{ h}$$

CALCULATING IV FLUID VOLUME

If you have an IV that is regulated at a particular flow rate (gtt/min) and you know the drop factor (gtt/mL) and the amount of time, you can determine the volume to be infused.

Apply the flow rate formula; V, volume, is unknown.

RULE

To calculate IV volume (V):

$$\frac{\text{V}}{\text{T}} \times \text{C} = \text{R}$$

Example:

When you start your shift at 0700, there is an IV bag of D_5W *infusing at the rate of 25 gtt/min*. The infusion set is calibrated for a drop factor of *15 gtt/mL*. How much can you anticipate that the patient will receive during your 8-hour shift?

$$8 \text{ h} = 8 \times 60 = 480 \text{ min}$$

$$\frac{\text{V}}{\text{T}} \times \text{C} = \text{R}: \frac{\text{V mL}}{480 \text{ min}} \times 15 \text{ gtt/mL} = 25 \text{ gtt/min}$$

$$\frac{\text{V } \cancel{\text{mL}}}{480 \text{ min}} \times \frac{15 \text{ gtt}}{1 \cancel{\text{mL}}} = \frac{25 \text{ gtt}}{1 \text{ min}}$$

$$\frac{15\text{V gtt}}{480 \text{ min}} = \frac{25 \text{ gtt}}{1 \text{ min}}$$

$$\frac{15\text{V}}{480} \times \frac{25}{1}$$

$$15\text{V} = 12\,000$$

$$\frac{15\text{V}}{15} = \frac{12\,000}{15}$$

$$\text{V} = 800 \text{ mL to be infused in 8 h}$$

If the IV is regulated in millilitres per hour, you can also calculate the total volume that will infuse over a specific time.

RULE

To calculate IV volume:
Total hours × mL/h = Total volume
Or use ratio-proportion:
Ratio for ordered mL/h = Ratio for X total volume per total hours

$$\frac{\text{mL}}{\text{h}} = \frac{\text{X Total mL}}{\text{Total h}}$$

Example:

Your patient's IV is running on an infusion pump set at the rate of 100 mL/h. How much will be infused during the next 8 hours?

$8 \cancel{h} \times 100 \text{ mL}/\cancel{h} = 800 \text{ mL}$

Or, use ratio-proportion:

$$\frac{100 \text{ mL}}{1 \text{ h}} = \frac{\text{X mL}}{8 \text{ h}}$$

X = 800 mL

QUICK REVIEW

- The formula to calculate IV infusion time, when mL is known:

  $\frac{\text{Total volume}}{\text{mL/h}} = \text{Total hours}$

  or use ratio-proportion: $\frac{\text{mL}}{\text{h}} = \frac{\text{Total mL}}{\text{X total h}}$
- The formula to calculate IV infusion time, when flow rate in gtt/min, drop factor, and volume are known: $\frac{V}{T} \times C = R$; "T" is the unknown.
- The formula to calculate total infusion volume, when mL/h is known:

  Total hours × mL/h = Total volume

  Or, use ratio-proportion: $\frac{\text{mL}}{\text{h}} = \frac{\text{X total mL}}{\text{Total h}}$
- The formula to calculate IV volume, when flow rate (gtt/min), drop factor, and time are known: $\frac{V}{T} \times C = R$; "V" is the unknown.

REVIEW SET 36

Calculate the infusion time and rate (as requested) for the following IV orders:

1. Order: *500 mL D_5W at 30 gtt/min*

   Drop factor: 10 gtt/mL

   Time: ________ h and ________ min
2. Order: *1000 mL Lactated Ringer's at 25 gtt/min*

   Drop factor: 10 gtt/mL

   Time: ________ h and ________ min

3. Order: *800 mL D_5 Lactated Ringer's at 25 gtt/min*

   Drop factor: 15 gtt/mL

   Time: ________ h

4. Order: *120 mL normal saline to run at 20 mL/h*

   Drop factor: 60 microdrops/mL

   Time: ________ h

   Flow rate: ______ gtt/min

5. Order: *80 mL D_5W to run at 20 mL/h*

   Drop factor: 60 microdrops/mL

   Time: ________ h

   Flow rate: ________ gtt/min

Calculate the completion time for the following IVs.

6. At 1600 h the nurse started an IV of 1200 mL D_5W at 27 gtt/min. The infusion set used is calibrated for a drop factor of 15 gtt/mL.

   Infusion time: ________ h

   Completion time: ________

7. At 1530 h the nurse starts 2000 mL of D_5W to run at 125 mL/h. The infusion set used is calibrated for a drop factor of 10 gtt/mL.

   Infusion time: ________ h

   Completion time: ________

Calculate the total volume (mL) to be infused per 24 hours.

8. An IV of D_5 Lactated Ringer's is infusing on an electronic infusion pump at 125 mL/h.

   Total volume: ________ mL/24 h

9. An IV is flowing at 12 gtt/min and the infusion set has a drop factor of 15 gtt/mL.

   Total volume: ________ mL/24 h

10. IV: D_5W

    Flow rate: 21 gtt/min

    Drop factor: 10 gtt/mL

    Total volume: ________ mL/24 h

Calculate IV volume for the following IVs.

11. *0.9% sodium chloride IV infusing at 65 mL/h for 4 h*

    Volume: ________ mL

12. *D_5W IV infusing at 150 mL/h for 2 h*

    Volume: ________ mL

13. *D_5LR IV at 75 mL/h for 8 h*

    Volume: ________ mL

14. *D_5 0.225% NaCl IV at 40 gtt/min for 8 h*

    Drop factor: 60 gtt/mL

    Infusion time: ________ min

    Volume: ________ mL

15. *0.45% NaCl IV at 45 gtt/min for 4 h*

    Drop factor: 10 gtt/mL

    Infusion time: ________ min

    Volume: ________ mL

After completing these problems, see pages 498–499 to check your answers.

CRITICAL THINKING SKILLS

It is important to know the equipment you are using. An example in which the nurse was unfamiliar with the IVPB setup follows.

error

Failing to follow manufacturer's directions when using a new IVPB system.

possible scenario

Suppose the physician ordered ceftriaxone sodium 1 g IV q12h for an older adult patient with streptococcus pneumonia. The medication was sent to the unit by pharmacy utilizing the ADD-Vantage system. Ceftriaxone sodium 1 g was supplied in a powder form and attached to a 50-mL IV bag of D_5W. The directions for preparing the medication were attached to the label. The nurse, who was unfamiliar with the new ADD-Vantage system, hung the IV medication, calculated the drip rate, and infused the 50 mL of fluid. The nurse cared for the patient for 3 days. During walking rounds on the third day, the oncoming nurse noticed that the ceftriaxone sodium powder remained in the vial and never was diluted in the IV bag. The nurse realized that the vial stopper inside of the IV bag was not open. Therefore, the medication powder was not mixed in the IV fluid during this shift for the past 3 days.

potential outcome

The omission by the nurse resulted in the patient missing 3 doses of the ordered IV antibiotic. The delay in the medication administration could have serious consequences for the patient, such as worsening of the pneumonia, septicemia, and even death, especially in older adults. The patient received one-half of the daily dose ordered by the physician for 3 days. The physician would be notified of the error and likely order additional diagnostic studies, such as chest X-ray, blood cultures, and an additional one-time dose of ceftriaxone sodium.

prevention

This error could easily have been avoided had the nurse read the directions for preparing the medication or consulted with another nurse who was familiar with the system.

PRACTICE PROBLEMS—CHAPTER 12

Compute the flow rate in drops per minute or millilitres per hour as requested. For these situations, hospital policy permits recalculating IVs when off-schedule with a maximum variation in rate of 25%.

1. Order: *ampicillin 500 mg dissolved in 200 mL D_5W IV to run for 2 h*

   Drop factor: 10 gtt/mL

   Flow rate: ________ gtt/min

2. Order: *1000 mL D_5W IV per 24h*

   Drop factor: 60 gtt/mL

   Flow rate: ________ gtt/min

3. Order: *1500 mL D_5LR IV to run for 12 h*

   Drop factor: 10 gtt/mL

   Flow rate: ________ gtt/min

4. Order: *200 mL D_5RL IV for 24 h*

   Drop factor: 60 gtt/mL

   Flow rate: ________ gtt/min

5. Order: *1 L $D_{10}W$ IV to run from 1000 to 1800 h*

   Drop factor: On electronic infusion pump

   Flow rate: ________ mL/h

6. See question 5. At 1100 h, 800 mL remains. Describe the appropriate nursing action now.

   ____

   ____

7. Order: *1000 mL NS followed by 2,000 mL D_5W IV to run for 24 h*

   Drop factor: 15 gtt/mL

   Flow rate: ________ gtt/min

8. Order: *2.5 L NS IV to infuse at 125 mL/h*

   Drop factor: 10 gtt/mL

   Flow rate: ________ gtt/min

9. Order: *1000 mL D_5W IV for 6 h*

   Drop factor: 15 gtt/mL

   After 2 hours, 800 mL remains. Describe the appropriate nursing action now. ________________

   ____

The IV tubing package in the accompanying figure is the IV system available in the hospital for manually regulated, straight gravity flow IV administration with macrodrop. The patient has an order for *500 mL D_5W IV q4h* written at 1515 h and the nurse starts the IV at 1530 h. Questions 10 through 20 refer to this situation.

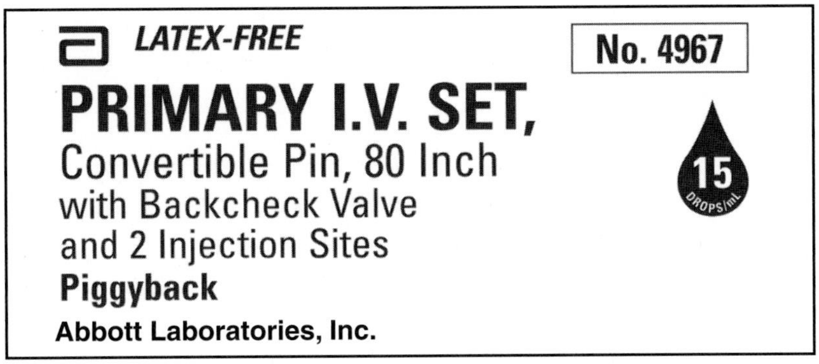

10. How much IV fluid will the patient receive in 24 hours? ________ mL
11. Who is the manufacturer of the IV infusion set tubing? ________
12. What is the drop factor calibration for the IV infusion set tubing? ________
13. What is the drop factor constant for the IV infusion set tubing? ________
14. Using the shortcut (drop factor constant) method, calculate the flow rate of the IV as ordered. Show your work.

    Shortcut method calculation: ________

    Flow rate: ________ gtt/min
15. Using the formula method, calculate the flow rate of the IV as ordered. Show your work.

    Formula method calculation: ________

    Flow rate: ________ gtt/min
16. At what time should the nurse anticipate the first IV bag of 500 mL D_5W will be completely infused? ________
17. How much IV fluid should be infused by 1730? ________ mL
18. At 1730 h the nurse notices that the IV has 210 mL remaining. After assessing the patient and confirming that her condition is stable, what should the nurse do? ________

    ____
19. After consulting the physician, the nurse decides to use an electronic controller to better regulate the flow rate. The physician orders an infusion of infuse 500 mL every 4 hours. The nurse should set the controller for ________ mL/h.
20. The next day the physician adds the order *ampicillin 250 mg in 50 mL D_5W IVPB to infuse in 30 min QID*. The patient is still on the IV controller. To infuse the IVPB, the nurse should set the controller for ________ mL/h.
21. List the components and concentration strengths of the fluid $D_{2.5}\frac{1}{2}$ NS.

    ____
22. Calculate the amount of dextrose and sodium chloride in D_5NS 500 mL.

    dextrose ________ g

    NaCl ________ g
23. Define a central line. ________

    ____

24. Define a primary line. ______________________________

____

25. Describe the purpose of a saline lock. ______________________________

____

26. A safe IV push infusion rate of protamine sulfate is 5 mg/min. What is a safe infusion time to administer 50 mg? ________ min

Protamine sulfate is available in a supply dosage of 10 mg/mL. To administer 50 mg IV push, prepare ________ mL and inject slowly IV at the rate of ________ mL/min or ________ mL/15 sec.

27. Describe the purpose of the patient-controlled analgesia pump. ______________________________

____

28. Identify two advantages of the syringe pump. ______________________________

____

29. List two complications of IV sites. ______________________________

____

30. How often should the IV site be monitored? ______________________________

____

31. Describe the purpose of the Y-set IV system. ______________________________

____

For each IV order in questions 32 through 43, use the drop factor to calculate the flow rate in gtt/min.

Order: *1 L hyperalimentation solution IV to infuse in 12 h*

32. Drop factor 10 gtt/mL Flow rate: ________ gtt/min

33. Drop factor 15 gtt/mL Flow rate: ________ gtt/min

34. Drop factor 60 gtt/mL Flow rate: ________ gtt/min

Order: *2 L D_5NS IV to infuse in 20 h*

35. Drop factor 10 gtt/mL Flow rate: ________ gtt/min

36. Drop factor 15 gtt/mL Flow rate: ________ gtt/min

37. Drop factor 60 gtt/mL Flow rate: ________ gtt/min

Order: *1000 mL of 0.45% NaCl IV @ 200 mL/h*

38. Drop factor 10 gtt/mL Flow rate: ________ gtt/min

39. Drop factor 15 gtt/mL Flow rate: ________ gtt/min

40. Drop factor 60 gtt/mL Flow rate: ________ gtt/min

Order: *540 mL D_5 0.33% NaCl IV @ 45 mL/h*

41. Drop factor 10 gtt/mL Flow rate: ________ gtt/min

42. Drop factor 15 gtt/mL Flow rate: ________ gtt/min

43. Drop factor 60 gtt/mL Flow rate: ________ gtt/min

44. You make rounds before your lunch break and find that a patient has 150 mL of IV fluid remaining. The flow rate is 25 gtt/min. The drop factor is 10 gtt/mL. What volume will be infused during the hour that you are at lunch? _________ mL What should you alert the relief nurse to watch for while you are off the unit? ______________________________

45. Your shift is 0700–1500 h. You make rounds at 0730 h and find an IV of D_5 0.45% NaCl is regulated on an electronic infusion pump at the ordered rate of 75 mL/h with 400 mL remaining. The order specifies a continuous infusion. At what time should you anticipate hanging the next IV bag? _________

46. Critical Thinking Skill: Describe the strategy you would implement to prevent this medication error.

possible scenario

Suppose the physician ordered *D_5LR at 125 mL/h* for an older adult patient just returning from the operating room following abdominal surgery. The nurse gathered the IV solution and IV tubing, which had a drop factor of 10 gtt/mL. The nurse did not check the package for the drop factor and assumed it was 60 gtt/mL. The manual rate was calculated this way:

$$\frac{125\ \cancel{mL}}{\cancel{60}\ min} \times \cancel{60}\ gtt/\cancel{mL} = 125\ gtt/min$$

The nurse infused the D_5LR at 125 gtt/min for 8 hours. While giving report to the oncoming nurse, the patient called for the nurse, complaining of shortness of breath. On further assessment the nurse heard crackles in the patient's lungs and noticed that the patient's third 1000-mL bottle of D_5LR this shift was nearly empty already. At this point the nurse realized the IV rate was in error. The nurse was accustomed to using the 60-gtt/mL IV set up and therefore calculated the drip rate using the 60 gtt/mL (microdrop) drop factor. However, the tubing used delivered a 10-gtt/mL (macrodrop) drop factor.

potential outcome

The patient developed signs of fluid overload and could have developed congestive heart failure due to the excessive IV rate. The physician would have been notified and likely ordered furosemide (a diuretic) to help eliminate the excess fluid. The patient likely would have been transferred to the ICU for closer monitoring.

prevention

____

____

Upon completion of these problems, see pages 499–501 to check your answers.

CHAPTER

13

Body Surface Area and Advanced Pediatric Calculations

LEARNING OBJECTIVES

1. Determine the body surface area (BSA) using a calculation formula or a nomogram scale.
2. Compute the safe amount of drug to be administered when ordered according to the BSA.
3. Calculate intermittent intravenous (IV) medications administered with IV infusion control sets.
4. Calculate the amount to mix proportionate IV additive medications into small-volume IV solutions.
5. Calculate the minimal and maximal dilution in which an IV medication can be safely prepared and delivered, such as via a syringe pump.
6. Calculate pediatric IV maintenance fluids.

The focus of this chapter is on additional and more advanced calculations used frequently by pediatric nurses. It will help you understand the unique drug and fluid management required by a growing child. Further, these concepts, which are most commonly related to children, are also applied to adults in special situations. Let us start by looking at the BSA method of calculating a dosage and checking for the accuracy and safety of a particular drug order.

BODY SURFACE AREA METHOD

The BSA is an important measure in calculating dosages for infants and children. BSA is also used for select adult populations, such as those undergoing open-heart surgery or radiation therapy, severe burn victims, and those with kidney disease. Regardless of age, chemotherapy drugs and an increasing number of other highly potent drug classifications are being prescribed based on BSA.

BSA is a mathematical estimate using the patient's *height* and *weight*. BSA is expressed in metres squared (**m²**). BSA can be determined by formula calculation or by using a chart, referred to as a *nomogram*, that estimates the BSA. Because drug dosages recommended by BSA measurement are potent, and because the formula calculation is the most accurate, we will begin with the formulas. In most situations, the prescribing practitioner will compute the BSA for drugs ordered by this method. However, the nurse who administers the drug is responsible for verifying safe dosage, which may require calculating the BSA.

BSA Formula

The BSA formula is based on the metric measurement of height in centimetres and weight in kilograms. This is easy to compute using the square root function on a calculator.

RULE

To calculate BSA in m² based on *metric measurement* of height and weight:

- **BSA (m²)** $= \sqrt{\dfrac{\text{ht (cm)} \times \text{wt (kg)}}{3600}}$

Next, we will apply the formula and see how the BSA measurements compare.

Example 1:

Use the metric formula to calculate the BSA of an infant whose length is 50 cm and weight is 6.8 kg.

$$\text{BSA (m}^2) = \sqrt{\frac{\text{ht (cm)} \times \text{wt (kg)}}{3600}} = \sqrt{\frac{50 \times 6.8}{3600}} = \sqrt{\frac{340}{3600}} = \sqrt{0.094} = 0.307 \text{ m}^2 = 0.31 \text{ m}^2$$

MATH TIP

To perform BSA calculations using the metric formula on most calculators, follow this sequence: multiply height in *cm* by weight in *kg*, divide by 3600, press =, then press $\sqrt{\ }$ to arrive at m². Round m² to hundredths (two decimal places). For example 1, enter 50 × 6.8 ÷ 3600 = 0.094, and press $\sqrt{\ }$ to arrive at 0.307, rounded to 0.31 m².

Or use the BSA formula based on household measurement.

$$\text{BSA (m}^2) = \sqrt{\frac{\text{ht (in)} \times \text{wt (lb)}}{3131}} = \sqrt{\frac{20 \times 15}{3131}} = \sqrt{\frac{300}{3131}} = \sqrt{0.095} = 0.309 \text{ m}^2 = 0.31 \text{ m}^2$$

Example 2:

Calculate the BSA of a child whose height is 105 cm and weight is 31.8 kg.

Metric:

$$\text{BSA (m}^2) = \sqrt{\frac{\text{ht (cm)} \times \text{wt (kg)}}{3600}} = \sqrt{\frac{105 \times 31.8}{3600}} = \sqrt{\frac{3339}{3600}} = \sqrt{0.927} = 0.963 \text{ m}^2 = 0.96 \text{ m}^2$$

Example 3:

Calculate the BSA of an adult whose height is 173 cm and weight is 88.8 kg.

Metric:

$$\text{BSA (m}^2) = \sqrt{\frac{\text{ht (cm)} \times \text{wt (kg)}}{3600}} = \sqrt{\frac{173 \times 88.8}{3600}} = \sqrt{\frac{15362.4}{3600}} = \sqrt{4.267} = 2.065 \text{ m}^2 = 2.07 \text{ m}^2$$

BSA Nomogram

Some practitioners use a chart called a *nomogram* that *estimates* the BSA by plotting the height and weight and simply connecting the dots with a straight line. Figure 13-1 shows the most well-known BSA chart, the West Nomogram. It is used for both children and adults for heights up to 240 cm, and weights up to 80 kg.

WEST NOMOGRAM

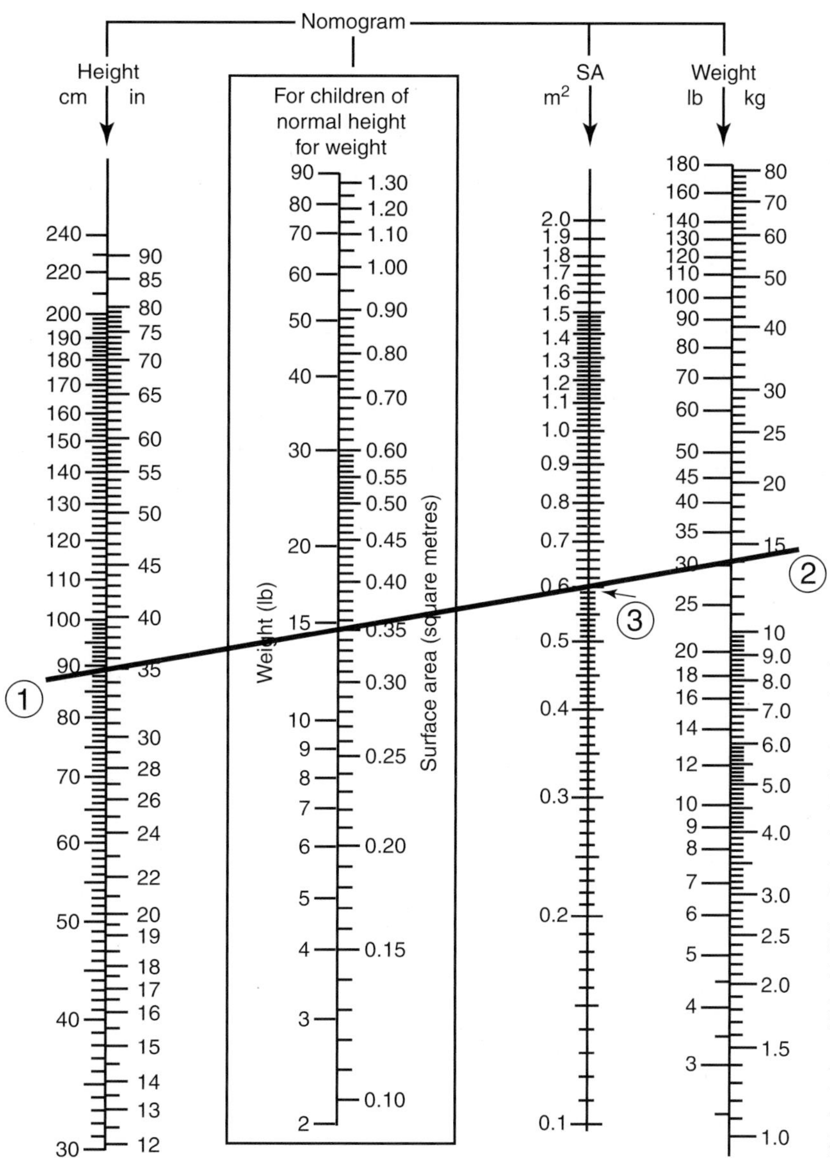

This chart was published in Nelson Textbook of Pediatrics, 16th ed., R. E. Behrman, R. M. Kliegman & H. B. Jenson, West Nomogram for Estimation of Body Surface Area, Copyright Elsevier, (2000).

FIGURE 13-1 Body surface area (BSA) is determined by drawing a straight line from the patient's height (1) in the far left column to her weight (2) in the far right column. Intersection of the line with the surface area (SA) column (3) is the estimated BSA (m^2). For infants and children of normal height and weight, BSA may be estimated from weight alone by referring to the enclosed area.

> **CAUTION**
>
> Notice that the increments of measurement and the spaces on the BSA nomogram are not consistent. Be sure you correctly read the numbers and the calibration values between them.

For a child of normal height for weight, the BSA can be determined on the West Nomogram using the weight alone. Notice the enclosed column to the centre left. Normal height and weight standards can be found on pediatric growth and development charts.

CAUTION

To use the normal column on the West Nomogram, you must be familiar with normal height and weight standards for children. If you are unsure, use both height and weight to estimate BSA. Do not guess.

QUICK REVIEW

- BSA is used to calculate select dosages across the life span, most often for children.
- BSA is calculated by height and weight and expressed in metres squared (m^2).
- The following metric formula is the preferred method of calculating BSA:

  Metric: $\text{BSA } (m^2) = \sqrt{\dfrac{\text{ht (cm)} \times \text{wt (kg)}}{3600}}$

- Nomograms can be used to estimate BSA, by correlating height and weight measures to m^2.

REVIEW SET 37

Use the formula method to determine the BSA. Round to two decimal places.

1. An adult measures 190 cm tall and weighs 105 kg. ________ m^2
2. A child measures 94 cm tall and weighs 18 kg. ________ m^2
3. A teenager measures 153 cm tall and weighs 46 kg. ________ m^2
4. An adult measures 175 cm tall and weighs 85 kg. ________ m^2
5. An adult measures 62 inches tall and weighs 140 lb. ________ m^2
6. A teenager measures 160 cm tall and weighs 64 kg. ________ m^2
7. A child measures 65 cm tall and weighs 15 kg. ________ m^2
8. A child measures 92 cm tall and weighs 24 kg. ________ m^2

Find the BSA on the West Nomogram (Figure 13-1) for a child of normal height and weight.

9. 4 lb ________ m^2
10. 42 lb ________ m^2
11. 17 lb ________ m^2

Find the BSA on the West Nomogram (Figure 13-1) for children with the following height and weight.

12. 41 inches and 32 lb ________ m^2
13. 140 cm and 30 kg ________ m^2
14. 80 cm and 11 kg ________ m^2
15. 106 cm and 25 kg ________ m^2

After completing these problems, see page 502 to check your answers.

BSA Dosage Calculations

Once the BSA is obtained, the drug dosage can be verified by consulting a reputable drug resource for the recommended dosage. Package inserts, the *Hospital Formulary*, or other dosage handbooks contain pediatric and adult dosages. Remember to carefully read the reference to verify if the drug dosage is calculated in *m^2 per dose* or *m^2 per day.*

RULE

To verify safe pediatric dosage based on BSA:

1. Determine BSA in m^2.
2. Calculate the safe dosage based on **BSA: $mg/m^2 \times m^2 = X$ mg**
3. Compare the ordered dosage to the recommended dosage, and decide if the dosage is safe.
4. If the dosage is safe, calculate the amount to give and administer the dose. If the dosage seems unsafe, consult with the ordering practitioner before administering the drug.

Note: Recommended dosage may specify mg/m^2, mcg/m^2, g/m^2, $units/m^2$, $microunits/m^2$, or mEq/m^2.

Example 1:

A child is 126 cm tall and weighs 23 kg. Drug order: *vincristine 1.8 mg IV at 1000*. Is this dosage safe for this child? The recommended dosage as noted on the package insert is 2 mg/m^2. Supply: See label, Figure 13-2.

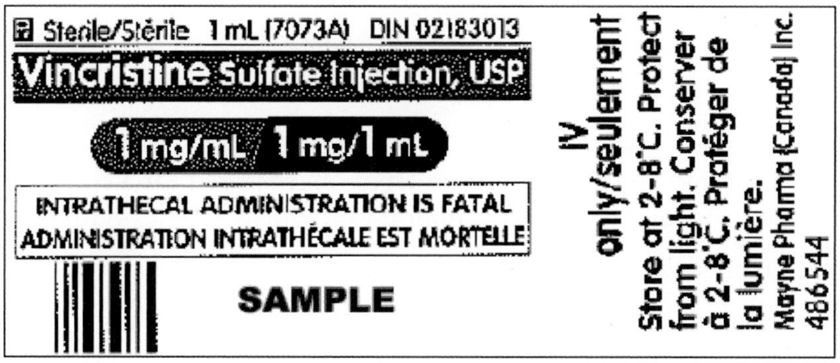

Mayne Pharma (Canada) Inc., Montreal, QUE

FIGURE 13-2 Vincristine Label

1. **Determine BSA.** The child's BSA is 0.9 m^2 (using the metric BSA formula).

$$\text{BSA } (m^2) = \sqrt{\frac{\text{ht (cm)} \times \text{wt (kg)}}{3600}} = \sqrt{\frac{126 \times 23}{3600}} = \sqrt{\frac{2898}{3600}} = \sqrt{0.805} = 0.897 \text{ m}^2 = 0.9 \text{ m}^2$$

2. **Calculate recommended dosage.** $mg/m^2 \times m^2 = 2 \text{ mg}/\cancel{m^2} \times 0.9 \cancel{m^2} = 1.8$ mg
3. **Decide if the dosage is safe.** The dosage ordered is 1.8 mg and 1.8 mg is the amount recommended by BSA. The dosage is safe. How much should you give?
4. **Calculate one dose.**

Step 1 Convert No conversion is necessary.

Step 2 Think You want to give more than 1 mL and less than 2 mL.

Step 3 Calculate $\frac{D}{H} \times Q = \frac{1.8 \cancel{mg}}{\cancel{1} \cancel{mg}} \times \cancel{1} \text{ mL} = 1.8 \text{ mL}$

Or, use ratio-proportion.

$$\frac{1 \text{mg}}{1 \text{mL}} = \frac{1.8 \text{ mg}}{X \text{ mL}}$$

X = 1.8 mL

Example 2:

A 2-year-old child with herpes simplex is 35 inches tall and weighs 30 lb. The drug order is *acyclovir 100 mg IV BID*. Is this order safe? The recommendation from the drug reference is 250 mg/m^2 q8h for children younger than 12 years and older than 6 months. Acyclovir is supplied as a 500-mg injection with directions to reconstitute with 10 mL sterile water for injection for a concentration of 50 mg/mL.

1. **Determine BSA.** The child's BSA is 0.6 m^2 (using the West Nomogram, Figure 13-1).
2. **Calculate recommended dosage.** $mg/m^2 \times m^2 = 250\ mg/\cancel{m^2} \times 0.6\ \cancel{m^2} = 150\ mg$
3. **Decide if the dosage is safe.** The dosage of 100 mg BID is not safe—the single dosage is too low. Further, the drug should be administered three times per day q8h, not BID or two times per day.
4. **Confer with the prescriber.**

QUICK REVIEW

- Safe dosage based on BSA: $mg/m^2 \times m^2$, compared to recommended dosage.

REVIEW SET 38

1. What is the dosage of one dose of interferon alpha-2b required for a child with a BSA of 0.82 m^2 if the recommended dosage is 2 million units/m^2? ________ units
2. What is the total daily dosage range of mitomycin required for a child with a BSA of 0.59 m^2 if the recommended dosage range is 10–20 mg/m^2/day? ________ mg/day to ________ mg/day
3. What is the dosage of a drug required for an adult with a BSA of 1.47 m^2 if the recommended dosage is 500 mg/m^2? ________ mg
4. What is the daily dosage of cyclophosphamide required for an adult with a BSA of 2.64 m^2 if the recommended dosage is 600 mg/m^2 for one dose on day 1? ________ mg/day
5. What is the dosage of acyclovir required for a child with a BSA of 1 m^2, if the recommended dosage is 250 mg/m^2? ________ mg
6. Child is 30 inches tall and weighs 25 pounds.

   Order: *acyclovir 122.5 mg IV q8h*

   Supply: acyclovir 500 mg with directions to reconstitute with 10 mL sterile water for injection for a final concentration of 50 mg/mL

   Recommended dosage from drug insert: 250 mg/m^2

   BSA = ________ m^2

   Recommended dosage for this child: ________ mg

   Is the ordered dosage safe? ________

   If safe, give ________ mL.

   If not safe, what should the nurse do? ____________________

7. Child is 114 cm tall and weighs 25 kg.

   Order: *methotrexate 2.9 mg IV daily*

   Supply: methotrexate 2.5 mg/mL

   Recommended dosage from drug insert: 3.3 mg/m^2

   BSA = ________ m^2

   Recommended dosage for this child: ________ mg

   Is the ordered dosage safe? ________

   If safe, give ________ mL.

   If not safe, what should the nurse do? ________________________________

8. Order: *diphenhydramine 22 mg IV q8h*. Child has BSA of 0.44 m^2. Recommended safe dosage of diphenhydramine is 150 mg/m^2/day in divided dosages every 8 hours.

   Recommended daily dosage for this child: ________ mg/day

   Recommended single dosage for this child: ________ mg/dose

   Is the ordered dosage safe? ________

   If not safe, what should the nurse do? ________________________________

9. Order: *quinidine 198 mg PO; daily for 5 days*. Child has BSA of 0.22 m^2. Recommended safe dosage of quinidine is 900 mg/m^2/day given in five daily doses.

   Recommended dosage for this child: ________ mg/dose

   Is the dosage ordered safe? ________

   If not safe, what should the nurse do? ________

   How much quinidine would this child receive over 5 days of therapy? ________ mg

10. Order: *deferoxamine mesylate IV per protocol*. Child has BSA of 1.02 m^2.

    Protocol: 600 mg/m^2 initially followed by 300 mg/m^2 at 4-hour intervals for 2 doses; then give 300 mg/m^2 q12h for 2 days. Calculate the total dosage received.

    Initial dosage: ________ mg

    Two q4h dosages: ________ mg

    Two days of q12h dosages: ________ mg

    Total dosage child would receive: ________ mg

11. Protocol: *fludarabine 10 mg/m² bolus over 15 minutes followed by a continuous IV infusion of 30.5 mg/m²/day*. Child has BSA of 0.81 m^2. The bolus dosage is ________ mg, and the continuous 24-hour IV infusion will contain ________ mg of fludarabine.

12. Order: *drug X 83.75 mg IV q12h* for a child with a BSA of 0.67 m^2. The recommended dosage range is 100–250 mg/m^2/day in two divided doses.

    Recommended daily dosage range for this child: ________ mg/day to ________ mg/day

    Recommended single dosage range for this child: ________ mg/dose to ________ mg/dose

    Is the ordered dosage safe? ________

    If not, what should the nurse do? ________________________________

13. Order: *daunorubicin 9.6 mg IV on day 1 and day 8 of cycle.*

    Protocol: 25–45 mg/m^2 on days 1 and 8 of cycle. Child has BSA of 0.32 m^2.

    Recommended dosage range for this child: ________ mg/dose to ________ mg/dose

    Is the ordered dosage safe? ________

    If not safe, what should the nurse do? ________________________________

Answer questions 14 and 15 based on the following information.

The recommended dosage of pegaspargase is 2500 units/m^2/dose IV daily × 14 days for adults and children with a BSA more than 0.6 m^2.

Supply: pegaspargase 750 units/mL with directions to dilute in 100 mL D_5W and give over 2 hours. The nurse will administer the drug via infusion pump.

14. Order: *Give pegaspargase 2050 units IV today at 1600 h*. Child is 100 cm tall and weighs 24 kg. The child's BSA is ________ m^2.

    The recommended dosage for this child is ________ units. Is the ordered dosage of pegaspargase safe? ________

    If yes, add ________ mL of pegaspargase for a total IV fluid volume of ________ mL. Set the IV infusion pump at ________ mL/h.

    If the order is not safe, what should the nurse do? ________

15. Order: *pegaspargase 4050 units IV stat* for an adult patient who is 162 cm tall and weighs 58.2 kg. The patient's BSA is ________ m^2. The recommended dosage of pegaspargase for this adult is ________ units.

    Is the ordered dosage of pegaspargase safe? ________

    If safe, the nurse should add ________ mL of pegaspargase for a total IV fluid volume of ________ mL. Set the infusion pump at ________ mL/h.

    If the order is not safe, what should the nurse do? ________________________________

After completing these problems, see page 502 to check your answers.

PEDIATRIC VOLUME CONTROL SETS

Volume control sets (see Figure 13-3) are most frequently used to administer hourly fluids and intermittent IV medications to children. The fluid chamber will hold 100–150 mL of fluid to be infused in a specified time period as ordered, usually in 60 minutes or less. The medication is added to the IV fluid in the chamber for a prescribed dilution volume.

The volume of fluid in the chamber is filled by the nurse every 1–2 hours or as needed. Only small, ordered quantities of fluid are added, and the clamp above the chamber is fully closed. The IV bag acts only as a reservoir to hold future fluid infusions. The patient is protected from receiving more volume than intended. This is especially important for children, because they can tolerate only a narrow range of fluid volume. This differs from standard IV infusions that run directly from the IV bag through the drip chamber and IV tubing into the patient's vein.

Volume control sets may also be used to administer intermittent IV medications to adults with fluid restrictions, such as for heart or kidney disease. An electronic controller or pump may also be used to regulate the flow rate. When used, the electronic device will alarm when the chamber empties.

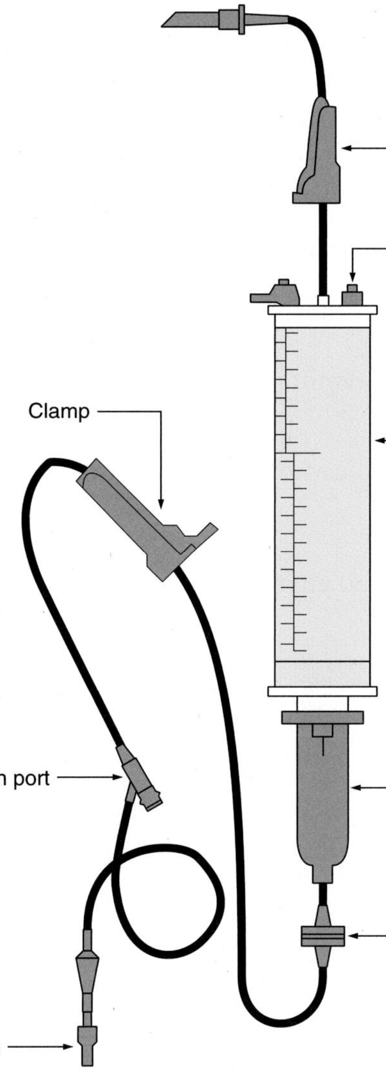

FIGURE 13-3 Volume Control Set

Intermittent IV Medication Infusion via Volume Control Set

Children receiving IV medications may have a saline lock in place of a continuous IV infusion. The nurse will inject the medication into the volume control set chamber, add an appropriate volume of IV fluid to dilute the drug, and attach the IV tubing to the child's IV lock to infuse over a specified period of time. After the chamber has emptied and the medication has infused, a flush of IV fluid is given to be sure all the medication has cleared the tubing. Realize that when the chamber empties, some medication still remains in the drip chamber, IV tubing, and the IV lock above the child's vein. There is no standard amount of fluid used to flush peripheral or central IV lines. Because tubing varies by manufacturer, the flush can vary from 15 mL to as much as 50 mL, according to the overall length of the tubing and extra extensions added. Verify the institution policy on the correct volume to flush peripheral and central IV lines in children. For the purpose of sample calculations, this text uses a 15-mL volume to flush a peripheral IV line, unless specified otherwise.

To calculate the IV flow rate for the volume control set, you must consider the total fluid volume of the medication, the IV fluid used for dilution, and the volume of IV flush fluid. Volume control sets are microdrip sets with a drop factor of 60 gtt/mL.

Example:

Order: *cefotaxime sodium 250 mg IV q6h in 50 mL $D_5\frac{1}{4}$ NS to infuse in 30 min followed by a 15-mL flush.* Child has a saline lock.

Supply: See label.

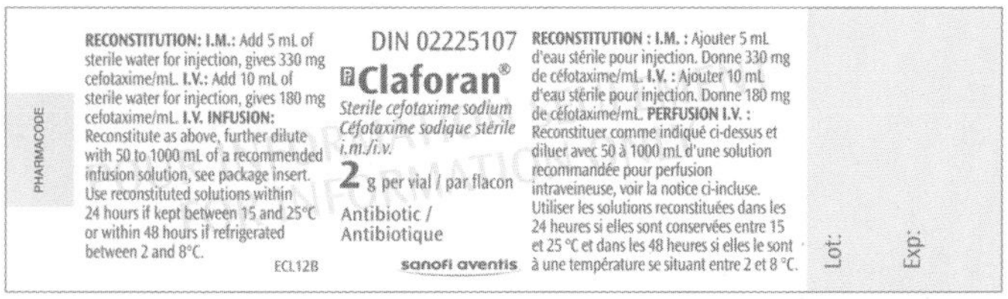

Instructions from package insert for IV use: Add 10 mL diluent for a total volume of 11 mL with a concentration of 180 mg/mL.

Step 1 Calculate the total volume of the intermittent IV medication and the IV flush. 50 mL + 15 mL = 65 mL

Step 2 Calculate the flow rate of the IV medication and the IV flush. Remember: The drop factor is 60 gtt/mL.

$$\frac{V}{T} \times C = \frac{65\text{ mL}}{\cancel{30}_{1}\text{ min}} \times \overset{2}{\cancel{60}}\text{ gtt/}\cancel{\text{mL}} = 130\text{ gtt/min}$$

Step 3 Calculate the volume of the medication to be administered.

$$\frac{D}{H} \times Q = \frac{250\ \cancel{\text{mg}}}{180\ \cancel{\text{mg}}} \times 1\text{ mL} = 1.39\text{ mL} = 1.4\text{ mL}$$

Step 4 Add 1.4 mL cefotaxime sodium 2 g to the chamber and fill with IV fluid to a volume of 50 mL. This provides the prescribed total volume of 50 mL in the chamber.

Step 5 Set the flow rate of the 50 mL of intermittent IV medication for 130 gtt/min. Follow with the 15-mL flush also set at 130 gtt/min. When complete, detach IV tubing, and follow saline lock policy.

The patient may also have an intermittent medication ordered as part of a continuous infusion at a prescribed IV volume per hour. In such cases, the patient is to receive the same fluid volume each hour, regardless of the addition of intermittent medications. This means that the total prescribed fluid volume must include the intermittent IV medication volume.

Example:

Order: *D_5NS IV at 30 mL/h for continuous infusion and methylprednisolone acetate 30 mg IV q8h over 30 min*

Supply: See label, Figure 13-4.

An infusion controller is in use with the volume control set.

Step 1 Calculate the dilution volume required to administer the methylprednisolone acetate at the prescribed continuous flow rate of 30 mL/h.

Think If 30 mL infuses in 1 hour, then $\frac{1}{2}$ of 30, or 15 mL, will infuse in $\frac{1}{2}$ hour or 30 minutes.

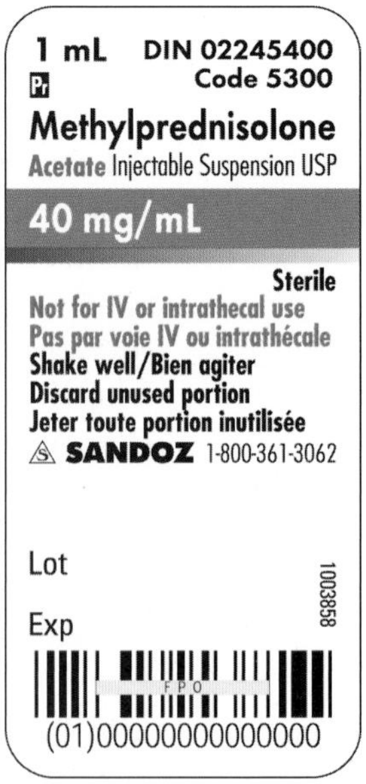

FIGURE 13-4
Gentamicin Label

Calculate Use ratio-proportion to verify your estimate.

$$\frac{30 \text{ mL}}{60 \text{ min}} \times \frac{X \text{ mL}}{30 \text{ min}}$$

$$60X = 900$$

$$\frac{60X}{60} = \frac{900}{60}$$

$$X = 15 \text{ mL in } 30 \text{ min}$$

Therefore, the IV fluid dilution volume required to administer 30 mg of methylprednisolone acetate in 30 minutes is 15 mL to maintain the prescribed, continuous infusion rate of 30 mL/h.

Step 2 Determine the volume of methyprednisolone acetate and IV fluid to add to the volume control chamber.

$$\frac{D}{H} \times Q = \frac{\overset{3}{\cancel{30} \cancel{\text{mg}}}}{\underset{4}{\cancel{40} \cancel{\text{mg}}}} \times 1 \text{ mL} = \frac{3}{4} \text{ mL} = 0.75 \text{ mL}$$

Add 0.75 mL methyprednisolone acetate and fill the chamber with D_5NS to the total volume of 15 mL.

Step 3 Set the controller to 30 mL/h in order to deliver 15 mL of intermittent IV methylprednisolone acetate solution in 30 minutes. Resume the regular IV, which will also flush out the tubing. The continuous flow rate will remain at 30 mL/h.

QUICK REVIEW

- Volume control sets have a drop factor of 60 gtt/mL.
- The total volume of the medication, IV dilution fluid, and the IV flush fluid must be considered to calculate flow rates when using volume control sets.
- Use ratio-proportion to calculate flow rates for intermittent medications when a continuous IV rate in mL/h is prescribed.

REVIEW SET 39

Calculate the IV flow rate to administer the following IV medications by using a volume control set, and determine the amount of IV fluid and medication to be added to the chamber. The ordered time includes the flush volume.

1. Order: *amikacin 125 mg IV q8h in 50 mL* $D_5\frac{1}{3}$ *NS over 45 min. Flush with 15 mL.*

   Supply: amikacin 250 mg/mL

   Flow rate: ________ gtt/min

   Add ________ mL medication and add IV fluid to make a total of ________ mL in the chamber.

2. Order: *cefuroxime sodium 500 mg IV q6h in 50 mL $D_5 \frac{1}{4}$ NS over 30 min. Flush with 15 mL.*

   Supply: cefuroxime sodium 750 mg vial. Reconstitute with 8.0 mL for injection to yield 90-mg/mL solution.

   Flow rate: ________ gtt/min

   Add ________ mL medication and add IV fluid to make a total of ________ mL in the chamber.

3. Order: *ampicillin 150 mg IV BID in 25 mL 0.9% NaCl over 20 min. Flush with 15 mL.*

   Supply: ampicillin 250 mg/3 mL

   Flow rate: ________ gtt/min

   Add ________ mL medication and add IV fluid to make a total of ________ mL in the chamber.

4. Order: *cefazolin sodium 0.6 g IV q12h in 50 mL D_5NS over 60 min on an infusion pump. Flush with 30 mL.*

   Supply: cefazolin sodium 1 g/10 mL

   Flow rate: ________ mL/h

   Add ________ mL medication and add IV fluid to make a total of ________ mL in the chamber.

5. Order: *clindamycin phosphate 150 mg IV q8h in 32 mL D_5NS over 60 min on an infusion pump. Flush with 28 mL.*

   Supply: clindamycin phosphate 150 mg/mL

   Flow rate: ________ mL/h

   Add ________ mL medication and add IV fluid to make a total of ________ mL in the chamber.

   Total IV volume after three doses are given is ________ mL.

   Calculate the amount of IV fluid to be added to the volume control chamber.

6. Order: *0.9% NaCl at 50 mL/h for continuous infusion with cefazolin sodium 250 mg IV q8h to be infused over 30 min by volume control set.*

   Supply: cefazolin 125 mg/mL

   Add ________ mL medication and add IV fluid to make a total of ________ mL in the chamber.

7. Order: *D_5W at 30 mL/h for continuous infusion with dexamethasone sodium phosphate 2 mg BID to be infused over 20 min by volume control set.*

   Supply: dexamethasone sodium phosphate 4 mg/mL

   Add ________ mL medication and add IV fluid to make a toal of ________ mL in the chamber.

8. Order: *D_5 0.225% NaCl IV at 85 mL/h with erythromycin 600 mg IV q6h to be infused over 40 min by volume control set.*

   Supply: erythromycin 50 mg/mL

   Add ________ mL medication and add IV fluid to make a total of ________ mL in the chamber.

9. Order: *D_5 0.33% NaCl IV at 66 mL/h with ceftazidime 720 mg IV q8h to be infused over 40 min by volume control set.*

   Supply: ceftazidime 1 g/10 mL

   Add ________ mL medication and add IV fluid to make a total of ________ mL in the chamber.

10. Order: *D_5 0.45% NaCl IV at 90 mL/h with cefotetan disodium 1 g IV q6h to be infused over 30 min by volume control set.*

    Supply: cefotetan disodium 1 g/vial. Add 10 mL to provide 10.5 mL of volume.

    Add ________ mL medication and add IV fluid to make a total of ________ mL in the chamber.

After completing these problems, see pages 502–503 to check your answers.

MINIMAL DILUTIONS FOR IV MEDICATIONS

Intravenous medications in infants and young children (or adults on limited fluids) are often ordered to be given in the smallest volume or *maximal safe concentration* to prevent fluid overload. Consult a pediatric reference, *Hospital Formulary*, or drug insert to assist you in problem solving. These types of medications are usually given via an electronic pump.

Many pediatric IV medications allow a dilution *range* or a minimum and maximum allowable concentration. A solution of *lower* concentration may be given if the patient can tolerate the added volume (called *minimal safe concentration, maximal dilution,* or *largest volume*). A solution of *higher* concentration (called *maximal safe concentration, minimal dilution,* or *smallest volume*) must not exceed the recommended dilution instructions. Recall that the greater the volume of diluent or solvent, the less concentrated the resulting solution. Likewise, less volume of diluent or solvent results in a more concentrated solution.

CAUTION

An excessively high concentration of an IV drug can cause vein irritation and potentially life-threatening toxic effects. Dilution calculations are critical skills.

Let us examine how to follow the drug reference recommendations for a minimal IV drug dilution, when a minimal and maximal range is given for an IV drug dilution.

RULE

Ratio for recommended drug dilution equals ratio for desired drug dilution.

Example 1:

The physician orders *vancomycin 40 mg IV q12h* for an infant who weighs 4000 g. What is the minimal amount of IV fluid in which the vancomycin can be safely diluted? The package insert is provided for your reference (Figure 13-5). It indicates that a "concentration of no more than 10 mg/mL is recommended." This is the *maximal safe concentration.*

$$\frac{10\ \text{mg}}{1\ \text{mL}} \times \frac{40\ \text{mg}}{X\ \text{mL}}$$

$$10X = 40$$

$$\frac{10X}{10} = \frac{40}{10}$$

$X = 4$ mL (This is the minimal amount of IV fluid.)

DOSAGE AND ADMINISTRATION
Each dose should be administered at a rate of no more than 10 mg/min or over a period of at least 60 minutes.

Intravenous Dosage
Adults: The usual intravenous dose is 500 mg every 6 hours or 1 g every 12 hours. Other patient factors such as age or obesity may call for modification of the usual intravenous daily dose.

Adults with Impaired Renal Function: To avoid toxic serum levels, dosage adjustment is required in patients with impaired renal function. Since accumulation in such patients has been reported to occur over several weeks of treatment, serum levels should be checked regularly.

The dosage calculation may be made by using the following nomogram if the creatinine clearance value is known for most patients with renal impairment or the elderly:

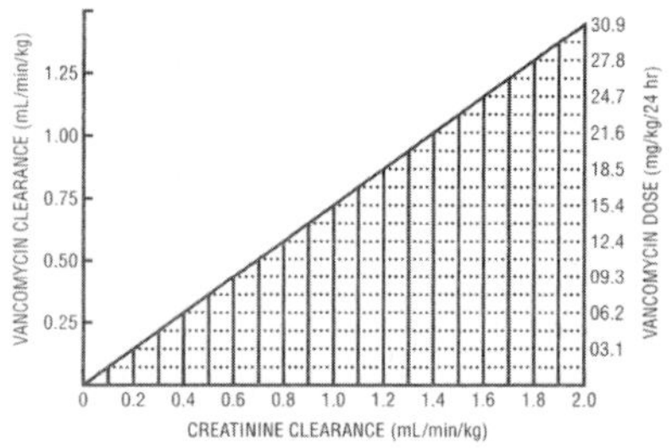

(Moellering et al. 1981)

For functionally anephric patients on dialysis, the nomogram is not valid. In order to achieve therapeutic serum levels promptly in such patients, a loading dose of 15 mg/kg of body weight should be given. The dose required to maintain stable serum levels is 1.9 mg/kg/24 h.

When only serum creatinine is available, the conversion of this value into estimated creatinine clearance may be accomplished by using the following formula based on sex, weight and age of the patient.

A steady state of renal function is represented by the serum creatinine.

Males: $\frac{\text{Weight (kg)} \times (140 - \text{age})}{72 \times \text{serum creatinine}}$

Females: 0.85 x above value

Neonates, Infants and Children: The dosage schedule which follows has been used. Infusions can be divided and incorporated in the child's 24-hour fluid requirement and should be infused over 60 minutes.

Infants and Neonates: It is suggested that an initial dose of 15 mg/kg be administered followed by 10 mg/kg every twelve hours for neonates in the first week of life and every eight hours thereafter up to the age of one month. Each dose should be given over 60 minutes. Close monitoring of serum concentrations of vancomycin may be warranted in these patients.

Children: The usual i.v. dosage of vancomycin is 10 mg/kg given every six hours.

The majority of patients with infections caused by organisms susceptible to the antibiotic demonstrate a therapeutic response by 48 to 72 hours. The total duration of therapy is determined by the type and severity of the infection and the clinical response of the patient. In staphylococcal endocarditis, therapy for three weeks or longer is recommended.

Oral Dose
Vancomycin, when administered orally, is to be used only in the treatment of staphylococcal enterocolitis, and/or pseudomembranous colitis associated with toxigenic *Clostridium difficile*.

Adults: The usual daily dose for antibiotic-associated colitis and/or staphylococcal enterocolitis is 125-500 mg orally every 6-8 hours for 7-10 days.

Children: The usual daily dosage is approximately 40 mg/kg in 3 or 4 divided doses for 7-10 days. The total daily dose should not exceed 2 g.

FIGURE 13-5 Portion of Vancomycin Package Insert

Example 2:

The physician orders *cefotaxime sodium 1.2 g IV q8h* for a child who weighs 36 kg. The recommended safe administration of cefotaxime sodium for intermittent IV administration is a final concentration of 20–60 mg/mL to infuse over 15–30 minutes. What is the minimal amount of IV fluid to safely dilute this dosage? (*Remember this represents the* ***maximal safe concentration.***)

Step 1 Convert 1.2 g = 1.2 × 1000 = 1200 mg

Step 2 Think 1200 is more than 10 times 60, in fact it is 20 times 60. So you need at least 20 mL to dilute the drug.

Step 3 Calculate

$$\frac{60\ \text{mg}}{1\ \text{mL}} \times \frac{1200\ \text{mg}}{X\ \text{mL}}$$

$$60X = 1200$$

$$\frac{60X}{60} = \frac{1200}{60}$$

$X = 20$ mL (minimal dilution for maximal safe concentration)

What is the maximal amount of IV fluid recommended to safely dilute this drug to the minimal safe concentration?

Step 1 Convert 1.2 g = 1.2 × 1000 = 1200 mg

Step 2 Think 1200 is more than 50 times 20; in fact, it is 60 times 20. So you can use up to 60 mL to dilute the drug.

Step 3 Calculate

$$\frac{20\ \text{mg}}{1\ \text{mL}} \times \frac{1200\ \text{mg}}{X\ \text{mL}}$$

$$20X = 1200$$

$$\frac{20X}{20} = \frac{1200}{20}$$

$X = 60$ mL (maximal dilution for minimal safe concentration)

CALCULATION OF DAILY VOLUME FOR MAINTENANCE FLUIDS

Another common pediatric IV calculation is to calculate 24-hour maintenance IV fluids for children.

RULE

Use this formula to calculate the daily rate of pediatric maintenance IV fluids:

- **100 mL/kg/day or 4 mL/kg/h for first 10 kg of body weight**
- **50 mL/kg/day or 2 mL/kg/h for 11–20 kg of body weight**
- **20 mL/kg/day or 1 mL/kg/h for each kilogram above 20 kg of body weight**

This formula uses the child's weight in kilograms to estimate the 24-hour total fluid need, including oral intake. It does not include replacement for losses, such as diarrhea, vomiting, or fever. This accounts only for fluid needed to maintain normal cellular metabolism and fluid turnover.

Pediatric IV solutions that run over 24 hours usually include a combination of glucose, saline, and potassium chloride and are *hypertonic* solutions (see Figure 12-1, page 315). Dextrose (glucose) for energy is usually concentrated between 5% and 12% for peripheral infusions. Sodium chloride is usually concentrated between 0.225% and 0.9% ($\frac{1}{4}$ NS up to NS). Further, 20 mEq per litre of potassium chloride (20 mEq KCl/L) is usually added to continuous pediatric infusions. Any dextrose and saline combination without potassium should be used only as an intermittent or short-term IV fluid in children. Be wary of isotonic solutions like 5% dextrose in water and 0.9% sodium chloride. They do not contribute enough electrolytes and can quickly lead to water intoxication.

CAUTION

A *red flag* should be raised if either plain 5% dextrose in water or 0.9% sodium chloride (normal saline) is running continuously on an infant or child. Consult the ordering practitioner immediately!

Let us examine the daily rate of maintenance fluids and the hourly flow rate for the children in the following examples.

Example 1:

Child who weighs 6 kg

$100 \text{ mL}/\cancel{\text{kg}}/\text{day} \times 6 \ \cancel{\text{kg}} = 600 \text{ mL/day or per 24 h}$

$$\frac{600 \text{ mL}}{24 \text{ h}} = 25 \text{ mL/h}$$

Example 2:

Child who weighs 12 kg

$100 \text{ mL}/\cancel{\text{kg}}/\text{day} \times 10 \ \cancel{\text{kg}} = 1000 \text{ mL/day (for first 10 kg)}$

$50 \text{ mL}/\cancel{\text{kg}}/\text{day} \times 2 \ \cancel{\text{kg}} = 100 \text{ mL/day (for the remaining 2 kg)}$

Total: 1000 mL/day + 100 mL/day = 1000 mL/day or per 24 h

$$\frac{1100 \text{ mL}}{24 \text{ h}} = 45.8 \text{ mL/h} = 46 \text{ mL/h}$$

Example 3:

Child who weighs 24 kg

100 mL/~~kg~~/day × 10 ~~kg~~ = 1000 mL/day (for first 10 kg)

50 mL/~~kg~~/day × 10 ~~kg~~ = 500 mL/day (for next 10 kg)

20 mL/~~kg~~/day × 4 ~~kg~~ = 80 mL/day (for the remaining 4 kg)

Total: 1000 mL/day + 500 mL/day + 80 mL/day = 1580 mL/day or per 24 h

$$\frac{1580 \text{ mL}}{24 \text{ h}} = 65.8 \text{ mL/h} = 66 \text{ mL/h}$$

QUICK REVIEW

- Minimal and maximal dilution volumes for some IV drugs are recommended to prevent fluid overload and to minimize vein irritation and toxic effects.
- The ratio for recommended dilution equals the ratio for desired drug dilution.
- When mixing IV drug solutions,
  - the *smaller* the added volume, the *stronger* or *higher* the resulting *concentration* (minimal dilution).
  - the *larger* the added volume, the *weaker (more dilute)* or *lower* the resulting *concentration* (maximal dilution).
- Daily volume of pediatric maintenance IV fluids based on body weight is:
  - 100 mL/kg/day for first 10 kg.
  - 50 mL/kg/day for next 10 kg.
  - 20 mL/kg/day for each kilogram above 20.

REVIEW SET 40

1. If a child is receiving chloramphenicol 400 mg IV q6h and the maximum concentration is 100 mg/mL, what is the minimum volume of fluid in which the medication can be safely diluted? ________ mL
2. If a child is receiving gentamicin sulfate 25 mg IV q8h and the minimal concentration is 1 mg/mL, what is the maximum volume of fluid in which the medication can be safely diluted? ________ mL
3. Calculate the total volume and hourly IV flow rate for a 25-kg child receiving maintenance IV fluids. Infuse ________ mL at ________ mL/h
4. Calculate the total volume and hourly IV flow rate for a 13-kg child receiving maintenance IV fluids. Infuse ________ mL at ________ mL/h
5. Calculate the total volume and hourly IV flow rate for a 77-lb child receiving maintenance fluids. Infuse ________ mL at ________ mL/h
6. Calculate the total volume and hourly IV flow rate for a 3500-g infant receiving maintenance fluids. Infuse ________ mL at ________ mL/h
7. A child is receiving 350 mg IV of a medication, and the minimal and maximal dilution range is 30–100 mg/mL. What is the minimum volume (maximal concentration) and the maximum volume (minimal concentration) for safe dilution? ________ mL (minimum volume); ________ mL (maximum volume)

8. A child is receiving 52 mg IV of a medication, and the minimal and maximal dilution range is 0.8–20 mg/mL. What is the minimum volume and the maximum volume of fluid for safe dilution? ________ mL (minimum volume); ________ mL (maximum volume)

9. A child is receiving 175 mg IV of a medication, and the minimal and maximal dilution range is 5–75 mg/mL. What is the minimum volume and the maximum volume of fluid for safe dilution? ________ mL (minimum volume); ________ mL (maximum volume)

10. You are making rounds on your pediatric patients and notice that a 2-year-old child who weighs 14 kg has 1000 mL of normal saline infusing at the rate of 50 mL/h. You decide to question this order. What is your rationale? ________________________________

____

After completing these problems, see pages 503–504 to check your answers.

PRACTICE PROBLEMS—CHAPTER 13

Calculate the volume for one dose of safe dosages. Refer to the BSA formulas or the West Nomogram on the next page as needed to answer questions 1 through 20.

1. Order: *vincristine 2 mg direct IV stat* for a child who weighs 85 pounds and is 50 inches tall.

   Recommended dosage of vincristine for children: 1.5–2 mg/m^2 1 time/week; inject slowly over a period of 1 minute.

   Supply: vincristine 1 mg/mL

   BSA (per formula) of this child: ________ m^2

   Recommended dosage range for this child: ________ mg to ________ mg

   Is the ordered dosage safe? ________

   If safe, give ________ mL/min or ________ mL/15 sec.

   If not, what should the nurse do? ________________________________

2. Use the BSA nomogram to calculate the safe oral dosage and amount to give of mercaptopurine for a child of normal proportions who weighs 11.4 kg.

   Recommended dosage: 80 mg/m^2/day once daily PO

   Supply: mercaptopurine 50 mg/mL

   BSA: ________ m^2

   Safe dosage: ________ mg

   Give: ________ mL

3. Use the BSA nomogram to calculate the safe IV dosage of sargramostim for a 1-year-old child who is 63.5 cm tall and weighs 9.1 kg. NOTE: Sargramostim is available in Canada only through the Special Access Program.

   Recommended dosage: 250 mcg/m^2/day once daily IV

   BSA: ________ m^2

   Safe dosage: ________ mcg

4. Sargramostim is available in a solution strength of 500 mcg/10 mL. Calculate one dose for the child in question 3.

   Give: ________ mL

5. Use the BSA nomogram to determine the BSA for a child who is 88.9 cm tall and weighs 18 kg.

   BSA: ________ m^2

Metric:

$$\text{BSA } (m^2) = \sqrt{\frac{\text{ht (cm)} \times \text{wt (kg)}}{3600}}$$

WEST NOMOGRAM

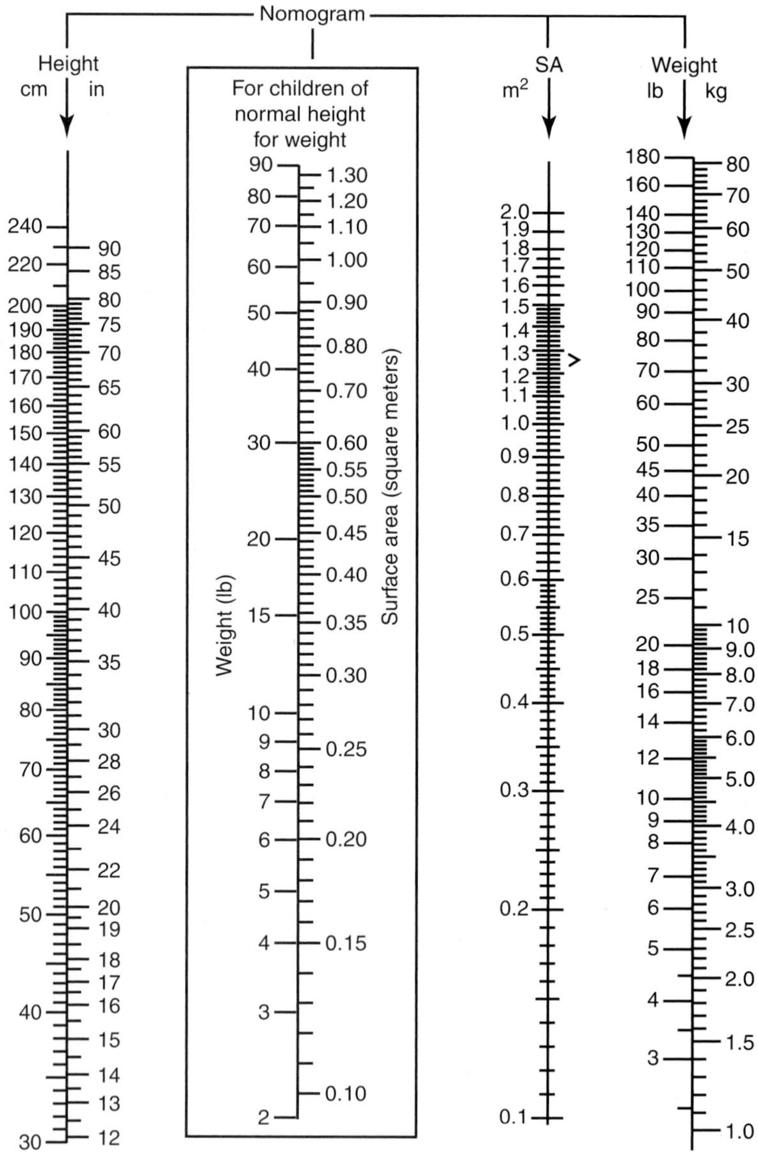

This chart was published in Nelson Textbook of Pediatrics, 16th ed., R. E. Behrman, R. M. Kliegman & H. B. Jenson, West Nomogram for Estimation of Body Surface Area, Copyright Elsevier, (2000).

West Nomogram for Estimation of Body Surface Area.

6. Use the BSA nomogram to determine the safe IM dosage of pegaspargase for a child who is 107 cm tall and weighs 20.5 kg. The recommended IM dosage is 2500 units/m^2/dose.

   NOTE: Pegaspargase is available in Canada only through the Special Access Program.

   BSA: ________ m^2

   Safe dosage: ________ units

7. Pegaspargase is reconstituted to 750 units per 1 mL. Calculate one dose for the child in question 6.

   Give: ________ mL

8. Should the pegaspargase in question 7 be given in one injection? ________

9. A child is 140 cm tall and weighs 43.5 kg. The recommended IV dosage of doxorubicin is 20 mg/m^2. Use the BSA formula to calculate the safe IV dosage of doxorubicin for this child.

   BSA: ________ m^2

   Safe dosage: ________ mg

10. Calculate the dose amount of doxorubicin for the child in question 9.

    Supply: doxorubicin 2 mg/mL

    Give: ________ mL

For questions 11 through 15, use the BSA formulas to calculate the BSA value.

11. Height: 60 cm Weight: 6 kg BSA: ________ m^2
12. Height: 68 in Weight: 170 lb BSA: ________ m^2
13. Height: 164 cm Weight: 58 kg BSA: ________ m^2
14. Height: 100 cm Weight: 17 kg BSA: ________ m^2
15. Height: 160 cm Weight: 63 kg BSA: ________ m^2
16. Height: 85 cm Weight: 11.5 kg BSA: ________ m^2
17. What is the safe dosage of one dose of interferon α-2b required for a child with a BSA of 0.28 m^2 if the recommended dosage is 2 million units/m^2? ________ units
18. What is the safe dosage of a drug required for an adult with a BSA of 2.17 m^2 if the recommended dosage is 500 mg/m^2? ________ mg or ________ g
19. What is the total daily dosage range of mitomycin required for a child with a BSA of 0.19 m^2 if the recommended dosage range is 10–20 mg/m^2/day? ________ to ________ mg/day
20. What is the total safe daily dosage of cyclophosphamide required for a adult with a BSA of 1.34 m^2 if the recommended dosage is 6 mg/m^2/day? ________ mg/day
21. After 5 full days of therapy receiving the recommended dosage, the patient in question 19 will have received a total of ________ mg of cyclophosphamide.
22. Order: *cefazolin 0.42 g IV q12h in 30 mL D_5NS over 30 min by volume control set on an infusion controller. Flush with 15 mL.*

    Supply: cefazolin 500 mg/5 mL

    Total IV fluid volume: ________ mL

    Flow rate: ________ mL/h

    Add ________ mL cefazolin and fill chamber to ________ mL with D_5NS.

23. After 7 days of IV therapy, the patient referred to in question 21 will have received a total of ________ mL of cefazolin.

24. Order: *clindamycin 285 mg IV q8h in 45 mL D_5NS over 60 min by volume control set on an infusion controller. Flush with 15 mL.*

    Supply: clindamycin 75 mg/0.5 mL

    Total IV fluid volume: ________ mL

    Flow rate: ________ mL/h

    Add ________ mL clindamycin and fill the chamber to ________ mL with D_5NS.

25. When the patient in question 24 has received 4 days therapy of clindamycin, he will have received a total IV medication volume of ________ mL.

26. Order: *D_5 0.33% NaCl IV at 65 mL/h with ampicillin 500 mg IV q6h to be infused over 20 min*

    You will use a volume control set and flush with 15 mL.

    Supply: ampicillin 250 mg/mL

    Add ________ mL of ampicillin and fill chamber to ________ mL with D_5 0.33% NaCl.

27. Order: *D_5 0.45% NaCl IV at 66 mL/h with ceftazidime 620 mg IV q8h to be infused over 40 min*

    You will use a volume control set and flush with 15 mL.

    Supply: ceftazidime 0.5 g/5 mL

    Add ________ mL ceftazidime and fill chamber to ________ mL with D_5 0.45% NaCl.

To calculate the daily volume of pediatric maintenance IV fluids, allow:

100 mL/kg/day for first 10 kg of body weight

50 mL/kg/day for next 10 kg of body weight

20 mL/kg/day for each kilogram of body weight above 20 kg

28. Calculate the total volume and hourly IV flow rate for a 21-kg child receiving maintenance fluids.

    Infuse ________ mL at ________ mL/h

29. Calculate the total volume and hourly IV flow rate for a 78-lb child receiving maintenance fluids.

    Infuse ________ mL at ________ mL/h

30. Calculate the total volume and hourly IV flow rate for a 15-kg child receiving maintenance fluids.

    Infuse ________ mL at ________ mL/h

31. Calculate the total volume and hourly IV flow rate for a 2-g infant receiving maintenance fluids.

    Infuse ________ mL at ________ mL/h

For questions 32 through 42, verify the safety of the following pediatric dosages ordered. If the dosage is safe, calculate one dose and the IV volume to infuse one dose.

Order for a child weighing 15 kg:

D_5 0.45% NaCl IV at 53 mL/h with ampicillin 275 mg IV q4h infused over 40 min by volume control set

Recommended dosage: ampicillin 100–125 mg/kg/day in six divided doses

Supply: ampicillin 1 g/10 mL

32. Safe daily dosage range for this child: ________ mg/day to ________ mg/day

    Safe single dosage range for this child: ________ mg/dose to ________ mg/dose

    Is the ordered dosage safe? ________ If safe, give ________ mL/dose.

    If not safe, describe the appropriate action. ________________________________

33. IV fluid volume to be infused in 40 min: ________ mL

    Add ________ mL ampicillin and fill chamber to ________ mL with D_5 0.45% NaCl.

Order for a child who weighs 12.3 kg:

D_5 0.33% NaCl IV at 46 mL/h. The child is to receive vancomycin 100 mg IV q6h to be infused over 6o min in 100 mL D_5W. by volume control set in 100 mL D_5W

Recommended dosage: vancomycin 10 mg/kg/dose given q6h

Supply: vancomycin 50 mg/ mL

34. Safe single dosage for this child: ________ mg/dose

    Is the ordered dosage safe? ________ If safe, give ________ mL/dose.

    If not safe, describe the appropriate action. ________________________________

35. IV fluid volume to be infused in 60 min: ________ mL

    Add ________ mL vancomycin and fill chamber to ________ mL with D_5W. Infuse over 60 min at a rate of 100 mL/h. Once the medication has been infused, read just the IV to the ordered rate.

Order for a child who weighs 22 kg:

D_5 0.225% NaCl IV at 50 mL/h with tranexamic acid 165 mg IV q8h to be infused over 30 min by volume control set

Recommended dosage: tranexamic acid 15–22.5 mg/kg/day in three divided doses q8h

Supply: tranexamic acid 100 mg/mL

36. Safe daily dosage range for this child: ________ mg/day to ________ mg/day

    Safe single dosage range for this child: ________ mg/dose to ________ mg/dose

    Is the ordered dosage safe? ________ If safe, give ________ mL/dose.

    If not safe, describe the appropriate action. ________________________________

37. IV fluid volume to be infused in 30 min: ________ mL

    Add ________ mL tranexamic acid and fill chamber to ________ mL with D_5 0.225% NaCl.

Order for a child who weighs 9 kg:

D_5 0.33% NaCl IV at 38 mL/h with ticarcillin disodium/clavulanate potassium 800 mg IV q4h to be infused over 40 min by volume control set

Recommended dosage: 200–300 mg/kg/day based on ticaricillin disodium content in six divided doses every 4 hours

Supply: ticarcillin disodium 200 mg/mL (when the vial is reconstituted with sterile water)

38. Safe daily dosage range for this child: ________ mg/day to ________ mg/day

    Safe single dosage range for this child: ________ mg/dose to ________ mg/dose

    Is the ordered dosage safe? ________ If safe, give ________ mL/dose.

    If not safe, describe the appropriate action. ________________________________

39. IV fluid volume to be infused in 40 min: ______ mL

Add ________ mL ticarcillin disodium and fill chamber to ________ mL with D_5 0.33% NaCl.

Order for a child who weighs 25 kg:

D_5NS IV at 60 mL/h with penicillin G sodium 525 000 units q4h to be infused over 20 min by volume control set

Recommended dosage: penicillin G sodium 100 000–250 000 units/kg/day in six divided doses q4h

Supply: penicillin G sodium 200 000 units/mL

40. Safe daily dosage for this child: ________ units/day to ________ units/day

Safe single dosage for this child: ________ units/dose to ________ units/dose

41. Is the ordered dosage safe? ________ If safe, give ________ mL/dose.

If not safe, describe the appropriate action. ________________________________

42. IV fluid volume to be infused in 20 min: ________ mL

Add ________ mL penicillin G sodium and fill chamber to ________ mL with D_5 NS.

After completing these problems, see pages 504–505 to check your answers.

CHAPTER

14

Advanced Adult Intravenous Calculations

LEARNING OBJECTIVES

1. Calculate and assess safe hourly heparin sodium dosage.
2. Calculate heparin sodium IV flow rate.
3. Calculate the flow rate and assess safe dosages for critical care IV medications administered over a specified time period.
4. Calculate the flow rate for primary IV and IV piggyback (IVPB) solutions for patients with restricted fluid intake requirements.

Nurses are becoming increasingly more responsible for the administration of intravenous (IV) medications in critical care areas as well as on general nursing units. Patients in life-threatening situations require thorough and timely interventions that frequently involve specialized, potent drugs. This chapter focuses on advanced adult IV calculations with special requirements that can be applied to patients across the life span.

IV HEPARIN SODIUM

Heparin sodium is an anticoagulant for the prevention of clot formation. It is measured in units (see Figure 14-1). IV heparin sodium is frequently ordered in *units per hour* and should be administered by an electronic infusion device. Because of the potential for hemorrhage or clots with incorrect dosage, careful monitoring of patients receiving heparin sodium is a critical nursing skill. The nurse is responsible for administering the correct dosage and for ensuring that the dosage is safe.

CAUTION

Heparin sodium order, dosage, vial, and amount to give should be checked by another nurse before the dose sodium is administered. Check institution policy.

Calculating Safe IV Heparin Sodium Flow Rate

When IV heparin sodium is ordered in units/h, use $\frac{D}{H} \times Q = R$ or ratio-proportion to calculate the flow rate in mL/h.

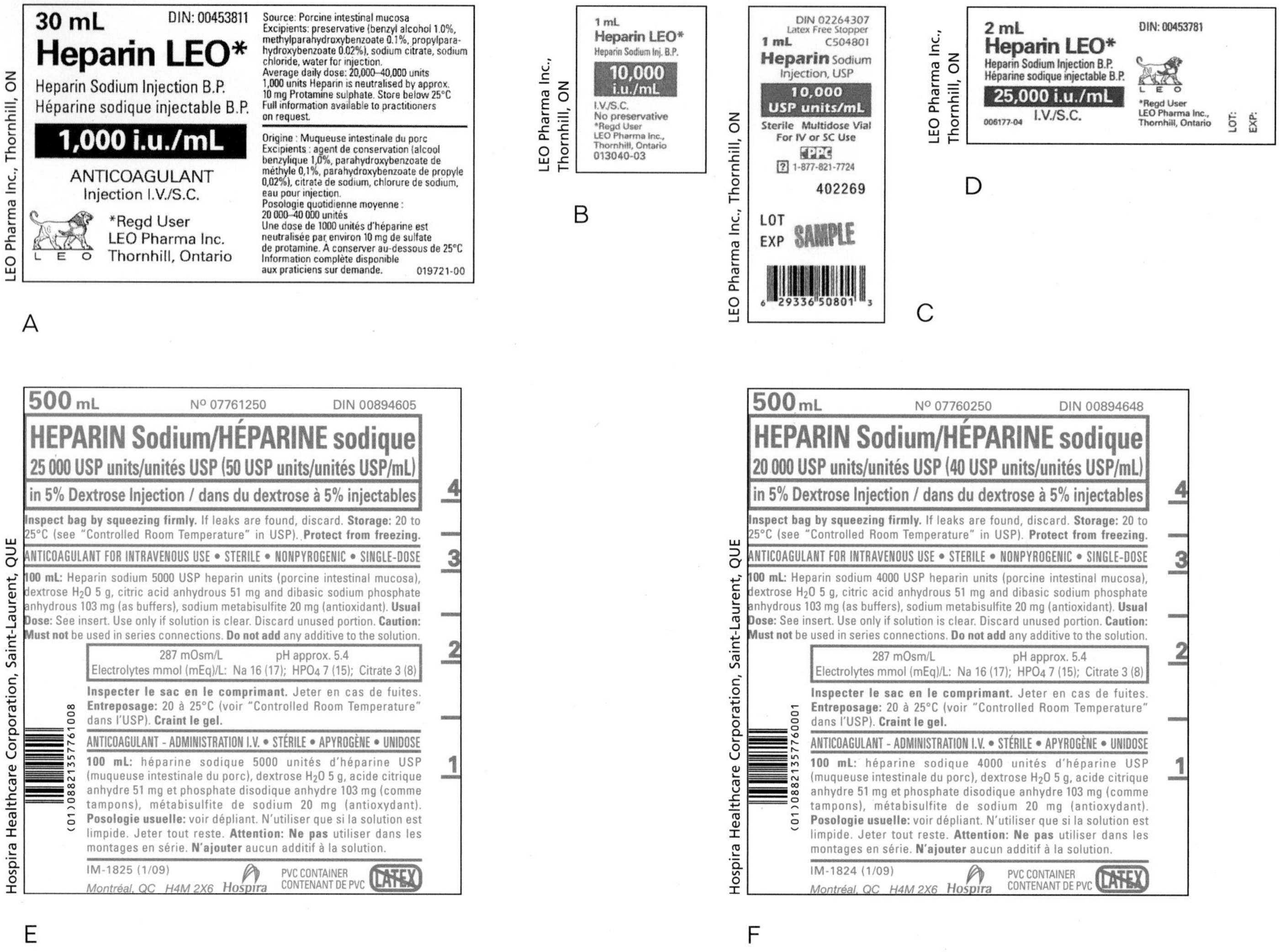

FIGURE 14-1 Various Heparin Sodium Dosage Strengths and Container Volumes and Commercially Premixed IV Solutions

RULE

To calculate IV heparin sodium flow rate in mL/h:

$$\frac{\text{D (units/h desired)}}{\text{H (units you have on hand)}} \times \text{Q (mL you have on hand)} = \text{R (mL/h)}$$

Or, ratio of supply dosage is equivalent to ratio of desired dosage rate:

$$\frac{\text{Supply units}}{\text{Supply mL}} = \frac{\text{Desired units/h}}{\text{X mL/h}}$$

Note: This rule applies to drugs ordered in units/h, milliunits/h, mg/h, mcg/h, g/h, or mEq/h.

Now we can apply the rule to some examples.

Example 1:

Order: *D_5W 500 mL with heparin sodium 25 000 units IV at 1000 units/h*

What is the flow rate in mL/h?

$$\frac{D}{H} \times Q = \frac{1000 \text{ units/h}}{25\,000 \text{ units}} \times 500 \text{ mL} = R \text{ (mL/h)}$$

MATH TIP

Units cancel out to leave mL/h in the $\frac{D}{H} \times Q = R$ formula.

$$\frac{1000 \cancel{\text{units}}/\text{h}}{\underset{50}{\cancel{25\,000}} \cancel{\text{units}}} \times \overset{1}{\cancel{500}} \text{ mL} = \frac{\overset{20}{\cancel{1000}}}{\underset{1}{\cancel{50}}} \text{ mL/h} = 20 \text{ mL/h}$$

Or, use ratio-proportion to calculate the flow rate in mL/h, which will administer 1000 units/h.

$$\frac{25\,000 \text{ units}}{500 \text{ mL}} = \frac{1000 \text{ units/h}}{\text{X mL}}$$

$$25\,000\text{X} = 500\,000$$

$$\frac{25\,000\text{X}}{25\,000} = \frac{500\,000}{25\,000}$$

$$\text{X} = 20 \text{ mL/h}$$

Look at the labels in Figure 14-1, representing the various supply dosages of heparin sodium you have available, including IV solutions with heparin sodium premixed. However, if you have to mix the solution, what label would you select to prepare the heparin sodium infusion as ordered? The best answer is label D: 2-mL vial of heparin sodium 25 000 units/mL. This is necessary because to add 25 000 units of heparin sodium to 500 mL of IV solution, you would need 1 mL of heparin sodium.

$$\frac{D}{H} \times Q = \frac{25\,000 \text{ units}}{25\,000 \text{ units}} \times 1 \text{ mL} = 1 \text{ mL}$$

However, notice that you could also select label A and prepare 25 mL of heparin sodium 1000 units/mL. Labels B and C do not have sufficient volume to fill the dosage required. (Of course, label E has the required solution premixed.)

Example 2:

Order: *D_5W 500 mL with heparin sodium 25 000 units IV at 850 units/h*

Calculate the flow rate in mL/h.

$$\frac{D}{H} \times Q = \frac{850 \cancel{\text{units}}/\text{h}}{\underset{50}{\cancel{25\,000}} \text{ units}} \times \overset{1}{\cancel{500}} \text{ mL} = \frac{\overset{17}{\cancel{850}}}{\underset{1}{\cancel{50}}} \text{ mL/h} = 17 \text{ mL/h}$$

Or, use ratio-proportion.

$$\frac{25\,000 \text{ units}}{500 \text{ mL}} = \frac{850 \text{ units/h}}{\text{X mL/h}}$$

$$25\,000\text{X} = 425\,000$$

$$\frac{25\,000\text{X}}{25\,000} = \frac{425\,000}{25\,000}$$

$$\text{X} = 17 \text{ mL/h}$$

Example 3:

D_5W 500 mL with heparin sodium 25 000 units IV is currently infusing at 850 units/h, or 17 mL/h. Based on laboratory results, it is determined that the patient's infusion must be increased by 120 units/h, so that it should now be infusing at 970 units/h.

Calculate the flow rate in mL/h.

$$\frac{D}{H} \times Q = \frac{970 \cancel{\text{units}}/h}{\underset{50}{\cancel{25\,000}} \cancel{\text{units}}} \times \overset{1}{\cancel{500}} \text{ mL} = \frac{970}{50} \text{ mL/h} = 19.4 \text{ mL/h} = 19 \text{ mL/h}$$

Or, use ratio-proportion.

$$\frac{25\,000 \text{ units}}{500 \text{ mL}} = \frac{970 \text{ units/h}}{X \text{ mL/h}}$$

$$25\,000X = 485\,000$$

$$\frac{25\,000X}{25\,000} = \frac{485\,000}{25\,000}$$

$$X = 19.4 = 19 \text{ mL/h}$$

You would need to increase the infusion from 17 mL/h (850 units/h) to 19 mL/h (970 units/h).

IV Heparin Sodium Protocol

Because patients vary significantly in weight, the IV heparin sodium dosage is individualized based on patient weight. Many institutions have standard protocols related to IV heparin administration. Figure 14-2 shows a sample protocol. Note that the bolus or loading dosage and the initial infusion dosage of heparin sodium are based on the patient's weight. Line 10 indicates that for this protocol, the standard heparin sodium bolus dosage is 80 units/kg and the infusion rate is 18 units/kg/h. When the patient's response to heparin therapy changes, as measured by the activated partial thromboplastin time (aPTT) measured in seconds, the heparin sodium dosage is adjusted as indicated in lines 11–15. These orders in Figure 14-2 are based on patient weight rounded to the nearest 10 kilograms. Some institutions use the patient's exact weight in kilograms. It is important to know the protocol for your clinical setting. Let us work through some examples of calculation of heparin sodium dosage based on patient weight and a standardized heparin sodium dosage protocol.

Example 1:

Protocol: *Bolus patient with heparin sodium 80 units/kg body weight and start drip at 18 units/kg/h*

Patient's weight: 50 kg

How many units of heparin sodium should the patient receive?

Step 1 Calculate the heparin sodium bolus dosage.

$$80 \text{ units}/\cancel{\text{kg}} \times 50 \cancel{\text{kg}} = 4000 \text{ units}$$

This patient should receive 4000 units IV heparin sodium as a bolus.

Step 2 Calculate the number of millilitres to administer for the bolus.

Supply: heparin sodium 1000 units/mL, as recommended by the protocol (see line 2, Figure 14-2)

Think: You want to give 4000 units, which is four times 1000 units/mL, so you want to give four times 1 mL or 4 mL.

$$\frac{D}{H} \times Q = \frac{\overset{4}{\cancel{4000}} \cancel{\text{units}}}{\underset{1}{\cancel{1000}} \cancel{\text{units}}} \times 1 \text{ mL} = 4 \text{ mL}$$

Administer 4 mL of heparin sodium for the bolus.

Standard Weight-Based Heparin Sodium Protocol

For all patients on heparin sodium drips:

1. Weight in KILOGRAMS. Required for order to be processed: _____ kg
2. Heparin sodium 25 000 units in 250 mL of $\frac{1}{2}$NS. Boluses to be given as 1000 units/mL.
3. aPTT q6h or 6 hours after rate change; daily after two consecutive therapeutic aPTTs.
4. CBC initially and repeat every _____ day(s).
5. Obtain aPTT and PT/INR on day 1 prior to initiation of therapy.
6. Guaiac stool initially then every _____ day(s) until heparin sodium discontinued. Notify if positive.
7. Neuro checks every _____ hours while on heparin sodium. Notify physician of any changes.
8. Discontinue aPTT and CBC once heparin sodium drip is discontinued, unless otherwise ordered.
9. Notify physician of any bleeding problems.
10. Bolus with 80 units/kg. Start drip at 18 units/kg/h.

11. If aPTT is less than 35 secs:	Rebolus with 80 units/kg and increase rate by 4 units/kg/h
12. If aPTT is 36–44 secs:	Rebolus with 40 units/kg and increase rate by 2 units/kg/h
13. If aPTT is 45–75 secs:	Continue current rate
14. If aPTT is 76–90 secs:	Decrease rate by 2 units/kg/h
15. If aPTT is more than 90 secs:	Hold heparin sodium for 1 h and decrease rate by 3 units/kg/h

FIGURE 14-2 Sample Orders for Patient on Heparin Sodium Therapy

Step 3 Calculate the infusion rate for the heparin sodium IV drip.

Protocol: *Start drip at 18 units/kg/h* (see line 10, Figure 14-2)

Supply: heparin sodium 25 000 units/250 mL (see line 2, Figure 14-2) or 100 units/mL

18 units/kg/h × 50 kg = 900 units/h

Think: You want to administer nine times 1 mL or 9 mL for the IV heparin sodium infusion.

$$\frac{D}{H} \times Q = \frac{\overset{9}{\cancel{900}}\ \cancel{\text{units}}/\text{h}}{\underset{1}{\cancel{100}}\ \cancel{\text{units}}} \times 1\ \text{mL} = 9\ \text{mL/h}$$

Example 2:

After 6 hours, the patient in Example 1 has an aPTT of 43 seconds. According to the protocol, you will *rebolus with 40 units/kg and increase the amount of IV heparin sodium by 2 units/kg/h* (see line 12, Figure 14-2).

You already know the patient's weight: 50 kg

Step 1 Calculate the heparin sodium rebolus dosage.

$40\ \text{units}/\cancel{\text{kg}} \times 50\ \text{kg} = 2000\ \text{units}$

Step 2 Calculate the number of millilitres to prepare.

Supply: heparin sodium 1000 units/mL, as recommended by the protocol

Think: You want to give two times 1 mL or 2 mL.

$$\frac{D}{H} \times Q = \frac{\overset{2}{\cancel{2000}}\ \cancel{\text{units}}}{\underset{1}{\cancel{1000}}\ \cancel{\text{units}}} \times 1\ \text{mL} = 2\ \text{mL}$$

Administer 2 mL of heparin sodium for the rebolus.

Step 3 Calculate the number of units the patient's IV heparin sodium will be increased.

2 units/kg/h × 50 kg = 100 units/h

Step 4 Calculate the new infusion rate.

Supply: heparin sodium 25 000 units/250 mL (see line 2, Figure 14-2) or 100 units/mL

Think: You want to administer 100 units/h and you have 100 units/mL, so you want to increase the infusion by 1 mL/h.

$$\frac{D}{H} \times Q = \frac{\overset{1}{\cancel{100}}\ \cancel{\text{units}}/\text{h}}{\underset{1}{\cancel{100}}\ \cancel{\text{units}}} \times 1\ \text{mL} = 1\ \text{mL/h}$$

9 mL/h + 1 mL/h = 10 mL/h

Reset the infusion rate to 10 mL/h.

QUICK REVIEW

- Use $\frac{D}{H} \times Q = R$ or ratio-proportion to calculate mL/h when you know units/h and units/mL.
- Many hospitals use standard protocols to initiate and maintain heparin sodium therapy.
- The protocols are based on patient weight in kilograms, and adjustments are made based on laboratory results (usually aPTT).

REVIEW SET 41

Calculate the flow rate.

1. Order: *1000 mL 0.45% NS with heparin sodium 25 000 units to infuse at 1000 units/h.*

   Flow rate: ________ mL/h

2. Order: *500 mL D_5W IV with heparin sodium 40 000 units to infuse at 1100 units/h.*

   Flow rate: ________ mL/h

3. Order: *500 mL 0.45% NS IV with heparin sodium 25 000 units to infuse at 500 units/h.*

   Flow rate: ________ mL/h

4. Order: *500 mL D_5W IV with heparin sodium 40 000 units to infuse at 1500 units/h.*

   Flow rate: ________ mL/h

5. Order: *1 L D_5W IV with heparin sodium 25 000 units to infuse at 1200 units/h.* On rounds, you assess the patient and observe that the infusion pump is set at 120 mL/h.

   At what rate should the pump be set? ________ mL/h

   What should your action be? ________________________________

6. Order: *500 mL D_5W with heparin sodium 25 000 units to infuse at 800 units/h*

   Flow rate: ________ mL/h

Questions 7 through 10 refer to a patient who weighs 75 kg and has IV heparin sodium ordered per the following Weight-Based Heparin Sodium Protocol.

Weight-Based Heparin Sodium Protocol:

Heparin sodium IV infusion: heparin sodium 25 000 units in 250 mL of $\frac{1}{2}$NS

IV boluses: Use heparin sodium 1000 units/mL

Bolus with heparin sodium 80 units/kg. Then initiate heparin sodium drip at 18 units/kg/h. Obtain aPTT every 6 hours and adjust dosage and rate as follows:

If aPTT is less than 35 seconds: Rebolus with 80 units/kg and increase rate by 4 units/kg/h.

If aPTT is 36–44 seconds: Rebolus with 40 units/kg and increase rate by 2 units/kg/h.

If aPTT is 45–75 seconds: Continue current rate.

If aPTT is 76–90 seconds: Decrease rate by 2 units/kg/h.

If aPTT is more than 90 seconds: Hold heparin sodium for 1 hour and then decrease rate by 3 units/kg/h.

7. Calculate the initial heparin sodium bolus dosage: ________ units

   Calculate the bolus dose: ________ mL

   Calculate the initial heparin sodium infusion rate: ________ units/h or ________ mL/h

8. At 0900 h, the patient's aPTT is 33 seconds. According to the protocol, what is the appropriate action?

   Rebolus with ________ units or ________ mL.

   Reset infusion rate to ________ units/h or ________ mL/h.

9. At 1500 h, the patient's aPTT is 40 seconds. According to the protocol, what is the appropriate action?

   Rebolus with ________ units or ________ mL.

   Reset infusion rate to ________ units/h or ________ mL/h.

10. At 2100 h, the patient's aPTT is 60 seconds. According to the protocol, what is the appropriate action? ________________________________

    The same method can be used to calculate flow rates for other medications ordered at a specified dosage unit per hour. Calculate flow rate for questions 11 through 15.

11. Order: *500 mL 0.9% NaCl IV with Humulin R insulin 500 units to infuse at 10 units/h.*

    Flow rate: ________ mL/h

12. Order: *1 L D_5W IV with potassium chloride 40 mEq to infuse at 2 mEq/h.*

    Flow rate: ________ mL/h

13. Order: *100 mL D_5W with diltiazem hydrochloride 125 mg to infuse at 5 mg/h*

    Flow rate: ________ mL/h

14. Order: *250 mL NS with diltiazem hydrochloride 125 mg to infuse at 10 mg/h*

    Flow rate: ________ mL/h

15. Order: *500 mL 0.9% NaCl with Humulin R insulin 300 units to infuse at 5 units/h*

    Flow rate: ________ mL/h

After completing these problems, see page 506 to check your answers.

CRITICAL CARE IV CALCULATIONS: CALCULATING FLOW RATE OF AN IV MEDICATION TO BE GIVEN OVER A SPECIFIED TIME PERIOD

With increasing frequency, medications are ordered for patients in critical care situations as a prescribed amount to be administered in a specified time period, such as *X mg per minute.* Such medications are usually administered by electronic infusion devices, programmed in millilitres per hour. Careful monitoring of patients receiving life-threatening therapies is a critical nursing skill.

IV Medication Ordered "Per Minute"

RULE

To determine the flow rate (mL/h) for IV medications ordered per minute (such as mg/min):

Step 1 **Calculate the dosage in mL/min:**

$$\frac{D}{H} \times Q = R \text{ (mL/min)}$$

Step 2 **Calculate the flow rate of the quantity to administer in mL/h:**

mL/min × 60 min/h = mL/h

Note: The order may specify mg/min, mcg/min, g/min, units/min, milliunits/min, or mEq/min.

In the formula $\frac{D}{H} \times Q = R$ (mL/min):

D = Dosage *desired:* mg/min

H = Dosage you *have* available

Q = *Quantity* of solution you have available

R = Flow *rate:* mL/min

Example 1:

Order: *lidocaine hydrochloride 2 g IV in 500 mL D_5W at 2 mg/min via infusion pump.* You must prepare and hang 500 mL of D_5W IV solution that has 2 g of lidocaine hydrochloride added to it. Then, you must regulate the flow rate so the patient receives 2 mg of the lidocaine every minute. Determine the flow rate in millilitres per hour.

Step 1 Calculate mL/min.

Apply the formula $\frac{D}{H} \times Q = R$ (mL/min).

D = dosage desired = 2 mg/min

H = dosage you have available = 2 g = 2 × 1000 = 2000 mg

Q = quantity of available solution = 500 mL

$$\frac{D}{H} \times Q = \frac{2 \text{ mg/min}}{2000 \text{ mg}} \times 500 \text{ mL} = R$$

MATH TIP

$$\frac{\cancel{mg}/min}{\cancel{mg}} \times mL = mL/min$$ because *mg* cancels out.

$$\frac{2 \cancel{\text{mg}}/\text{min}}{\underset{4}{\cancel{2000}} \cancel{\text{mg}}} \times \frac{\overset{1}{\cancel{500}} \text{ mL}}{1} = \frac{2}{4} \text{ mL/min} = 0.5 \text{ mL/min}$$

Step 2 Determine the flow rate (mL/h).

mL/min × 60 min/h = mL/h

0.5 mL/min × 60 min/h = X mL/h

MATH TIP

$$\frac{mL}{\cancel{min}} \times \frac{\cancel{min}}{h} = mL/h$$ because *min* cancels out.

$$\frac{0.5 \text{ mL}}{\cancel{\text{min}}} \times \frac{60 \cancel{\text{min}}}{\text{h}} = 30 \text{ mL/h}$$

Or, you can use ratio-proportion.

$$\frac{0.5 \text{ mL}}{1 \text{ min}} = \frac{X \text{ mL}}{60 \text{ min}}$$

X = 30 mL (per 60 min or 30 mL/h)

MATH TIP

In the original ratio, $\frac{X \text{ mL}}{60 \text{ min}}$ means X mL/60 min or X mL/h.

Regulate the flow rate to 30 mL/h to deliver 2 mg/min of the drug.

Example 2:

Order: *nitroglycerin 125 mg IV in 500 mL D_5W to infuse at 42 mcg/min*

Calculate the flow rate in millilitres per hour to program the infusion pump.

Step 1 Calculate mL/min.

Convert mg to mcg: 1 mg = 1000 mcg; 125 mg = 125 × 1000 = 125 000 mcg

$$\frac{D}{H} \times Q = \frac{42 \text{ mcg/min}}{125\,000 \text{ mcg}} \times 500 \text{ mL} = \frac{42}{250} \text{ mL/min} = 0.168 \text{ mL/min} = 0.17 \text{ mL/min}$$

(125 000 reduces to 250; 500 reduces to 1)

Step 2 Calculate mL/h. You know that 1 h = 60 min.

mL/min × 60 min/h = mL/h

0.17 mL/min × 60 min/h = 10.2 mL/h = 10 mL/h

Or, you can use ratio-proportion.

$$\frac{0.17 \text{ mL}}{1 \text{ min}} \quad \frac{X \text{ mL}}{60 \text{ min}}$$

X = 10.2 mL = 10 mL

Rate is 10 mL/60 min or 10 mL/h.

Regulate the flow rate to 10 mL/h to deliver 42 mcg/min of the drug.

IV Medication Ordered "Per Kilogram Per Minute"

The physician may also order the amount of medication in an IV solution that a patient should receive in a specified time period per kilogram of body weight. An electronic infusion device is usually used to administer these orders.

> **RULE**
>
> **To calculate flow rate (*mL/h*) for IV medications ordered by weight per minute (such as *mg/kg/min*):**
>
> **Step 1** Convert to like units, such as mg to mcg.
>
> **Step 2** Calculate desired dosage per minute.
>
> **Step 3** Calculate the desired dosage in mL/min: $\frac{D}{H} \times Q = R$ (mL/min).
>
> **Step 4** Calculate the flow rate of the quantity to administer in mL/h.
>
> **Note: The order may specify mg/kg/min, mcg/kg/min, g/kg/min, units/kg/min, milliunits/kg/min, or mEq/kg/min.**

Example:

Order: *250 mL of IV solution with 225 mg of a medication to infuse at 3 mcg/kg/min via infusion pump* for a person who weighs 50 kg.

Determine the flow rate (mL/h).

Step 1 Convert mg to mcg: 1 mg = 1000 mcg; 225 mg = 225 × 1000 = 225 000 mcg

Step 2 Calculate desired mcg/min.

3 mcg/kg/min × 50 kg = 150 mcg/min

Step 3 Calculate mL/min.

$$\frac{D}{H} \times Q = \frac{150 \text{ mcg/min}}{225\,000 \text{ mcg}} \times 250 \text{ mL} = \frac{150}{900} \text{ mL/min} = 0.166 \text{ mL/min} = 0.17 \text{ mL/min}$$

(225 000 reduces to 900; 250 reduces to 1)

Step 4 Calculate mL/h. You know that 1 h = 60 min.

$$\text{mL/min} \times 60\ \text{min/h} = 0.17\ \text{mL}/\cancel{\text{min}} \times 60\ \cancel{\text{min}}/\text{h} = 10.2\ \text{mL/h} = 10\ \text{mL/h}$$

Or you can use ratio-proportion.

$$\frac{0.17\ \text{mL}}{1\ \text{min}} \times \frac{X\ \text{mL}}{60\ \text{min}}$$

X = 10.2 mL = 10 mL

Rate is 10 mL/60 min or 10 mL/h.

Regulate the flow rate to 10 mL/h to deliver 150 mcg/min of the drug.

Titrating IV Drugs

Sometimes IV medications may be ordered to be administered at an initial dosage over a specified time period and then continued at a different dosage and time period. These situations are common in obstetrics and critical care. Medications, such as magnesium sulfate, dopamine, isoproterenol hydrochloride, and oxytocin, are ordered to be *titrated* or *regulated* to obtain measurable physiologic responses. Dosages will be adjusted until the desired effect is achieved. In some cases, a loading or bolus dose is infused and monitored closely. Most IV medications that require titration usually start at the lowest dosage and are increased or decreased as needed. An upper titration limit is usually set and is not exceeded unless the desired response is not obtained. A new drug order is then required.

Let us look at some of these situations.

RULE

To calculate flow rate (mL/h) for IV medications ordered over a specific time period (e.g., mg/min):

Step 1 Calculate mg/mL.
Step 2 Calculate mL/h.

Note: The order may specify mg/min, mcg/min, g/min, units/min, milliunits/min, or mEq/min; or mg/h, mcg/h, g/h, units/h, milliunits/h, or mEq/h.

Example 1:

Order: *RL IV 1000 mL with magnesium sulfate 20 g. Start with a bolus of 4 g/30 min, then maintain a continuous infusion at 2 g/h.*

1. What is the flow rate in millilitres per hour for the bolus order?

Step 1 Calculate the bolus dosage in g/mL.

There are 20 g in 1000 mL. How many millilitres are necessary to infuse 4 g?

Desired = 4 g Have = 20 g per 1000 mL (Q)

$$\frac{D}{H} \times Q = \frac{4\ \cancel{g}}{\underset{1}{\cancel{20}}\ g} \times \overset{50}{\cancel{1000}}\ \text{mL} = 200\ \text{mL}$$

Or you can use ratio-proportion.

$$\frac{20\ \text{g}}{1000\ \text{mL}} \times \frac{4\ \text{g}}{X\ \text{mL}}$$

20X = 4000

$$\frac{20X}{20} = \frac{4000}{20}$$

X = 200 mL

Therefore, 200 mL contain 4 g, to be administered over 30 min.

Step 2 Calculate the bolus rate in millilitres per hour.

What is the flow rate in millilitres per hour to infuse 200 mL (which contain 4 g of magnesium sulfate)? Remember 1 h = 60 min.

$$\frac{\text{Total mL}}{\text{Total min}} \times 60 \text{ min/h} = \frac{200 \text{ mL}}{\overset{}{\underset{1}{\cancel{30}\ \cancel{\text{min}}}}} \times \frac{\overset{2}{\cancel{60}\ \cancel{\text{min}}}}{1 \text{ h}} = 400 \text{ mL/h}$$

Or you can use ratio-proportion.

$$\frac{200 \text{ mL}}{30 \text{ min}} \times \frac{X \text{ mL}}{60 \text{ min}}$$

30X = 12 000

$$\frac{30X}{30} = \frac{12\ 000}{30}$$

X = 400 mL

Rate is 400 mL/60 min or 400 mL/h.

Set the infusion pump at 400 mL/h tok deliver the bolus of 4 g/30 min as ordered.

Now calculate the continuous IV rate in millilitres per hour.

2. What is the flow rate in millilitres per hour for the continuous infusion of magnesium sulfate of 2 g/h? You know from the bolus dosage calculation that 200 mL contains 4 g.

Desired = 2 g/h Have = 4 g per 200 mL (Q)

$$\frac{D}{H} \times Q = \frac{2\ \cancel{g}/h}{\underset{1}{\cancel{4}}\ \cancel{g}} \times \overset{50}{\cancel{200}} \text{ mL} = 100 \text{ mL/h}$$

Or you can use ratio-proportion.

$$\frac{4 \text{ g}}{200 \text{ mL}} \times \frac{2 \text{ g/h}}{X \text{ mL/h}}$$

4X = 400

$$\frac{4X}{4} = \frac{400}{4}$$

X = 100 mL/h

After the bolus has infused in the first 30 min, reset the infusion pump to 100 mL/h to deliver the continuous infusion of 2 g/h.

Let us look at an example using oxytocin (a drug used to induce or augment labour), measured in units and milliunits.

Example 2:

A patient care order is written to induce labour: *LR 1000 mL IV with oxytocin 20 units. Begin a continuous infusion IV at 1 milliunit/min, increase by 1 milliunit/min q15–30 min to a maximum of 20 milliunits/min.*

1. What is the flow rate in millilitres per hour to deliver 1 milliunit/min?

In this example, the medication is measured in units (instead of g or mg).

Step 1 Calculate milliunits/mL.

Convert: 1 unit = 1000 milliunits; 20 units = 20 × 1000 = 20 000 milliunits

Desired = 1 milliunit

Have = 20 000 milliunits per 1000 mL (Q)

$$\frac{D}{H} \times Q = \frac{1 \text{ }\cancel{\text{milliunit}}}{\underset{20}{\cancel{20\,000}} \text{ }\cancel{\text{milliunit}}} \times \overset{1}{\cancel{1000}} \text{ mL} = \frac{1}{20} \text{ mL} = 0.05 \text{ mL}$$

Or you can use ratio-proportion.

$$\frac{20\,000 \text{ milliunits}}{1000 \text{ mL}} = \frac{1 \text{ milliunit}}{X \text{ mL}}$$

$$20\,000X = 1000$$

$$\frac{20\,000X}{20\,000} = \frac{1000}{20\,000}$$

$$X = 0.05 \text{ mL}$$

Therefore, 0.05 mL contains 1 milliunit of oxytocin, or there is 1 milliunit/0.05 mL.

Step 2 Calculate mL/h.

What is the flow rate in millilitres per hour to infuse 0.05 mL/min (which is 1 milliunit oxytocin/min)?

$$\frac{\text{Total mL}}{\text{Total min}} \times 60 \text{ min/h} = \frac{0.05 \text{ mL}}{1 \text{ }\cancel{\text{min}}} \times \frac{60 \text{ }\cancel{\text{min}}}{1 \text{ h}} = 3 \text{ mL/h}$$

Or you can use ratio-proportion.

$$\frac{0.05 \text{ mL}}{1 \text{ min}} = \frac{X \text{ mL}}{60 \text{ min}}$$

$$X = 3 \text{ mL}$$

Rate is 3 mL/60 min or 3 mL/h.

Set the infusion pump at 3 mL/h to infuse oxytocin 1 milliunit/min as ordered.

2. What is the maximum flow rate in millilitres per hour that the oxytocin infusion can be set for the titration as ordered? Notice that the order allows a maximum of 20 milliunits/min. You know from the bolus dosage calculation that there is 1 milliunit per 0.05 mL.

Desired = 20 milliunits/min

Have = 1 milliunit per 0.05 mL (Q)

$$\frac{D}{H} \times Q = \frac{20 \text{ }\cancel{\text{milliunits}}\text{/min}}{1 \text{ }\cancel{\text{milliunit}}} \times 0.05 \text{ mL} = 1 \text{ mL/min}$$

Now convert mL/min to mL/h, so you can program the electronic infusion device.

$$\text{mL/min} \times 60 \text{ min/h} = 1 \text{ mL/}\cancel{\text{min}} \times 60 \text{ }\cancel{\text{min}}\text{/h} = 60 \text{ mL/h}$$

Or you can use ratio-proportion.

You know that 1 milliunit/min is infused at 3 mL/h.

$$\frac{3\text{ mL/h}}{1\text{ milliunit/min}} \times \frac{X\text{ mL/h}}{20\text{ milliunits/min}}$$

$X = 60\text{ mL/h}$

Rate of 60 mL/h will deliver 20 milliunits/min.

Verifying Safe IV Medication Dosage Recommended "Per Minute"

It is also a critical nursing skill to be sure that patients are receiving safe dosages of medications. Therefore, you must also be able to convert IVs with additive medications to **mg/h** or **mg/min** to check safe or normal dosage ranges.

RULE

To check safe dosage of IV medications ordered in mL/h:
Step 1 Calculate mg/h.
Step 2 Calculate mg/min.
Step 3 Compare recommended dosage and ordered dosage to decide if the dosage is safe.
Note: The ordered and recommended dosages may specify mg/min, mcg/min, g/min, units/min, milliunits/min, or mmol/min.

Example:

The recommended dosage of lidocaine hydrochloride is 1–4 mg/min as indicated in the Hospital Formulary. The patient care order is for *500 mL D_5W IV with lidocaine hydrochloride 1 g to infuse at 30 mL/h.* Is the lidocaine hydrochloride dosage within the safe range?

Step 1 Calculate mg/h.

Convert: 1 g = 1000 mg

Desired = Unknown X mg/h Have = 1000 mg per 500 mL (Q)

$$\frac{D}{H} \times Q = \frac{X\text{ mg/h}}{\cancel{1000}_{2}\text{ mg}} \times \overset{1}{\cancel{500}}\text{ mL} = 30\text{ mL/h}$$

$$\frac{X}{2} = 30$$

$$\frac{X}{2} \times \frac{30}{1}$$

X = 60 mg/h (You know the answer is in mg/h because "X" is measured in mg/h.)

Or you can use ratio-proportion.

$$\frac{1000\text{ mg}}{500\text{ mL}} \times \frac{X\text{ mg/h}}{30\text{ mL/h}}$$

$500X = 30\,000$

$$\frac{500X}{500} = \frac{30\,000}{500}$$

$X = 60\text{ mg/h}$

Sixty milligrams are administered in 1 hour when the flow rate is 30 mL/h.

Step 2 Calculate mg/min. THINK: It is obvious that 60 mg/h is the same as 60 mg/60 min or 1 mg/1 min.

$1 \text{ h} = 60 \text{ min}$

$$\frac{\text{mg/h}}{60 \text{ min/h}} = \text{mg/min}$$

$$\frac{\overset{1}{\cancel{60}} \text{ mg/}\cancel{\text{h}}}{\underset{1}{\cancel{60}} \text{ min/}\cancel{\text{h}}} = 1 \text{ mg/min}$$

Or you can use ratio-proportion.

$$\frac{60 \text{ mg}}{60 \text{ min}} = \frac{X \text{ mg}}{1 \text{ min}}$$

$60X = 60$

$$\frac{60X}{60} = \frac{60}{60}$$

$X = 1 \text{ mg}$

Rate is 1 mg/min.

Step 3 Compare ordered and recommended dosages.

One milligram per minute is within the safe range of 1–4 mg/min. The dosage is safe.

Likewise, IV medications ordered as mL/h and recommended in mg/kg/min require verification of their safety or normal dosage range.

RULE

To check safe dosage of IV medications recommended in mg/kg/min and ordered in mL/h:
Step 1 Convert to like units, such as mg to mcg.
Step 2 Calculate recommended mg/min.
Step 3 Calculate ordered mg/h.
Step 4 Calculate ordered mg/min.
Step 5 Compare ordered and recommended dosages. Decide if the dosage is safe.
Note: The ordered and recommended dosages may specify mg/kg/min, mcg/kg/min, g/kg/min, units/kg/min, milliunits/kg/min, or mmol/kg/min.

Example:

The recommended dosage range of nitroglycerin for adults is 0.3–10 mcg/kg/min. The patient has an order for *100 mL D_5W IV with nitroglycerin 420 mg to infuse at 1 mL/h.* The patient weighs 70 kg. Is the nitroglycerin dosage within the normal range?

Step 1

Convert mg to mcg: $420 \text{ mg} = 420 \times 1000 = 420\,000 \text{ mcg}$

Step 2 Calculate recommended mcg/min range.

$0.3 \text{ mcg/}\cancel{\text{kg}}\text{/min} \times 70 \cancel{\text{kg}} = 21 \text{ mcg/min}$ *minimum*

$10 \text{ mcg/}\cancel{\text{kg}}\text{/min} \times 70 \cancel{\text{kg}} = 700 \text{ mcg/min}$ *minimum*

Step 3 Calculate ordered mcg/h.

Desired = Unknown X mcg/h   Have = 42 000 mcg per 100 mL (Q)

$$\frac{D}{H} \times Q = \text{Rate}$$

$$\frac{X\ \cancel{mcg}/h}{\underset{420}{\cancel{42\,000}}\ \cancel{mcg}} \times \overset{1}{\cancel{100}}\ mL = 1\ mL/h$$

$$\frac{X}{420} = 1$$

$$\frac{X}{420} \times \frac{1}{1}$$

X = 420 mcg/h (You know the answer is in mcg/h because "X" is measured in mcg/h.)

Or you can use ratio-proportion.

$$\frac{420\,000\ mcg}{100\ mL} = \frac{X\ mcg/h}{1\ mL/h}$$

$$100\ X = 420\,000$$

$$\frac{100\ X}{100} = \frac{420\,000}{100}$$

$$X = 4200\ mcg/h$$

Step 4 Calculate ordered mcg/min: 4200 mcg/h = 4200 mcg/60 min

$$\frac{4200\ mcg}{60\ min} = 70\ mcg/min$$

Step 5 Compare ordered and recommended dosages. Decide if the dosage is safe. Seventy micrograms per minute is within the allowable range of 21–700 mcg/min. The ordered dosage is safe.

QUICK REVIEW

- For IV medications ordered in mg/min:
  Step 1 Calculate mL/min, and then
  Step 2 Calculate mL/h.
- To check safe dosages of IV medications recommended in mg/min and ordered in mL/h:
  Step 1 Calculate mg/h.
  Step 2 Calculate mg/min.
  Step 3 Compare recommended and ordered dosages. Decide if the dosage is safe.
- To check safe dosage of IV medications recommended in mg/kg/min and ordered in mL/h:
  Step 1 Convert to like units, such as mg to mcg.
  Step 2 Calculate recommended mg/min.
  Step 3 Calculate ordered mg/h.
  Step 4 Calculate ordered mg/min.
  Step 5 Compare ordered and recommended dosages. Decide if the dosage is safe.

REVIEW SET 42

Compute the flow rate for each of these medications administered by infusion pump.

1. Order: *lidocaine hydrochloride 2 g IV per 1000 mL D_5W at 4 mg/min*

   Rate: ________ mL/min and ________ mL/h

2. Order: *procainamide hydrochloride 0.5 g IV per 250 mL D_5W at 2 mg/min*

   Rate: ________ mL/min and ________ mL/h

3. Order: *isoproterenol hydrochloride 2 mg IV per 500 mL D_5W at 6 mcg/min*

   Rate: ________ mL/min and ________ mL/h

4. Order: *Medication "X" 450 mg IV per 500 mL NS at 4 mcg/kg/min*

   Weight: 90 kg

   Give: ________ mcg/min

   Rate: ________ mL/min and ________ mL/h

5. Order: *dopamine hydrochloride 800 mg in 500 mL NS IV at 15 mcg/kg/min*

   Weight: 70 kg

   Give: ________ mcg/min

   Rate: ________ mL/min and ________ mL/h

Refer to this patient care order for questions 6 through 8.

Order: *500 mL D_5W IV with dobutamine hydrochloride 500 mg to infuse at 15 mL/h.* The patient weighs 56.8 kg. Recommended range: 2.5–10 mcg/kg/min

6. What mcg/min range of dobutamine hydrochloride should this patient receive? ________ to ________ mcg/min
7. What mg/min range of dobutamine hydrochloride should this patient receive? ________ to ________ mg/min
8. Is the dobutamine hydrochloride as ordered within the safe range? ________

Refer to this patient care order for questions 9 and 10.

Order: *500 mL D_5W IV with procainamide hydrochloride 2 g to infuse at 60 mL/h.* Normal range: 2–6 mg/min

9. How many mg/min of procainamide hydrochloride is the patient receiving? ________ mg/min
10. Is the dosage of procainamide hydrochloride within the normal range? ________
11. Order: *magnesium sulfate 20 g IV in LR 500 mL. Start with a bolus of 2 g to infuse over 30 min. Then maintain a continuous infusion at 1 g/h.*

    Rate: ________ mL/h for bolus

    ________ mL/h for continuous infusion

12. A patient care order is written to induce labour as follows:

    oxytocin 15 units 250 mL. Begin a continuous infusion at the rate of 1 milliunit/min.

    Rate: ________ mL/h

Refer to this order for question 13.

Order: *1000 mL of D_5W IV with aminophylline 10 mg to infuse at 150 mL/h.*

13. How many mg/min of aminophylline is the patient receiving? ________ mg/min

After completing these problems, see pages 506–507 to check your answers.

LIMITING INFUSION VOLUMES

Calculating IV rates to include the IVPB volume may be necessary to limit the total volume of IV fluid a patient receives. To do this, you must calculate the flow rate for both the regular IV and the IVPB. In such instances of restricted fluids, the IVPBs are to be included as part of the total prescribed IV volume and time.

RULE

Follow these six steps to calculate the flow rate of an IV, which includes IVPB. Calculate:

Step 1 *IVPB flow rate:* $\frac{V}{T} \times C = R$

or use $\frac{\text{mL/h}}{\text{Drop factor constant}} = R$

Step 2 *Total IVPB time:* Time for 1 dose × number of doses in 24 h

Step 3 *Total IVPB volume:* Volume of 1 dose × number of doses in 24 h

Step 4 *Total regular IV volume:* Total volume − IVPB volume = regular IV volume

Step 5 *Total regular IV time:* Total time − IVPB time = regular IV time

Step 6 *Regular IV flow rate:* $\frac{V}{T} \times C = R$

or use $\frac{\text{mL/h}}{\text{Drop factor constant}} = R$

Example 1:

Order: *3000 mL D_5LR for 24 h with cefazolin sodium 1 g IVPB/100 mL D_5W q6h to run 1 h. Limit total fluids to 3000 mL daily.*

The drop factor is 10 gtt/mL.

NOTE: The order intends that the patient will receive a maximum of 3000 mL in 24 hours. Remember, when fluids are restricted, the piggybacks are to be *included* in the total 24-hour intake, not added to it.

Step 1 Calculate the flow rate of the IVPB.

$$\frac{V}{T} \times C = \frac{100\ \cancel{\text{mL}}}{\underset{6}{\cancel{60}}\ \text{min}} \times \overset{1}{\cancel{10}}\ \text{gtt}/\cancel{\text{mL}} = \frac{100\ \text{gtt}}{6\ \text{min}} = 16.6\ \text{gtt/min} = 17\ \text{gtt/min}$$

or $\frac{\text{mL/h}}{\text{Drop factor constant}} = \text{gtt/min}$ (Drop factor constant is 6.)

$$\frac{100\ \text{mL/h}}{6} = 16.6\ \text{gtt/min} = 17\ \text{gtt/min}$$

Set the flow rate for the IVPB at 17 gtt/min to infuse 1 g cefazolin sodium in 100 mL over 1 h or 60 min.

Step 2 Calculate the total time the IVPB will be administered.

q6h = 4 times/24 h; 4 × 1 h = 4 h

Step 3 Calculate the total volume of the IVPB.

100 mL × 4 = 400 mL IVPB per 24 hours

Step 4 Calculate the volume of the regular IV fluids to be administered between IVPB. Total volume of regular IV minus total volume of IVPB: 3000 mL − 400 mL = 2600 mL.

Step 5 Calculate the total regular IV fluid time or the time between IVPB. Total IV time minus total IVPB time: 24 h − 4 h = 20 h

Step 6 Calculate the flow rate of the regular IV.

$$\text{mL/h} = \frac{2600\text{ mL}}{20\text{ h}} = 130\text{ mL/h}$$

$$\frac{V}{T} \times C = \frac{130\ \cancel{\text{mL}}}{\overset{}{\cancel{60}}_{6}\text{ min}} \times \overset{1}{\cancel{10}}\text{ gtt/}\cancel{\text{mL}} = \frac{130\text{ gtt}}{6\text{ min}} = 21.6\text{ gtt/min} = 22\text{ gtt/min}$$

$$\text{or } \frac{\text{mL/h}}{\text{Drop factor constant}} = \text{gtt/min (Drop factor constant is 6.)}$$

$$\frac{130\text{ mL/h}}{6} = 21.6\text{ gtt/min} = 22\text{ gtt/min}$$

Set the regular IV of D_5LR at the flow rate of 22 gtt/min. Then after 5 hours, switch to the cefazolin IVPB at the flow rate of 17 gtt/min for 1 hour. Repeat this process four times in 24 hours.

Example 2:

Order: *2000 mL NS IV for 24 h with 80 mg gentamicin sulfate in 80 mL IVPB q8h to run for 30 min. Limit fluid intake to 2000 mL daily.*

Drop factor: 15 gtt/mL

Calculate the flow rate for the regular IV and for the IVPB.

Step 1 IVPB flow rate:

$$\frac{V}{T} \times C = \frac{80\ \cancel{\text{mL}}}{\cancel{30}_{2}\text{ min}} \times \overset{1}{\cancel{15}}\text{ gtt/}\cancel{\text{mL}} = \frac{80\text{ gtt}}{2\text{ min}} = 40\text{ gtt/min}$$

Step 2 Total IVPB time: q8h = 3 times/24 h; 3 × 30 min = 90 min $= \frac{90}{60} = 1\frac{1}{2}$ h

Step 3 Total IVPB volume: 80 mL × 3 = 240 mL

Step 4 Total regular IV volume: 2000 mL − 240 mL = 1760 mL

Step 5 Total regular IV time: 24 h − $1\frac{1}{2}$ h = $22\frac{1}{2}$ h = 22.5 h

Step 6 Regular IV flow rate:

$$\text{mL/h} = \frac{1760\text{ mL}}{22.5\text{ h}} = 78.2 = 78\text{ mL/h}$$

$$\frac{V}{T} \times C = \frac{78 \cancel{mL}}{\cancel{60}_4 \text{ min}} \times \cancel{15}^1 \text{ gtt}/\cancel{mL} = \frac{78 \text{ gtt}}{4 \text{ min}} = 19.5 \text{ gtt/min} = 20 \text{ gtt/min}$$

$$\text{or } \frac{\text{mL/h}}{\text{Drop factor constant}} = \text{R (Drop factor constant is 4.)}$$

$$\frac{78 \text{ mL/h}}{4} = 19.5 \text{ gtt/min} = 20 \text{ gtt/min}$$

Set the regular IV of NS at the flow rate of 20 gtt/min. After $7\frac{1}{2}$ hours, switch to the gentamicin sulfate IVPB at the flow rate of 40 gtt/min for 30 minutes. Repeat this process 3 times in 24 hours.

Patients receiving a primary IV at a specific rate via an infusion controller or pump may require that the infusion rate be altered when a secondary (piggyback) medication is being administered. To do this, calculate the flow rate of the secondary medication in millilitres per hour as you would for the primary IV, and reset the infusion device.

Some infusion controllers or pumps allow you to set the flow rate for the secondary IV independent of the primary IV. Upon completion of the secondary infusion, the infusion device automatically returns to the original flow rate. If this is not the case, be sure to manually readjust the primary flow rate after the completion of the secondary set.

QUICK REVIEW

- To calculate the flow rate of a regular IV with an IVPB and restricted fluids, calculate:

Step 1 IVPB flow rate
Step 2 Total IVPB time
Step 3 Total IVPB volume
Step 4 Total regular IV volume
Step 5 Total regular IV time
Step 6 Regular IV flow rate

REVIEW SET 43

Calculate the flow rates for the IV and IVPB orders. These patients are on limited fluid volume (restricted fluids).

1. Orders: *3000 mL NS IV for 24 h*

   Limit total IV fluids to 3000 mL daily

   penicillin G sodium 1 000 000 units IVPB q4h in 100 mL NS to run over 30 min

   Drop factor: 10 gtt/mL

   IVPB flow rate: ________ gtt/min

   IV flow rate: ________ gtt/min

2. Orders: *1000 mL D_5W IV for 24 h*

   Limit total IV fluids to 1000 mL daily

   gentamicin sulfate 40 mg QID in 40 mL IVPB to run over 1 h

   Drop factor: 60 gtt/mL

   IVPB flow rate: ________ gtt/min

   IV flow rate: ________ gtt/min

3. Orders: *3000 mL D_5 LR IV for 24 h*

   Limit total IV fluids to 3000 mL daily

   ampicillin sodium 0.5 g q6h IVPB in 50 mL D_5W to run over 30 min

   Drop factor: 15 gtt/mL

   IVPB flow rate: ________ gtt/min

   IV flow rate: ________ gtt/min

4. Orders: *2000 mL $\frac{1}{2}$ NS IV for 24 h*

   Limit total IV fluids to 2000 mL daily

   Amikacin sulfate 500 mg/50 mL NS IVPB q6h to run over 1 h

   Drop factor: 60 gtt/mL

   IVPB flow rate: ________ gtt/min

   IV flow rate: ________ gtt/min

5. Orders: *1000 mL LR IV for 24 h*

   Limit total IV fluids to 1000 mL daily

   cefazolin sodium 250 mg IVPB/50 mL D_5W q8h to run over 1 h

   Drop factor: 60 gtt/mL

   IVPB flow rate: ________ gtt/min

   IV flow rate: ________ gtt/min

6. Orders: *2400 mL of D_5 LR for 24 h*

   Limit total IV fluids to 2400 mL daily

   cefazolin sodium 1 g IVPB q6h in 50 mL D_5W to run over 30 min

   Drop factor: On infusion pump

   IVPB flow rate: ________ mL/h

   IV flow rate: ________ mL/h

7. Orders: *2000 mL NS for 24 h*

   Limit total IV fluids to 2000 mL daily

   gentamicin sulfate 100 mg IVPB q8h in 100 mL D_5W to run over 30 min

   Drop factor: On infusion controller

   IVPB flow rate: ________ mL/h

   IV flow rate: ________ mL/h

8. Orders: *3000 mL D_5 0.45% NS to run 24 h*

   Limit total IV fluids to 3000 mL daily

   ranitidine hydrochloride 50 mg q6h in 50 mL D_5W to infuse over 15 min

   Drop factor: On infusion controller

   IVPB flow rate: ________ mL/h

   IV flow rate: ________ mL/h

9. Orders: *1500 mL D_5 NS to run 24 h*

   Limit total IV fluids to 1500 mL daily

   cefazolin sodium 500 mg IVPB/50 mL D_5W q8h to run over 1 h

   Drop factor: 20 gtt/mL

   IVPB flow rate: ________ gtt/min

   IV flow rate: ________ gtt/min

10. Orders: *2700 mL NS IV for 24 h*

    Limit total IV fluids to 2700 mL daily

    gentamicin sulfate 60 mg in 60 mL D_5W IVPB q8h to run over 30 min

    Drop factor: On infusion pump

    IVPB flow rate: ________ mL/h

    IV flow rate: ________ mL/h

After completing these problems, see pages 507–509 to check your answers.

CRITICAL THINKING SKILLS

The importance of knowing the therapeutic dosage of a given medication is a critical nursing skill. Let us look at an example in which the order was unclear, and the nurse did not verify the order with the appropriate person.

error

Failing to clarify an order.

possible scenario

Suppose the physician ordered a heparin infusion for a patient with thrombophlebitis who weighs 100 kg. The facility uses the Standard Weight-Based Heparin Protocol as seen in Figure 14-2, page 391. The patient care order was written this way:

heparin 25 000 units in 250 mL $\frac{1}{2}$ NS IV at 18 000/h.

The order was difficult to read and the nurse asked a co-worker to help her decipher it. They both agreed that it read 18 000 units per hour. The nurse calculated mL/h to be:

$$\frac{18\,000 \text{ units}}{25\,000 \text{ units}} \times 250 \text{ mL} = 180 \text{ mL/h}$$

She proceeded to start the heparin drip at 180 mL/h. The patient's aPTT prior to initiation of the infusion was 37 seconds. Six hours into the infusion, an aPTT was drawn according to protocol. The nurse was shocked when the results returned and were 95 seconds, which is abnormally high. She called the physician, who asked, "What is the rate of the heparin drip?" The nurse replied, "I have the infusion set at 180 mL/h so the patient receives the prescribed amount of 18 000 units per hour." The physician was astonished and replied, "I ordered the drip at 1800 units per hour, not 18 000 units per hour."

(continues)

(continued)

potential outcome

The physician would likely have discontinued the heparin; ordered protamine sulfate, the antidote for heparin overdosage; and obtained another aPTT. The patient may have started to show signs of abnormal bleeding, such as blood in the urine, bloody nose, and increased tendency to bruise.

prevention

When the physician wrote the order for 1800 U/h, the U looked like a 0 and the nurse misinterpreted the order as 18 000. The nurse missed three opportunities to prevent this error. The order as written is unclear, unsafe, and incomplete. Contacting the physician and requesting a clarification of the order are appropriate actions for several reasons. First, the writing is unclear, which is an automatic caution to contact the prescribing practitioner for clarification. Guessing about the exact meaning of an order is dangerous, as this scenario demonstrates. Clearly this indicates how easily U can be misinterpreted as an extra 0 and the potential consequences. The Institute for Safe Medication Practices (ISMP Canada) recommends writing out *units* to avoid errors.

Second, the Standard Weight-Based Heparin Protocol recommends a safe heparin infusion rate of 1800 units/h or 18 mL/h (with a supply dosage of 25 000 units/250 mL = 100 units/mL) for an individual weighing 100 kg. It is the responsibility of the individual administering a medication to be sure the Rights of medication administration are observed. The first three Rights are that the "*right* patient must receive the *right* drug in the *right* amount." The order of 18 000 units as understood by the nurse was unsafe. The patient was overdosed by 10 times the recommended amount of heparin.

Third, if the nurse clearly interpreted the order as 18 000, then no units were specified, which is a medication error that requires contact with the physician for correction. An incomplete order must not be filled.

PRACTICE PROBLEMS—CHAPTER 14

You are working on the day shift 0700–1500 h. You observe that one of the patients assigned to you has an IV infusion with a volume control set. His patient care orders include:

D_5W IV at 50 mL/h for continuous infusion

piperacillin sodium 1 g IV q6h

You prepare the piperacillin sodium to a concentration of *1 g per 5.5 mL*. Instructions are to pre-add piperacillin sodium to volume control set, and infuse over 30 minutes. Answer questions 1 through 5.

1. What is the drop factor of the volume control set? ________ gtt/mL
2. What amount of piperacillin sodium will you add to the chamber? ________ mL
3. How much D_5W IV fluid will you add to the chamber with the piperacillin sodium? ________ mL
4. To maintain the flow rate at 50 mL/h, you will time the IV piperacillin sodium to infuse at ________ gtt/min.
5. The medication administration record indicates that the patient received his last dose of IV piperacillin sodium at 0600 h. How many doses of piperacillin sodium will you administer during your shift? ________
6. Order: *heparin sodium 25 000 units in 250 mL 0.45% NS to infuse at 1200 units/h*

   Drop factor: On infusion controller

   Flow rate: ________ mL/h.

7. Order: *thiamine hydrochloride 100 mg per L D_5W IV to infuse at 5 mg/h*

   Drop factor: On infusion pump

   Flow rate: ________ mL/h

8. Order: *magnesium sulfate 4 g in 500 mL D_5W at 500 mg/h*

   Drop factor: On infusion pump

   Flow rate: ________ mL/h

9. A patient is to receive *D_5W 500 mL with heparin sodium 20 000 units at 1400 units/h.*

   Set the infusion pump at ________ mL/h.

10. At the rate of 4 mL/min, how long will it take to administer 1.5 L of IV fluid? ________ h and ________ min

11. Order: *lidocaine hydrochloride drip IV to run at 4 mg/min*

    Supply: 500 mL D_5W with lidocaine 2 g added

    Drop factor: On infusion pump

    Flow rate: ________ mL/h

12. Order: *lidocaine hydrochloride 1 g IV in 250 mL D_5W at 3 mg/min*

    Drop factor: On infusion controller

    Flow rate: ________ mL/h

13. Order: *procainamide hydrochloride 1 g in 500 mL D_5W to infuse at 2 mg/min*

    Drop factor: On infusion pump

    Flow rate: ________ mL/h

14. Order: *dobutamine hydrochloride 250 mg in 250 mL D_5W to infuse at 5 mcg/kg/min*

    Weight: 80 kg

    Drop factor: On infusion controller

    Flow rate: ________ mL/h

15. Your patient has *1 L D_5W with 2 g lidocaine hydrochloride added infusing at 75 mL/h.* The recommended continuous IV dosage of lidocaine hydrochloride is 1–4 mg/min. Is this dosage safe?

    ____

16. Order: *Restricted fluids: 3000 mL D_5 NS IV for 24 h*

    amikacin sulfate 1 g IVPB in 100 mL NS q6h to run 1 h

    Drop factor: 10 gtt/mL

    Flow rate: ________ gtt/min IVPB and ________ gtt/min primary IV

17. Order: *Restricted fluids: 3000 mL D_5W IV for 24 h*

    ampicillin sodium 500 mg in 50 mL D_5W IVPB QID for 30 min

    Drop factor: On infusion pump

    Flow rate: ________ mL/h IVPB and ________ mL/h primary IV

18. Order: *50 mg nitroglycerin IV in 500 mL D_5W to infuse at 3 mcg/kg/min*

    Weight: 125 lb

    Drop factor: On infusion pump

    Flow rate: ________ mL/h

19. Order: *potassium chloride 40 mEq/L of 5% D_5W*

    Situation: IV discontinued with 800 mL remaining

    How much potassium chloride infused? ________

20. A patient's infusion rate is 125 mL/h. The rate is equivalent to ________ mL/min.

21. Order: *1500 mL $\frac{1}{2}$ NS to run at 100 mL/h.* Calculate the infusion time. ________ h

    Calculate the information requested for questions 22 and 23, assuming that the drop factor for the infusion set is 60 gtt per mL.

22. Order: *potassium chloride 40 mEq/L D_5W IV to infuse at 2 mEq/h*

    Rate: ________ mL/h

    Rate: ________ gtt/min

23. Order: *heparin sodium 50 000 units/L D_5W to infuse at 3750 units/h*

    Rate: ________ mL/h

    Rate: ________ gtt/min

24. If the minimal dilution for tobramycin sulfate is 5 mg/mL and you are giving 37 mg, what is the least amount of fluid in which you could safely dilute the dosage? ________ mL

25. Order: *oxytocin 10 units in 500 mL NS. Infuse 4 milliunits/min for 20 min, followed by 6 milliunits/min for 20 min. Use electronic infusion pump.*

    Rate: ________ mL/h for first 20 min

    Rate: ________ mL/h for next 20 min

26. Order: *magnesium sulfate 20 g IV in 500 mL of LR solution. Start with a bolus of 3 g to infuse over 30 min. Then maintain a continuous infusion at 2 g/h.*

    You will use an electronic infusion pump.

    Rate: ________ mL/h for bolus

    Rate: ________ mL/h for continuous infusion

27. Order: *oxytocin 15 units in 500 mL of LR solution. Infuse at 1 milliunit/min*

    You will use an electronic infusion pump.

    Rate: ________ mL/h

28. Order: *heparin sodium drip 40 000 units/L D_5W to infuse at 1400 units/h*

    Drop factor: On infusion pump

    Flow rate: ________ mL/h

    Refer to this order for questions 29 and 30.

    Order: *magnesium sulfate 4 g in 500 mL D_5W at 500 mg/h on an infusion pump*

29. What is the solution concentration? ________ mg/mL

30. What is the hourly flow rate? ________ mL/h

Calculate the drug concentration of the following IV solutions as requested.

31. A solution containing 80 units of oxytocin in 1000 mL of D_5W: ________ milliunits/mL

32. A solution containing 200 mg of nitroglycerin in 500 mL of D_5W: ________ mg/mL

33. A solution containing 4 mg of isoproterenol hydrochloride in 1000 mL of D_5W: ________ mcg/mL

34. A solution containing 2 g of lidocaine hydrochloride in 500 mL of D_5W: ________ mg/mL

Refer to this patient care order for questions 35 through 37.

Order: *rocuronium bromide IV 1 mg/kg/min* to control respirations for a ventilated patient. The patient weighs 100 kg.

35. The available rocuronium bromide 10 mg is dissolved in 100 mL NS. This available solution concentration is ________ mg/mL, which is equivalent to ______ mcg/mL.

36. The IV is infusing at the rate of 1 mcg/kg/min on an infusion pump. The hourly rate is ________ mL/h.

Refer to this patient care order for questions 37 through 42.

Order: *Restricted fluids: 3000 mL/24 h. Primary IV of D_5LR running via infusion pump. ampicillin sodium 3 g IVPB q6h in 100 mL of D_5W over 30 min gentamicin sulfate 170 mg IVPB q8h in 50 mL of D_5W to infuse in 1 h.*

37. Calculate the IVPB flow rates. ampicillin sodium: ________ mL/h; gentamicin sulfate: ________ mL/h

38. Calculate the total IVPB time. ________ h

39. Calculate the total IVPB volume. ________ mL

40. Calculate the total regular IV volume. ________ mL

41. Calculate the total regular IV time. ________ h

42. Calculate the regular IV flow rate. ________ mL/h

43. A 86.4-kg patient in kidney failure receives *dopamine hydrochloride 800 mg in 500 mL of D_5W IV at 4 mcg/kg/min*. As the patient's blood pressure drops, the nurse titrates the drip to *12 mcg/kg/min* as ordered.

    What is the initial flow rate? ________ mL/h

    After titration, what is the flow rate? ________ mL/h

Questions 44 through 48 refer to your patient who has left leg deep vein thrombosis. He has orders for IV heparin sodium therapy. He weighs 100 kg. On admission his aPTT is 25 seconds. You initiate therapy at 1130 h on 5/10/xx. Follow the "Standard Weight-Based Heparin Sodium Protocol" on the next page. Record your answers on the "Standard Weight-Based Heparin Sodium Protocol Worksheet" on page 414.

44. What does the protocol indicate for the standard bolus dosage of heparin sodium? ________ units/kg

45. Calculate the dosage of heparin sodium that should be administered for the bolus for this patient. ________ units (Record on the worksheet.)

    What does the protocol indicate as the required solution concentration (supply dosage) of heparin sodium to use for the bolus? ________ units/mL

    Calculate the dose volume of heparin sodium that should be administered for the bolus for this patient. ________ mL (Record on the worksheet.)

46. What does the protocol indicate for the initial infusion rate? ________ units/kg/h

    Calculate the dosage of heparin sodium this patient should receive each hour. ________ units/h (Record on the worksheet.)

    What does the protocol indicate as the required solution concentration (supply dosage) of heparin sodium to use for the initial infusion? ________ units/mL

    Calculate the heparin sodium solution volume this patient should receive each hour to provide the correct infusion for his weight. ________ mL/h (Record on the worksheet.)

47. According to the protocol, how often should the patient's aPTT be checked? ________ h

    At 1730 h, the patient's aPTT is 37 seconds. Rebolus with heparin sodium ________ units (________ mL) (Record on the worksheet.)

    How much should you change the infusion rate? ________ increase or ________ decrease heparin sodium ________ units/h and ________ mL/h (Record on the worksheet.)

    The new infusion rate will be heparin sodium ________ mL/h (Record on the worksheet.)

48. At 2330 h, the patient's aPPT is 77 seconds. What should you do now?

    ____

    The infusion rate will be heparin sodium ________ mL/h (Record on the worksheet.)

Standard Weight-Based Heparin Sodium Protocol

For all patients on heparin drips:

1. Weight in KILOGRAMS. Required for order to be processed: ________ kg
2. Heparin sodium 25 000 units in 250 mL of $\frac{1}{2}$NS. Boluses to be given as 1000 units/mL.
3. aPTT q6h or 6 hours after rate change; daily after two consecutive therapeutic aPTTs.
4. CBC initially and repeat every ________ day(s).
5. Obtain aPTT and PT/INR on day 1 prior to initiation of therapy.
6. Guaiac stool initially then every ________ day(s) until heparin sodium discontinued. Notify if positive.
7. Neuro checks every ________ hours while on heparin sodium. Notify physician of any changes.
8. D/C aPTT and CBC once heparin sodium drip is discontinued, unless otherwise ordered.
9. Notify physician of any bleeding problems.
10. Bolus with 80 units/kg. Start drip at 18 units/kg/h.
11. If aPTT is less than 35 secs: Rebolus with 80 units/kg and increase rate by 4 units/kg/h
12. If aPTT is 36–44 secs: Rebolus with 40 units/kg and increase rate by 2 units/kg/h
13. If aPTT is 45–75 secs: Continue current rate
14. If aPTT is 76–90 secs: Decrease rate by 2 units/kg/h
15. If aPTT is more than 90 secs: Hold heparin sodium for 1 h and decrease rate by 3 units/kg/h

STANDARD WEIGHT-BASED HEPARIN SODIUM PROTOCOL WORKSHEET

Round Patient's Total Body Weight to Nearest 10 kg: _______ kg

DO NOT Change the Weight Based on Daily Measurements

FOUND ON THE ORDER FORM

Initial Bolus (80 units/kg) _______ units _______ mL

Initial Infusion Rate (18 units/kg/h) _______ units/h _______ mL/h

Make adjustments to the heparin sodium drip rate as directed by the order form.

ALL DOSES ARE ROUNDED TO THE NEAREST 100 UNITS

Date	Time	aPTT	Bolus	Rate Change		New Rate	RN 1	RN 2
				units/h	mL/h			

If aPTT is	Then
less than 35 secs:	Rebolus with 80 units/kg and increase rate by 4 units/kg/h
36–44 secs:	Rebolus with 40 units/kg and increase rate by 2 units/kg/h
45–75 secs:	Continue current rate
76–90 secs:	Decrease rate by 2 units/kg/h
more than 90 secs:	Hold heparin sodium for 1 h and decrease rate by 3 units/kg/h

Signatures	Initials

49. Critical Thinking Skill: Describe the strategy you would implement to prevent this medication error.

possible scenario

Suppose the physician writes patient care order to induce labour, as follows: *oxytocin 20 units added to 1 L of LR beginning at 1 milliunit/min, then increase by 1 milliunit/min q15–30 min to a maximum of 20 milliunits/min until adequate labour is reached.* The labour and delivery unit stocks oxytocin ampoules 10 units per mL in boxes of 50 ampoules. The nurse preparing the IV solution misread the order as "20 mL of oxytocin added to 1 litre of lactated Ringer's . . ." and pulled 20 ampoules of oxytocin from the supply shelf. Another nurse, seeing this nurse drawing up medication from several ampoules, asked what the nurse was preparing. When the nurse described the IV solution being prepared, he suddenly realized he had misinterpreted the order.

potential outcome

The amount of oxytocin that was being drawn up (20 mL) to be added to the IV solution would have been 10 units/mL $\times$ 20 mL = 200 units of oxytocin, 10 times the ordered amount of 20 units. Starting this oxytocin solution, even at the usual slow rate, would have delivered an excessively high amount of oxytocin that could have led to fatal consequences for both the fetus and labouring mother. What should the nurse have done to avoid this type of error?

prevention

____

____

After completing these problems, see pages 509–512 to check your answers.

SECTION 4 SELF-EVALUATION

Chapter 12: Intravenous Solutions, Equipment, and Calculations

1. Which of the following IV solutions is normal saline?
_________ 0.45% NaCl _________ 0.9% NaCl _________ D_5W

2. What is the solute and concentration of 0.9% NaCl? _________

3. What is the solute and concentration of 0.45% NaCl? _________

Use the following information to answer questions 4 and 5.

Order: *1000 mL of D_5 0.33% NaCl IV solution*

4. The IV solution contains _________ g dextrose.

5. The IV solution contains _________ g sodium chloride.

6. An order specifies *500 mL 0.45% NS IV*. The IV solution contains _________ g sodium chloride.

Refer to this patient care order for questions 7 and 8.

Order: *750 mL D_{10} 0.9% NaCl IV*

7. The IV solution contains _________ g dextrose.

8. The IV solution contains _________ g sodium chloride.

9. Are most electronic infusion devices calibrated in gtt/min, mL/h, mL/min, or gtt/mL?
____

Use the following information to answer questions 10 and 11.

Mrs. Wilson has an order to receive *2000 mL of IV fluids over 24 h*. The IV tubing is calibrated for a drop factor of 15 gtt/mL.

10. Calculate the "watch count" flow rate for Mrs. Wilson's IV. _________ gtt/min

11. An infusion controller becomes available, and you decide to use it to regulate Mrs. Wilson's IV. Set the controller at _________ mL/h.

12. Mrs. Hawkins returns from the delivery room at 1530 h with 400 mL D_5LR infusing at 24 gtt/min with your hospital's standard macrodrop infusion control set calibrated at 15 gtt/mL. You anticipate that Mrs. Hawkins's IV will be complete at _________ (hours).

13. You start your shift at 1500 h. On your nursing rounds, you find that Mr. Johnson has an IV of $D_5 \frac{1}{2}$ NS infusing at 32 gtt/min. The tubing is calibrated for 10 gtt/mL. Mr. Johnson will receive _________ mL during your 8-hour shift.

Use the following information to answer questions 14 through 16.

As you continue on your rounds, you find Mr. Boyd with an infiltrated IV and decide to restart it and regulate it on an electronic infusion pump. The orders specify:
1000 mL NS IV with 20 mEq KCl q8h
cefazolin sodium 250 mg IVPB/100 mL NS q8h over 30 min
Limit IV total fluids to 3000 mL daily

14. Interpret Mr. Boyd's IV and medication order. ____
____

15. Regulate the electronic infusion pump for Mr. Boyd's standard IV at ________ mL/h.

16. Regulate the electronic infusion pump for Mr. Boyd's IVPB at ________ mL/h.

17. Order: *D_5LR 1200 mL IV @ 100 mL/h.* You start this IV at 1530 h and regularly observe the IV and the patient. The IV has been infusing as scheduled, but during your nursing assessment at 2200 h, you find 650 mL remaining. The flow rate is 100 gtt/min using a microdrip infusion set. Describe your action now. ________________________________

____

Chapter 13: Body Surface Area and Advanced Pediatric Calculations

Calculate the hourly maintenance IV rate for the children described in questions 18 through 21. Use the following recommendations:

First 10 kg of body weight: 100 mL/kg/day

Second 10 kg of body weight: 50 mL/kg/day

Each additional kilogram over 20 kg of body weight: 20 mL/kg/day

18. An 18.2-kg child requires ________ mL/day for maintenance IV fluids.

19. The infusion rate for the same 18.2-kg child is ________ mL/h.

20. An 1185-g infant requires ________ mL/day for maintenance IV fluids.

21. The infusion rate for the same 1185-g infant is ________ mL/h.

Use the BSA formula method (next page) to answer questions 22 and 23.

22. Height: 76 cm Weight: 11 kg BSA: ________ m^2

23. Height: 155 cm Weight: 39 kg BSA: ________ m^2

Questions 24 through 30 refer to the following situation.

A child who is 71 cm tall and weighs 11.4 kg will receive one dosage of cisplatin IV. The recommended dosage is 37–75 mg/m^2 once every 2–3 weeks. The order reads *cisplatin 18.5 mg IV @ 1 mg/min today at 1500 h.* You have available a 50-mg vial of cisplatin. Reconstitution directions are to add 50 mL of sterile water to yield 1 mg/mL. Minimal dilution instructions require 2 mL of IV solution for every 1 mg of cisplatin.

24. According to the nomogram (next page), the child's BSA is ________ m^2.

25. The safe dosage range for this child is ________ to ________ mg.

26. Is this dosage safe? ________

27. If safe, you will prepare ________ mL. If not, describe your action. ________________

____

28. How many mL of IV fluid are required for safe dilution of the cisplatin? ________ mL

29. Given the ordered rate of 1 mg/min, set the infusion pump at ________ mL/h.

30. How long will this infusion take? ________ min

WEST NOMOGRAM

$$BSA(m^2) = \sqrt{\frac{ht(cm) \times wt(kg)}{3600}}$$

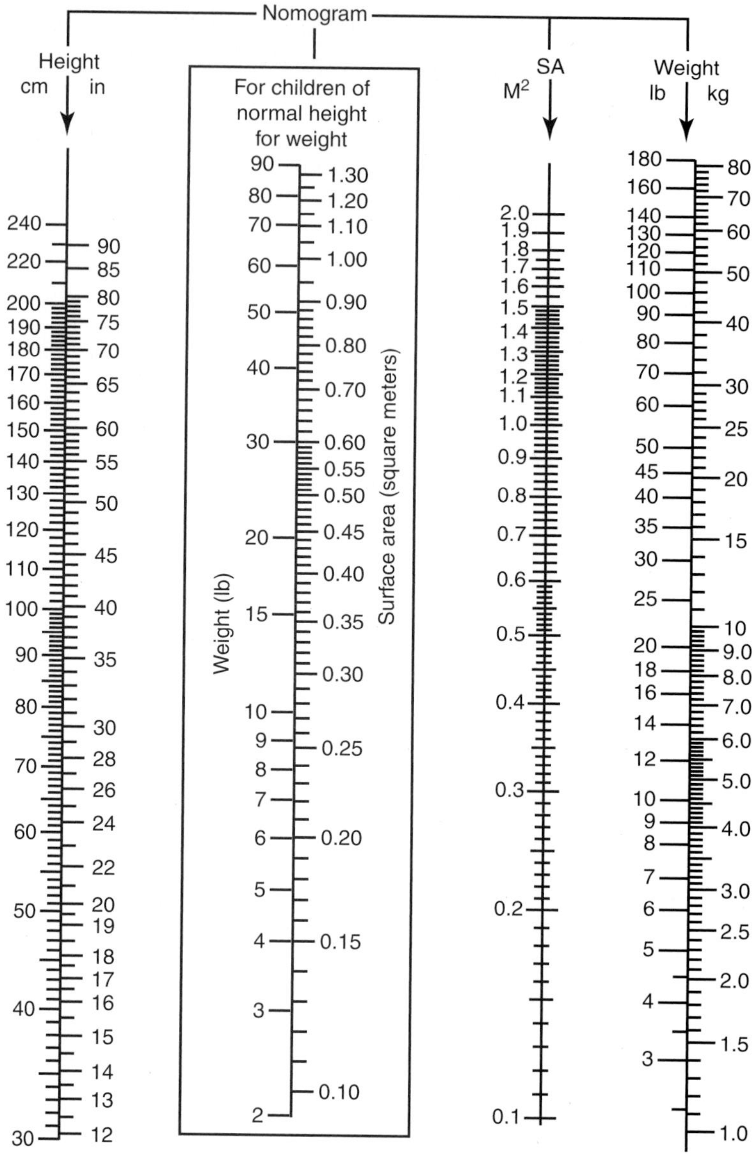

West Nomogram for Estimation of Body Surface Area.

This chart was published in Nelson Textbook of Pediatrics, 16th ed., R. E. Behrman, R. M. Kliegman & H. B. Jenson, West Nomogram for Estimation of Body Surface Area, Copyright Elsevier, (2000).

Questions 31 through 34 refer to the following situation.

Order: *vincristine sulfate 1.6 mg IV stat*. The child is 127 cm tall and weighs 18.2 kg. The label on page 419 represents the vincristine sulfate solution you have available. The recommended dosage of vincristine sulfate is 2 mg/m^2 daily.

31. According to the nomogram, the child's BSA is ________ m^2.
32. The recommended safe dosage for this child is ________ mg.
33. Is the dosage ordered safe? ________
34. If safe, you will prepare ________ mL vincristine sulfate to add to the IV. If not safe, describe your action. ____
____

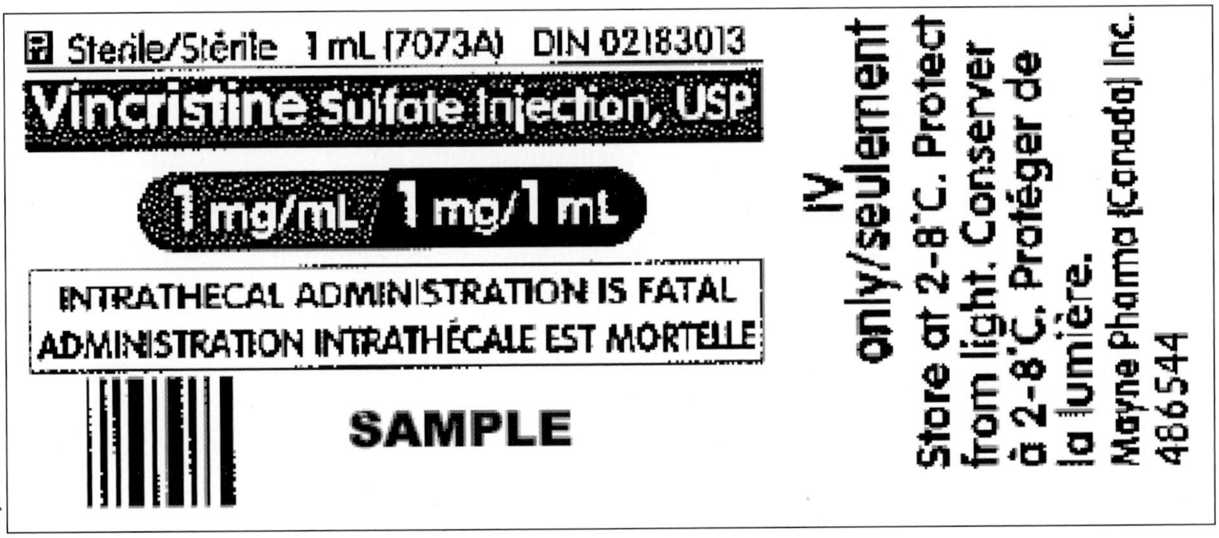

Mayne Pharma (Canada) Inc., Montreal, QUE

35. Order: *NS IV for continuous infusion at 40 mL/h with cefazolin sodium 250 mg IV q8h over 30 min by volume control set*

    Available: cefazolin sodium 125 mg/mL

    Add _______ mL NS and _______ mL cefazolin sodium to the chamber to infuse at 40 mL/h.

Order: *metoclopramide hydrochloride 75 mg IV q3h × 3 doses* for a 25-kg child receiving chemotherapy. Recommended dose is 0.5–1.5/mg/dose (not to exceed 2 mg/kg/dose). Metoclopramide hydrochloride is available as a 30 mL vial containing 150 mg.

36. Calculate the recommended dosage range of metoclopramide hydrochloride. ________ mg to ________ mg
37. Is this dose safe. If yes, administer ________ mL. If not, describe your action. ________

Chapter 14: Advanced Adult Intravenous Calculations

Use the following information to answer questions 38 through 41.

Mr. Smith is on restricted fluids. His IV order is: *1500 mL NS IV/24 h with 300 000 units penicillin G sodium IVPB 100 mL NS q4h over 30 min*. The infusion set is calibrated at 60 gtt/mL.

38. Set Mr. Smith's regular IV at ________ gtt/min.
39. Set Mr. Smith's IVPB at ________ gtt/min.
40. Later during your shift, an electronic infusion pump becomes available. You decide to use it to regulate Mr. Smith's IVs. Regulate Mr. Smith's regular IV at ________ mL/h.
41. Regulate Mr. Smith's IVPB at ________ mL/h.
42. Order: *potassium chloride 40 mEq/L D_5W IV @ 2 mEq/h.*

    Regulate the infusion pump at ________ mL/h.
43. Order: *nitroglycerin 25 mg/L D_5W IV @ 5 mcg/min*

    Regulate the infusion pump at ________ mL/h.

Refer to the following patient care order for questions 44 through 47.

Order: *Induce labour with oxytocin 15 units/L LR IV continuous infusion @ 2 milliunits/min; increase by 1 milliunit/min q30 min to a maximum of 20 milliunits/min*

44. The initial concentration of oxytocin is ________ milliunits/mL.

45. The initial oxytocin order will infuse at the rate of ________ mL/min.

46. Regulate the electronic infusion pump at ________ mL/h to initiate the order.

47. The infusion pump will be regulated at a maximum of ________ mL/h to infuse the maximum of 20 milliunits/min.

Use the following information to answer questions 48 and 49.

Order for Ms. Hill, who weighs 68 kg: *dopamine hydrochloride 400 mg/0.5 L D_5W at 4 mcg/kg/min titrated to 12 mcg/kg/min to stabilize blood pressure*

48. Regulate the electronic infusion pump for Ms. Hill's IV at ________ mL/h to initiate the order.

49. Anticipate that the maximum flow rate for Ms. Hill's IV to achieve the maximum safe titration would be ________ mL/h.

50. Mr. Black has a new order for *heparin sodium 10 000 units in 500 mL NS IV at 750 units/h*. Regulate the infusion pump at ________ mL/h.

After completing these problems, refer to pages 513–515 to check your answers. Give yourself 2 points for each correct answer.

Perfect score = 100% My score = ________

Minimum mastery score = 86 (43 correct)

Essential Skills Evaluation

This evaluation is designed to assess your mastery of essential dosage calculation skills. It is similar to the type of entry-level test given by hospitals and healthcare agencies during orientation for new graduates and new employees. It excludes the advanced calculation skills presented in Chapters 13 and 14.

You are assigned to give "Team Medications" on a busy Adult Medical Unit. The following labels represent the medications available in the medication cart to fill the orders given in questions 1 through 17. Calculate the amount you will administer for one dose. Assume that all tablets are scored. Draw an arrow on the appropriate syringe to indicate how much you will prepare for parenteral medications.

1. Order: *promethazine hydrochloride 12.5 mg IM q3h prn*

   Give: ______ mL

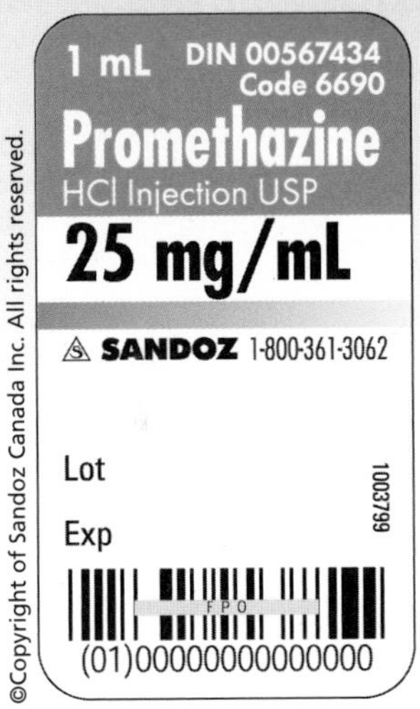

1 mL DIN 00567434
Code 6690
Promethazine
HCl Injection USP
25 mg/mL
SANDOZ 1-800-361-3062
Lot
Exp
1003799
(01)00000000000000
©Copyright of Sandoz Canada Inc. All rights reserved.

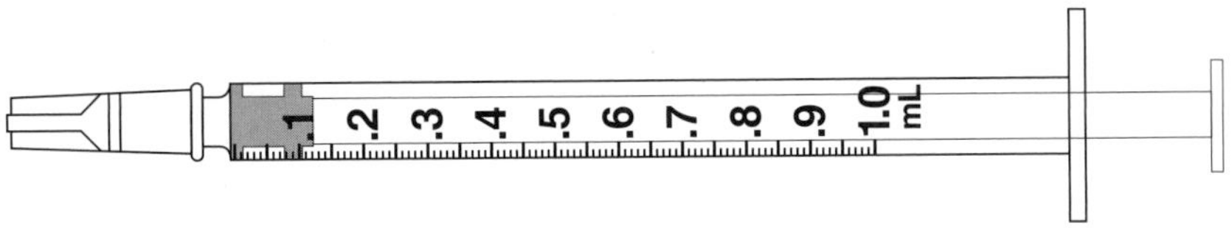

.1 .2 .3 .4 .5 .6 .7 .8 .9 1.0 mL

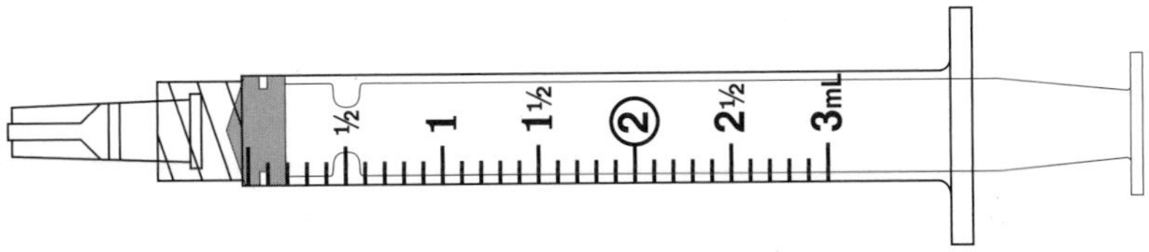

½ 1 1½ 2 2½ 3mL

2. Order: *chlorpromazine hydrochloride 35 mg IM stat*

   Give: ______ mL

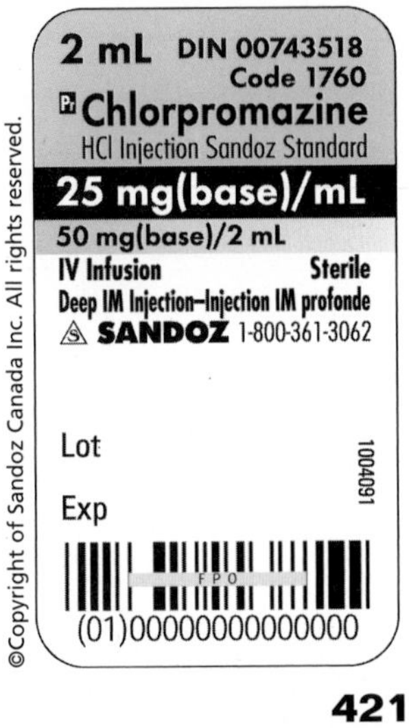

2 mL DIN 00743518
Code 1760
Chlorpromazine
HCl Injection Sandoz Standard
25 mg(base)/mL
50 mg(base)/2 mL
IV Infusion Sterile
Deep IM Injection–Injection IM profonde
SANDOZ 1-800-361-3062
Lot
Exp
1004091
(01)00000000000000
©Copyright of Sandoz Canada Inc. All rights reserved.

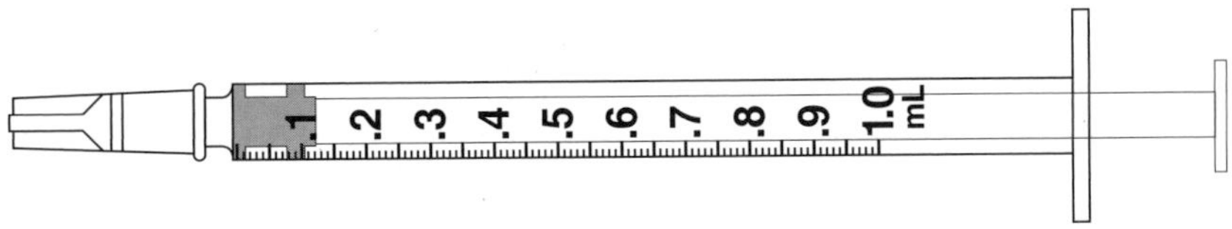

.1 .2 .3 .4 .5 .6 .7 .8 .9 1.0 mL

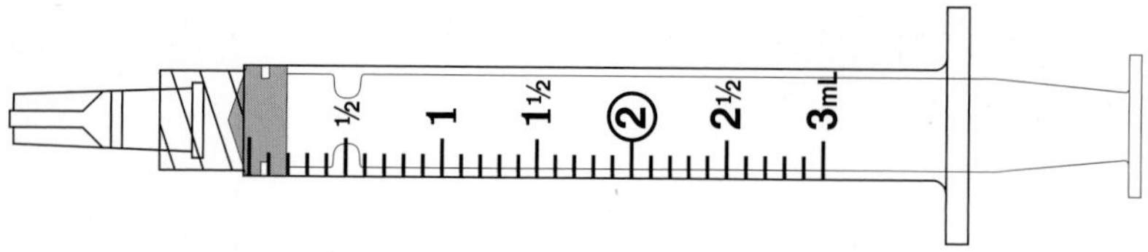
½
1
1½
2
2½
3mL

3. Order: *diazepam 7.5 mg IV push (administer slowly, at 5 mg/min)*

   Give: ______ mL at ______ mL/min or ______ mL/15 sec

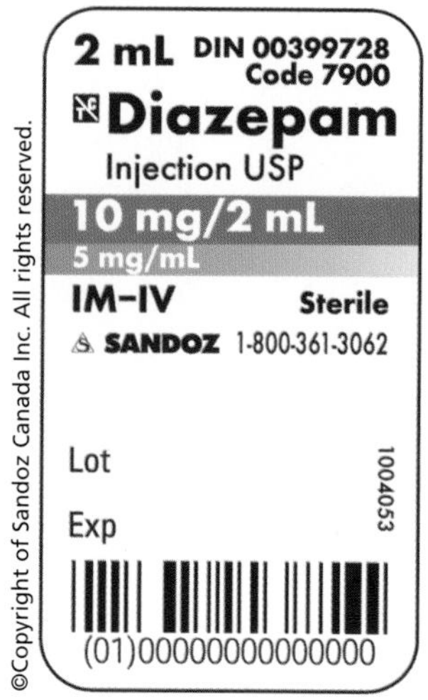
2 mL DIN 00399728
Code 7900
Diazepam
Injection USP
10 mg/2 mL
5 mg/mL
IM–IV Sterile
SANDOZ 1-800-361-3062
Lot
Exp
1004053
(01)00000000000000
©Copyright of Sandoz Canada Inc. All rights reserved.

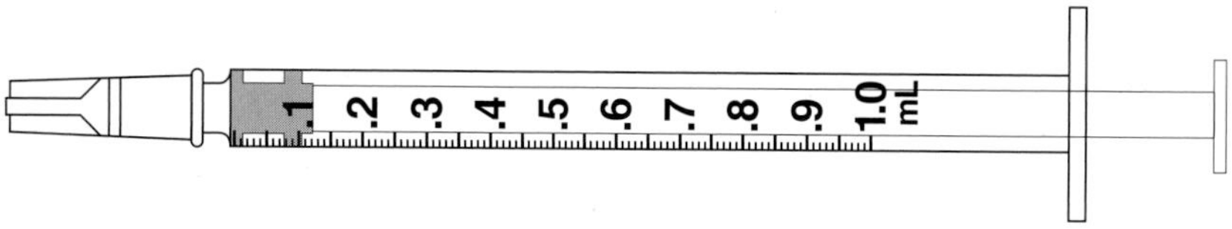
.1 .2 .3 .4 .5 .6 .7 .8 .9 1.0 mL

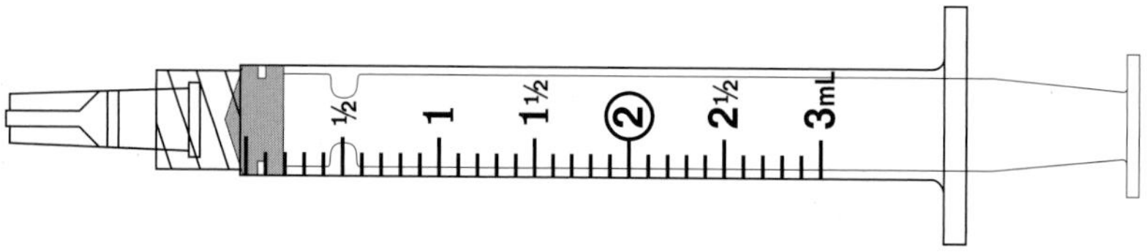
½
1
1½
2
2½
3mL

4. Order: *glycopyrrolate 200 mcg IV stat*

   Give: ______ mL

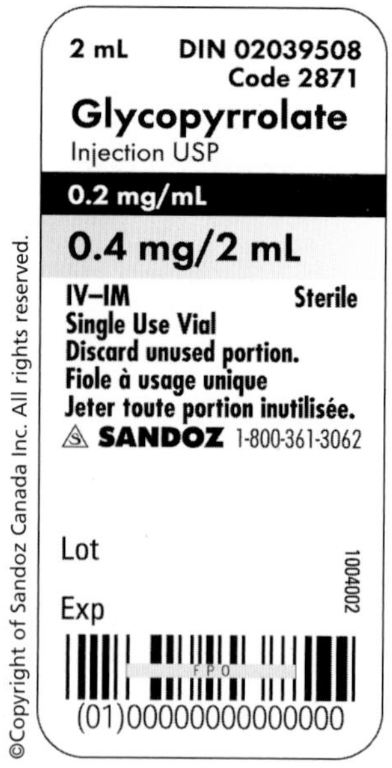
2 mL DIN 02039508
Code 2871
Glycopyrrolate
Injection USP
0.2 mg/mL
0.4 mg/2 mL
IV–IM Sterile
Single Use Vial
Discard unused portion.
Fiole à usage unique
Jeter toute portion inutilisée.
SANDOZ 1-800-361-3062
Lot
Exp
1004002
(01)00000000000000
©Copyright of Sandoz Canada Inc. All rights reserved.

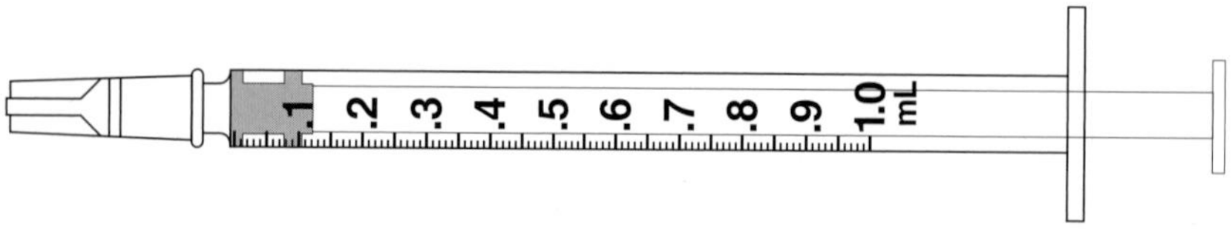
.1 .2 .3 .4 .5 .6 .7 .8 .9 1.0 mL

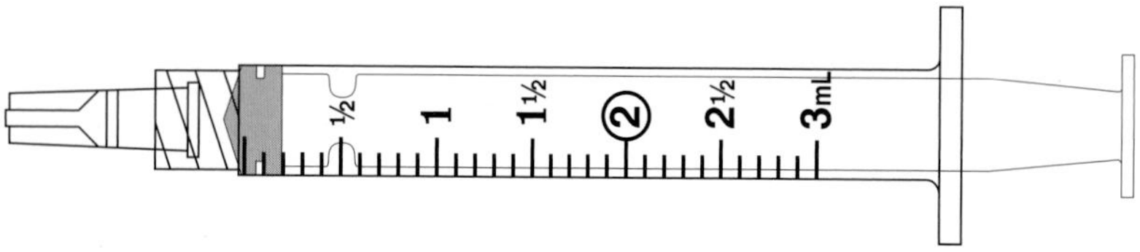
½
1
1½
2
2½
3mL

5. Order: *hydrocodone bitartrate and acetaminophen 7.5 mg PO q3h prn, pain*

   Dosage is based on hydrocodone.

   Give: ______ tablet(s)

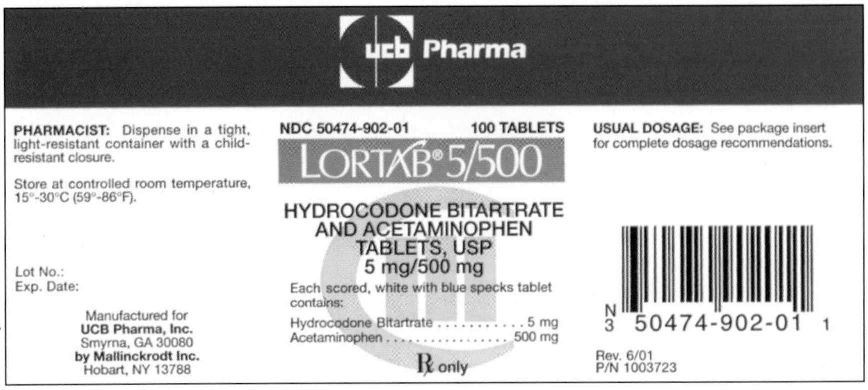

Courtesy UCB Pharma

6. Order: *digoxin 0.125 mg IV qAM*

   Give: ______ mL

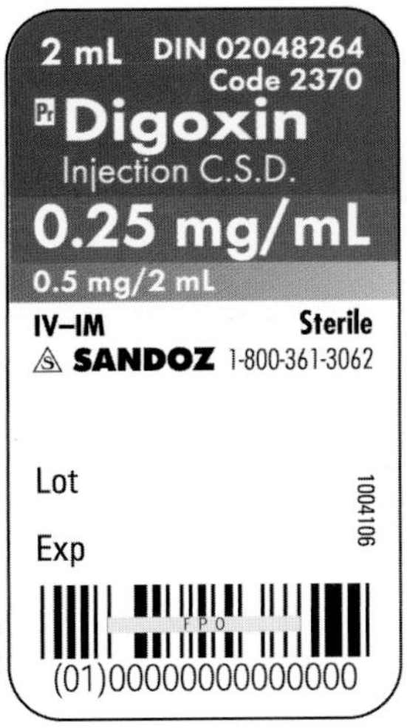

©Copyright of Sandoz Canada Inc. All rights reserved.

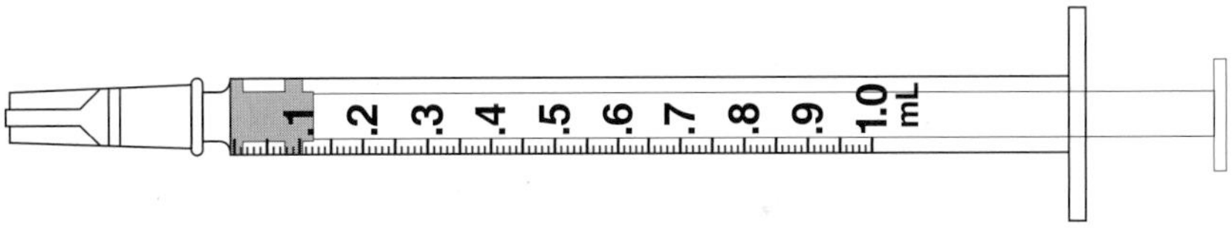

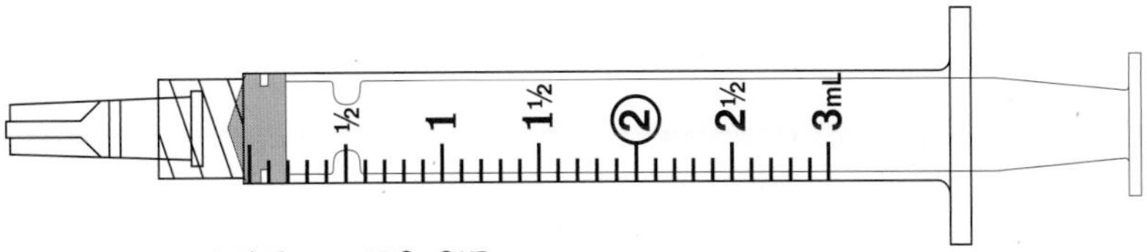

7. Order: *phenobarbital 7.5 mg PO QID*

   Give: ______ tablet(s)

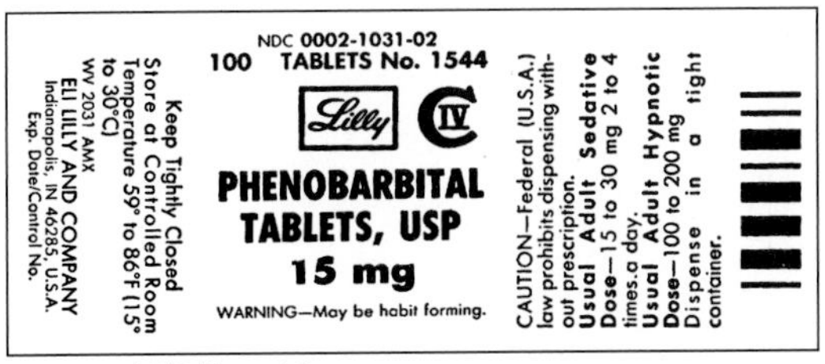

Courtesy of Eli Lilly and Company

8. Order: *amikacin sulfate 350 mg IM BID*

   Give: ______ mL

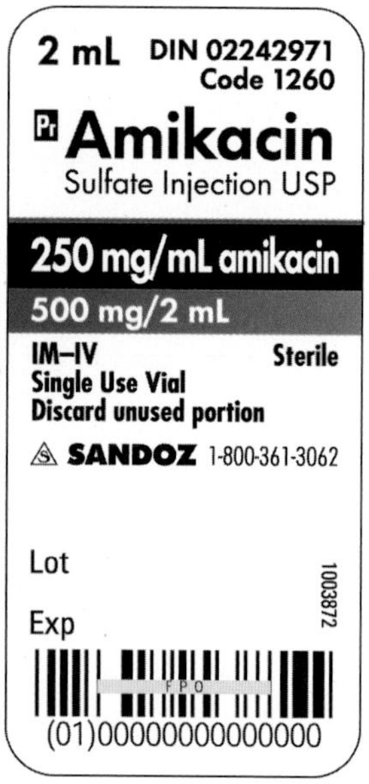

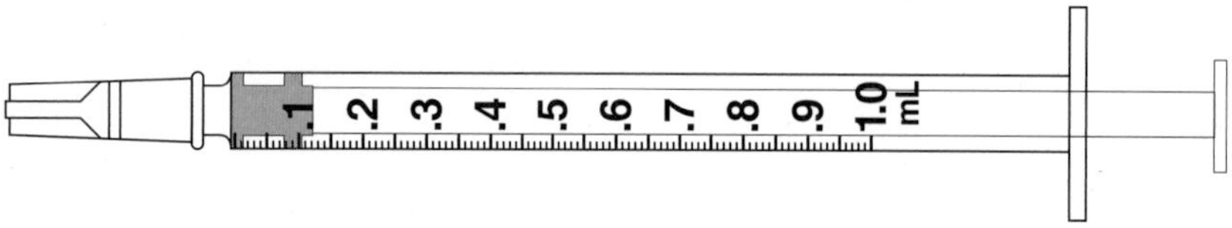

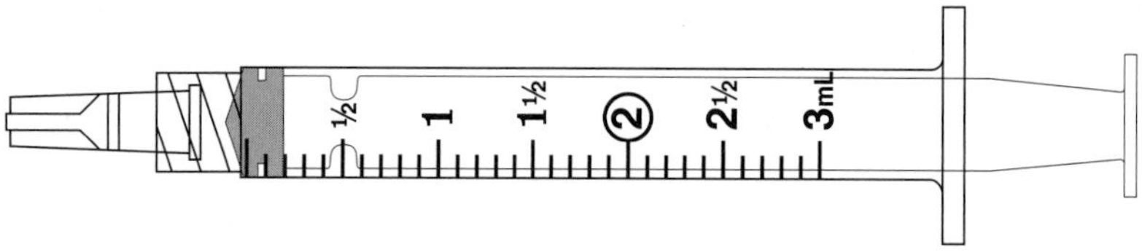

9. Order: *Humulin N 100-unit insulin 46 units with Humulin R 100-unit insulin 22 units subcutaneous stat*

   You will give _____ units total.

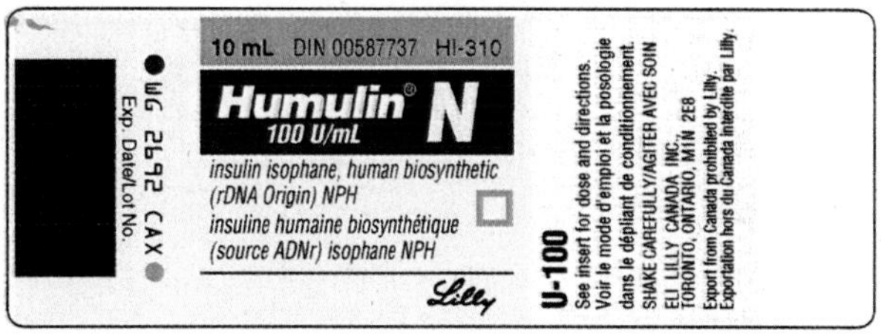

Humalog and Humulin are trademarks of Eli Lilly and Company and are used with permission. Eli Lilly Canada Inc., Toronto, ON

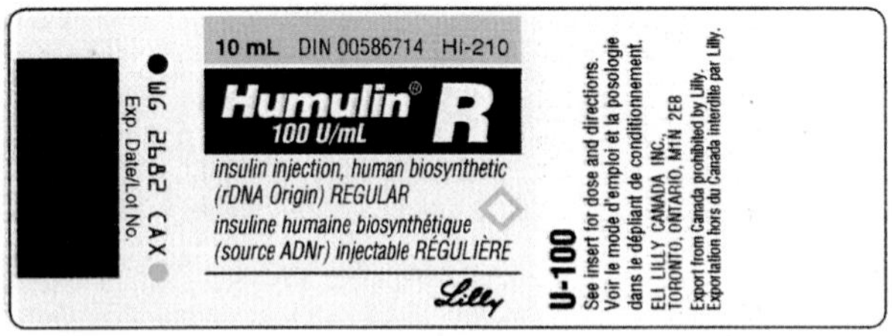

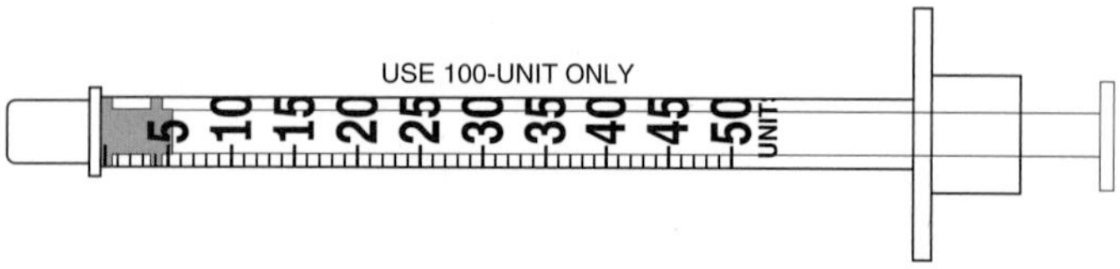

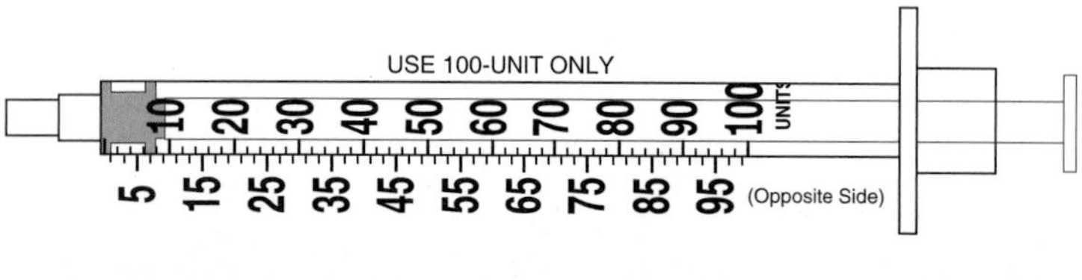

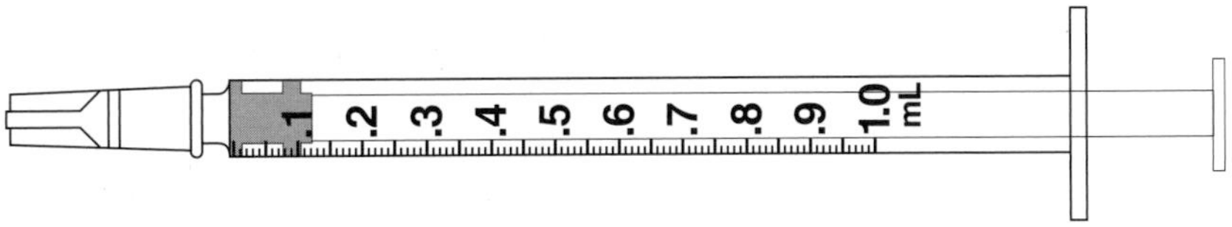
.1 .2 .3 .4 .5 .6 .7 .8 .9 1.0 mL

10. Order: *levothyroxine sodium 0.5 mg PO qAM*

Give: _____ tablet(s)

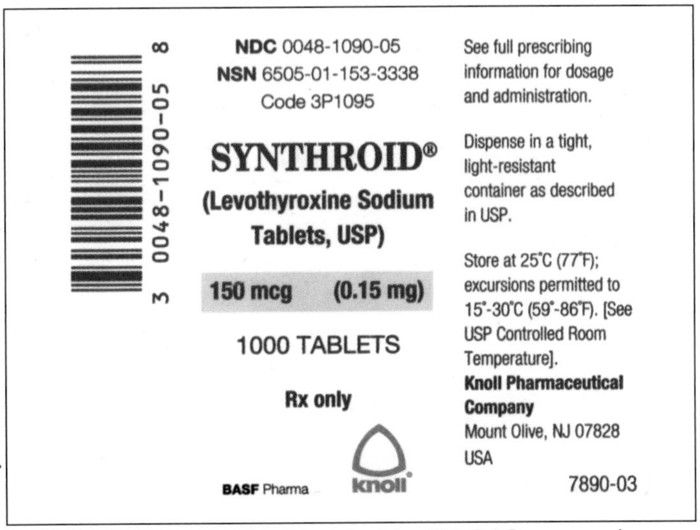
3 0048-1090-05 8
NDC 0048-1090-05
NSN 6505-01-153-3338
Code 3P1095
SYNTHROID®
(Levothyroxine Sodium Tablets, USP)
150 mcg (0.15 mg)
1000 TABLETS
Rx only
BASF Pharma
knoll
See full prescribing information for dosage and administration.
Dispense in a tight, light-resistant container as described in USP.
Store at 25°C (77°F); excursions permitted to 15°-30°C (59°-86°F). [See USP Controlled Room Temperature].
Knoll Pharmaceutical Company
Mount Olive, NJ 07828
USA
7890-03
Courtesy Knoll Pharmaceutical Company

11. Order: *verapamil hydrochloride SR 240 mg each morning plus 120 mg each evening, with food*

Give: _____ tablet(s) for the morning dose and _____ for the evening dose

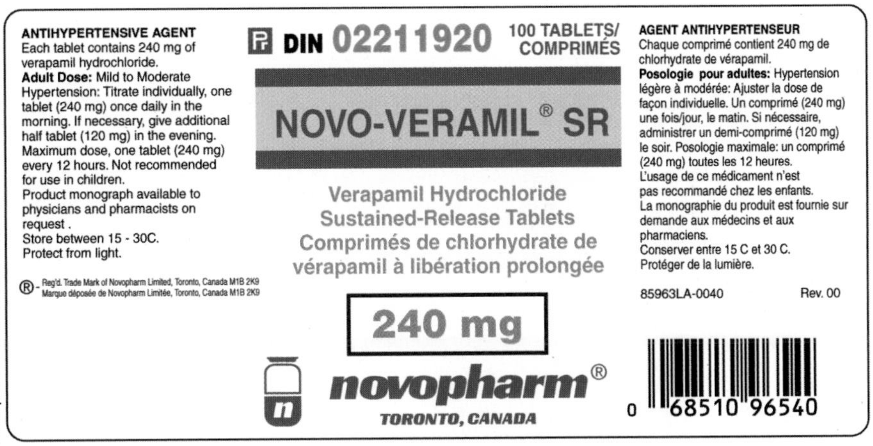
ANTIHYPERTENSIVE AGENT
Each tablet contains 240 mg of verapamil hydrochloride.
Adult Dose: Mild to Moderate Hypertension: Titrate individually, one tablet (240 mg) once daily in the morning. If necessary, give additional half tablet (120 mg) in the evening. Maximum dose, one tablet (240 mg) every 12 hours. Not recommended for use in children.
Product monograph available to physicians and pharmacists on request.
Store between 15 - 30C.
Protect from light.
® - Reg'd. Trade Mark of Novopharm Limited, Toronto, Canada M1B 2K9
Marque déposée de Novopharm Limitée, Toronto, Canada M1B 2K9
Pr DIN 02211920
100 TABLETS/ COMPRIMÉS
NOVO-VERAMIL® SR
Verapamil Hydrochloride Sustained-Release Tablets
Comprimés de chlorhydrate de vérapamil à libération prolongée
240 mg
novopharm®
TORONTO, CANADA
AGENT ANTIHYPERTENSEUR
Chaque comprimé contient 240 mg de chlorhydrate de vérapamil.
Posologie pour adultes: Hypertension légère à modérée: Ajuster la dose de façon individuelle. Un comprimé (240 mg) une fois/jour, le matin. Si nécessaire, administrer un demi-comprimé (120 mg) le soir. Posologie maximale: un comprimé (240 mg) toutes les 12 heures.
L'usage de ce médicament n'est pas recommandé chez les enfants.
La monographie du produit est fournie sur demande aux médecins et aux pharmaciens.
Conserver entre 15 C et 30 C.
Protéger de la lumière.
85963LA-0040 Rev. 00
0 68510 96540
Novopharm Limited, Toronto, ON

12. Order: *Novo-Naprox-EC (Naproxen EC) 500 mg PO BID*

Give: _____ tablet(s)

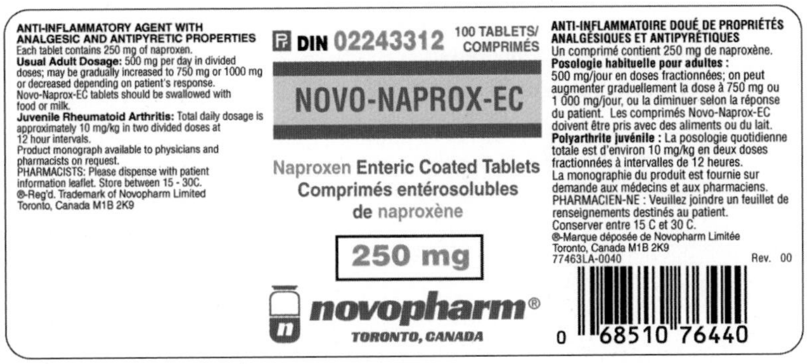
ANTI-INFLAMMATORY AGENT WITH ANALGESIC AND ANTIPYRETIC PROPERTIES
Each tablet contains 250 mg of naproxen.
Usual Adult Dosage: 500 mg per day in divided doses; may be gradually increased to 750 mg or 1000 mg or decreased depending on patient's response. Novo-Naprox-EC tablets should be swallowed with food or milk.
Juvenile Rheumatoid Arthritis: Total daily dosage is approximately 10 mg/kg in two divided doses at 12 hour intervals.
Product monograph available to physicians and pharmacists on request.
PHARMACISTS: Please dispense with patient information leaflet. Store between 15 - 30C.
®-Reg'd. Trademark of Novopharm Limited Toronto, Canada M1B 2K9
Pr DIN 02243312
100 TABLETS/ COMPRIMÉS
NOVO-NAPROX-EC
Naproxen Enteric Coated Tablets
Comprimés entérosolubles de naproxène
250 mg
novopharm®
TORONTO, CANADA
ANTI-INFLAMMATOIRE DOUÉ DE PROPRIÉTÉS ANALGÉSIQUES ET ANTIPYRÉTIQUES
Un comprimé contient 250 mg de naproxène.
Posologie habituelle pour adultes : 500 mg/jour en doses fractionnées; on peut augmenter graduellement la dose à 750 mg ou 1 000 mg/jour, ou la diminuer selon la réponse du patient. Les comprimés Novo-Naprox-EC doivent être pris avec des aliments ou du lait.
Polyarthrite juvénile : La posologie quotidienne totale est d'environ 10 mg/kg en deux doses fractionnées à intervalles de 12 heures.
La monographie du produit est fournie sur demande aux médecins et aux pharmaciens.
PHARMACIEN-NE : Veuillez joindre un feuillet de renseignements destinés au patient.
Conserver entre 15 C et 30 C.
®-Marque déposée de Novopharm Limitée Toronto, Canada M1B 2K9
77463LA-0040 Rev. 00
0 68510 76440
Novopharm Limited, Toronto, ON

13. Order: *promethazine hydrochloride 20 mg IM stat*

Give: ______ mL

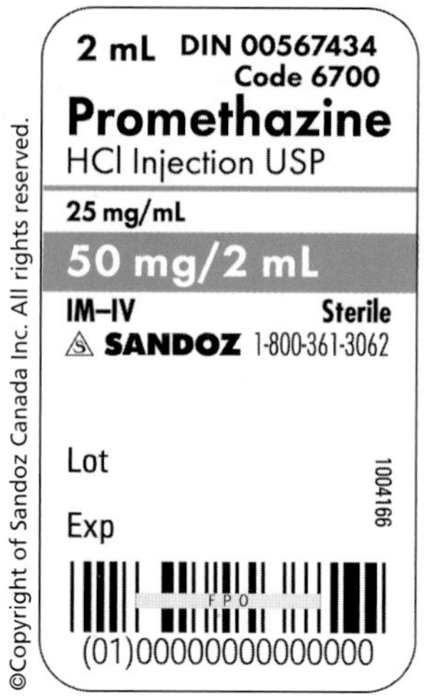
2 mL DIN 00567434
Code 6700
Promethazine
HCl Injection USP
25 mg/mL
50 mg/2 mL
IM–IV Sterile
SANDOZ 1-800-361-3062
Lot
Exp
1004166
(01)00000000000000
©Copyright of Sandoz Canada Inc. All rights reserved.

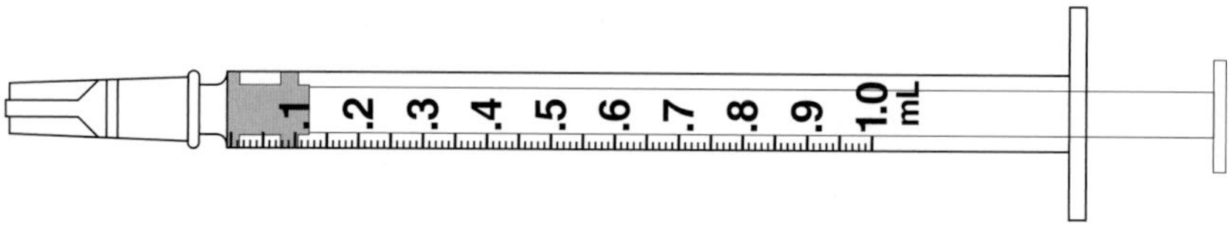
.1 .2 .3 .4 .5 .6 .7 .8 .9 1.0 mL

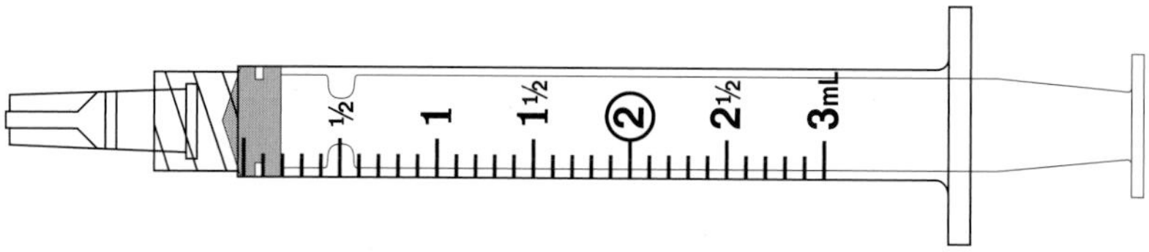
½ 1 1½ 2 2½ 3mL

14. Order: *morphine hydrochloride 15 mg PO q4h*

Give: ______ mL

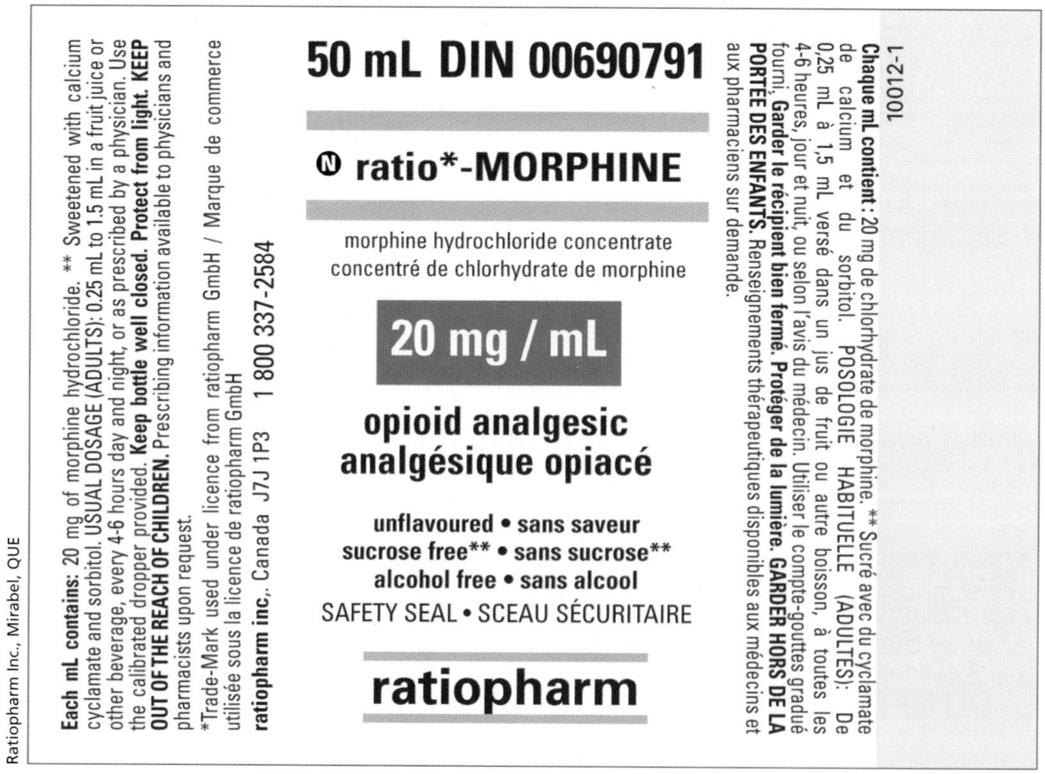
Ratiopharm Inc., Mirabel, QUE
Each mL contains: 20 mg of morphine hydrochloride. ** Sweetened with calcium cyclamate and sorbitol. USUAL DOSAGE (ADULTS): 0.25 mL to 1.5 mL in a fruit juice or other beverage, every 4-6 hours day and night, or as prescribed by a physician. Use the calibrated dropper provided. Keep bottle well closed. Protect from light. KEEP OUT OF THE REACH OF CHILDREN. Prescribing information available to physicians and pharmacists upon request.
*Trade-Mark used under licence from ratiopharm GmbH / Marque de commerce utilisée sous la licence de ratiopharm GmbH
ratiopharm inc., Canada J7J 1P3 1 800 337-2584
50 mL DIN 00690791
ratio*-MORPHINE
morphine hydrochloride concentrate
concentré de chlorhydrate de morphine
20 mg / mL
opioid analgesic
analgésique opiacé
unflavoured • sans saveur
sucrose free** • sans sucrose**
alcohol free • sans alcool
SAFETY SEAL • SCEAU SÉCURITAIRE
ratiopharm
Chaque mL contient : 20 mg de chlorhydrate de morphine. ** Sucré avec du cyclamate de calcium et du sorbitol. POSOLOGIE HABITUELLE (ADULTES): De 0,25 mL à 1,5 mL versé dans un jus de fruit ou autre boisson, à toutes les 4-6 heures, jour et nuit, ou selon l'avis du médecin. Utiliser le compte-gouttes gradué fourni. Garder le récipient bien fermé. Protéger de la lumière. GARDER HORS DE LA PORTÉE DES ENFANTS. Renseignements thérapeutiques disponibles aux médecins et aux pharmaciens sur demande.
10012-1

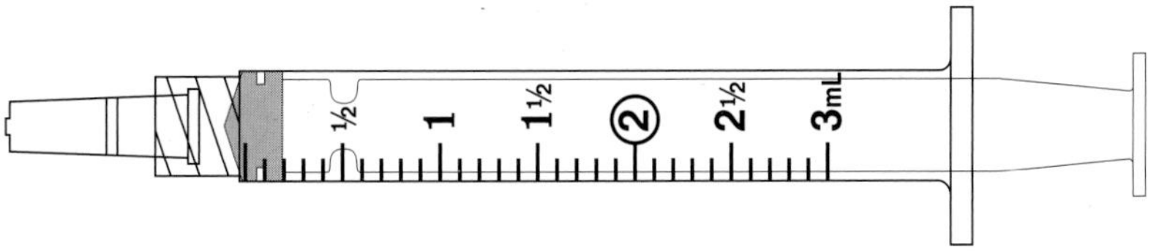
½
1
1½
2
2½
3mL

15. Order: *amoxicillin/clavulanate potassium 100 mg PO q8h*

Give: ______ mL

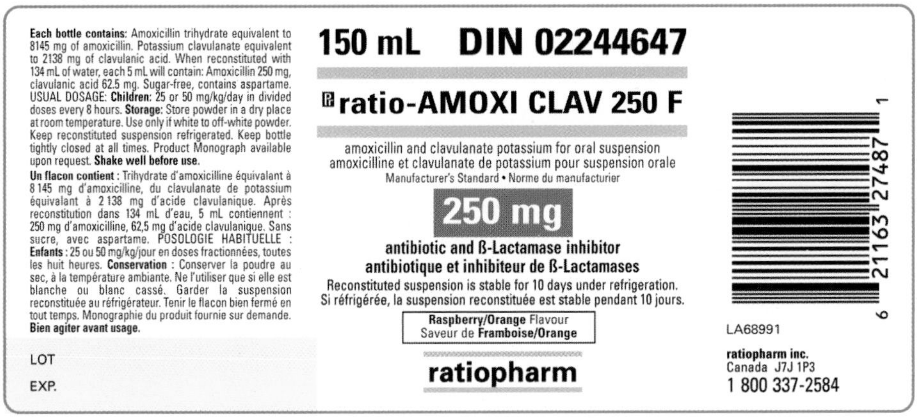
Each bottle contains: Amoxicillin trihydrate equivalent to 8145 mg of amoxicillin. Potassium clavulanate equivalent to 2138 mg of clavulanic acid. When reconstituted with 134 mL of water, each 5 mL will contain: Amoxicillin 250 mg, clavulanic acid 62.5 mg. Sugar-free, contains aspartame. USUAL DOSAGE: Children: 25 or 50 mg/kg/day in divided doses every 8 hours. Storage: Store powder in a dry place at room temperature. Use only if white to off-white powder. Keep reconstituted suspension refrigerated. Keep bottle tightly closed at all times. Product Monograph available upon request. Shake well before use.
Un flacon contient : Trihydrate d'amoxicilline équivalant à 8 145 mg d'amoxicilline, du clavulanate de potassium équivalant à 2 138 mg d'acide clavulanique. Après reconstitution dans 134 mL d'eau, 5 mL contiennent : 250 mg d'amoxicilline, 62,5 mg d'acide clavulanique. Sans sucre, avec aspartame. POSOLOGIE HABITUELLE : Enfants : 25 ou 50 mg/kg/jour en doses fractionnées, toutes les huit heures. Conservation : Conserver la poudre au sec, à la température ambiante. Ne l'utiliser que si elle est blanche ou blanc cassé. Garder la suspension reconstituée au réfrigérateur. Tenir le flacon bien fermé en tout temps. Monographie du produit fournie sur demande. Bien agiter avant usage.
LOT
EXP.
150 mL DIN 02244647
ratio-AMOXI CLAV 250 F
amoxicillin and clavulanate potassium for oral suspension
amoxicilline et clavulanate de potassium pour suspension orale
Manufacturer's Standard • Norme du manufacturier
250 mg
antibiotic and ß-Lactamase inhibitor
antibiotique et inhibiteur de ß-Lactamases
Reconstituted suspension is stable for 10 days under refrigeration.
Si réfrigérée, la suspension reconstituée est stable pendant 10 jours.
Raspberry/Orange Flavour
Saveur de Framboise/Orange
ratiopharm
ratiopharm inc.
Canada J7J 1P3
1 800 337-2584

Ratiopharm Inc., Mirabel, QUE

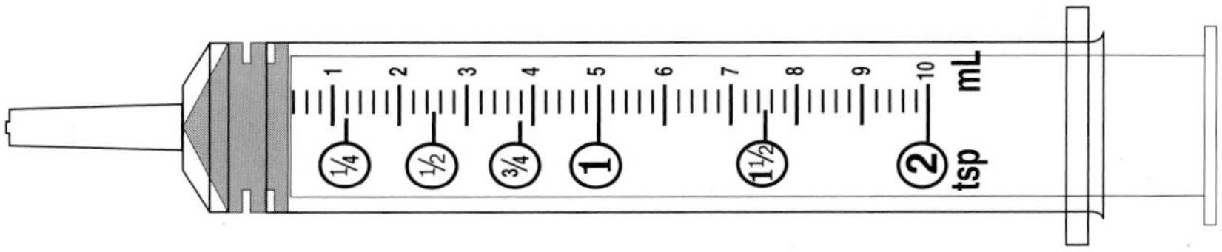
1
2
3
4
5
6
7
8
9
10
mL
¼
½
¾
1
1½
2
tsp

16. Order: *atropine sulfate 0.6 mg IM stat*

Give: ______ mL

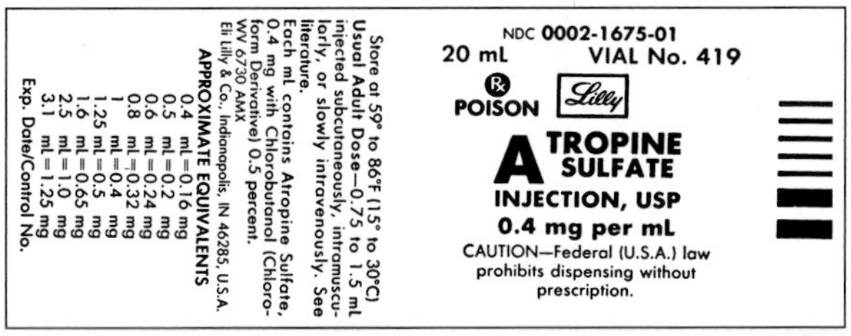
Store at 59° to 86°F (15° to 30°C)
Usual Adult Dose—0.75 to 1.5 mL injected subcutaneously, intramuscularly, or slowly intravenously. See literature.
Each mL contains Atropine Sulfate, 0.4 mg with Chlorobutanol (Chloroform Derivative) 0.5 percent.
WV 6730 AMX
Eli Lilly & Co., Indianapolis, IN 46285, U.S.A.
APPROXIMATE EQUIVALENTS
0.4 mL = 0.16 mg
0.5 mL = 0.2 mg
0.6 mL = 0.24 mg
0.8 mL = 0.32 mg
1 mL = 0.4 mg
1.25 mL = 0.5 mg
1.6 mL = 0.65 mg
2.5 mL = 1.0 mg
3.1 mL = 1.25 mg
Exp. Date/Control No.
NDC 0002-1675-01
20 mL VIAL No. 419
POISON
Lilly
ATROPINE SULFATE
INJECTION, USP
0.4 mg per mL
CAUTION—Federal (U.S.A.) law prohibits dispensing without prescription.

Courtesy of Eli Lilly and Company

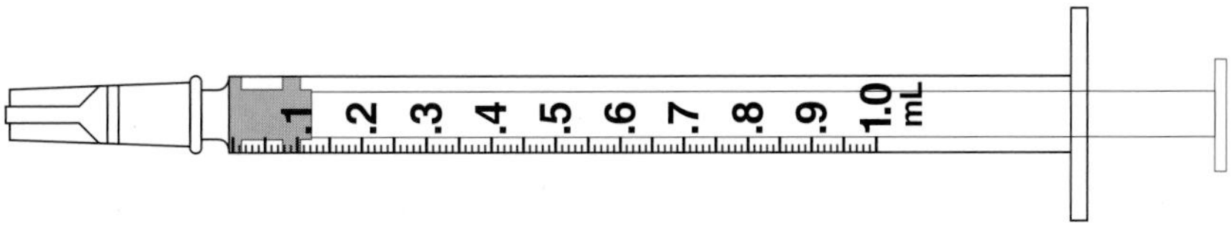
.1
.2
.3
.4
.5
.6
.7
.8
.9
1.0
mL

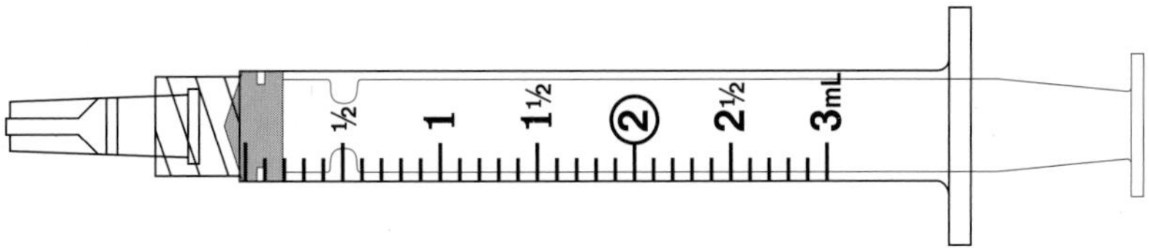
½
1
1½
2
2½
3mL

17. Order: *ranitidine hydrochloride 35 mg in 100 mL D_5W IVPB over 20 min (drop factor: 15gtt/mL)*

    Add _____ mL ranitidine to the IV fluid, and set the flow rate to _____ gtt/min.

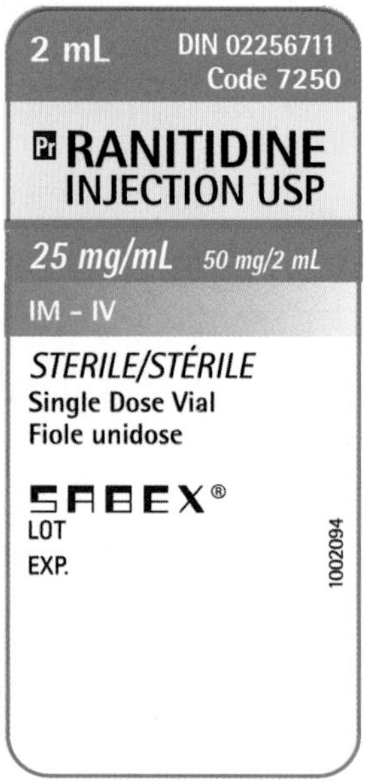

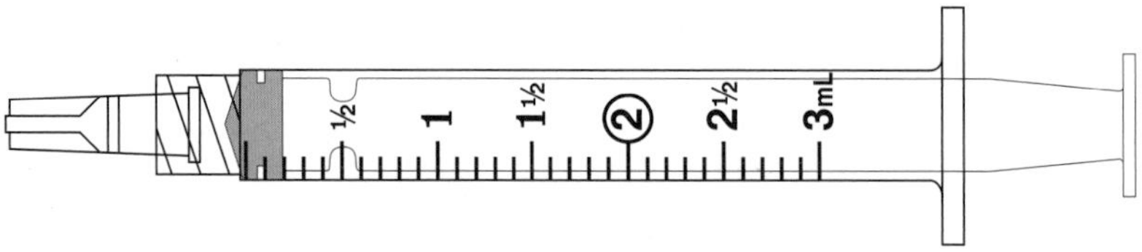

Refer to the medication administration record (MAR) on the next page to answer questions 18 through 22.

Mrs. Betty Smedley in Room 217A is assigned to your team. She is hospitalized with osteoarthritis. The medications available from the pharmacy are noted on the MAR.

18. Mrs. Smedley had her last dose of acetaminophen at 2110 h. It is now 0215 h, and her temperature is 39°C. Is acetaminophen indicated? _____

    Explain: ____

    ____

19. How much acetaminophen should she receive for each dose? _____ tablet(s)

20. Mrs. Smedley had 60 mg IM of ketorolac tromethamine at 1500 h. At 2130 h, she is complaining of severe pain again. How much ketorolac tromethamine will you give her now? Give _____ mL.

21. Mrs. Smedley is complaining of itching. What prn medication would you select, and how much will you administer? Select _____, and give _____ capsule or tablet.

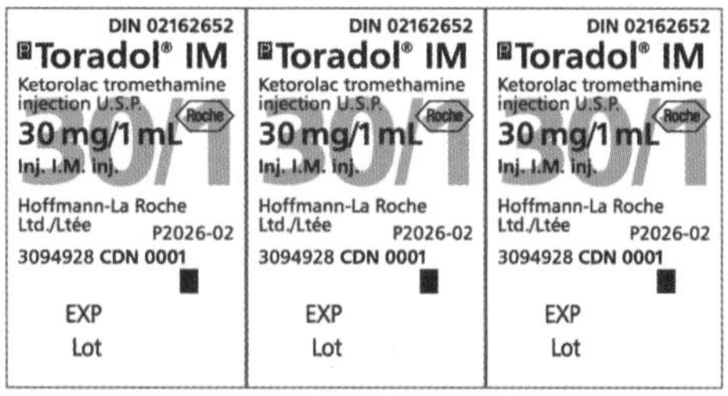

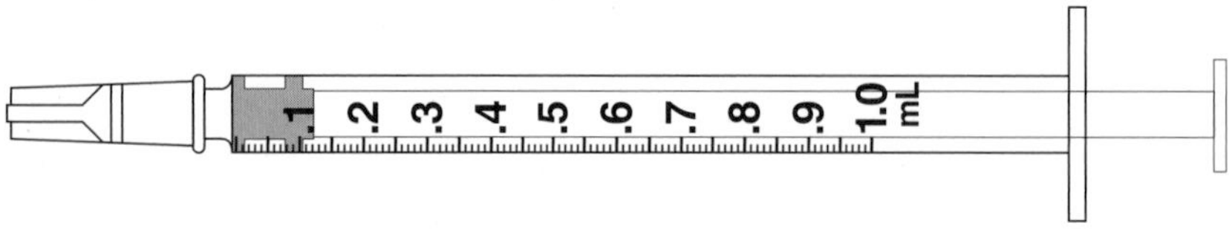

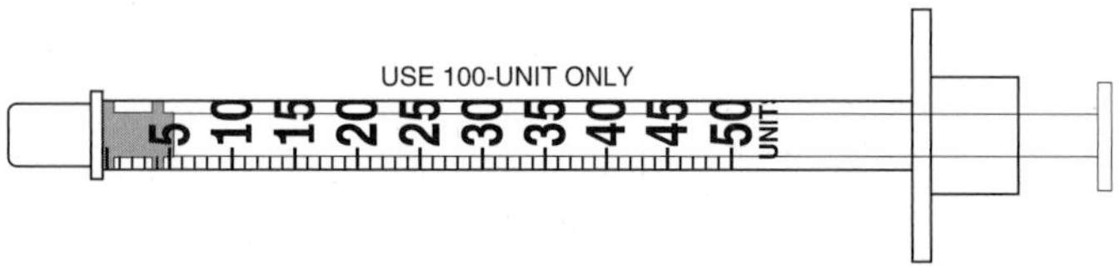

15/09/xx
18:26
CHECKED BY:

MEDICATION ADMINISTRATION RECORD

PAGE: 1
REPT: PHR20B

2ND 241
217A 532729
Smedley, Betty

DIAGNOSIS: 71590
ALLERGIES: NKA
NOTES:

DIET: Regular
ADMIT: 15/09/xx
WT: 70 kg

DX: OSTEOARTHRITIS-UNSPEC

ADMINISTRATION PERIOD: 0730 15/09/xx TO 0729 16/09/xx

ORDER # DRUG NAME, STRENGTH, DOSAGE FORM **DOSE RATE ROUTE SCHEDULE**	**START**	**STOP**	**TIME PERIOD** 0730 to 1529	**TIME PERIOD** 1530 to 2329	**TIME PERIOD** 2330 to 0729
NURSE:					
• • • PRN's FOLLOW • • •			• • • PRN's FOLLOW • • •		
264077 acetaminophen 325 mg TABLET PRN **650 mg** ORAL Q4H/PRN FOR TEMP over 38.3 C	0930 15/09/xx		0930 GP	2110 GP	
264147 ketorolac tromethamine 60 mg PRN **60 mg** IM PRN GIVE 60 mg FOR BREAKTHROUGH PAIN X1 DOSE THEN 30 mg Q6H/PRN	1500 15/09/xx		60 mg 1500 MS		
264148 ketorolac tromethamine 60 mg PRN **30 mg** IM Q6H/PRN GIVE 6 HOURS AFTER 60 mg DOSE FOR BREAK-THROUGH PAIN.	1500 15/09/xx				
264151 droperidol 2.5 mg/mL AMPOULE PRN **SEE NOTE** IV Q6H/PRN DOSE IS 0.625 MG TO 1.25 MG (0.5-1.0 ML) FOR NAUSEA	1500 15/09/xx				
264152 diphenhydramine 50 mg CAPSULE PRN **50 mg** ORAL Q4H/PRN FOR ITCHING	1500 15/09/xx				
264153 naloxone hydrochloride 0.4 mg/mL AMPOULE PRN **0.4 MG** IV PRN FOR RR less than 8 AND IF PATIENT IS UNAROUSABLE	1500 15/09/xx				
NURSE:					
NURSE:					

INITIALS	SIGNATURE	INITIALS	SIGNATURE	NOTES	
GP	G. Pickar, RN				
MS	M. Smith, RN				

217A Betty Smedley AGE: 73 SEX: F PHYSICIAN: J. Physician, MD

22. Mrs. Smedley's respiratory rate (R.R.) is 7, and she is difficult to arouse. What medication is indicated? ___________________. Draw an arrow on the syringe to indicate how much of this medication you will give.

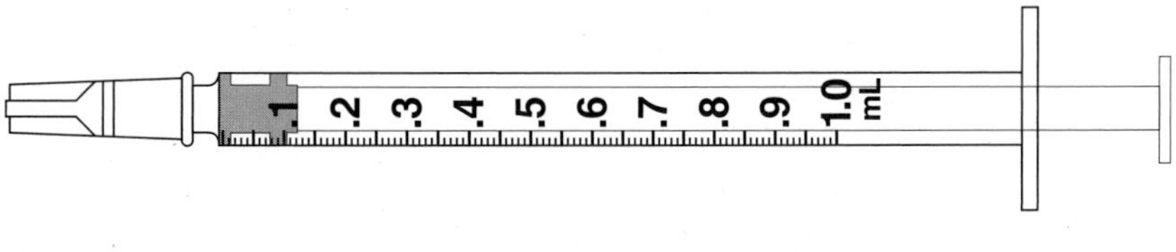

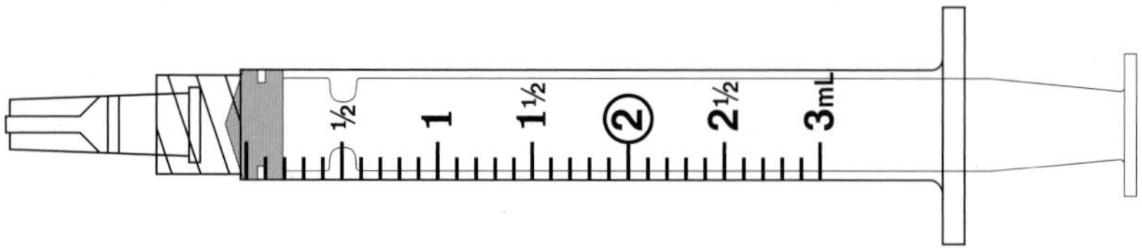

Refer to the following MAR to answer questions 23 through 27.

PAGE ____ of ____

MEDICATION ADMINISTRATION RECORD

ORIGINAL ORDER DATE	DATE STARTED / RENEWED	MEDICATION - DOSAGE	ROUTE	SCHEDULE 2300–0700	SCHEDULE 0700–1500	SCHEDULE 1500–2300	DATE 10-3-xx 2300–0700	10-3-xx 0700–1500	10-3-xx 1500–2300	DATE 11-3-xx 2300–0700	11-3-xx 0700–1500	11-3-xx 1500–2300	DATE 12-3-xx 2300–0700	12-3-xx 0700–1500	12-3-xx 1500–2300	DATE 13-3-xx 2300–0700	13-3-xx 0700–1500	13-3-xx 1500–2300
10-03-xx	10-3	theophylline 100 mg IV (available theophylline in D5W 800 mg/250 mL (0.8 mg/mL)) x 30 min q6h	IV PB	2400 0600	1200	1800		GP 1200	MS 1800	JJ2400 JJ0600								
10-03-xx	10-3	hydrocortisone 125 mg q8h	IV	2400 0600	1200	1800		GP 1200	MS 1800	JJ2400 JJ0600								
10-03-xx	10-3	sucralfate 1 g	PO	1145	0745	1745 2200		GP0745 GP1145	MS1745 MS2200									
10-03-xx	10-3	humulin R	SUB-CUT		0730 1130			GP0730 GP1130	MS1730									
		per sliding scale: Blood sugar Units																
		0-8 0 units																
		8.1-12 2 units																
		12.1-14 4 units																
		14.1-16 6 units																
		16.1-18 8 units																
		18.1-20 10 units																
		more than 20 call MD stat																

PRN

INJECTION SITES

B - RIGHT ARM
C - RIGHT ABDOMEN
D - RIGHT ANTERIOR THIGH
G - LEFT ARM
H - LEFT ABDOMEN
J - LEFT ANTERIOR THIGH
L - LEFT BUTTOCKS
M - RIGHT BUTTOCKS

DATE GIVEN	TIME	INT.	ONE - TIME MEDICATION - DOSAGE	RT.

SIGNATURE OF NURSE ADMINISTERING MEDICATIONS

SCHEDULE	DATE	DATE	DATE	DATE
2300–0700		JJ J.Jones LPN		
0700–1500	GP G.Pickar,RN			
1500–2300	MS M.Smith,RN			

DATE GIVEN	TIME	INT.	MEDICATION-DOSAGE-CONT.	RT.
			RECOPIED BY:	
			CHECKED BY:	

LITHO IN U.S.A. K6508 (7-92) D395538

Beck, John
ID #76834-21

ALLERGIES:

602-31 (7-xx) (MPC# 1355)

1
ORIGINAL COPY

PRINTED BY STANDARD REGISTER U.S.A. ZIPSET ®

John Beck, 19 years old, has diabetes mellitus. He is admitted to the medical unit with asthma. You are administering his medications. The MAR on page 430 is in the medication notebook on the medication cart. The label represents the infusion set available. Questions 23 through 27 refer to John.

23. Theophylline is available in a premixed D5W solution strength of 0.8 mg/mL. Deliver _____ mL of premixed theophylline in D5W over _____min. Set the flow rate at _____ gtt/min.

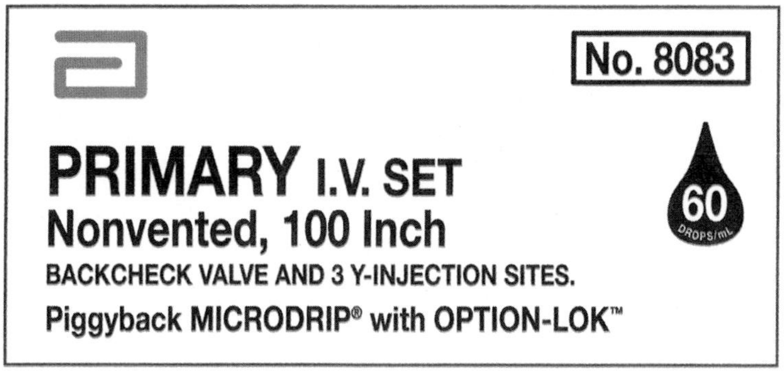

Courtesy of Abbott Laboratories, Inc.

24. An infusion pump becomes available, and you decide to use it for Mr. Beck IV. It is calibrated in millilitres per hour. To administer the theophylline by infusion pump, set the pump at _____ mL/h.

25. Reconstitute the hydrocortisone sodium succinate with _____ mL diluent, and give _____ mL.

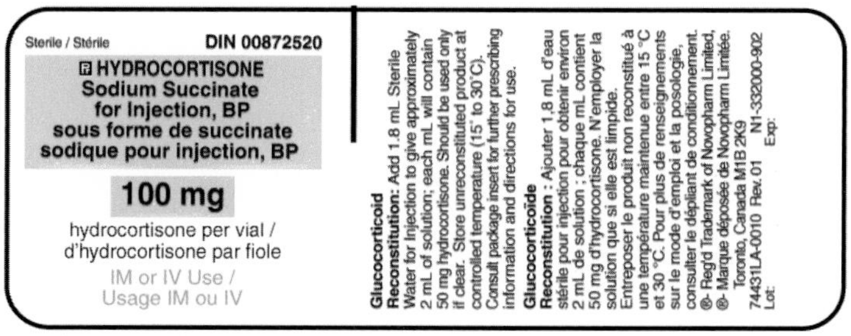

Novopharm Limited, Toronto, ON

26. Mealtimes and bedtime are 0800, 1200, 1800, and 2200. Administer _____ tablet(s) of Apo-sucralfate per dose each day at _____, _____, _____, and _____ hours.

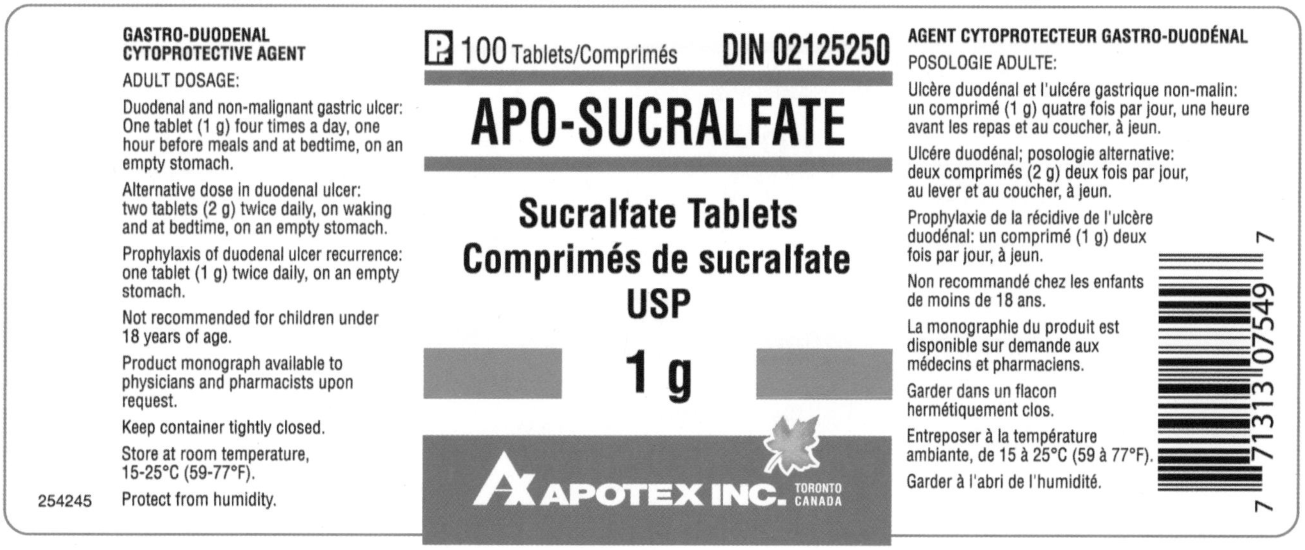

Apotex Inc., Weston, ON

27. At 0730 h, Mr. Beck blood sugar is 20 mmol/L. You will give him _____ units of insulin by the _____ route. Draw an arrow on the appropriate syringe to indicate the correct dosage.

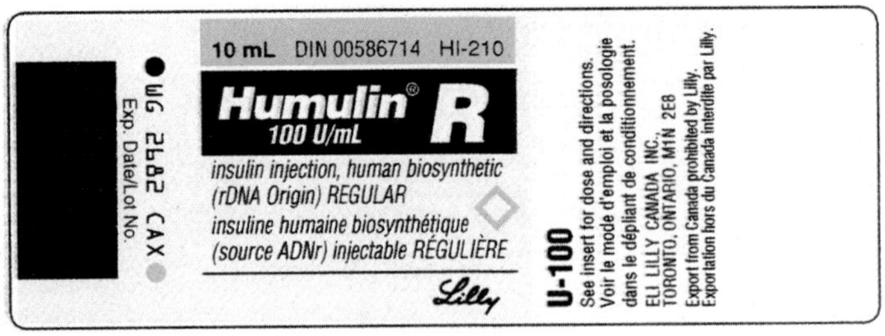

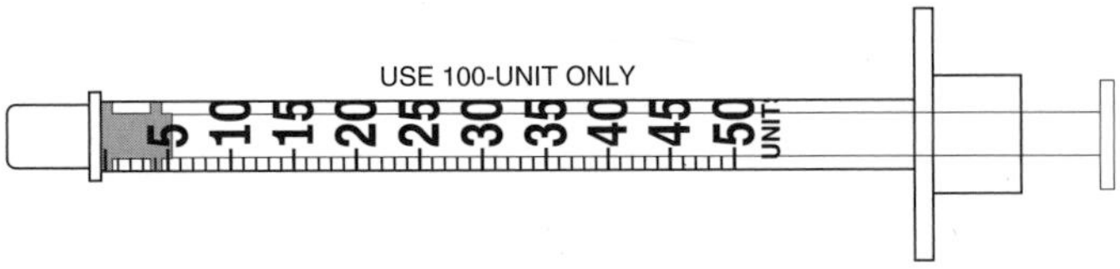

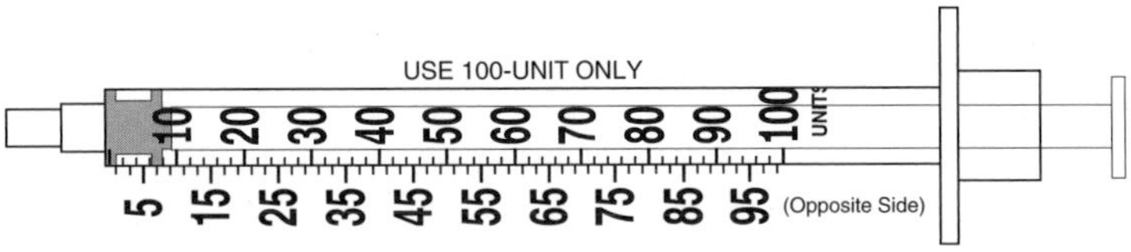

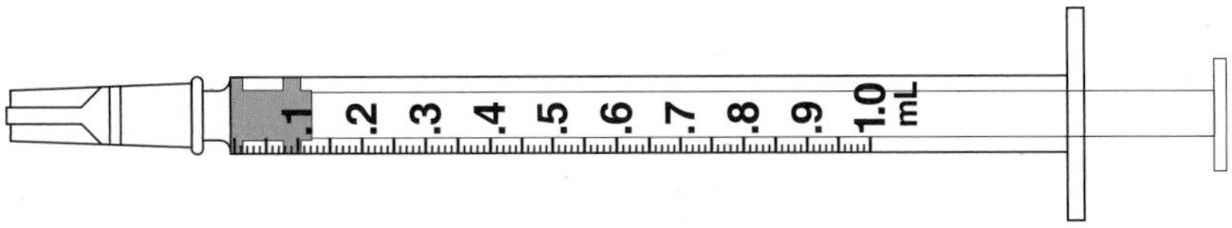

Jimmy Bryan is brought to the clinic by his mother. He is a 6.8 kg baby with an ear infection. Questions 28 through 31 refer to Jimmy.

28. The physician orders *amoxicillin trihydrate 91 mg PO q8h* for Jimmy. Recommended dose is 40 mg/kg/day divided q8h for 10 days.

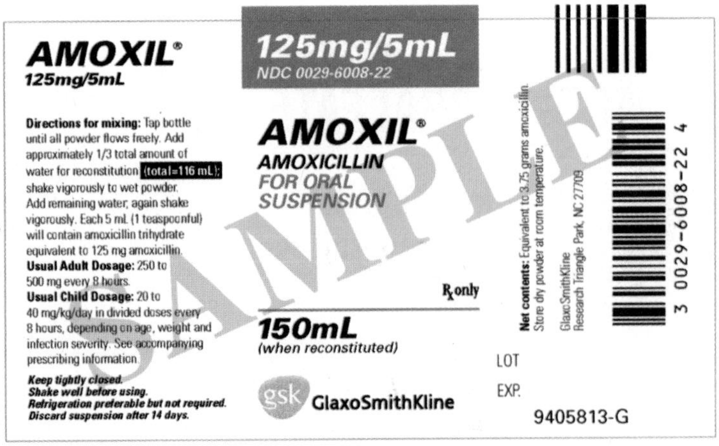

Is Jimmy's amoxicillin trihydrate order safe and reasonable? ______________

Explain: ____

29. The physician asks you to give Jimmy one dose of the amoxicillin trihydrate stat. How many mL of water will be used to reconstitute the solution? _____mL

30. Once reconstituted, you would administer _____mL to Jimmy.

31. The physician also asks you to instruct Jimmy's mother about administering the medication at home. Tell Jimmy's mother to give the baby medication up to the _____ mL line of the oral syringe for each dose. How often will she give Jimmy his dose? ____________________

32. Jill Jones is a 16-year-old, 50-kg teenager with a duodenal ulcer and abdominal pain. Order: *ranitidine hydrochloride 50 mg q6h in 50 mL D_5W to be infused in 20 min*

    The recommended ranitidine hydrochloride dosage is 2–6 mg/kg/day in four divided doses. Available is ranitidine hydrochloride for injection, 25 mg/mL. The label represents the infusion set available. What is the safe single dosage range for this adolescent? _____ mg/dose to _____ mg/dose. Is this ordered dosage safe? _____

    If safe, add _____ mL ranitidine hydrochloride, and set the flow rate at _____ gtt/min.

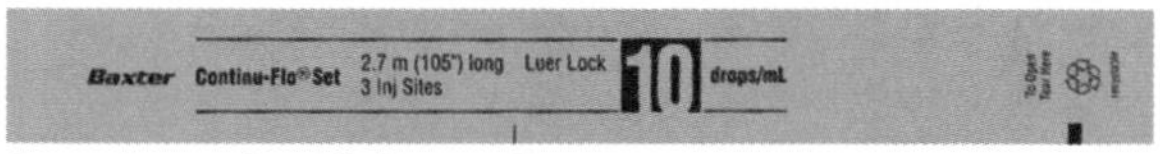
Baxter Continu-Flo® Set
2.7 m (105") long Luer Lock
3 Inj Sites
10
drops/mL

Baxter Corporation, Mississauga, ON

33. The doctor writes a new patient care order for strict intake and output assessment for a child. During your 8-hour shift, in addition to his IV fluids of 200 mL D_5NS, he consumed the following oral fluids:

    gelatin—120 mL

    water—90 mL × 2

    apple juice—500 mL

    What is his total fluid intake during your shift? _____ mL

Use the following information to answer questions 34 through 36.

Order for a child with severe otitis media (inner ear infection) who weighs 18.2 kg: *amoxicillin/clavulanate potassium 240 mg PO q8h.* The following amoxicillin/clavulanate potassium label represents the dosage you have available. Recommended amoxicillin/clavulanate potassium dosage is 40 mg/kg/day q8h in divided doses.

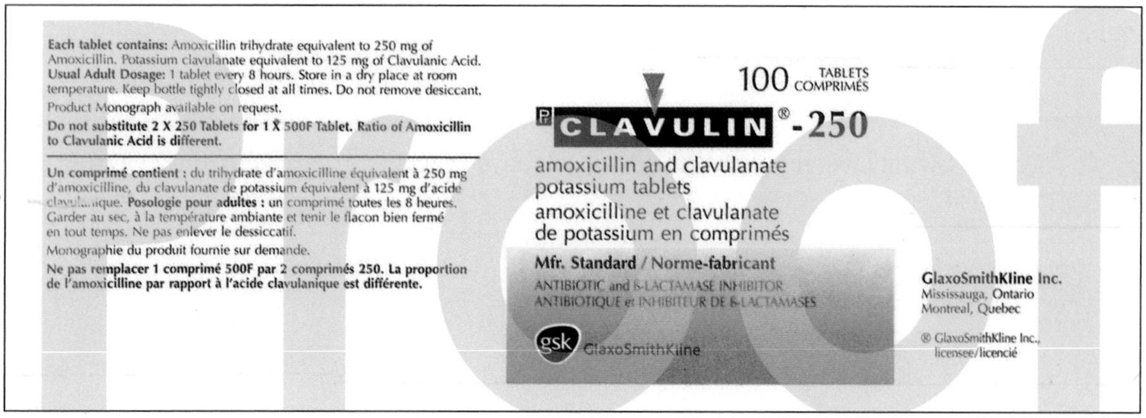
Each tablet contains: Amoxicillin trihydrate equivalent to 250 mg of Amoxicillin. Potassium clavulanate equivalent to 125 mg of Clavulanic Acid. Usual Adult Dosage: 1 tablet every 8 hours. Store in a dry place at room temperature. Keep bottle tightly closed at all times. Do not remove desiccant.
Product Monograph available on request.
Do not substitute 2 X 250 Tablets for 1 X 500F Tablet. Ratio of Amoxicillin to Clavulanic Acid is different.
Un comprimé contient : du trihydrate d'amoxicilline équivalent à 250 mg d'amoxicilline, du clavulanate de potassium équivalent à 125 mg d'acide clavulanique. Posologie pour adultes : un comprimé toutes les 8 heures. Garder au sec, à la température ambiante et tenir le flacon bien fermé en tout temps. Ne pas enlever le dessiccatif.
Monographie du produit fournie sur demande.
Ne pas remplacer 1 comprimé 500F par 2 comprimés 250. La proportion de l'amoxicilline par rapport à l'acide clavulanique est différente.
100 TABLETS COMPRIMÉS
CLAVULIN®-250
amoxicillin and clavulanate potassium tablets
amoxicilline et clavulanate de potassium en comprimés
Mfr. Standard / Norme-fabricant
ANTIBIOTIC and ß-LACTAMASE INHIBITOR
ANTIBIOTIQUE et INHIBITEUR DE ß-LACTAMASES
gsk GlaxoSmithKline
GlaxoSmithKline Inc.
Mississauga, Ontario
Montreal, Quebec
® GlaxoSmithKline Inc., licensee/licencié

34. Is the ordered dosage safe? _____

35. If it is safe, how much would you administer to the child? _____ tablets per dose. If it is not safe, what would you do next? ____________________

36. The physician has ordered *washed, packed red blood cells 2 units (600 mL) IV to infuse in 4 h.* The IV tubing has a drop factor of 15 gtt/mL. You will regulate the IV flow rate at _____ gtt/min.

Use the following information to answer questions 37 and 38.

A child who weighs 28 kg has an elevated temperature. For hyperthermia in children, the recommended dosage of acetaminophen is 10–15 mg/kg PO q4h, not to exceed five doses per day.

37. What is the safe single dosage range of acetaminophen for this child? _____ mg/dose to _____ mg/dose

38. If the physician orders the maximum safe dosage and acetaminophen is available as a suspension of 160 mg/5 mL, how many millilitres will you give per dose? _____ mL

Use the following information to answer questions 39 and 40 for a child who weighs 23.6 kg.

Order: *diphenhydramine hydrochloride 25 mg IV q6h*

Supply: diphenhydramine hydrochloride 50 mg/mL

Recommended dosage: 5 mg/kg/day in four divided doses

39. A safe single dosage for this child is _____ mg/dose. Is the order safe? _____

40. If safe, administer _____ mL. If not safe, what should you do? _____________________________

____

Use the following information to answer questions 41 through 44.

At 1430 h, a patient is started on *meperidine hydrochloride PCA IV pump at 10 mg q10 min.* The meperidine hydrochloride syringe in the pump contains 300 mg/30 mL.

41. The patient can receive _____ mL every 10 minutes.

42. If the patient attempts five doses this hour, he would receive _____ mg and _____ mL of meperidine.

43. Based on the amount of meperidine hydrochloride in the syringe in the patient-controlled analgesia pump, how many total doses can the patient receive? _____ dose(s)

44. If the patient receives five doses every hour, the meperidine hydrochloride will be empty at _____ hours. Convert this time to traditional AM/PM time. _____

45. Order: *sodium nitroprusside 100 mg stat in 250 mL D_5W IVPB, infuse over 30 min*

    Regulate the electronic infusion pump at _____ mL/h.

Use the following information to answer questions 46 through 49.

Order: *ceftazidime 0.5 g IV q8h*

The following label represents the drug you have available. You reconstitute the drug at 1400 h on 30/01/11.

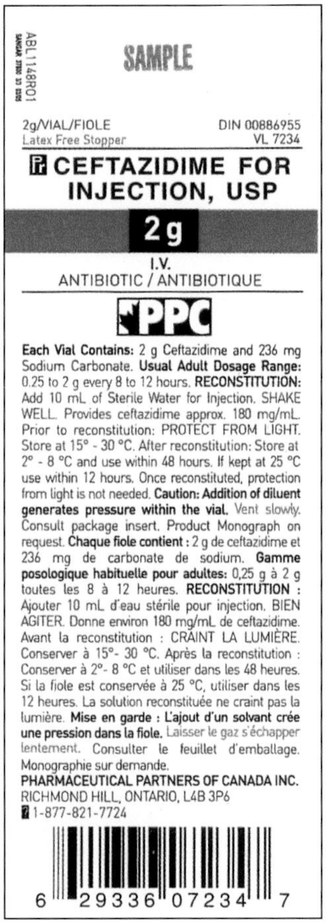

Pharmaceutical Partners of Canada Inc., Richmond Hill, ON

46. The total volume of ceftazidime after reconstitution is _____ mL.
47. The resulting dosage strength of ceftazidime is _____ mg/mL.
48. Give _____ mL of ceftazidime.
49. Prepare a reconstitution label for ceftazidime.

50. Critical Thinking Skill: Describe the strategy you would implement to prevent this medication error.

possible scenario

Order: *dexamethasone sodium phosphate 4 mg IV q6h*

Day 1 Supply: dexamethasone sodium phosphate 4 mg/mL

Student nurse prepared and administered 1 mL.

Day 2 Supply: dexamethasone sodium phosphate 10 mg/mL

Student nurse prepared 1 mL.

potential outcome

Day 2, the student's instructor asked the student to recheck the order, think about the action, check the calculation, and provide the rationale for the amount prepared. The student was alarmed at the possibility of administering 2.5 times the prescribed dosage. The student insisted that the pharmacy should consistently supply the same unit dosage. The instructor advised the student of the possibility that different pharmacy technicians could be involved, or possibly the original supply dosage was not available.

prevention

____

____

After completing these problems, see pages 515–519 to check your answers. Give yourself 2 points for each correct answer.

Perfect score = 100 My score = ______

Mastery score = 90 or higher (45 correct)

Comprehensive Skills Evaluation

This evaluation is a comprehensive assessment of your mastery of the concepts presented in all 14 chapters of *Dosage Calculations.*

Donna Smith, a 46-year-old patient of Dr. J. Physician, has been admitted to the Telemetry Unit with complaints of an irregular heartbeat, shortness of breath, and chest pain. Usually chest pain is relieved by nitroglycerin 0.3 mg SL q8h. Questions 1 through 14 refer to the admitting orders on the next page for Mrs. Smith. The labels shown represent available medications and infusion set.

Mrs. Smith is also on isosorbide dinitrate 20 mg TID.

1. Mrs. Smith complains of chest pain. How many tablets of nitroglycerin will you give Mrs. Smith and how often?

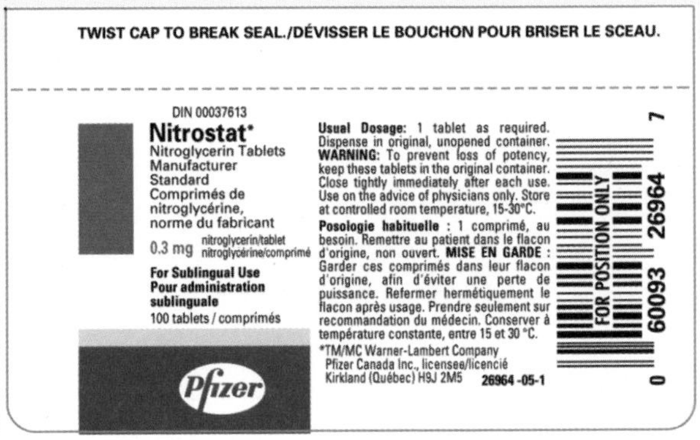

TWIST CAP TO BREAK SEAL./DÉVISSER LE BOUCHON POUR BRISER LE SCEAU.
DIN 00037613
Nitrostat*
Nitroglycerin Tablets Manufacturer Standard
Comprimés de nitroglycérine, norme du fabricant
0.3 mg nitroglycerin/tablet nitroglycérine/comprimé
For Sublingual Use
Pour administration sublinguale
100 tablets / comprimés
Pfizer
Usual Dosage: 1 tablet as required. Dispense in original, unopened container. WARNING: To prevent loss of potency, keep these tablets in the original container. Close tightly immediately after each use. Use on the advice of physicians only. Store at controlled room temperature, 15-30°C.
Posologie habituelle : 1 comprimé, au besoin. Remettre au patient dans le flacon d'origine, non ouvert. MISE EN GARDE : Garder ces comprimés dans leur flacon d'origine, afin d'éviter une perte de puissance. Refermer hermétiquement le flacon après usage. Prendre seulement sur recommandation du médecin. Conserver à température constante, entre 15 et 30 °C.
*TM/MC Warner-Lambert Company
Pfizer Canada Inc., licensee/licencié
Kirkland (Québec) H9J 2M5 26964-05-1
FOR POSITION ONLY
0 60093 26964 7

2. Oral nitroglycerin is usually administered by the SL or buccal route. "SL" is the medical abbreviation for ____________ Explain: ____________

   What is the difference between SL and buccal? ____________

3. How much and at what rate will you administer Mrs. Smith's first dose of furosemide? Draw an arrow on the appropriate syringe to indicate how much you will prepare. The recommended direct intravenous (IV) administration rate for furosemide is 40 mg/2 min. Give: ________ mL at the rate of ________ mL/min or ________ mL/15 sec

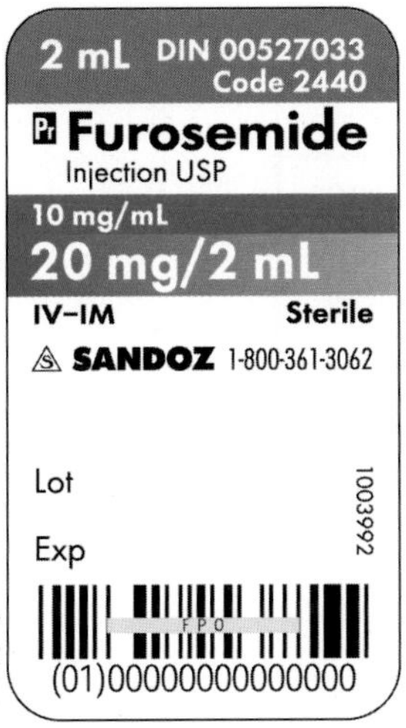

2 mL DIN 00527033
Code 2440
Furosemide
Injection USP
10 mg/mL
20 mg/2 mL
IV–IM
Sterile
SANDOZ 1-800-361-3062
Lot
Exp
1003992
FPO
(01)00000000000000

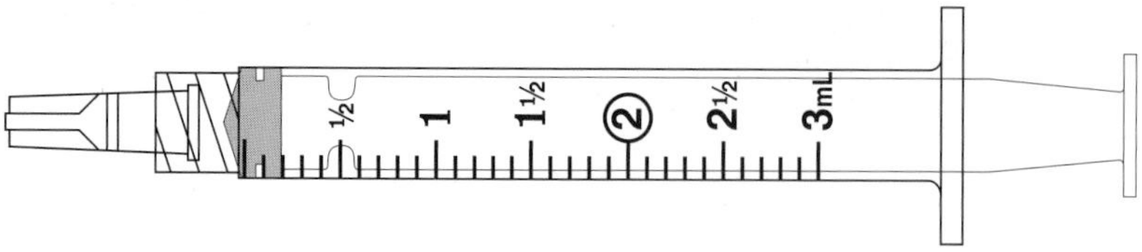

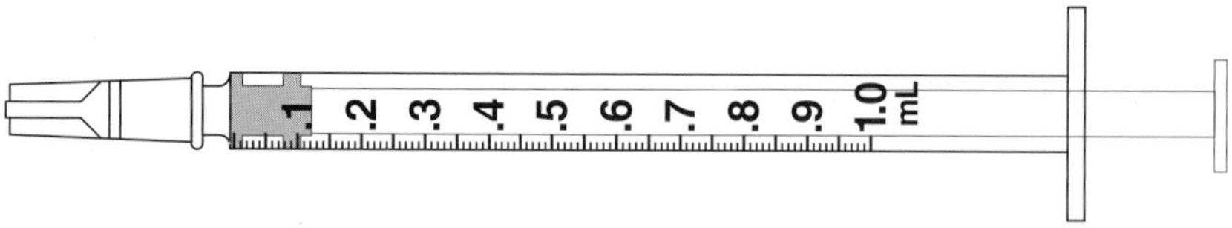

ENTERED	FILLED	CHECKED	VERIFIED
			—

NOTE: A NON-PROPRIETARY DRUG OF EQUAL QUALITY MAY BE DISPENSED - IF THIS COLUMN IS NOT CHECKED!

DATE	TIME WRITTEN	PLEASE USE BALL POINT - PRESS FIRMLY	✓	TIME NOTED	NURSES SIGNATURE
03/09/xx	1600	Admit to telemetry unit	✓		
		Bedrest with bathroom privileges	✓		
		nitroglycerin 0.3 mg SL q8h stat followed by 0.3-mg q 3-5	✓		
		min for another 2 doses X 3 for angina pain	✓		
		furosemide 20 mg IV Push stat, then 20 mg PO BID	✓	1610 GP	
		digoxin 0.25 mg IV on admission then PO daily X 3 days			
		KCl 10 mEq per L D5 1/2 NS iv @ 80 mL/h	✓		
		acetaminophen 1 g q4h prn for headache	✓		
		Labwork: Electrolytes and CBC in am	✓		
		Soft diet, advance as tolerated	✓		
		Dr. J. Physician			

AUTO STOP ORDERS: UNLESS REORDERED, FOLLOWING WILL BE D/C'D AT 0800 ON:

DATE	ORDER		
		☐ CONT ☐ D/C	PHYSICIAN SIGNATURE
		☐ CONT ☐ D/C	PHYSICIAN SIGNATURE
		☐ CONT ☐ D/C	PHYSICIAN SIGNATURE

CHECK WHEN ANTIBIOTICS ORDERED ☐ Prophylactic ☐ Empiric ☐ Therapeutic

Allergies: None Known

Chest Pain
CLIENT DIAGNOSIS

HEIGHT 152 cm WEIGHT 50 kg

Smith, Donna
ID #257-226-3

FORM 959-708 (6-XX) **PHYSICIAN'S ORDER** Reynolds + Reynolds LITHO IN U.S.A. K41814 (7-90) D339360

1

4. After the initial dose of furosemide, how much will you administer for each subsequent dose?

   Give: __________ tablet(s)

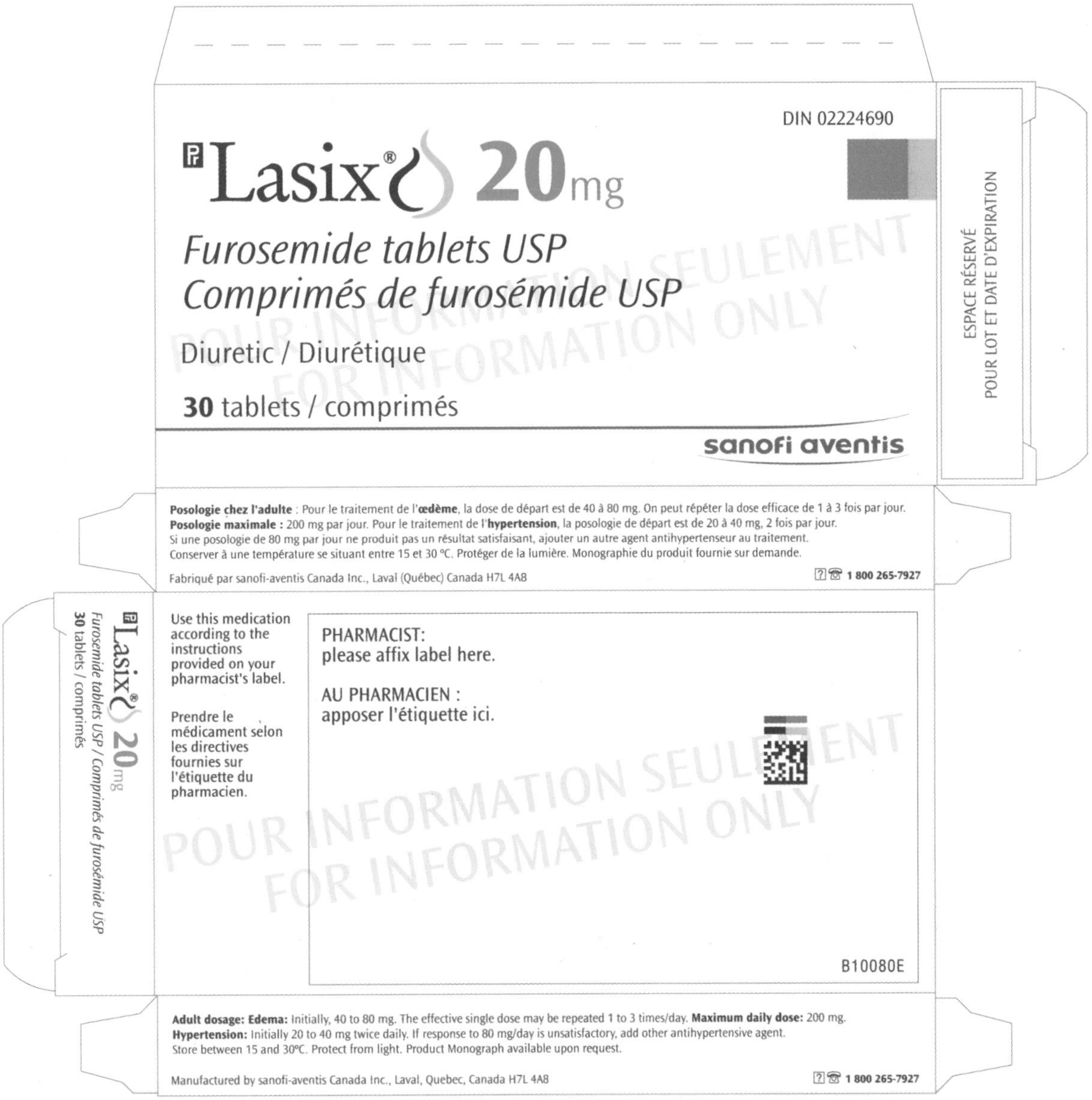

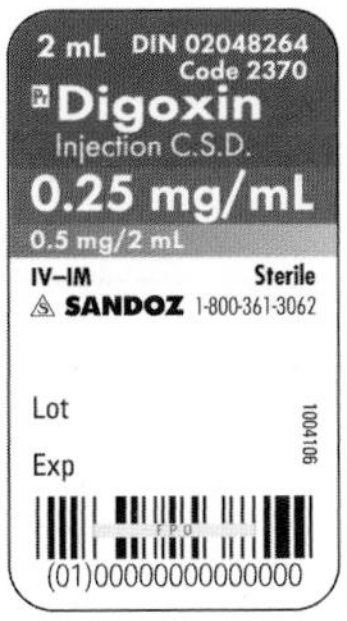

5. How much and at what rate will you administer the IV digoxin on admission? Draw an arrow on the syringe to indicate how much you will prepare. The recommended direct IV rate for digoxin is 0.25 mg in 4 mL normal saline (NS) administered IV at the rate of 0.25 mg/5 min.

   Give: __________ mL at the rate of __________ mL/min or __________ mL/15 sec

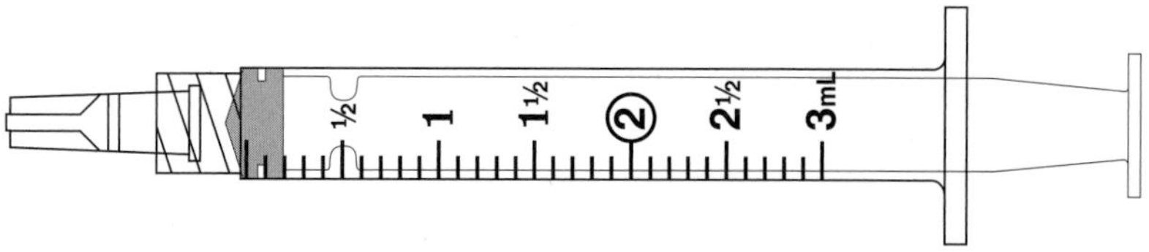

6. How many digoxin tablets would you need for a 3-day supply of this PO order, when the medication label indicates that each tablet has 0.125 mg? __________ tablet(s)

7. Calculate the "watch count" flow rate for the IV fluid ordered. __________ gtt/min

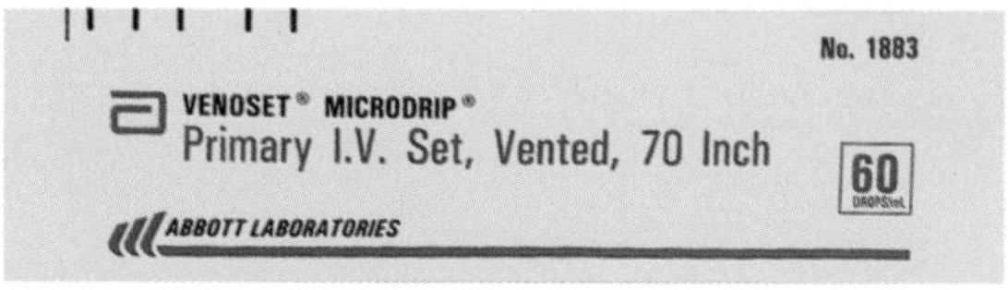

Courtesy of Abbott Laboratories, Inc.

8. How many mEq of potassium chloride will Mrs. Smith receive per hour? __________ mEq/h

9. At the present infusion rate, how much $D_5 \frac{1}{2}$ NS will Mrs. Smith receive in a 24-hour period? __________ mL/day

10. The IV is started at 1630 h. Estimate the time and date that you should plan to hang the next litre of $D_5 \frac{1}{2}$ NS. __________ hours __________ date

11. Mrs. Smith has a headache. How much acetaminophen will you administer?

    Give: __________ tablet(s)

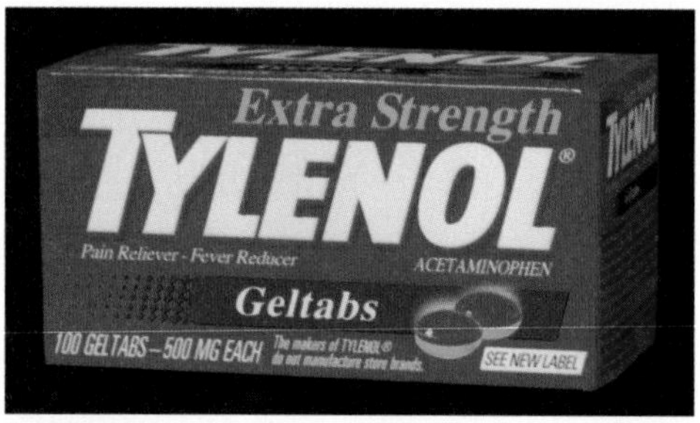

Courtesy of McNeil Consumer and Specialty Pharmaceuticals

12. You have located an infusion controller for Mrs. Smith's IV. At what rate will you set the controller? __________ mL/h

13. Compare the patient care order and the labels to determine which of Mrs. Smith's medications are ordered by their generic or chemical names. ______________________________

    ____

Despite your excellent care, Mrs. Smith's condition worsens. She is transferred into the coronary care unit (CCU) with the following medical orders. Questions 14 through 19 refer to these orders. Mrs. Smith weighs 50 kg.

ENTERED	FILLED	CHECKED	VERIFIED
			–

NOTE: A NON-PROPRIETARY DRUG OF EQUAL QUALITY MAY BE DISPENSED - IF THIS COLUMN IS NOT CHECKED!

DATE	TIME WRITTEN	PLEASE USE BALL POINT - PRESS FIRMLY	✓	TIME NOTED	NURSES SIGNATURE
04/09/xx	2230	Transfer to CCU	✓		
		NPO	✓		
		Discontinue nitroglycerin SL	✓		
		Lidocaine hydrochloride bolus 50 mg IV stat, then begin lidocaine hydrochloride drip 2 g in 500 mL D_5W (premixed solution) @ 2 mg/min by infusion pump	✓		
		Increase lidocaine hydrochloride to 4 mg/min if PVCs (premature ventricular contractions) persist	✓	2235	MS
		Dopamine hydrochloride 400 mg (1600 mcg/mL) IVPB in 250 mL D_5W (premixed solution) @ 500 mcg/kg/min by infusion pump	✓		
		Increase KCl to 20 mEq per L D_5W 1/2 NS IV @ 50 mL/h	✓		
		Increase furosemide to 40 mg IV q12h	✓		
		O_2 @ 30% after ABGs (arterial blood gases)	✓		
		Labwork: Electrolytes stat and in am and ABGs stat & prn	✓		
		Dr. J. Physician			

AUTO STOP ORDERS: UNLESS REORDERED, FOLLOWING WILL BE D/C'D AT 0800 ON:

DATE	ORDER		PHYSICIAN SIGNATURE
		☐ CONT ☐ D/C	PHYSICIAN SIGNATURE
		☐ CONT ☐ D/C	PHYSICIAN SIGNATURE
		☐ CONT ☐ D/C	

CHECK WHEN ANTIBIOTICS ORDERED ☐ Prophylactic ☐ Empiric ☐ Therapeutic

Allergies: None Known

Chest Pain
CLIENT DIAGNOSIS

HEIGHT 152 cm WEIGHT 50 kg

Smith, Donna
ID #257-226-3

FORM 959-706 (8-XX) PHYSICIAN'S ORDER Reynolds + Reynolds LITHO IN U.S.A. K41914 (7-00) D339360

1

14. Available is lidocaine hydrochloride 10 mg/mL. How much lidocaine hydrochloride will you give for the bolus? Draw an arrow on the appropriate syringe to indicate the amount you will give.

Give: __________ mL

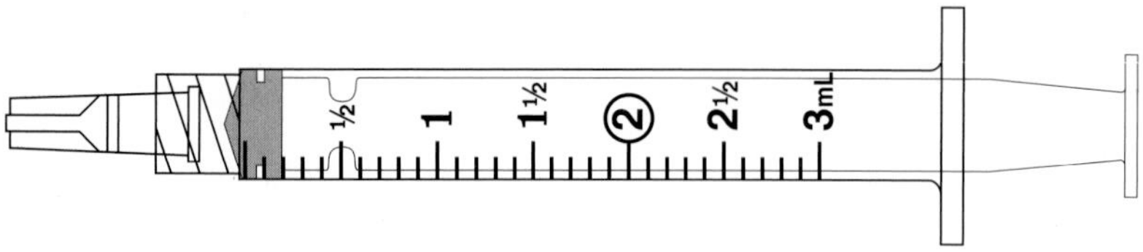

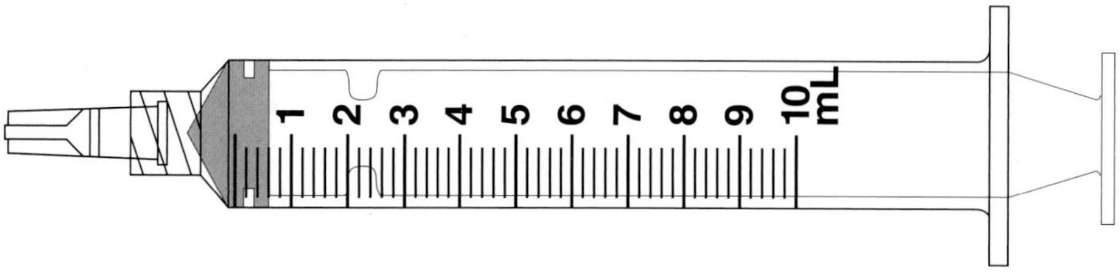

15. The infusion pump is calibrated to administer millilitres per hour. At what rate will you initially set the infusion pump for the lidocaine hydrochloride drip? __________ mL/h

16. The dose of dopamine hydrochloride ordered for Mrs. Smith is 500 mcg/mL. The recommended dosage of dopamine hydrochloride is 5–10 mcg/kg/min. Is the dose ordered for Mrs. Smith safe?

____

17. Calculate the rate for the infusion pump for the dopamine hydrochloride drip. __________ mL/h

18. How much dopamine hydrochloride will Mrs. Smith receive per hour? __________ mcg/h or __________ mg/h

19. Mrs. Smith is experiencing increasing amounts of PVCs. To increase her lidocaine hydrochloride drip to 4 mg/min, you will now change the IV infusion pump setting to __________ mL/h.

20. Julie Thomas is a 6-year-old child who weighs 15 kg. She is in the hospital for fever of unknown origin. Julie complains of burning on urination and her urinalysis shows *E. coli* bacterial infection. The doctor prescribes gentamicin sulfate 38 mg IV q8h to be administered by volume control set on an infusion pump in 100 mL 0.9% NS followed by 15 mL flush over 1 hour. The recommended dosage of gentamicin sulfate is 7.5 mg/kg/day IV divided in three doses.

Is the patient care order safe? __________ Explain:

____

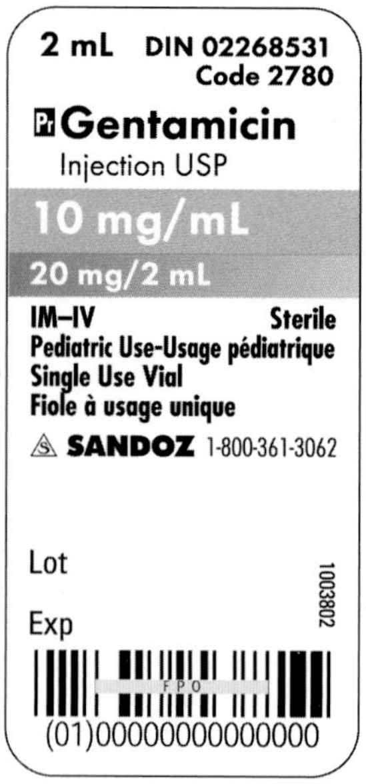

If safe, add __________ mL gentamicin sulfate and __________ mL 0.9% NS to the chamber, and set the flow rate for __________ mL/h.

21. Order: *diltiazem hydrochloride 125 mg in 100 mL D_5W IV @ 15 mg/h*

    Set the IV pump at __________ mL/h.

22. Jamie Smith is hospitalized with a staphylococcal bone infection. He weighs 30 kg.

    Orders: *$D_5 \frac{1}{2}$ NS IV @ 50 mL/h for continuous infusion*

    vancomycin hydrochloride 300 mg IV q6h

    Supply: vancomycin hydrochloride 500 mg/10 mL with instructions to "add to volume control set and infuse over 60 min."

    Recommended dosage: vancomycin hydrochloride 40 mg/kg/day IV in four equally divided doses

    Is this patient care order safe? __________ Explain: ______________________________

    If safe, how much vancomycin hydrochloride will you add to the chamber? __________ mL

    How much IV fluid will you add to the chamber with the vancomycin hydrochloride? __________ mL

    How much IV fluid will Jamie receive in 24 hours? __________ mL

    Questions 23 to 25 refer to the following patient care order.

    Order: meperidine hydrochloride 60 mg and atropine sulfate 0.12 mg

    Supply: meperidine sulfate 75 mg/mL atropine sulfate 0.3 mg/mL

    The two drugs are compatible and can be mixed in the same syringe. Both are available in ampules.

23. Give __________ mL meperidine sulfate
24. Give __________ mL atropine sulfate
25. The two drugs are compatible. How much in total will be administered? __________ mL

Use the related patient care orders and labels to answer questions 26 through 30. Select and mark the dose volume on the appropriate syringe, as indicated.

26. Order: *cefazolin sodium 500 mg IV q6h in 50 mL D_5W IV by volume control set over 30 min. Follow with 15 mL IV flush.*

    Reconstitute with __________ mL diluent to provide 334 mg/mL.

27. If necessary, prepare a reconstitution label for the cefazolin sodium.

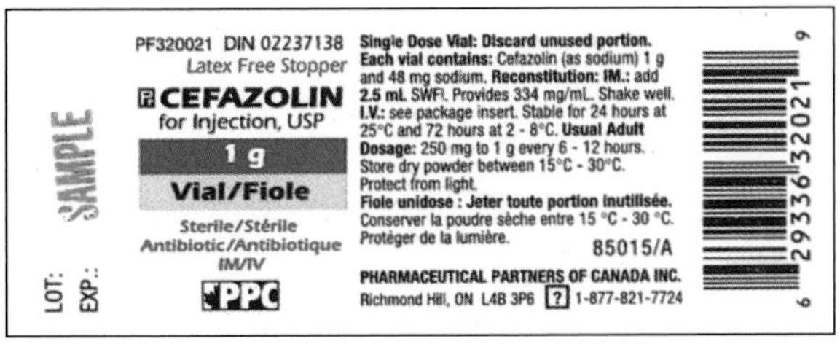

Pharmaceutical Partners of Canada Inc., Richmond Hill, ON

28. Add _____ mL cefazolin sodium and _____ mL D_5W to the chamber.

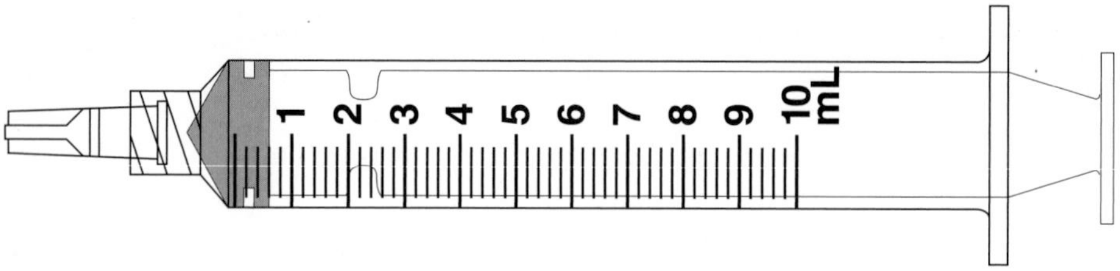
1
2
3
4
5
6
7
8
9
10
mL

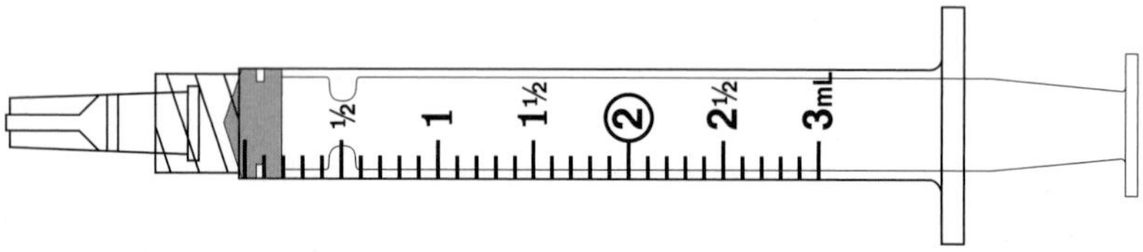
½
1
1½
2
2½
3mL

29. The IV cefazolin sodium is regulated on an infusion pump. Set the volume control set flow rate at __________ mL/h.

30. Order: *heparin sodium 10 000 units IV in 500 mL D_5W to infuse @ 1200 units/h.*

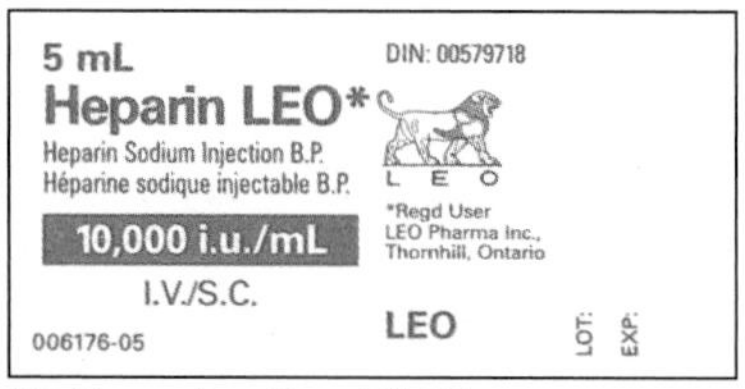
5 mL
DIN: 00579718
Heparin LEO*
Heparin Sodium Injection B.P.
Héparine sodique injectable B.P.
L E O
10,000 i.u./mL
*Regd User
LEO Pharma Inc.,
Thornhill, Ontario
I.V./S.C.
006176-05
LEO
LOT:
EXP.:

LEO Pharma Inc., Thornhill, ON

Add __________ mL heparin sodium to the IV solution. Set the flow rate to __________ mL/h on an IV infusion pump.

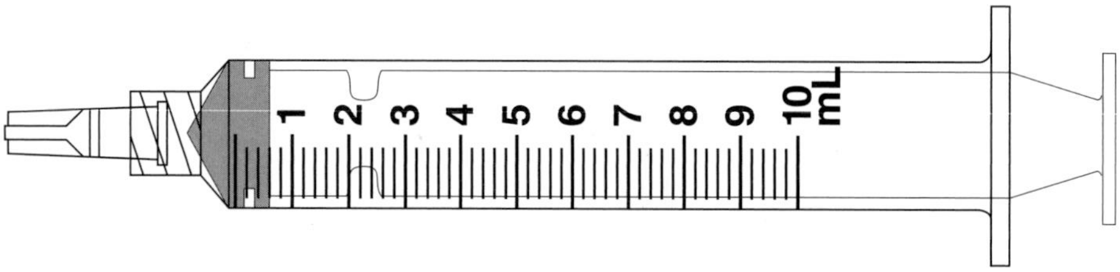
1
2
3
4
5
6
7
8
9
10
mL

Questions 31 and 32 refer to a patient who weighs 56.8 kg and has IV heparin sodium ordered per the following Weight-Based Heparin Sodium Protocol.

Weight-Based Heparin Sodium Protocol:

Heparin sodium IV infusion: *heparin sodium 25 000 units in 250 mL of $\frac{1}{2}$ NS*

IV boluses: Use heparin sodium 1000 units/mL

Bolus with heparin sodium 80 units/kg. Then initiate heparin sodium drip at 18 units/kg/h. Obtain, aPTT, every 6 hours and adjust dosage and rate as follows:

If aPTT is less than 35 seconds: Rebolus with 80 units/kg and increase rate by 4 units/kg/h.

If aPTT is 36–44 seconds: Rebolus with 40 units/kg and increase rate by 2 units/kg/h.

If aPTT is 45–75 seconds: Continue current rate.

If aPTT is 76–90 seconds: Decrease rate by 2 units/kg/h.

If aPTT is more than 90 seconds: Hold heparin sodium for 1 hour and then decrease rate by 3 units/kg/h.

31. Calculate the initial heparin sodium bolus dosage: __________ units

    Calculate the bolus dose: __________ mL

    Calculate the initial heparin sodium infusion rate: __________ units/h or __________ mL/h

32. At 0930 h, the patient's aPTT is 77 seconds. According to the protocol, what will your action be?

    ____

    ____

    Reset infusion rate to __________ units/h or __________ mL/h.

33. Order: *Humulin R 100-unit insulin SC ac per sliding scale and blood sugar level. The patient's blood sugar at 1730 h is 13.2 mmol/L.*

Sliding Scale	Insulin Dosage
BS: 0–8	0 units
BS: 8.1–14	8 units
BS: 14.1–19	13 units
BS: 19.1–22	18 units
BS: more than22.1	Call MD

Give: __________ units, which equals __________ mL. (Mark dose on appropriate syringe.)

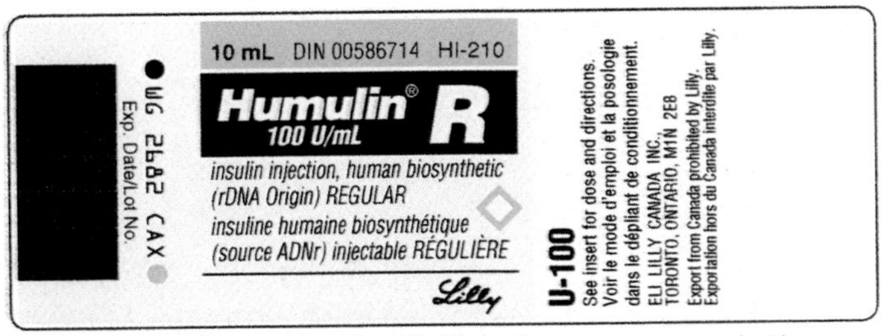

Humalog and Humulin are trademarks of Eli Lilly and Company and are used with permission. Eli Lilly Canada Inc., Toronto, ON

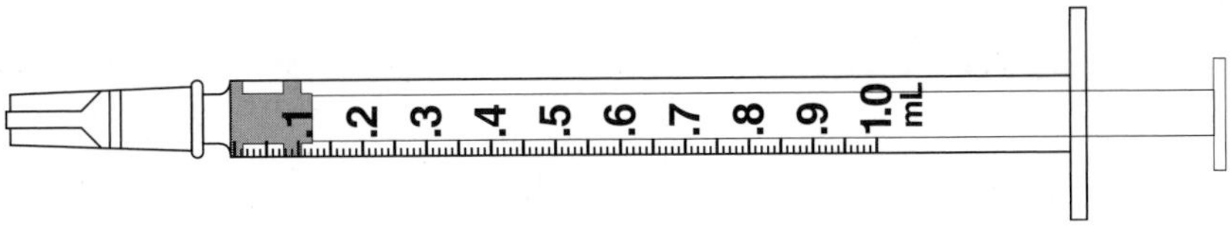

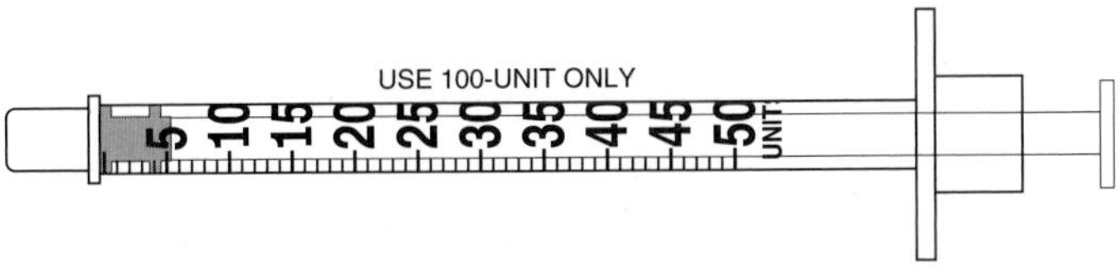

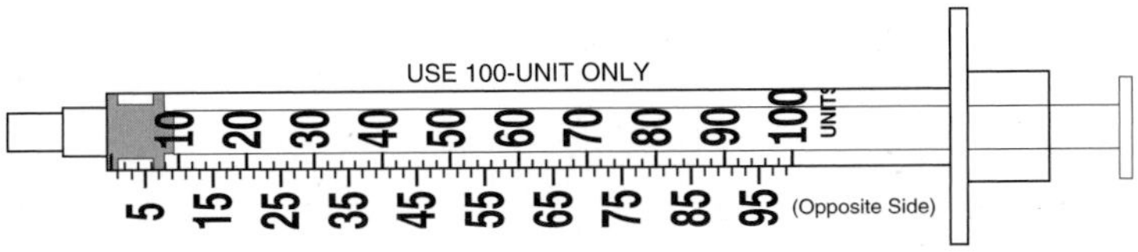

34. Order: *Humulin R 100-unit insulin 15 units with Humulin N 100-unit insulin 45 units SC at 0730 h*

    You will give a total of __________ units insulin. (Mark dose on appropriate syringe, designating regular and NPH insulin.)

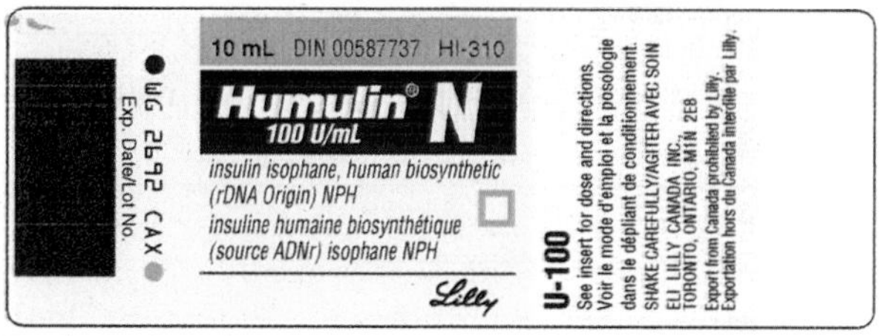

Humalog and Humulin are trademarks of Eli Lilly and Company and are used with permission. Eli Lilly Canada Inc., Toronto, ON

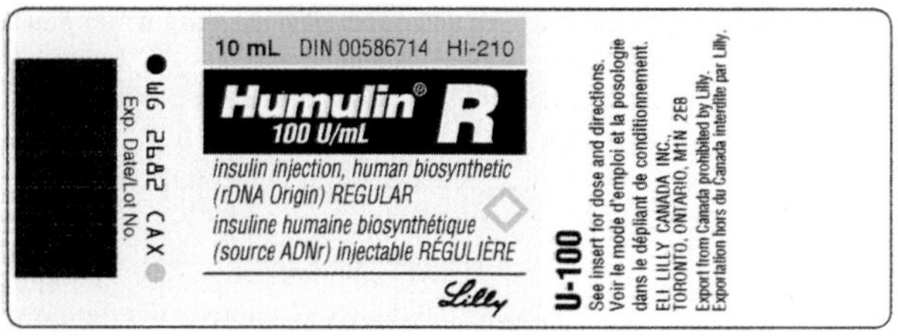

Humalog and Humulin are trademarks of Eli Lilly and Company and are used with permission. Eli Lilly Canada Inc., Toronto, ON

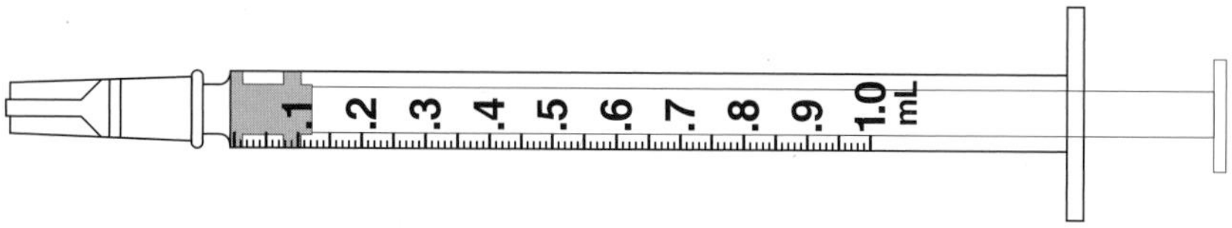

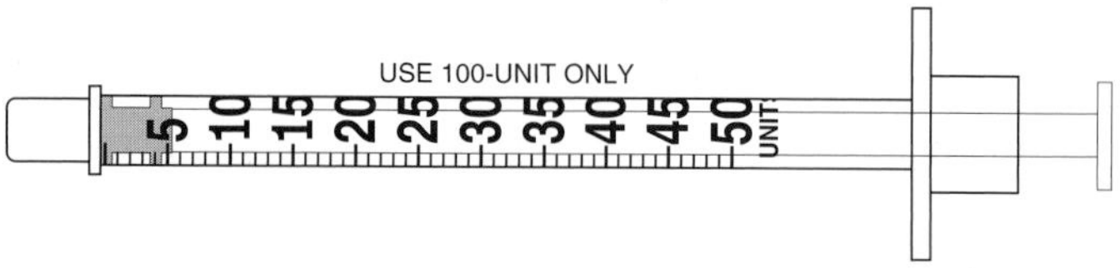

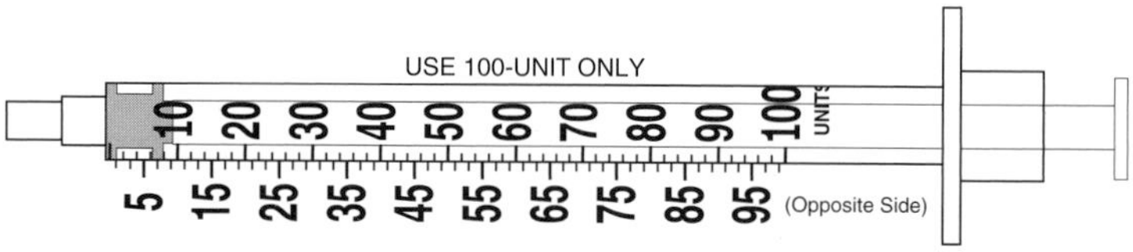

35. A patient with diabetes is receiving an insulin drip of *Humulin R 100-unit insulin 300 units in 150 mL NS infusing at 10 mL/h.* How many units/h of insulin is this patient receiving? __________ units/h

Questions 36 and 37 refer to an infant who weighs 7.3 kg and is admitted to the pediatric unit with vomiting and diarrhea of 3 days' duration.

Order: *$\frac{1}{4}$ strength Isomil 80 mL q3h for four feedings; if tolerated, increase Isomil to $\frac{1}{2}$ strength 80 mL q3h for four feedings*

Supply: Isomil Ready-to-Feed formula in 235-mL cans

36. Prepare sufficient quantity of the 1/4 strength Isomil for four feedings. __________ Isomil and __________ water

37. The child is not tolerating the oral feedings. Calculate this child's allowable daily and hourly IV maintenance fluids using the following recommendation. __________ mL/day or __________ mL/h

    Daily rate of pediatric maintenance IV fluids:

    100 mL/kg for first 10 kg of body weight

    50 mL/kg for next 10 kg of body weight

    20 mL/kg for each kilogram above 20 kg of body weight

Use the following information and order to answer questions 38 and 39.

$$BSA(m^2) = \sqrt{\frac{ht(cm) \times wt(kg)}{300}}$$

Order: mitomycin 28 mg IV Push stat

Recommended dosage is 10–20 mg/m²/single IV dose.

Patient is 157.5 cm tall and weighs 46.8 kg.

Mitomycin is available in a 20-mg vial with directions to reconstitute with 40 mL sterile water for injection to make a total volume of 40 mL. The dose is injected slowly over 10 minutes.

38. The patient's BSA is __________ m².

39. What is the recommended dosage of mitomycin for this patient? __________ mg to __________ mg

Is the ordered dosage safe? __________

What is the concentration of mitomycin after reconstitution? __________ mg/mL

If the order is safe, administer __________ mL mitomycin at the rate of __________ mL/min or __________ mL/15 sec.

40. A child's IV is 1 L D_5 0.33% NaCl. Calculate the amount of solute in this IV solution. __________ g dextrose and _____ g NaCl.

Use the following patient care order and label for the available drug to answer questions 41 and 42.

Order: *vancomycin hydrochloride 500 mg IV q6h in IV fluid for total volume of 100 mL to infuse over 1 h via volume control set. Reconstitute 500-mg vial with 10 mL sterile water for injection.*

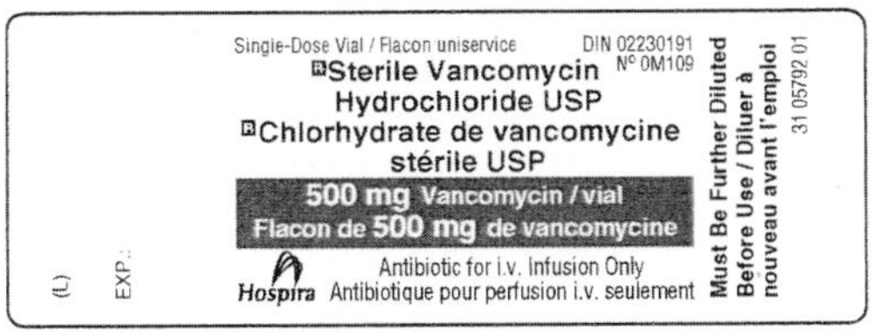

Hospira Healthcare Corporation, Saint-Laurent, QUE

41. Add __________ mL vancomycin hydrochloride and __________ mL IV fluid to the chamber.

42. The minimal dilution (maximal concentration) of vancomycin hydrochloride is 10 mg/mL. Is the ordered amount of IV fluid sufficient to safely dilute the vancomycin hydrochloride? __________
Explain: __________

____

____

Use the following information to answer questions 43 and 44.

Order: *penicillin G sodium 400 000 units IVPB q6h* for a child who weighs 10 kg. Recommended dosage for children: Give penicillin G sodium 100 000–400 000 units/kg/day in divided doses q6h; dilute with 50 mL NS and infuse over 30 minutes.

Pharmaceutical Partners of Canada Inc., Richmond Hill, ON

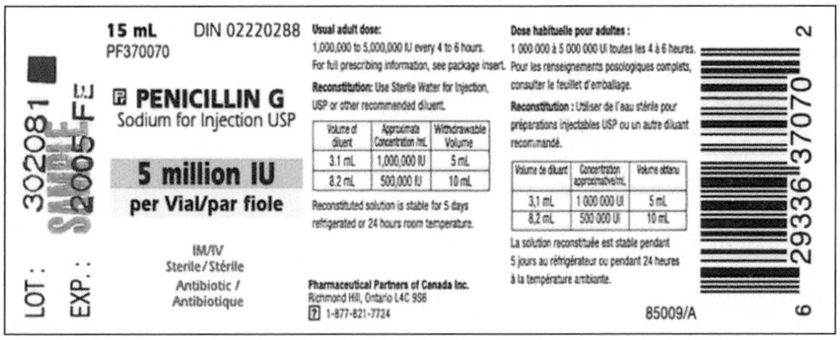

43. How many units per day of penicillin G sodium is this child ordered to receive? __________ units/day

Is the ordered dosage safe? __________ Explain: ______________________________

If safe, reconstitute with __________ mL diluent for a concentration of __________ units/mL, and prepare a reconstitution label.

Prepare to give __________ mL.

If not safe, what should you do? ______________________________

44. The child's IV is infusing on an electronic infusion pump. If the dosage is safe, set the IV flow rate at __________ mL/h.

Use the following patient situation to answer questions 45 through 48.

A patient has been admitted to the hospital with fever and chills, productive cough with yellow-green sputum, shortness of breath, malaise, and anorexia. Laboratory tests and X-rays confirmed a diagnosis of pneumonia. The patient is complaining of nausea. The physician writes the following orders. The labels represent the drugs you have available.

NS 1000 mL IV @ 125 mL/h

ceftazidime 1500 mg IVPB q8h in 100 mL NS over 30 min

promethazine hydrochloride 25 mg IV push q4h prn nausea & vomiting

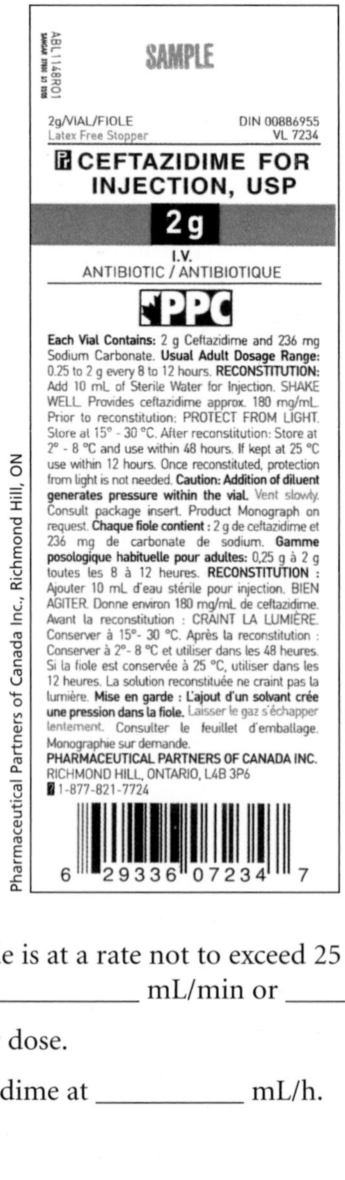

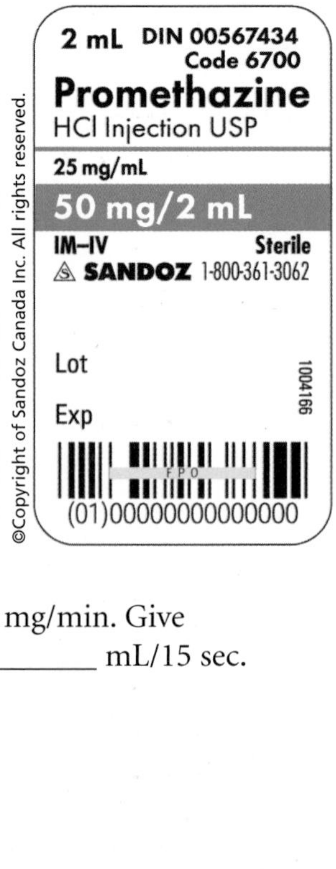

45. You can start the primary IV at 1:15 PM on an infusion pump. When do you estimate (using international time) the primary IV will be completely infused and have to be replaced? __________ hours

46. The recommendation for direct IV administration of promethazine hydrochloride is at a rate not to exceed 25 mg/min. Give __________ mL promethazine at the rate of __________ mL/min or __________ mL/15 sec.

47. You will give __________ mL ceftazidime per dose.

48. Set the IVPB flow rate for each dose of ceftazidime at __________ mL/h.

49. Critical Thinking Skill: Describe the strategy you would implement to prevent this medication error.

possible scenario

A student nurse was preparing for medication administration. One of the orders on the medication administration record was written as *digoxin 0.125 mg OD.* The student nurse crushed the digoxin tablet. Prior to giving the medication, the nursing instructor checked the medications that the student had prepared. The instructor asked the student to explain the rationale for crushing the digoxin tablet. The student explained to the instructor that the digoxin order was for the right eye and the student planned to add a small amount of sterile water to the crushed tablet and put it in the patient's eye.

potential outcome

What is wrong with the digoxin order? ______________________________

What could be the result? ______________________________

prevention

____

____

50. Critical Thinking Skill: Describe the strategy you would implement to prevent this medication error.

possible scenario

Order: *quinine sulfate 300 mg PO bedtime*

Supply: quinidine sulfate 300 mg tablets

A student nurse administering medications noted the difference between the order and the supply drug, and queried the staff nurse about the order and what had been administered. The staff nurse at first dismissed it as only the brand name versus the generic name of the drug. Later the nurse realized that the student was exactly right to question the order and the drug supplied, and admitted to the student that the patient had been receiving the wrong drug all week.

potential outcome

The student referred to a drug reference book and compared the therapeutic and adverse effects of both drugs. The quinine sulfate was correctly ordered for leg cramps. Quinidine sulfate is an anti-arrhythmic heart medication. The student reviewed the patient's record and noted that the patient had been experiencing serious hypotension (an adverse effect of quinidine) for the past several days.

prevention

____

____

After completing these problems, see pages 520–524 to check your answers. Give yourself 2 points for each correct answer.

Perfect score = 100 My score = __________

Mastery score = 90 or higher (45 correct)

Answers to Mathematics Diagnostic Evaluation from pages 3–5

1) 1517.63 **2)** 20.74 **3)** 100.66 **4)** \$323.72 **5)** 46.11 **6)** 754.5 **7)** 16.91 **8)** 19,494.7 **9)** \$173.04 **10)** 403.26 **11)** 36 **12)** 2500 **13)** $\frac{2}{3}$ **14)** 6.25 **15)** $\frac{4}{5}$ **16)** 40% **17)** 0.4% **18)** 0.05 **19)** 1:3 **20)** 0.02 **21)** $1\frac{1}{4}$ **22)** $6\frac{13}{24}$ **23)** $1\frac{11}{18}$ **24)** $\frac{3}{5}$ **25)** $14\frac{7}{8}$ **26)** $\frac{1}{100}$ **27)** 0.009 **28)** 320 **29)** 3 **30)** 0.05 **31)** 4 **32)** 0.09 **33)** 0.22 **34)** 25 **35)** 4 **36)** 0.75 **37)** 3 **38)** 500 **39)** 18.24 **40)** 2.4 **41)** $\frac{1}{5}$ **42)** 1:50 **43)** 5 tablets **44)** 2 milligrams **45)** 30 kilograms **46)** 3.3 pounds **47)** $6\frac{1}{4}$ = 6.25 centimetres **48)** 7.5 centimetres **49)** 90% **50)** 5:1

Selected Solutions—Mathematics Diagnostic Evaluation

3)
$$\begin{array}{r} 9.50 \\ 17.06 \\ 32.00 \\ 41.11 \\ \underline{0.99} \\ 100.66 \end{array}$$

6)
$$\begin{array}{r} 1{,}005.0 \\ \underline{-250.5} \\ 754.5 \end{array}$$

10)
$$\begin{array}{r} 17.16 \\ \underline{23.5} \\ 8580 \\ 5148 \\ \underline{3432} \\ 403.260 \end{array} = 403.26$$

12)
$$0.001\overline{)2.500.} \quad \text{(quotient } 2500.\text{)} = 2500$$

19)
$$\frac{33\frac{1}{3}}{100} = \frac{\frac{100}{3}}{100} = \frac{100}{3} \div \frac{100}{1} = \frac{\cancel{100}}{3} \times \frac{1}{\cancel{100}} = \frac{1}{3} = 1:3$$

23)
$$1\frac{5}{6} - \frac{2}{9} = \frac{11}{6} - \frac{2}{9} = \frac{66}{36} - \frac{8}{36} = \frac{58}{36} = \frac{29}{18} = 1\frac{11}{18}$$

25)
$$4\frac{1}{4} \times 3\frac{1}{2} = \frac{17}{4} \times \frac{7}{2} = \frac{119}{8} = 14\frac{7}{8}$$

29)
$$\frac{0.02 + 0.16}{0.4 - 0.34}$$
$$\begin{array}{r} 0.02 \\ \underline{+0.16} \\ 0.18 \end{array} \qquad \begin{array}{r} 0.40 \\ \underline{-0.34} \\ 0.06 \end{array}$$
$$\frac{0.18}{0.06} = 0.06.\overline{)0.18.} \quad \text{(quotient } 3.\text{)} = 3$$

32)
$$\frac{1}{2}\% = 0.5\% = 0.005 \qquad \begin{array}{r} 18 \\ \underline{\times\ 0.005} \\ 0.090 \end{array} = 0.09$$

34)
$$\frac{\frac{1}{1000}}{\frac{1}{100}} \times 250 = \frac{1}{\cancelto{10}{1000}} \times \frac{\cancelto{1}{100}}{1} \times \frac{250}{1} = \frac{250}{10} = 25$$

45)
$$66 \text{ pounds} \times \frac{1 \text{ kilogram}}{2.2 \text{ pounds}} =$$
$$66\ \cancel{\text{pounds}} \times \frac{1 \times 10 \text{ kilogram}}{2.2 \times 10\ \cancel{\text{pounds}}} =$$
$$\frac{\cancelto{60}{660}}{\cancelto{2}{22}} \text{ kilograms} = 30 \text{ kilograms}$$

46)
$$\begin{array}{r} 2.2 \\ \underline{\times\ 1.5} \\ 110 \\ \underline{22} \\ 3.30 \end{array}$$
$$1.5\ \cancel{\text{kilograms}} \times \frac{2.2 \text{ pounds}}{1\ \cancel{\text{kilograms}}}$$
$$= 1.5 \times 2.2 \text{ pounds} = 3.3 \text{ pounds}$$

48)
$$3\ \cancel{\text{inches}} \times \frac{2.5 \text{ centimetres}}{1\ \cancel{\text{inch}}} = 3 \times 2.5 \text{ centimetres}$$
$$= 7.5 \text{ centimetres}$$

49)
$$\begin{array}{r} 50 \\ \underline{-5} \\ 45 \end{array} \qquad \frac{45}{50} = \frac{9}{10} = 90\%$$

Answers to Review Set 1 from pages 13–14

1) $\frac{6}{6}, \frac{7}{5}$ **2)** $\frac{1}{4}, \frac{1}{14}$ **3)** $1\frac{2}{9}, 1\frac{1}{4}, 5\frac{7}{8}$ **4)** $\frac{3}{4} = \frac{6}{8}, \frac{1}{5} = \frac{2}{10}, \frac{3}{9} = \frac{1}{3}$ **5)** $\frac{13}{2}$ **6)** $\frac{6}{5}$ **7)** $\frac{32}{3}$ **8)** $\frac{47}{6}$ **9)** 2 **10)** 1 **11)** $3\frac{1}{3}$ **12)** $1\frac{1}{3}$ **13)** $\frac{6}{8}$ **14)** $\frac{4}{16}$ **15)** $\frac{4}{10}$ **16)** $\frac{6}{9}$ **17)** $\frac{1}{100}$ **18)** $\frac{1}{10\,000}$ **19)** $\frac{5}{9}$ **20)** $\frac{3}{10}$ **21)** $\frac{2}{5}$ bottle **22)** 600 mL on Day 2; 900 mL on Day 3; 1350 mL on Day 4 **23)** $\frac{1}{20}$ of the class are men **24)** $\frac{9}{10}$ of the questions were answered correctly **25)** $\frac{1}{4}$

Selected Solutions—Review Set 1

7) $10\frac{2}{3} = \frac{(3 \times 10) + 2}{3} = \frac{32}{3}$

12) $\frac{100}{75} = 1\frac{25}{75} = 1\frac{1}{3}$

21) 300 mL − 180 mL = 120 mL remaining

$\frac{\cancel{120}^{\,2}}{\cancel{300}_{\,5}} = \frac{2}{5}$ bottle remaining

23)

$$\begin{array}{r} 57 \\ +3 \\ \hline 60 \end{array}$$

60 people in class

The men represent $\frac{3}{60}$ or $\frac{1}{20}$ of the class.

25) $\frac{1}{8} = \frac{3}{24}; \frac{1}{6} = \frac{4}{24}; \frac{1}{4} = \frac{6}{24}$

therefore, $\frac{1}{4}$ is the largest fraction

Answers to Review Set 2 from pages 16–17

1) $8\frac{7}{15}$ **2)** $1\frac{5}{12}$ **3)** $17\frac{5}{24}$ **4)** $1\frac{1}{24}$ **5)** $32\frac{5}{6}$ **6)** $1\frac{1}{3}$ **7)** $5\frac{53}{72}$ **8)** 43 **9)** $5\frac{118}{119}$ **10)** $2\frac{8}{15}$ **11)** $\frac{1}{2}$ **12)** $4\frac{5}{6}$ **13)** $\frac{1}{24}$ **14)** $63\frac{2}{3}$ **15)** $\frac{1}{6}$ **16)** $1\frac{2}{5}$ **17)** $7\frac{1}{16}$ **18)** $7\frac{2}{9}$ **19)** $1\frac{1}{4}$ **20)** $9\frac{1}{2}$ **21)** $\frac{1}{12}$ **22)** $1\frac{1}{2}$ tablets daily **23)** $4\frac{11}{12}$ cups of fluid **24)** $2\frac{11}{12}$ km left to walk **25)** $112\frac{1}{4}$ apples eaten

Selected Solutions—Review Set 2

1) $7\frac{4}{5} + \frac{2}{3} = 7\frac{12}{15}$

$$\begin{array}{r} 7\frac{12}{15} \\ +\frac{10}{15} \\ \hline 7\frac{22}{15} = 8\frac{7}{15} \end{array}$$

3) $4\frac{2}{3} + 5\frac{1}{24} + 7\frac{1}{2} = 4\frac{16}{24}$

$$\begin{array}{r} 4\frac{16}{24} \\ 5\frac{1}{24} \\ +7\frac{12}{24} \\ \hline 16\frac{29}{24} = 17\frac{5}{24} \end{array}$$

4) $\frac{3}{4} + \frac{1}{8} + \frac{1}{6} = \frac{18}{24} + \frac{3}{24} + \frac{4}{24} =$

$\frac{18 + 3 + 4}{24} = \frac{25}{24} = 1\frac{1}{24}$

12) $8\frac{1}{12} - 3\frac{1}{4} = 8\frac{1}{12} - 3\frac{3}{12} = 7\frac{13}{12}$

$$\begin{array}{r} 7\frac{13}{12} \\ -3\frac{3}{12} \\ \hline 4\frac{10}{12} = 4\frac{5}{6} \end{array}$$

20) $27 - 17\frac{1}{2} = 26\frac{2}{2}$

$$\begin{array}{r} 26\frac{2}{2} \\ -17\frac{1}{2} \\ \hline 9\frac{1}{2} \end{array}$$

litres

21) $1 - \left(\frac{2}{3} + \frac{1}{4}\right) = 1 - \left(\frac{8 + 3}{12}\right) = 1 - \frac{11}{12} = \frac{1}{12}$

22) $\frac{1}{2} \times 3 = \frac{3}{2} = 1\frac{1}{2}$ tablets daily

23) $1\frac{1}{2} + 1 + \frac{2}{3} + 1\frac{3}{4} = \frac{3}{2} + 1 + \frac{2}{3} + \frac{7}{4} =$

$\frac{18}{12} + \frac{12}{12} + \frac{8}{12} + \frac{21}{12} = \frac{59}{12} = 4\frac{11}{12}$ cups of fluid

24) $1\frac{1}{4} + 1\frac{1}{3} + 1\frac{1}{2} + 1 = \frac{5}{4} + \frac{4}{3} + \frac{3}{2} + \frac{1}{1} =$

$\frac{15}{12} + \frac{16}{12} + \frac{18}{12} + \frac{12}{12} = \frac{61}{12}$ km walked

$8 \text{ km} - \frac{61}{12} \text{ km} = \frac{96}{12} - \frac{61}{12} = \frac{35}{12} = 2\frac{11}{12}$ km left to walk

25) $54\frac{1}{2} + 57\frac{3}{4} = \frac{218}{4} + \frac{231}{4} = \frac{449}{4} = 112\frac{1}{4}$ apples eaten

Answers to Review Set 3 from pages 22–23

1) $\frac{1}{40}$ **2)** $\frac{36}{125}$ **3)** $\frac{35}{48}$ **4)** $\frac{3}{100}$ **5)** 3 **6)** $1\frac{2}{3}$ **7)** $\frac{4}{5}$ **8)** $6\frac{8}{15}$ **9)** $\frac{1}{2}$ **10)** $23\frac{19}{36}$ **11)** $\frac{3}{32}$ **12)** 3 **13)** $1\frac{34}{39}$ **14)** $\frac{3}{14}$ **15)** $\frac{1}{11}$ **16)** $\frac{1}{2}$ **17)** $\frac{1}{30}$ **18)** $3\frac{1}{3}$ **19)** $\frac{3}{20}$ **20)** $1\frac{1}{9}$ **21)** 60 calories **22)** 560 sec **23)** 20 doses **24)** $31\frac{1}{2}$ tablets **25)** 1275 millilitres

Selected Solutions—Review Set 3

3) $\frac{5}{8} \times 1\frac{1}{6} = \frac{5}{8} \times \frac{7}{6} = \frac{35}{48}$

5) $\dfrac{\frac{1}{6}}{\frac{1}{4}} \times \dfrac{3}{\frac{2}{3}} = \left(\frac{1}{6} \times \frac{4}{1}\right) \times \left(\frac{3}{1} \times \frac{3}{2}\right) = \frac{\cancel{4}^{2}}{\cancel{6}_{3}} \times \frac{9}{2} = \frac{\cancel{18}^{3}}{\cancel{6}_{1}} = 3$

15) $\frac{1}{33} \div \frac{1}{3} = \frac{1}{33} \times \frac{3}{1} = \frac{3}{33} = \frac{1}{11}$

18) $2\frac{1}{2} \div \frac{3}{4} = \frac{5}{2} \div \frac{3}{4} = \frac{5}{\cancel{2}_{1}} \times \frac{\cancel{4}^{2}}{3} = \frac{10}{3} = 3\frac{1}{3}$

24) $3 \times 7 = 21$ doses

$21 \times 1\frac{1}{2} = 21 \times \frac{3}{2} = \frac{63}{2} = 31\frac{1}{2}$ tablets

25) $850 \div \frac{2}{3} = \frac{\cancel{850}^{425}}{1} \times \frac{3}{\cancel{2}_{1}} = 1275$ millilitres

Answers to Review Set 4 from pages 29–30

1) 0.2, two tenths **2)** $\frac{17}{20}$, 0.85 **3)** $1\frac{1}{20}$, one and five hundredths **4)** $\frac{3}{500}$, six thousandths **5)** 10.015, ten and fifteen thousandths **6)** $1\frac{9}{10}$, one and nine tenths **7)** $5\frac{1}{10}$, 5.1 **8)** 0.8, eight tenths **9)** $250\frac{1}{2}$, two hundred fifty and five tenths **10)** 33.03, thirty-three and three hundredths **11)** $\frac{19}{20}$, ninety-five hundredths **12)** 2.75, two and seventy-five hundredths **13)** $7\frac{1}{200}$, 7.005 **14)** 1000.005, one thousand and five thousandths **15)** $4085\frac{3}{40}$, 4085.075 **16)** 0.0170 **17)** 0.25, twenty-five hundreths **18)** 0.75, seventy-five hundreths **19)** $\frac{9}{200}$ **20)** 0.120 **21)** 0.063 **22)** False **23)** False **24)** True **25)** 0.8 gram and 1.25 grams

Selected Solutions—Review Set 4

4) $0.006 = \frac{6}{1000} = \frac{3}{500}$

8) $\frac{4}{5} = 5\overline{)4.0}$ = 0.8

14) $1000\frac{1}{200} = \frac{2000001}{200} = 200\overline{)2000001.00}$ = 1000.005

```
      1000.005
200)2000001.00
    200
    0001000
       1000
```

25) 0.8 g is greater than 0.5 g and less than 2 g. Therefore, it is a safe dosage.

0.25 g is less than 0.5 g. Therefore, it is NOT a safe dosage.

2.5 g is greater than 2 g. Therefore, it is NOT a safe dosage.

1.25 g is greater than 0.5 g and less than 2 g. Therefore, it is a safe dosage.

Answers to Review Set 5 from pages 31–32

1) 22.585 **2)** 44.177 **3)** 12.309 **4)** 11.3 **5)** 175.199 **6)** 25.007 **7)** 0.518 **8)** \$9.48 **9)** \$18.91 **10)** \$22.71 **11)** 6.403 **12)** 0.27 **13)** 4.15 **14)** 1.51 **15)** 10.25 **16)** 2.517 **17)** 374.35 **18)** 604.42 **19)** 27.449 **20)** 23.619 **21)** 0.697 gram **22)** 7.5 mg **23)** \$2058.06 **24)** 3 kg **25)** 8.1 h

Selected Solutions—Review Set 5

2)
$$\begin{array}{r} 7.517 \\ 3.200 \\ 0.160 \\ \underline{33.300} \\ 44.177 \end{array}$$

9)
$$\begin{array}{r} \overset{8\ 9\,10}{\$1\not{9}.\not{0}\not{0}} \\ \underline{-0.09} \\ \$18.91 \end{array}$$

22) $30 \text{ mg} - (7.5 \text{ mg} + 15 \text{ mg}) = \begin{array}{r} 30.0 \text{ mg} \\ \underline{-\ 22.5 \text{ mg}} \\ 7.5 \text{ mg} \end{array}$

25)
$$\begin{array}{r} 3 \text{ h } 20 \text{ min} \\ 40 \text{ min} \\ 3 \text{ h } 30 \text{ min} \\ 24 \text{ min} \\ \underline{12 \text{ min}} \\ 6 \text{ h } 126 \text{ min} \end{array} = 8 \text{ h } 6 \text{ min (60 minutes/hour)}$$
$$= 8\frac{6}{60} = 8\frac{1}{10} = 8.1 \text{ h}$$

Answers to Review Set 6 from pages 38–39

1) 5.83 **2)** 2.20 **3)** 42.75 **4)** 0.15 **5)** 75 100.75 **6)** 32.86 **7)** 2.78 **8)** 348.58 **9)** 400 **10)** 3.74 **11)** 5 **12)** 2.98 **13)** 5.45 **14)** 272.67 **15)** 1.5 **16)** 50 020 **17)** 562.50. = 56 250 **18)** 16.0. = 160 **19)** .025. = 0.025 **20)** .032.005 = 0.032005 **21)** 23.2.5 = 232.5 **22)** 71.7.717 = 71.7717 **23)** 83.1.6 = 831.6 **24)** 0.33. = 33 **25)** 14.106. = 14 106

Selected Solutions—Review Set 6

8) $23.2 \times 15.025 = 348.58$

12) $45.5 \div 15.25 = 2.9836 = 2.98$

Answers to Practice Problems—Chapter 1 from pages 39–41

1) $\frac{7}{20}$ **2)** 0.375 **3)** LCD = 21 **4)** LCD = 55 **5)** LCD = 18 **6)** LCD = 15 **7)** $3\frac{7}{15}$ **8)** $7\frac{29}{60}$ **9)** $\frac{1}{2}$ **10)** $2\frac{7}{24}$ **11)** $\frac{7}{27}$ **12)** $10\frac{1}{8}$ **13)** $4\frac{4}{17}$ **14)** $\frac{39}{80}$ **15)** $5\frac{1}{55}$ **16)** $5\frac{5}{18}$ **17)** $2\frac{86}{87}$ **18)** $\frac{3}{20}$ **19)** $\frac{1}{3125}$ **20)** $\frac{1}{4}$ **21)** $1\frac{5}{7}$ **22)** $16\frac{1}{32}$ **23)** 60.27 **24)** 66.74 **25)** 42.98 **26)** 4833.92 **27)** 190.8 **28)** 19.17 **29)** 9.48 **30)** 7.7 **31)** 42.75 **32)** 300 **33)** 12 930.43 **34)** 3200.63 **35)** 2 **36)** 150.96 **37)** 9716 **38)** 0.5025 **39)** 0.25. = 25 **40)** 5750 **41)** 0.025 **42)** 11.5.25 = 115.25 **43)** 0.16 mg **44)** $\frac{1}{8}$ **45)** 0.35 mg **46)** \$915.08 **47)** \$1.46 **48)** 2.5 tablets **49)** 800 mL **50)** 2.95 kilograms

Selected Solutions—Practice Problems—Chapter 1

43) $4\ tab \times \frac{0.4\ mg}{1\ \not{tab}} = 0.16\ mg$

44) $\left(1\ assignment - \frac{1}{2}\ assignment\ completed\right) = \frac{1}{2}\ assignment\ remaining$

$\frac{1}{2}\ assignment\ remaining \div 4\ students = \frac{1}{2}\ assignment \times \frac{1}{4\ students} = \frac{1}{8}\ assignment\ remaining\ per\ student$

45) $\frac{0.1\ mg}{\not{tab}} \times 3.5\ tab = 0.35\ mg$

46) $(\$17.43/\text{h} \times 40 \text{ h}) + (6.25 \text{ h} \times \$17.43 \times 2)$

$= \$697.20 + \$217.875$ (round off routinely)

$= \$697.20 + \$217.88 = \$915.08$

47) \$98.76/12 catheters = \$8.23 per catheter

$\$975 \div (12 \times 12) = \frac{\$975}{144} = \$6.77\ per\ catheter$

\$8.23 − \$ 6.77 = \$1.46 is saved per catheter

48) $1.25\ mg \div \frac{0.5\ mg}{tablet} = 1.25\ mg \times \frac{1\ tablet}{0.5\ mg} = 2.5\ tablets$ or $2\frac{1}{2}$ tablets

49) $\frac{2}{\not{3}_1}\ of\ \overset{400}{\not{1200}}\ mL = 2 \times 400\ mL = 800\ mL$

50)
$$\begin{array}{r} 6.65 \text{ kg} \\ \underline{-\ 3.70 \text{ kg}} \\ 2.95 \text{ kg} \end{array}$$

Answers to Review Set 7 from page 48

1) $\frac{1}{50}$ **2)** $\frac{3}{5}$ **3)** $\frac{1}{3}$ **4)** 0.5 **5)** 0.15 **6)** 0.07 **7)** 0.24 **8)** 25% **9)** 12.5% **10)** 70% **11)** 50% **12)** $\frac{9}{20}$ **13)** $\frac{1}{200}$ **14)** $\frac{1}{100}$ **15)** $\frac{2}{3}$ **16)** 0.03 **17)** 0.33 **18)** 0.01 **19)** 4:25 **20)** 1:4 **21)** 1:2 **22)** 0.9 **23)** $\frac{200}{400}$ **24)** 0.25% **25)** 0.5

Selected Solutions—Review Set 7

1) $\frac{3}{150} = \frac{\overset{1}{\cancel{3}}}{\underset{50}{\cancel{150}}} = \frac{1}{50}$

3) $\frac{\overset{1}{\cancel{0.05}}}{\underset{3}{\cancel{0.15}}} = \frac{1}{3}$

5) $\frac{\frac{1}{1000}}{\frac{1}{150}} = \frac{1}{\underset{100}{\cancel{1000}}} \times \frac{\overset{15}{\cancel{150}}}{1} = \frac{15}{100} = 0.15. = 0.15$

9) $0.08 : 0.64 = \frac{0.08}{0.64} = \frac{1}{8} = 0.125;$

$0.125 = \frac{125}{1000} = \frac{12.5}{100} = 12.5\%$

13) $0.5\% = \frac{0.5}{100} = 0.5 \div 100 = 0.00.5 = 0.005$

$= \frac{5}{1000} = \frac{1}{200}$

16) $2.94\% = \frac{2.94}{100} = 2.94 \div 100 = 0.02.94 = 0.029 = 0.03$

22) Convert to decimals and compare:

0.9% = 0.009

0.9 = 0.900 (largest)

1:9 = 0.111

1:90 = 0.011

Answers to Review Set 8 from page 50

1) 1.3 **2)** 4.75 **3)** 56 **4)** 0.43 **5)** 26.67 **6)** 15 **7)** 0.8 **8)** 2.38 **9)** 37.5 **10)** 112.5 **11)** 8 pills **12)** 720 millilitres **13)** \$3530.21 **14)** 300 g **15)** 700 calories

Selected Solutions—Review Set 8

1) $0.0025 \times 520 = 1.3$

8) $0.07 \times 34 = 2.38$

11) 0.4×20 pills = 8 pills

13) 80% of \$17 651.07 = 0.8 × \$17 651.07 = \$14 120.86

\$17 651.07 total bill
−14 120.86 paid by insurance co.
\$3530.21 paid by client

14) 0.4×750 g = 300 g

15) 0.2×3500 calories = 700 calories

Answers to Practice Problems—Chapter 2 from pages 50–52

1) 0.4, 40%, 2:5 **2)** $\frac{1}{20}$, 5%, 1:20 **3)** 0.17, $\frac{17}{100}$, 17:100 **4)** 0.25, $\frac{1}{4}$, 25% **5)** 0.06, $\frac{3}{50}$, 3:50 **6)** 0.17, 17%, 1.6 **7)** 0.5, $\frac{1}{2}$, 1:2 **8)** 0.01, $\frac{1}{100}$, 1% **9)** $\frac{9}{100}$, 9%, 9:100 **10)** 0.38, 38%, 3:8 **11)** 0.67, $\frac{2}{3}$, 67% **12)** 0.33, 33%, 1:3 **13)** $\frac{13}{25}$, 52%, 13:25 **14)** 0.45, $\frac{9}{20}$, 45% **15)** 0.86, 86%, 6:7 **16)** 0.3, $\frac{3}{10}$, 30% **17)** 0.02, 2%, 1:50 **18)** $\frac{3}{50}$, 6%, 3:50 **19)** $\frac{1}{25}$, 4%, 1:25 **20)** 0.1, $\frac{1}{10}$, 1:10 **21)** 0.04 **22)** 1:40 **23)** 7.5% **24)** $\frac{1}{2}$ **25)** 3:4 **26)** 262.5 **27)** 3.64 **28)** 1.99 **29)** 1:4 **30)** $\frac{1}{10}$ **31)** 84 **32)** 16 **33)** 1 **34)** 1.1 **35)** 100 **36)** 35.33 **37)** 0.75 **38)** 21 **39)** 120 **40)** 90 **41)** 138 nurses; 46 maintenance/cleaners; 92 technicians; 92 others; **42)** 25 grams protein; 6.25 grams fat **43)** 231 points **44)** 60 min **45)** 50 millilitres **46)** 27 milligrams **47)** 283.5 milligrams **48)** 3 kg **49)** \$10.42 **50)** 6 total doses

Selected Solutions—Practice Problems—Chapter 2

41) $\frac{3}{8} \times 368 = 138$ nurses

$\frac{1}{8} \times 368 = 46$ maintenance/cleaners

$\frac{1}{4} \times 368 = 92$ technicians and 92 others

42) $125 \times 0.2 = 25$ grams protein

$125 \times 0.05 = 6.25$ grams fat

$$\begin{array}{r} 125 \\ \times 0.2 \\ \hline 25.0 \end{array} = 25$$

$$\begin{array}{r} 125 \\ \times 0.05 \\ \hline 6.25 \end{array} = 6.25$$

44) $\frac{27 \text{ minutes}}{\cancel{90}_{9} \text{ } \cancel{\text{calories}}} \times \cancel{200}^{20} \text{ } \cancel{\text{calories}} =$

$\frac{540 \text{ minutes}}{9} = 60$ min

46) $60 \times 0.45 = 27$ milligrams

$$\begin{array}{r} 60 \\ \times 0.45 \\ \hline 300 \\ 240 \\ \hline 27.00 \end{array} = 27$$

47) $\frac{6.75 \text{ mg}}{1 \cancel{\text{min}}} \times 42 \cancel{\text{min}} =$

$6.75 \text{ mg} \times 42 = 283.5$ mg of medication

48) $60 \text{ kg} \times 0.05 = 3$ kg

49) $0.17 \times \$12.56 = 2.14$;

$$\begin{array}{r} \$12.56 \\ -2.14 \\ \hline \$10.42 \end{array}$$

50) 10% of 150 = $0.10 \times 150 = 15$;

150 mg first dose
−15
135 mg second dose
−15
120 mg third dose
−15
105 mg fourth dose
−15
90 mg fifth dose
−15
75 mg sixth dose
6 total doses

Answers to Review Set 9 from page 56

1) metric **2)** volume **3)** weight **4)** length **5)** $\frac{1}{1000}$ or 0.001 **6)** 1000 **7)** 10 **8)** kilogram **9)** milligram **10)** 1000 **11)** 1 **12)** 1000 **13)** 10 **14)** 0.3 g **15)** 1.33 mL **16)** 5 kg **17)** 1.5 mm **18)** 10 mg **19)** microgram **20)** millilitre **21)** millimole **22)** gram **23)** millimetre **24)** kilogram **25)** centimetre

Answers to Review Set 10 from pages 58–59

1) one thousand units **2)** 10 milliequivalents **3)** 30 mEq **4)** 1500 units **5)** False **6)** units, official abbreviation is "u", but its use is not recommended **7)** international unit, official abbreviation is "IU" but its use is not recommended; recommended to be written as "units" to reduce errors **8)** milliequivalents **9)** 0.1

Answers to Review Set 11 from pages 63–64

1) 2:57 AM **2)** 0310 h **3)** 1622 h **4)** 8:01 PM **5)** 11:02 AM **6)** 0033 h **7)** 0216 h **8)** 4:42 PM **9)** 11:56 PM **10)** 0420 h **11)** 1931 h **12)** 2400 h or 0000 h **13)** 0645 h **14)** 9:15 AM **15)** 9:07 PM **16)** 6:23 PM **17)** 5:40 AM **18)** 1155 h **19)** 2212 h **20)** 2106 h **21)** "zero-six-twenty-three hours" **22)** "zero-zero-forty-one hours" **23)** "nineteen-zero-three hours" **24)** "twenty-three-eleven hours" **25)** 4 h **26)** 7 h **27)** 8 h 30 min **28)** 12 h 15 min **29)** 14 h 50 min **30)** 4 h 12 min **31)** 4 h 48 min **32)** 3 h 41 min **33)** 16 h 38 min **34)** False **35)** a. AM; b. PM; c. AM; d. PM

Selected Solutions—Review Set 11

28)
$$\begin{array}{r} 2150\text{ h} \\ -\ 0935\text{ h} \\ \hline 1215\text{ h} \end{array} = 12\text{ h }15\text{ min}$$

30) 2316 h = 11:16 PM, 0328 h = 3:28 AM

11:16 PM → 3:16 AM = 4 h

$$3{:}16\text{ AM} \rightarrow 3{:}28\text{ AM} = \begin{array}{r} 12\text{ min} \\ \hline 4\text{ h }12\text{ min} \end{array}$$

32) 4:35 PM → 7:35 PM = 3 h

$$7{:}35\text{ PM} \rightarrow 8{:}16\text{ PM} = \begin{array}{r} 41\text{ min} \\ \hline 3\text{ h }41\text{ min} \end{array}$$

Answers to Practice Problems—Chapter 3 from pages 64–66

1) milli **2)** micro **3)** centi **4)** kilo **5)** 1 milligram **6)** 1 kilogram **7)** 1 microgram **8)** 1 centimetre **9)** metre **10)** gram **11)** litre **12)** milligram **13)** microgram **14)** unit **15)** milliequivalent **16)** millilitre **17)** kilometre **18)** millimetre **19)** gram **20)** centimetre **21)** litre **22)** metre **23)** kilogram **24)** international unit **25)** 500 mg **26)** 0.5 L **27)** 0.05 mg **28)** three hundred seventy-five units **29)** two and six tenths millilitres **30)** twenty milliequivalents **31)** four tenths of a litre **32)** seventeen hundredths of a milligram **33)** 250 mL **34)** 0.15 mg **35)** 1500 g **36)** 100 mg **37)** 1.5 cm **38)** 200 mcg **39)** 500 mL **40)** 0.256g **41)** 150 mg **42)** 1330 h **43)** 0004 h **44)** 2400 h or 0000 h **45)** 0620 h **46)** zero zero forty-one hours **47)** eleven fifteen hours **48)** zero six twenty-three hours

49) Critical Thinking Skill: Prevention. This type of error can be prevented by avoiding the use of a decimal point or extra zero when not necessary. In this instance, the decimal point and zero serve no purpose and can easily be misinterpreted, especially if the decimal point is difficult to see. Question any order that is unclear or unreasonable.

50) Critical Thinking Skill: Prevention. This was an example of a near miss. The original nurse may have prevented the near miss by carefully comparing the order and the stock solution. If the nurse transcribed the units as part of the calculation process, the confusion between *mg* and *mL* may have been noticed earlier. When using stock supplies, extra diligence by the nurse is frequently required. The nurse always should follow up on her or his sense of "it doesn't seem reasonable" and question any order that seems out of the ordinary. In addition to double-checking calculations with a colleague when the policy of the institution requires it, the nurse should also double-check calculations with a colleague if the nurse feels uncertain.

Answers to Review Set 12 from page 70

1) 0.5 **2)** 15 **3)** 0.008 **4)** 0.01 **5)** 0.06 **6)** 0.3 **7)** 0.0002 **8)** 1200 **9)** 2.5 **10)** 65 **11)** 5 **12)** 1500 **13)** 0.25 **14)** 2000 **15)** 5 **16)** 1000 **17)** 1000 **18)** 0.001 **19)** 0.023 **20)** 0.00105 **21)** 0.018 **22)** 400 **23)** 0.025 **24)** 0.5 **25)** 10 000

Selected Solutions—Review Set 12

2)
$$\text{mg} = 0.015\ \cancel{\text{g}} \times \frac{1000\text{ mg}}{1\ \cancel{\text{g}}}$$
$$= 0.015 \times 1000\text{ mg} = 0.015.$$
$$= 15\text{ mg}$$

3)
$$\text{g} = 8\ \cancel{\text{mg}} \times \frac{1\text{ g}}{1000\ \cancel{\text{mg}}}$$
$$= \frac{8\text{ g}}{1000} = 0.008.0$$
$$= 0.008\text{ g}$$

7)
$$\text{g} = 0.2\ \cancel{\text{mg}} \times \frac{1\text{ g}}{1000\ \cancel{\text{mg}}}$$
$$= \frac{0.2\text{ g}}{1000} = 0.000.2$$
$$= 0.0002\text{ g}$$

9)
$$\text{g} = 0.0025\ \cancel{\text{kg}} \times \frac{1000\text{ g}}{1\ \cancel{\text{kg}}}$$
$$= 0.0025 \times 1000\text{ g} = 0.002.5$$
$$= 2.5\text{ g}$$

20)
$$\text{kg} = 1.05\ \cancel{\text{g}} \times \frac{1\text{ kg}}{1000\ \cancel{\text{g}}}$$
$$= \frac{1.05\text{ kg}}{1000} = 0.001.05$$
$$= 0.00105\text{ kg}$$

23)
$$\text{kg} = 25\ \cancel{\text{g}} \times \frac{1\text{ kg}}{1000\ \cancel{\text{g}}}$$
$$= \frac{25\text{ kg}}{1000} = 0.025.0$$
$$= 0.025\text{ kg}$$

Answers to Review Set 13 from page 72

1) 2 mL **2)** 1.2 mL **3)** 1 mL **4)** 0.72 mL **5)** 1.9 mL **6)** 5 mL **7)** 2.5 mL

Selected Solutions—Review Set 13

1) $\frac{0.8\ \cancel{g}}{1\ \cancel{g}} \times 2.5\text{ mL} = 2\text{ mL}$

2) $\frac{200\ \cancel{mg}}{250\ \cancel{mg}} \times 1.5\text{ mL} = 1.2\text{ mL}$

3) $\frac{0.2\ \cancel{g}}{1\ \cancel{g}} \times 5\text{ mL} = 1\text{ mL}$

4) $\frac{300\ \cancel{mcg}}{500\ \cancel{mcg}} \times 1.2\text{ mL} = 0.72\text{ mL}$

5) $\frac{1250\ \cancel{units}}{1000\ \cancel{units}} \times 1.5\text{ mL} = 1.875\text{ mL} = 1.9\text{ mL}$

6) $\frac{50\ \cancel{mEq}}{200\ \cancel{mEq}} \times 20\text{ mL} = 5\text{ mL}$

7) $\frac{0.25\ \cancel{mg}}{0.2\ \cancel{mg}} \times 2\text{ mL} = 2.5\text{ mL}$

Answers to Review Set 14 from page 76–77

1) 0.25 **2)** 1000 **3)** 0.7 **4)** 514.29 **5)** 3 **6)** 0.63 **7)** 10 **8)** 0.67 **9)** 1.25 **10)** 16.67 **11)** 0.75 **12)** 6 **13)** 108 nurses **14)** 81.82 milligrams/hour **15)** 10 g

Selected Solutions—Review Set 14

2) $\frac{0.5}{2} \times \frac{250}{X}$ (cross-multiply)

$0.5X = 500$

$\frac{\cancel{0.5}X}{\cancel{0.5}} = \frac{500}{0.5}$

$X = 1000$

4) $\frac{1200}{X} \times 12 = 28$

$\frac{1200}{X} \times \frac{12}{1} = 28$

$\frac{14\,400}{X} \times \frac{28}{1}$ (cross-multiply)

$28X = 14\,400$

$\frac{\cancel{28}X}{\cancel{28}} = \frac{14\,400}{28}$

$X = 514.285$

$X = 514.29$

5) $\frac{250}{1} \times \frac{750}{X}$ (cross-multiply)

$250X = 750$

$\frac{\cancel{250}X}{\cancel{250}} = \frac{750}{250}$

$X = 3$

8) $\frac{\frac{1}{100}}{1} \times \frac{\frac{1}{150}}{X}$ (cross-multiply)

$\frac{1}{100}X = \frac{1}{150}$

$\frac{\cancel{\frac{1}{100}}X}{\cancel{\frac{1}{100}}} = \frac{\frac{1}{150}}{\frac{1}{100}}$

$X = \frac{1}{150} \div \frac{1}{100}$

$X = \frac{1}{\cancel{150}_{3}} \times \frac{\cancel{100}^{2}}{1}$

$X = \frac{2}{3} = 0.666 = 0.67$

12) $\frac{25\%}{30\%} = \frac{5}{X}$

$\frac{0.25}{0.3} \times \frac{5}{X}$ (cross-multiply)

$0.25X = 1.5$

$\frac{\cancel{0.25}X}{\cancel{0.25}} = \frac{1.5}{0.25}$

$X = 6$

13) $\frac{45}{100} \times \frac{X}{240}$ (cross-multiply)

$100X = 10\,800$

$\frac{\cancel{100}X}{\cancel{100}} = \frac{10\,800}{100}$

$X = 108$

15) $\frac{X}{500\text{ mL}} \times \frac{5\text{g}}{250\text{ mL}}$ (cross-multiply)

$5 \times 500 = 250X$

$\frac{2500}{250} = \frac{\cancel{250}X}{\cancel{250}}$

$X = 10\text{ g}$

Answers to Review Set 15 from pages 78–79

1) 2 tablets **2)** 1.5 mL **3)** 10 mL **4)** 3 tablets **5)** 0.5 tablets **6)** 2 **7)** 2.5 **8)** 0.8 **9)** 0.7 **10)** 7.5 **11)** 0.6 **12)** 1.5 **13)** 3 **14)** 30 **15)** 1.6 **16)** 3 **17)** 0.5 **18)** 2 **19)** 2 **20)** 2.4 **21)** 2 **22)** 8 **23)** 1.6 **24)** 16 **25)** 7

Solutions—Review Set 15

7) $\frac{300\text{ mg}}{5\text{ mL}} \times \frac{150\text{ mg}}{\text{X mL}}$

$300\text{X} = 750$

$\frac{\cancel{300}\text{X}}{\cancel{300}} = \frac{750}{300}$

$\text{X} = 2.5\text{ mL}$

10) $\frac{8\text{ mEq}}{5\text{ mL}} \times \frac{12\text{ mEq}}{\text{X mL}}$

$8\text{X} = 60$

$\frac{\cancel{8}\text{X}}{\cancel{8}} = \frac{60}{8}$

$\text{X} = 7.5\text{ mL}$

11) $\frac{4\text{ mg}}{1\text{ mL}} \times \frac{2.4\text{ mg}}{\text{X mL}}$

$4\text{X} = 2.4$

$\frac{\cancel{4}\text{X}}{\cancel{4}} = \frac{2.4}{4}$

$\text{X} = 0.6\text{ mL}$

14) $\frac{80\text{ mg}}{15\text{ mL}} \times \frac{160\text{ mg}}{\text{X mL}}$

$80\text{X} = 2400$

$\frac{\cancel{80}\text{X}}{\cancel{80}} = \frac{2400}{80}$

$\text{X} = 30\text{ mL}$

18) $\frac{15\text{ mg}}{1\text{ tab}} \times \frac{30\text{ mg}}{\text{X tab}}$

$15\text{X} = 30$

$\frac{\cancel{15}\text{X}}{\cancel{15}} = \frac{30}{15}$

$\text{X} = 2\text{ tab}$

21) $\frac{75\text{ mcg}}{1\text{ tab}} \times \frac{150\text{ mcg}}{\text{X}}$

$75\text{X} = 150$

$\frac{\cancel{75}\text{X}}{\cancel{75}} = \frac{150}{75}$

$\text{X} = 2\text{ tab}$

23) $\frac{125\text{ mg}}{2\text{ mL}} \times \frac{100\text{ mg}}{\text{X mL}}$

$125\text{X} = 200$

$\frac{125\text{ X}}{125} = \frac{200}{125}$

$\text{X} = 1.6\text{ mL}$

24) $\frac{2.5\text{ mg}}{5\text{ mL}} \times \frac{8\text{ mg}}{\text{X mL}}$

$2.5\text{X} = 40$

$\frac{2.5\text{X}}{2.5} = \frac{40}{2.5}$

$\text{X} = 16\text{ mL}$

Answers to Practice Problems—Chapter 4 from pages 80–82

1) 45 **2)** 2 **3)** 2 **4)** 2.5 **5)** 2.5 **6)** 16 **7)** 1.4 **8)** 0.7 **9)** 2.3 **10)** 0.13 **11)** 1.6 **12)** 1.5 **13)** 2.5 **14)** 2.5 **15)** 1.6 **16)** 7.5 **17)** 8 **18)** 2 **19)** 8 **20)** 3 **21)** 1.4 **22)** 15 **23)** 12

24) Critical Thinking: Prevention. This type of calculation error occurred because the nurse set up the proportion incorrectly. In this instance, the nurse mixed up the units, *mg* and *mL* in the denominators. The *mg* unit should be in each numerator of the proportion, and the *mL* unit should be in each denominator. This type of error can be avoided by using either the formula or the dimensional analysis method of medication calculation. For example:

$$mL = 50\,\cancel{mg} \times \frac{5\ mL}{125\,\cancel{mg}}$$

$$= \frac{\overset{2}{\cancel{50}} \times 5\ mL}{\underset{5}{\cancel{125}}}$$

$$= 2\ mL$$

The child should receive 2 mL of the Amoxicillin suspension.

25) Critical Thinking Skill: Prevention. The nurse did not set up the problem correctly with all the information needed. If the nurse were to use the formula $\frac{\text{D}}{\text{H}} \times \text{Q}$, the nurse would have written: $\frac{2\text{ g}}{1000\text{ mg}} \times 10\text{ mL}$

Then the nurse could have added the conversion factor to convert grams to milligrams. The problem would then look like this: $\frac{2\,\cancel{\text{g}}}{1000\,\cancel{\text{mg}}} \times 10\text{ mL} \times \frac{1000\,\cancel{\text{mg}}}{1\,\cancel{\text{g}}}$

The nurse could have easily seen then that the answer would correctly result with *mL* as the units left when the other units cancel out each other. Then the arithmetic could have been completed and answer found to be 10 mL. The nurse could then double check by asking the question, “Is this dosage reasonable?” Since the nurse knows there are *1000 mg in 1 g* and that the dosage required is 2 g, then it is easily obvious that more than one vial of the medication will be necessary for this prescribed dose.

Selected Solutions—Practice Problems—Chapter 4

1) $\text{mL} = \frac{5\text{ mL}}{3.33\ \cancel{g}} \times \frac{30\ \cancel{g}}{1\text{ dose}} = 45.045\text{ mL/dose} = 45\text{ mL/dose}$

2) $\text{mL} = \frac{20\text{ mL}}{5\,000\,000\ \cancel{\text{units}}} \times \frac{500\,000\ \cancel{\text{units}}}{1\text{ dose}} = 2\text{ mL/dose}$

6) $\text{mL} = \frac{5\text{ mL}}{12.5\ \cancel{\text{mg}}} \times \frac{40\ \cancel{\text{mg}}}{1\text{ dose}} = 16\text{ mL/dose}$

7) $\text{mL} = \frac{2\text{ mL}}{500\,000\ \cancel{\text{units}}} \times \frac{350\,000\ \cancel{\text{units}}}{1\text{ dose}} = 1.4\text{ mL /dose}$

8) $\text{mL} = \frac{1\text{ mL}}{5\ \cancel{\text{mg}}} \times \frac{3.5\ \cancel{\text{mg}}}{1\text{ dose}} = 0.7\text{ mL/dose}$

9) $\text{mL} = \frac{2\text{ mL}}{80\ \cancel{\text{mg}}} \times \frac{90\ \cancel{\text{mg}}}{1\text{ dose}} = 2.25\text{ mL/dose} = 2.3\text{ mL/dose}$

13) $\text{mL} = \frac{10\text{ mL}}{2\ \cancel{g}} \times \frac{1\ \cancel{g}}{1000\ \cancel{\text{mg}}} \times \frac{500\ \cancel{\text{mg}}}{1\text{ dose}} = 2.5\text{ mL/dose}$

16) $\text{mL} = \frac{15\text{ mL}}{20\ \cancel{\text{mEq}}} \times \frac{10\ \cancel{\text{mEq}}}{1\text{ dose}} = 7.5\text{ mL/dose}$

18) $\text{tablets} = \frac{1\text{ tablet}}{0.075\ \cancel{\text{mg}}} \times \frac{1\ \cancel{\text{mg}}}{1000\ \cancel{\text{mcg}}} \times \frac{150\ \cancel{\text{mcg}}}{1\text{ dose}} = 2\text{ tablets/dose}$

Answers to Section 1—Self-Evaluation from pages 83–85

1) 3.05 **2)** 4002.5 **3)** LCD = 12 **4)** LCD = 110 **5)** $\frac{11}{2}$ **6)** $\frac{47}{63}$ **7)** 1 **8)** $\frac{1}{2}$ **9)** 45.78 **10)** 0.02 **11)** 59.24 **12)** 0.09 **13)** $\frac{2}{3}$ **14)** $\frac{1}{2}$ **15)** 0.64 **16)** $\frac{1}{10}, \frac{1}{6}, \frac{1}{5}, \frac{1}{3}, \frac{1}{2}$ **17)** 0.009, 0.125, 0.1909, 0.25, 0.3 **18)** 1:3 **19)** 0.01 **20)** 0.04 **21)** 0.9% **22)** $\frac{1}{3}$ **23)** $\frac{1}{20}$ **24)** 1:200 **25)** $\frac{2}{3}$ **26)** 75% **27)** 40% **28)** 1.21 **29)** 1.3 **30)** 4 **31)** 20 000 **32)** 3.3 **33)** 0.5 mL **34)** four hundred fifty milligrams **35)** twenty-five hundredths of a litre **36)** (7.13 kg) = 7130 g = 7 130 000 mg = 7 130 000 000 mcg **37)** 0.000000925 kg = 0.000925 g = 0.925 mg = (925 mcg) **38)** 0.000125 kg = 0.125 g = (125 mg) = 125 000 mcg **39)** 0.0164 kg = (16.4 g) = 16 400 mg = 16 400 000 mcg **40)** 0.02 g **41)** 5.62 cm **42)** 11 590 g **43)** 6 **44)** 2335 h **45)** 6:44 PM **46)** 1 capsule **47)** 0.8 mL **48)** 20 mL **49)** 0.5 mL **50)** 7 mL

Selected Solutions—Section 1—Self-Evaluation

13) $\frac{1}{150} \div \frac{1}{100} = \frac{1}{150} \times \frac{100}{1} = \frac{\overset{2}{\cancel{100}}}{\underset{3}{\cancel{150}}} = \frac{2}{3}$

15) $\frac{16\%}{\frac{1}{4}} = 16\% \times \frac{4}{1} = 0.16 \times 4 = 0.64$

26) $3{:}4 = \frac{3}{4} = 4\overline{)3.0}$ giving $0.75 = 75\%$

29) $\frac{0.3}{2.6} \times \frac{0.15}{X}$ (cross-multiply)

$0.3\text{ X} = 2.6 \times 0.15$

$0.3\text{ X} = 0.39$

$\frac{\cancel{0.3}\text{ X}}{\cancel{0.3}} = \frac{0.39}{0.3}$

$\text{X} = 1.3$

31) $\frac{10\%}{\frac{1}{2}\%} \times 1000 = \text{X}$

$\frac{0.1}{0.005} \times \frac{1000}{1} = \text{X}$

$\frac{100}{0.005} = \text{X}$

$X = 20\,000$

47) $\text{mL} = 60\ \cancel{\text{mg}} \times \frac{1\text{ ml}}{75\ \cancel{\text{mg}}}$

$= \frac{60\text{ ml}}{75}$

$= \frac{4\text{ ml}}{5}$

$= 0.8\text{ mL}$

Answers to Review Set 16 from pages 98–100

1) 1 mL syringe (tuberculin) **2)** a. yes; b. Round 1.25 to 1.3 and measure on the mL scale as 1.3 mL. **3)** No **4)** 0.5 mL **5)** a. False; b. The size of the drop varies according to the diameter of the tip of the dropper. **6)** No **7)** Measure the oral liquid in a 3-mL oral syringe, which is not intended for injections. **8)** 5 **9)** Discard the excess prior to injecting the client. **10)** To prevent needlestick injury.

11)

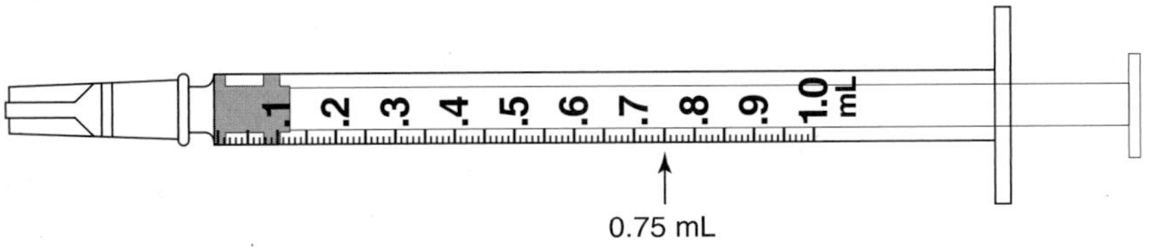
.1 .2 .3 .4 .5 .6 .7 .8 .9 1.0 mL
0.75 mL

12)

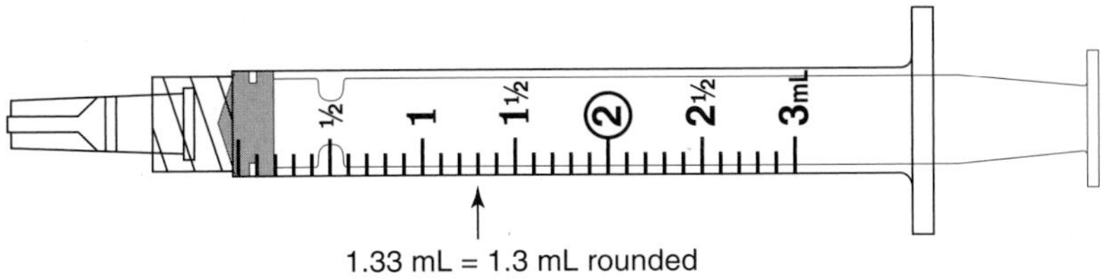
½ 1 1½ 2 2½ 3mL
1.33 mL = 1.3 mL rounded

13)

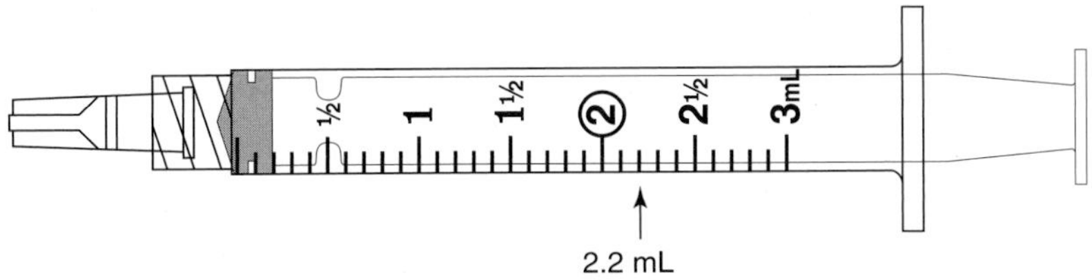
½ 1 1½ 2 2½ 3mL
2.2 mL

14)

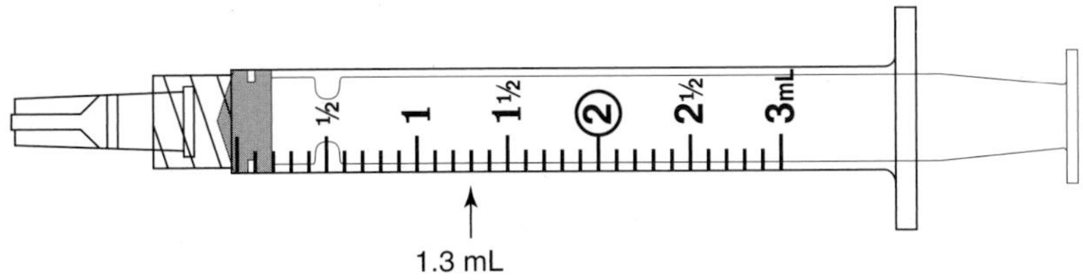
½ 1 1½ 2 2½ 3mL
1.3 mL

15)

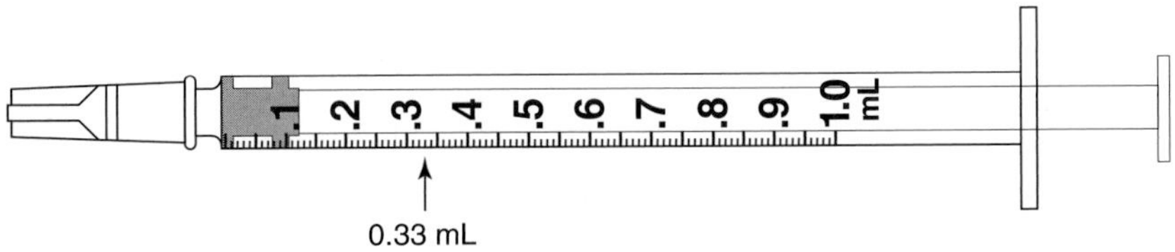
.1 .2 .3 .4 .5 .6 .7 .8 .9 1.0 mL
0.33 mL

16)

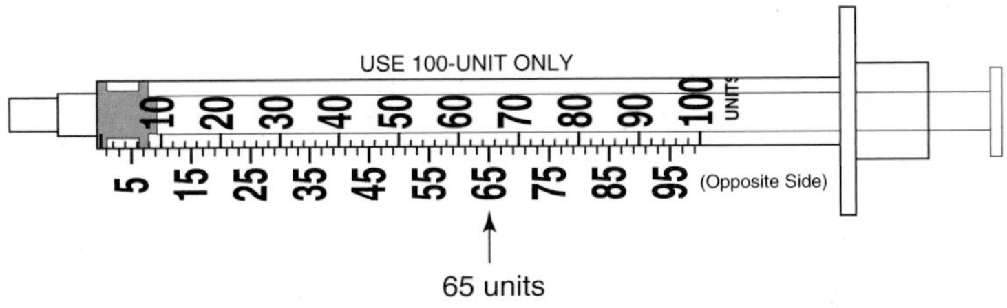
USE 100-UNIT ONLY
10 20 30 40 50 60 70 80 90 100 UNITS
5 15 25 35 45 55 65 75 85 95 (Opposite Side)
65 units

17)

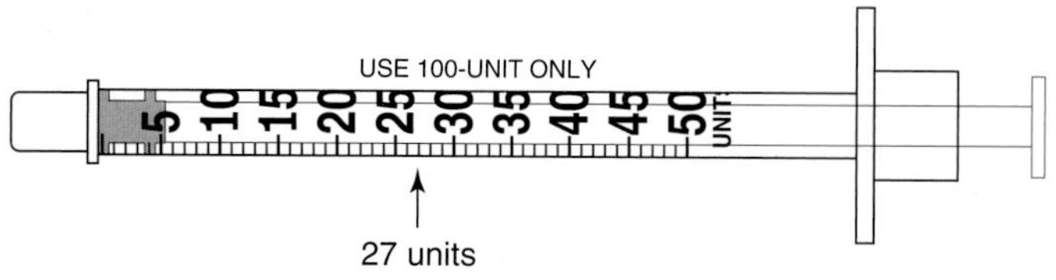

18)

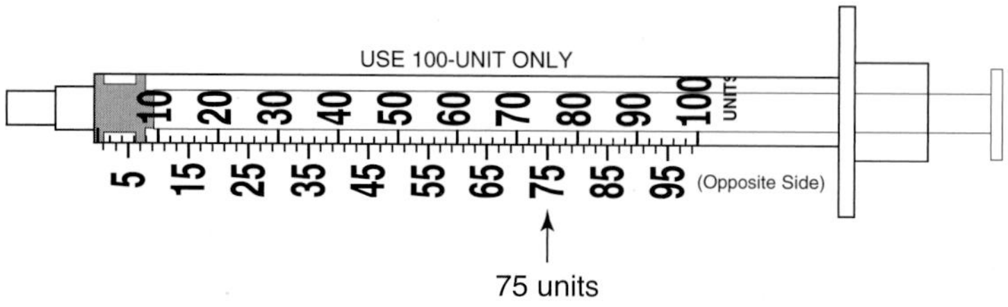

19)

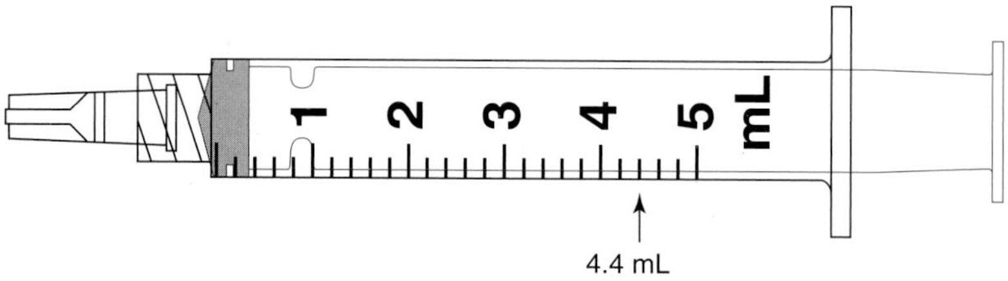

20)

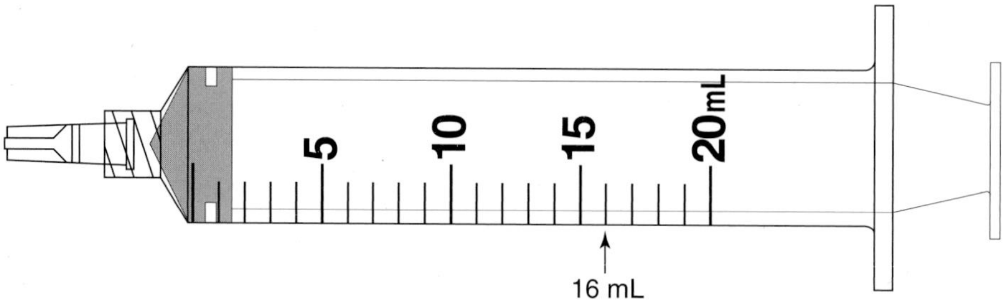

21) 0.2 mL **22)** 1 mL **23)** 0.2 mL

Answers to Practice Problems—Chapter 5 from pages 101–104

1) 1 **2)** hundredths or 0.01 **3)** No. The tuberculin syringe has a maximum capacity of 1 mL. **4)** Round to 1.3 mL and measure at 1.3 mL. **5)** 30 mL **6)** 1 mL; if drug is ordered by mouth an oral syringe or calibrated oral device should be used. **7)** 0.75 **8)** False **9)** False **10)** True **11)** To prevent accidental needlesticks during intravenous administration **12)** top ring **13)** 10 **14)** True **15)** standard 3-mL, 1-mL, and insulin

16)

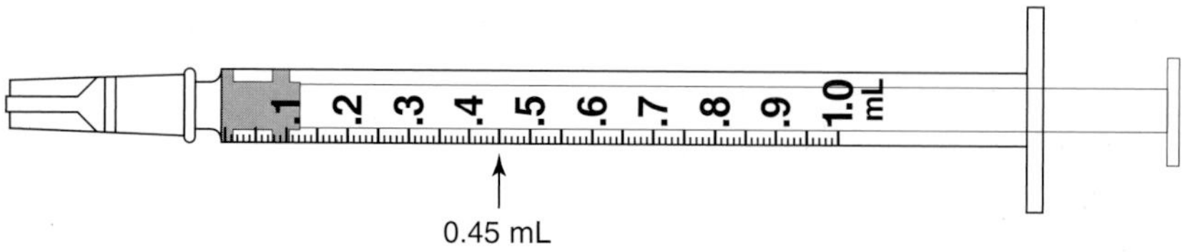

17)

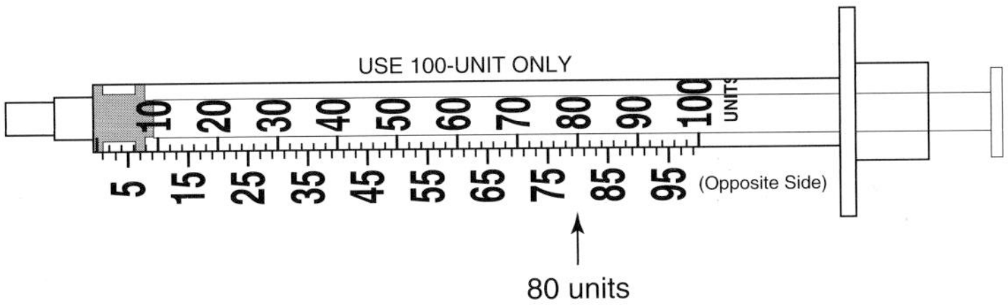
USE 100-UNIT ONLY
10 20 30 40 50 60 70 80 90 100 UNITS
5 15 25 35 45 55 65 75 85 95 (Opposite Side)
80 units

18)

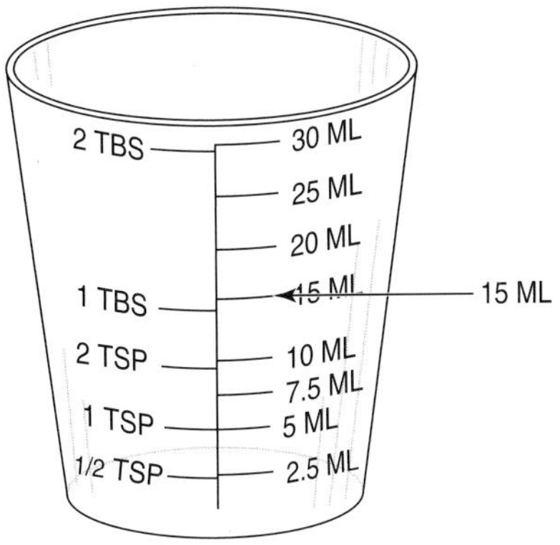
2 TBS
30 ML
25 ML
20 ML
1 TBS
15 ML
15 ML
2 TSP
10 ML
7.5 ML
1 TSP
5 ML
1/2 TSP
2.5 ML

19)

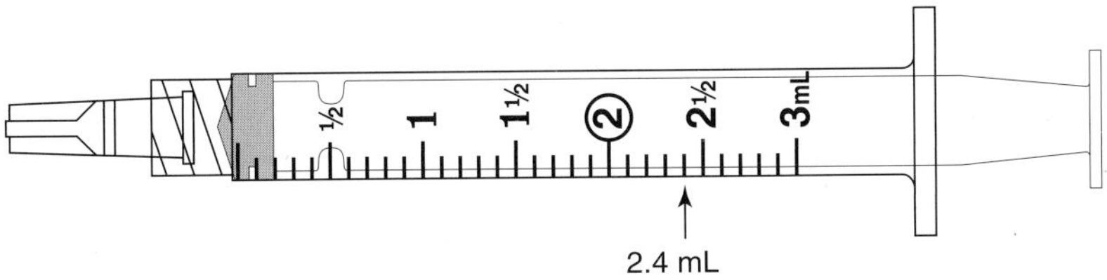
½ 1 1½ 2 2½ 3mL
2.4 mL

20)

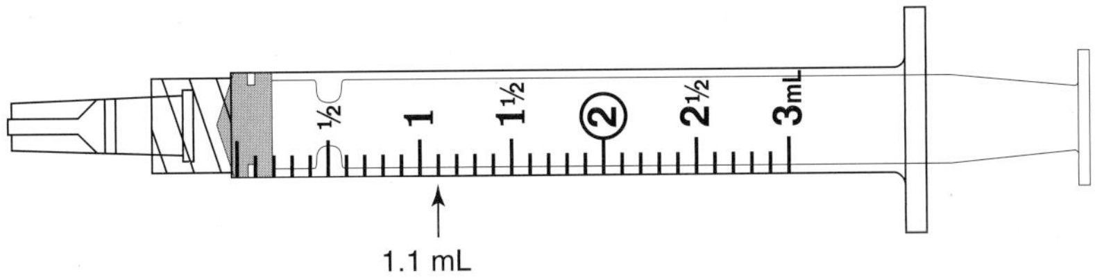
½ 1 1½ 2 2½ 3mL
1.1 mL

21)

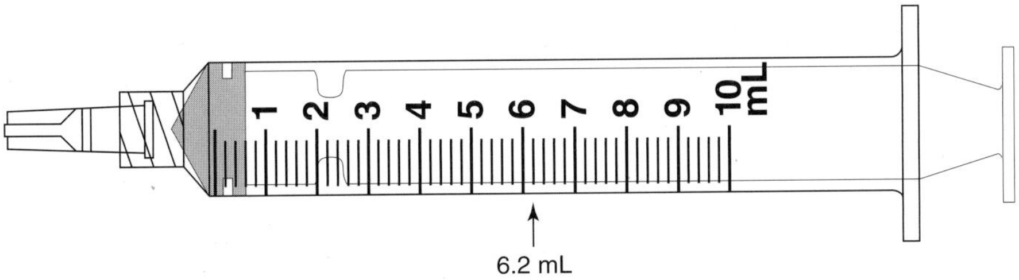
1 2 3 4 5 6 7 8 9 10 mL
6.2 mL

22)

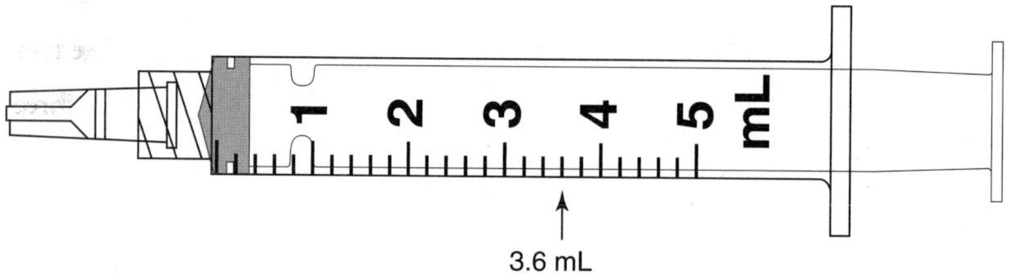

23)

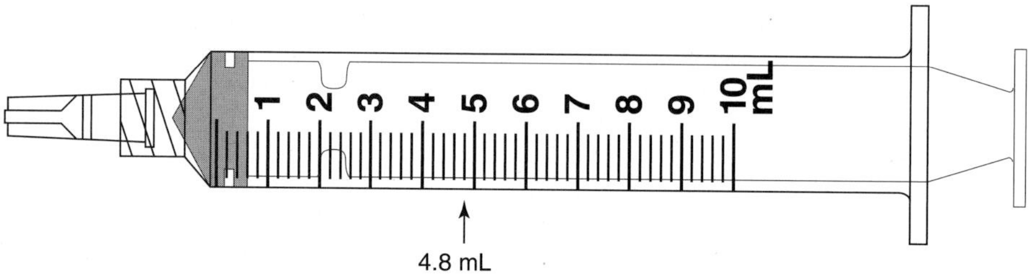

24)

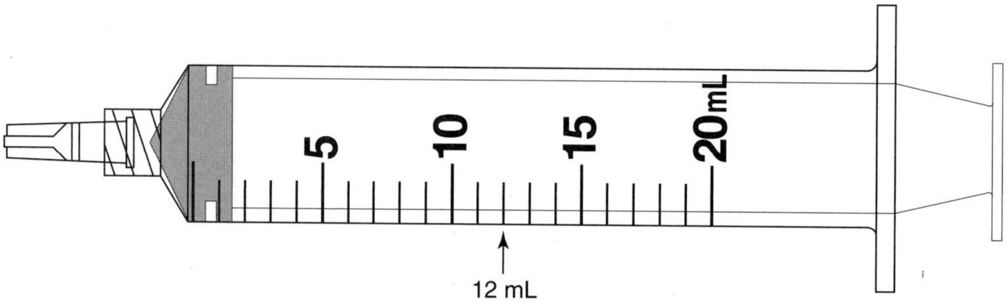

25) Critical Thinking Skill: Prevention. This error could have been avoided by following the principle of not putting oral drugs in syringes intended for injection. Instead, place the medication in an oral syringe to which a needle cannot be attached. In addition, the medication should have been labelled for oral use only. The medication was ordered orally, not by injection. The alert nurse would have noticed the discrepancy. Finally, but certainly as important, a medication should be prepared just before administration and should be administered only by the nurse who prepared it.

26) Critical Thinking Skill: Prevention. The nurse needs to recognize the difference between an oral and a parenteral syringe. Look at the syringe markings that are typically for oral measurement and the absence of the luer lock hub, found on parenteral injection syringes. The nurse must remove the cap on the oral syringe prior to administering the medication, so that the child cannot choke on the cap.

Answers to Review Set 17 from pages 110–111

1) Give 250 milligrams of naproxen orally two times a day. **2)** Give 30 units of Humulin N insulin subcutaneously every day 30 minutes before breakfast. **3)** Give 500 milligrams orally of cefaclor orally immediately, and then give 250 milligrams orally every 8 hours. **4)** Give 25 micrograms of levothyroxine orally once a day. **5)** Give 10 milligrams of lorazepam intramuscularly every 4 hours as necessary for agitation. **6)** Give 500 milligrams of cefazolin intravenously per piggyback as per protocol **7)** Give 10 millilitres of aluminum hydroxide orally at bedtime. **8)** Give two drops of 1%

atropine sulfate ophthalmic in the right eye every 15 minutes for four applications. **9)** Give 15 mg of morphine sulfate intramuscularly every 3–4 hours as needed for pain. **10)** Give 0.25 milligram of Lanoxin orally once a day. **11)** Give 250 milligrams of tetracycline orally four times a day. **12)** Give 0.6 mg of nitroglycerin sublingually immediately. **13)** Give two drops of Cortisporin otic suspension in both ears three times a day and at bedtime. **14)** The abbreviation TID means three times a day with no specific interval between times. An attempt is made to give the three doses during waking hours. The abbreviation q8h means every 8 hours. These doses would be given around the clock at 8-hour intervals. For example, administration times for TID might be 0800 h, 1200 h, 1700 h; administration times for q8h could be 0800 h, 1600 h, 2400 h. **15)** Contact the physician for clarification. **16)** No, QID orders are given four times in 24 hours with no specific interval between times indicated in order, typically during waking hours; whereas q4h orders are given six times in 24 hours at 4-hour intervals. **17)** Determined by hospital or institution policy. **18)** Patient, drug, dosage, route, frequency, date and time written, signature of physician/writer. **19)** Specific jurisdictional documents on practice standards, information from the Institute for Safe Medication Practices (ISMP), and current Canadian nursing practice textbooks. **20)** The *right patient* must receive the *right drug* for the *right reason* in the *right amount* by the *right route* in the *right site* at the *right time* and the *right frequency*, followed by the right documentation.

Answers to Review Set 18 from page 116

1) subcutaneous injection **2)** once **3)** cephalexin **4)** 30 min before breakfast **5)** milliequivalent **6)** cephalexin and potassium chloride **7)** acetaminophen **8)** twice **9)** In the "One-Time Medication Dosage" section, lower left corner. **10)** 6 AM, 12 noon, 6 PM, 12 midnight **11)** 9 AM **12)** 7:30 AM, 11:30 AM, 4:30 PM, 9 PM **13)** 9 AM, 5 PM **14)** every 4 hours, as needed for severe pain **15)** 09/09/xx at 0900 h or 9 AM **16)** sublingual, under the tongue **17)** once a day **18)** 125 mcg **19)** nitroglycerin, oxycodone and acetaminophen (Percocet), meperidine hydrochloride, promethazine (Phenergan)

Answers to Practice Problems—Chapter 6 from pages 117–121

1) nasogastric **2)** per rectum **3)** before meals **4)** sublingual **5)** three times a day **6)** every 4 hours **7)** when necessary **8)** by mouth, orally **9)** tablet **10)** immediately **11)** freely, as desired **12)** intramuscular **13)** after meals **14)** NPO **15)** gtt **16)** mL **17)** hs **18)** g **19)** QID **20)** qh **21)** SUBCUT **22)** IV **23)** BID **24)** q3h **25)** q12h **26)** cap **27)** kg **28)** Give 60 milligrams of keterolac intramuscularly immediately and every 6 hours. **29)** Give 300 000 units of procaine penicillin G intramuscularly four times a day. **30)** Give 1 tablet of Mylanta orally 1 hour before and 1 hour after meals, at bedtime, and every 2 hours during the night as needed for gastric upset. **31)** Give 25 milligrams of chlordiazepoxide orally every 6 hours when necessary for agitation. **32)** Give 5000 units of heparin subcutaneously immediately. **33)** Give 50 milligrams of meperidine hydrochloride intramuscularly every 3–4 hours when necessary for pain. **34)** Give 0.25 milligram of digoxin orally every day. **35)** Give 2 drops of 10% Neosynephrine ophthalmic to the left eye every 30 minutes for two applications. **36)** Give 40 milligrams of furosemide intramuscularly immediately. **37)** Give 4 milligrams of betamethasone intravenously twice a day. **38)** 20 units **39)** SUBCUT, subcutaneous **40)** Give 500 milligrams of ciprofloxacin hydrochloride orally every 12 hours. **41)** 0800 h, 1200 h, 1800 h **42)** digoxin (Lanoxin) 0.125 mg PO **43)** Give 150 milligrams of ranitidine tablets orally twice daily with breakfast and supper. **44)** Vancomycin **45)** 12 h **46)** Critical Thinking Skill: Prevention. This error could have been avoided by paying careful attention to the ordered frequency and by writing the frequency on the MAR.

Answers to Review Set 19 from pages 136–138

1) E **2)** D **3)** C **4)** A **5)** B **6)** F **7)** G **8)** 2.5 mL **9)** IM or IV **10)** A, C, D, E, F **11)** 4 mg/2 mL **12)** 2 tablets **13)** penicillin G sodium **14)** 5 000 000 units per vial; reconstituted to 250 000 units/mL, 500 000 units/mL, or 1 000 000 units/mL **15)** IM or IV **16)** 02220288 **17)** Pharmaceutical Partners of Canada **18)** 2% **19)** 2 g per 100 mL **20)** 20 mg/mL

Answers to Practice Problems—Chapter 7 from pages 139–143

1) 8.4% **2)** 00261998 **3)** $\frac{84\text{ mg}}{\text{mL}}$ **4)** cefixime **5)** "Tap the bottle several times to loosen powder contents prior to reconstitution. Add 33 mL of water in two portions. Mix well after each addition." **6)** Sanofi Aventis **7)** 2 mL **8)** $\frac{50\text{ mg}}{2\text{ mL}}$ **9)** 1 mL **10)** multiple **11)** tobramycin **12)** 00533688 **13)** injection solution **14)** 1 mL **15)** intramuscular **16)** Novopharm Limited **17)** tablet **18)** Store between 15°C and 25°C (as per label) **19)** 07/2008 **20)** 2 mEq per mL **21)** I **22)** H **23)** H **24)** oral **25)** 1003992 **26)** 2% **27)** 2 g per 100 mL, or 20 mg per mL

28) Critical Thinking Skill: Prevention. The nurse should have recognized that the patient was still complaining of signs and symptoms that the medication was ordered to treat. If the order was difficult to read, the physician should have been called to clarify the order. Was the dosage of 100 mg a usual dosage for Celexa? The nurse should have consulted a drug guide to ensure that the dosage was appropriate. Also, if the patient wasn't complaining of depression, the nurse should have questioned why Celexa was ordered.

Answers to Section 2—Self-Evaluation from pages 144–146

1)

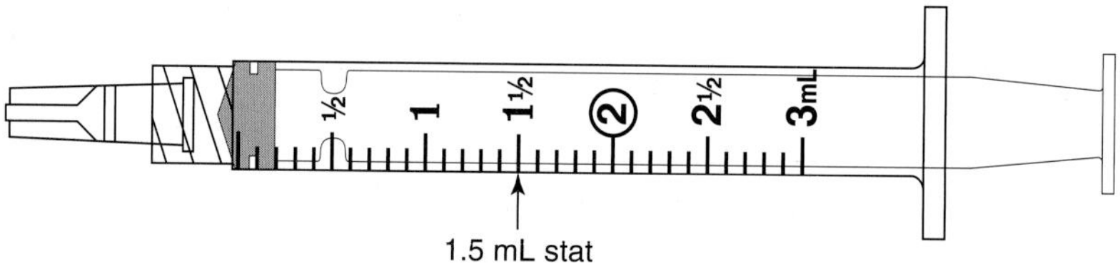

2)

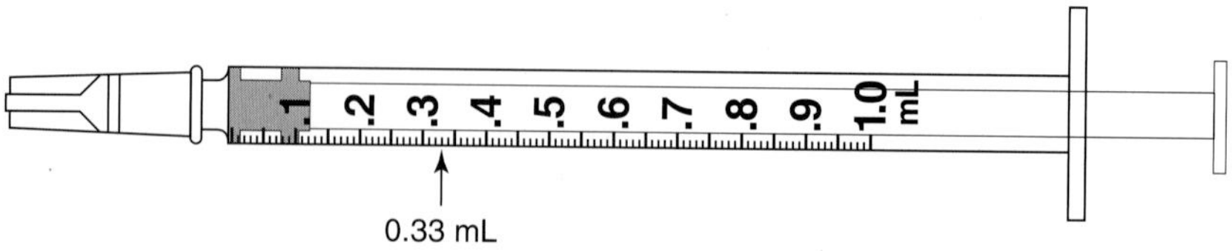

3)

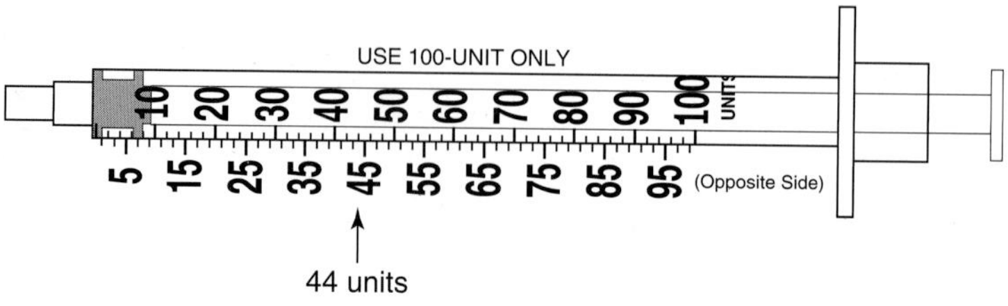

4)

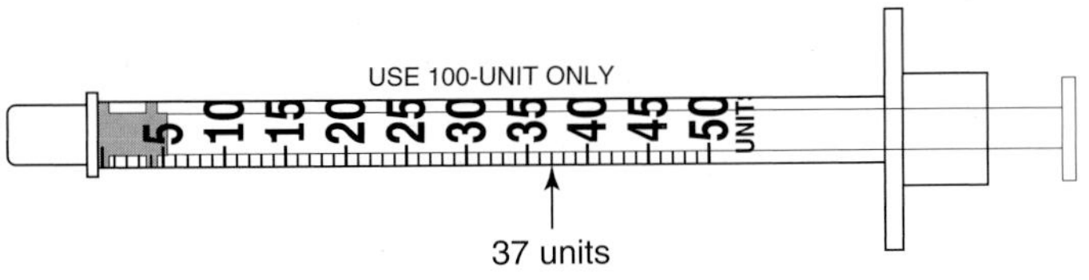

5)

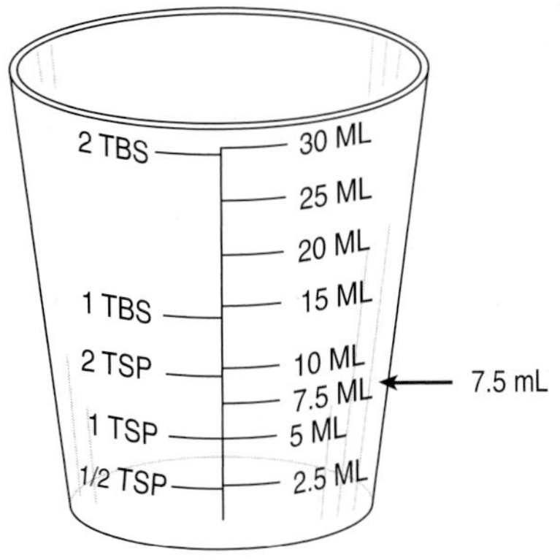

6) neomycin and polymixin B compounds and hydrocortisone **7)** Use in ears only. **8)** 10 mL **9)** Give 2 drops of Cortisporin otic solution in both ears every 15 minutes for 3 doses. **10)** 10 000 units per mL **11)** 00579718 **12)** Give 3750 units of heparin subcutaneously every 8 hours. **13)** Novo-Trimel **14)** 200 mg of sulfamethoxazole and 40 mg of trimethoprim in every 5 mL

15) a. 2.5 mL

b.

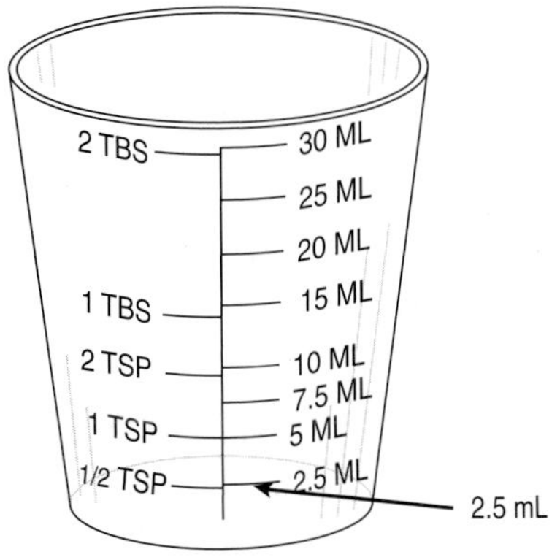

16) Give 250 mg of Amoxil by mouth three times per day.

Answers to Review Set 20 from pages 158–160

1) 1 **2)** 1 **3)** $1\frac{1}{2}$ **4)** $\frac{1}{2}$ **5)** $\frac{1}{2}$ **6)** 2 **7)** 2 **8)** 2 **9)** $1\frac{1}{2}$ **10)** 2 **11)** 1 **12)** $\frac{1}{2}$ **13)** 2 **14)** 2 **15)** 2 **16)** 2 **17)** 2.5, 3 **18)** 10 and 5; 1 of each (or 3 of 5 mg or $1\frac{1}{2}$ of 10 mg); 4 **19)** 30, 1.5 **20)** 60, 1 **21)** B, 1 caplet **22)** A, 1 tablet **23)** F, 1 tablet **24)** G, 2 tablets **25)** C, 1 tablet **26)** E, 2 capsules **27)** D, 2 tablets **28)** H, 1 tablet

Selected Solutions—Review Set 20

1) Order: 0.1 g = 0.1 × 1000 = 100 mg

Supply: 100 mg/tab

$$\frac{D}{H} \times Q = \frac{\overset{1}{\cancel{100 \text{ mg}}}}{\underset{1}{\cancel{100 \text{ mg}}}} \times 1 \text{ tab} = 1 \text{ tab}$$

5) Order: 0.125 mg

Supply: 0.25 mg/tab = 0.250 mg/tab

$$\frac{D}{H} \times Q = \frac{\overset{1}{\cancel{0.125 \text{ mg}}}}{\underset{2}{\cancel{0.250 \text{ mg}}}} \times 1 \text{ tab} = \frac{1}{2} \text{ tab}$$

10) Order: 5 mg = 5.0 mg

Supply: 2.5 mg/tab

$$\frac{D}{H} \times Q = \frac{\overset{2}{\cancel{5.0 \text{ mg}}}}{\underset{1}{\cancel{2.5 \text{ mg}}}} \times 1 \text{ tab} = 2 \text{ tab}$$

14) Order: 0.1 mg = 0.1 × 1000 = 100 mcg

Supply: 50 mcg/tab

$$\frac{D}{H} \times Q = \frac{\overset{2}{\cancel{100 \text{ mg}}}}{\underset{1}{\cancel{50 \text{ mg}}}} \times 1 \text{ tab} = 2 \text{ tab}$$

Answers to Review Set 21 from pages 166–169

1) 7.5 **2)** Give one 0.5 mg and one 1 mg (or 3 of the 0.5 mg) **3)** 16.7 **4)** 4 **5)** 5 **6)** 2 **7)** 1.25 **8)** 7.5 **9)** 3 **10)** 2.5 **11)** 22.5 **12)** 15 **13)** 10 **14)** 20 **15)** 5 **16)** 15 **17)** 7.5 **18)** 30 **19)** 15 **20)** 5 **21)** 2 **22)** B; 2.5 mL **23)** C; 2 mL **24)** A; 5 mL **25)** 4 mL **26)** 0.75 **27)** 10; 45 **28)** 3 mL

Selected Solutions—Review Set 21

4) Order: 100 mg

Supply: $\frac{125 \text{ mg}}{5 \text{ mL}}$

$$\frac{D}{H} \times Q = \frac{\overset{4}{\cancel{100 \text{ mg}}}}{\underset{5}{\cancel{125 \text{ mg}}}} \times 5 \text{ mL} = \frac{\overset{4}{\cancel{20}}}{\underset{1}{\cancel{5}}} \text{ mL} = 4\text{mL}$$

6) Order: 25 mg

Supply: $\frac{62.5 \text{ mg}}{5 \text{ mL}}$

$$\frac{D}{H} \times Q = \frac{25 \cancel{\text{mg}}}{62.5 \cancel{\text{mg}}} \times 5 \text{ mL} = \frac{125}{62.5} \text{ mL} = 2 \text{ mL}$$

7) Order: 4 mg

Supply: $\frac{3.2 \text{ mg}}{\text{mL}}$

$$\frac{D}{H} \times Q = \frac{\overset{1}{\cancel{4 \text{ mg}}}}{\underset{0.8}{\cancel{3.2 \text{ mg}}}} \times 1 \text{ mL} = 1.25 \text{ mL}$$

11) Order: 0.24 g = 0.24 × 1000 = 240 mg

Supply: $\frac{80 \text{ mg}}{7.5\text{mL}}$

$$\frac{D}{H} \times Q = \frac{\overset{3}{\cancel{240 \text{ mg}}}}{\underset{1}{\cancel{80 \text{ mg}}}} \times 7.5 \text{ mL} = 22.5 \text{ mL}$$

15) Order: 0.25 mg = 0.25 × 1000 = 250 mcg

Supply: $\frac{50 \text{ mcg}}{1 \text{ mL}}$

$$\frac{D}{H} \times Q = \frac{\overset{5}{\cancel{250 \text{ mcg}}}}{\underset{1}{\cancel{50 \text{ mcg}}}} \times 1 \text{ mL} = 5 \text{ mL}$$

17) Order: 375 mg

Supply: $\frac{250 \text{ mg}}{5 \text{ mL}}$

$$\frac{D}{H} \times Q = \frac{375 \cancel{\text{mg}}}{\underset{50}{\cancel{250 \text{ mg}}}} \times \overset{1}{\cancel{5}} \text{ mL} = \frac{375}{50} \text{ mL} = 7.5 \text{ mL}$$

19) Order: 1.2 g = 1.2 × 1000 = 1200 mg

Supply: $\frac{400 \text{ mg}}{5 \text{ mL}}$

$$\frac{D}{H} \times Q = \frac{\overset{3}{\cancel{1200 \text{ mg}}}}{\underset{1}{\cancel{400 \text{ mg}}}} \times 5 \text{ mL} = 15 \text{ mL}$$

20) Order: 0.25 g = 0.25 × 1000 = 250 mg

Supply: $\frac{125 \text{ mg}}{2.5 \text{ mL}}$

$$\frac{D}{H} \times Q = \frac{\overset{2}{\cancel{250 \text{ mg}}}}{\underset{1}{\cancel{125 \text{ mg}}}} \times 2.5 \text{ mL} = 5 \text{ mL}$$

21) Order: 100 mg

Supply: $\frac{250 \text{ mg}}{5 \text{ mL}}$

$$\frac{D}{H} \times Q = \frac{100 \cancel{\text{mg}}}{\underset{50}{\cancel{250 \text{ mg}}}} \times \overset{1}{\cancel{5}} \text{ mL} = \frac{\overset{2}{\cancel{100}}}{\underset{1}{\cancel{50}}} \text{ mL} = 2 \text{ mL}$$

Answers to Practice Problems—Chapter 8 from pages 171–182

1) $\frac{1}{2}$ **2)** 3 **3)** $\frac{1}{2}$ **4)** 0.38 **5)** 10 **6)** 2 **7)** 8 mL **8)** $1\frac{1}{2}$ **9)** 2 **10)** $\frac{1}{2}$ **11)** $1\frac{1}{2}$ **12)** 1 **13)** $1\frac{1}{2}$ **14)** 1 **15)** 5; $1\frac{1}{2}$ **16)** 7.5 **17)** $1\frac{1}{2}$ **18)** 2 **19)** 2.5 **20)** 0.75; 1 **21)** $\frac{1}{2}$ **22)** 2 **23)** 2 **24)** 2 **25)** 2 **26)** 15 and 30; one of each or 2 of 15 mg or $1\frac{1}{2}$ of 30 mg **27)** 3 **28)** 1.6 **29)** 3 **30)** B, 1 tablet **31)** A; 1 tablet **32)** C; 1 tablet **33)** H; 2 tablets **34)** C, 1 tablet **35)** G; 2 tablets **36)** F; 1 tablet **37)** M; 4 tablets **38)** I; $\frac{1}{2}$ tablet **39)** E; 30 mL **40)** K; 1 tablet **41)** J; 2 tablets **42)** O; 1 tablet **43)** Q; 2 tablets **44)** P; 4 tablets **45)** R; 1 tablet **46)** S; 1 tablet

47) Critical Thinking Skill: Prevention. This medication error could have been prevented if the nurse had more carefully read the patient care order as well as the medication label. The patient care order misled the nurse by noting the volume first and then the drug dosage. If confused by the order, the nurse should have clarified the intent with the physician. By focusing on the volume, the nurse failed to follow the steps in dosage calculation. Had the nurse noted 250 mg as the desired dosage and the supply (or on-hand) dosage as 125 mg per 5 mL, the correct amount to be administered would have been clear. Slow down and take time to compare the order with the labels. Calculate each dose carefully before preparing and administering both solid- and liquid-form medications.

Selected Solutions—Practice Problems—Chapter 8

2) Order: 45 mg

Supply: 15 mg/tab

$$\frac{D}{H} \times Q = \frac{\overset{3}{\cancel{45}}\text{ mg}}{\underset{1}{\cancel{15}}\text{ mg}} \times 1\text{ tab} = 3\text{ tab}$$

3) Order: 0.075 mg = 0.075 × 1000 = 75 mcg

Supply: 150 mcg/tab

$$\frac{D}{H} \times Q = \frac{\overset{1}{\cancel{75\text{ mcg}}}}{\underset{2}{\cancel{150\text{ mcg}}}} \times 1\text{ tab} = \frac{1}{2}\text{ tab}$$

8) Order: 120 mg

Supply: 80 mg/tab

$$\frac{D}{H} \times Q = \frac{\overset{3}{\cancel{120}}\text{ mg}}{\underset{2}{\cancel{80}}\text{ mg}} \times 1\text{ tab} = 1\frac{1}{2}\text{ tab}$$

18) Order: 0.25 mg = 0.250 mg

Supply: 0.125 mg/tab

$$\frac{D}{H} \times Q = \frac{\overset{2}{\cancel{0.250\text{ mg}}}}{\underset{1}{\cancel{0.125\text{ mg}_1}}} \times 1\text{ tab} = 2\text{ tab}$$

26) Order: 45 mg

Supply: 10-mg, 15-mg, and 30-mg tablets

Select: One 15-mg tablet and one 30-mg tablet for 45 mg total

Alternative choices: give 3 of the 15 mg tablets OR give $1\frac{1}{2}$ of the 30 mg tablets to provide 45 mg total

Remember: If you have a choice, give whole tablets and as few as possible.

Answers to Review Set 22 from pages 190–196

1) 0.67

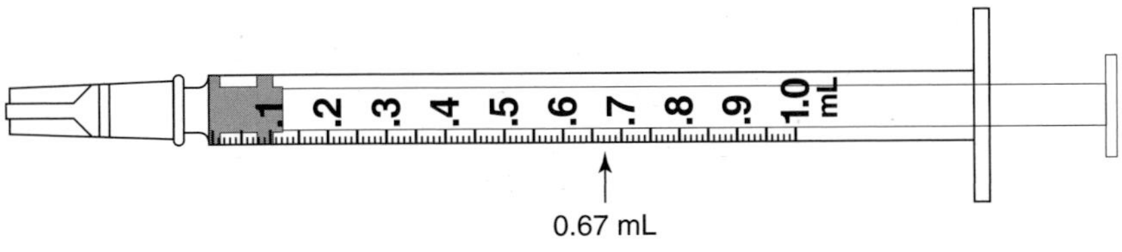

2) 7.2

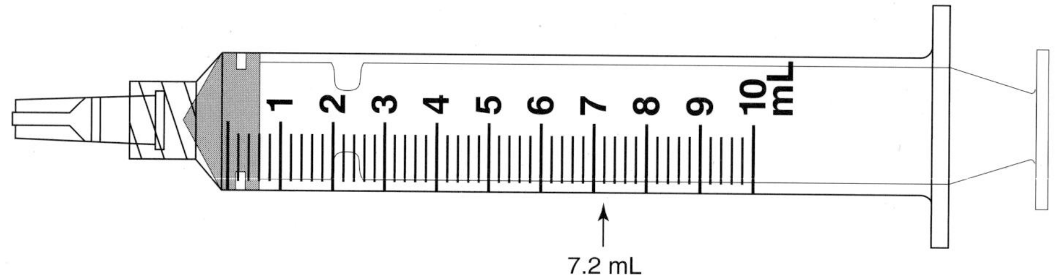

3) 0.4

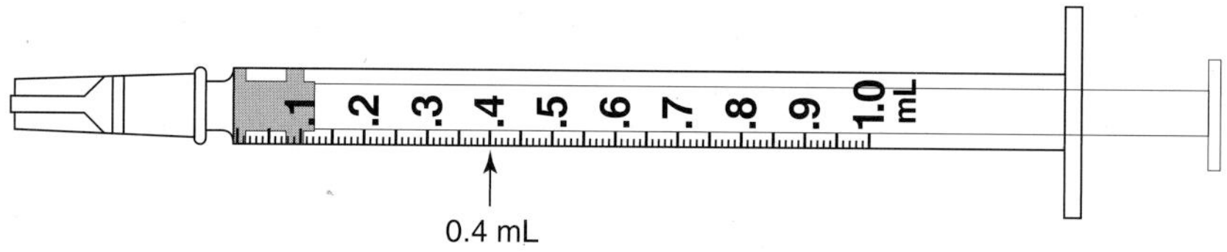

4) 0.15

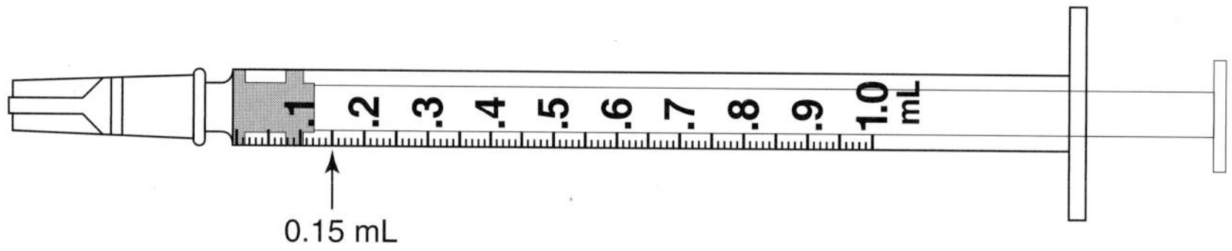

5) 2

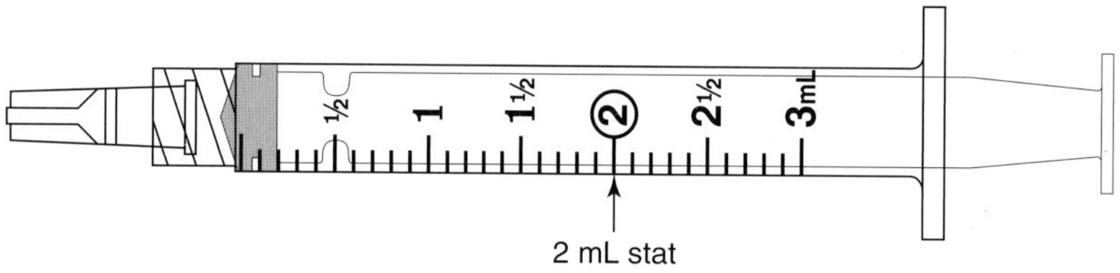

6) 0.35

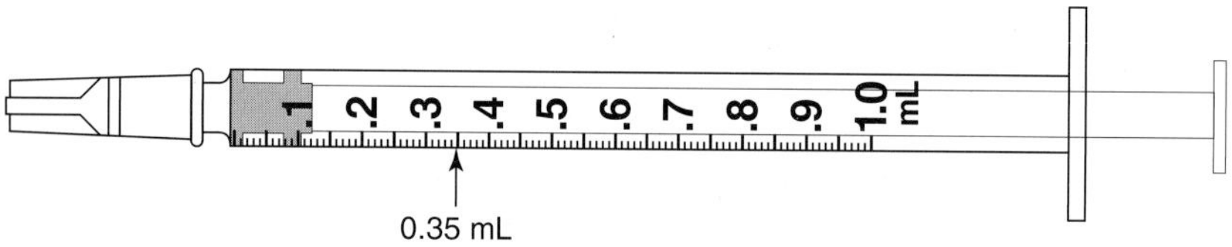

7) 0.5

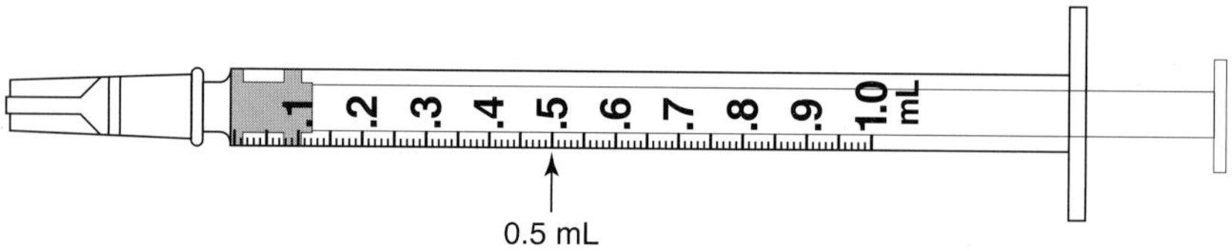

8) 0.7

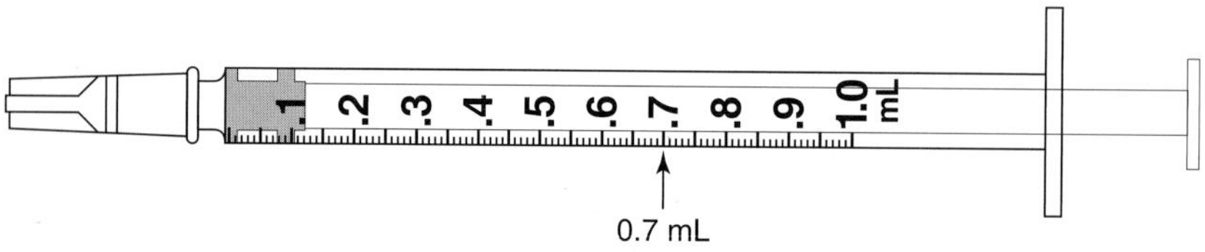

9) 4

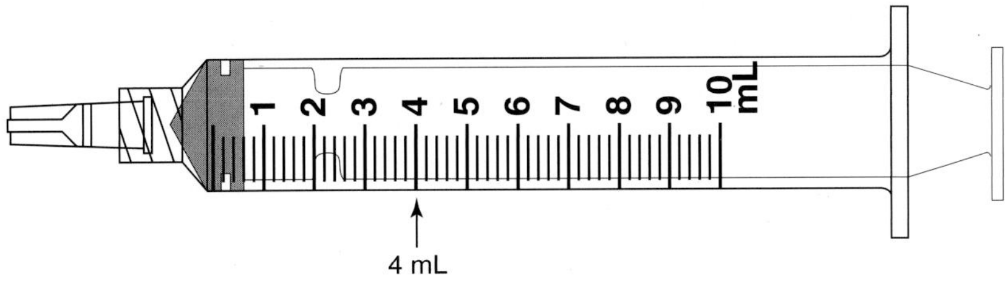

10) 1

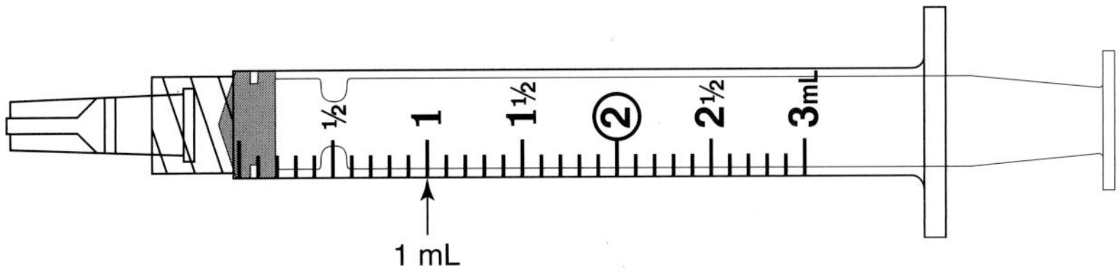

11) 1.2

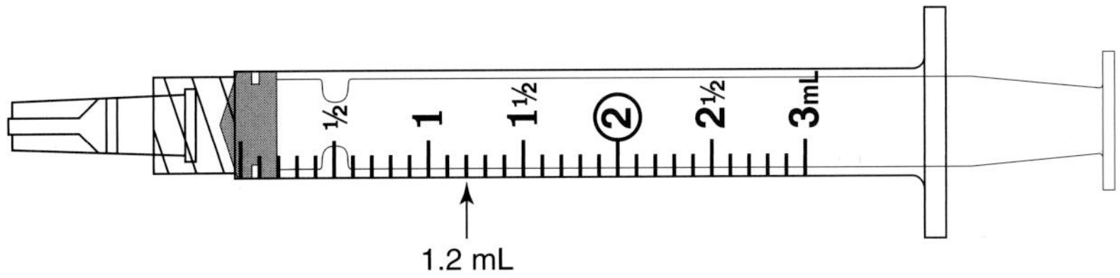

12) 0.4

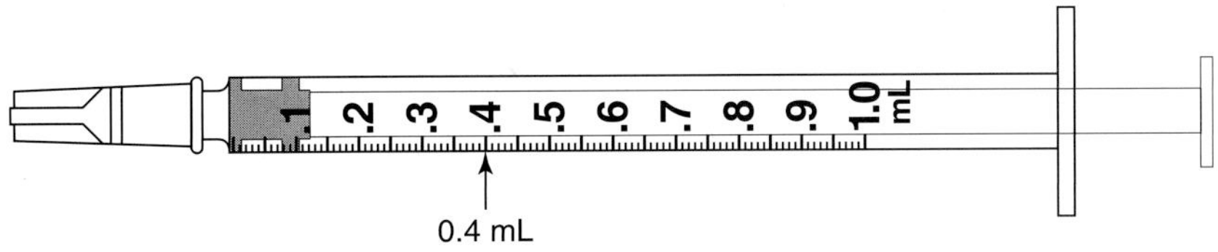

13) 2.5

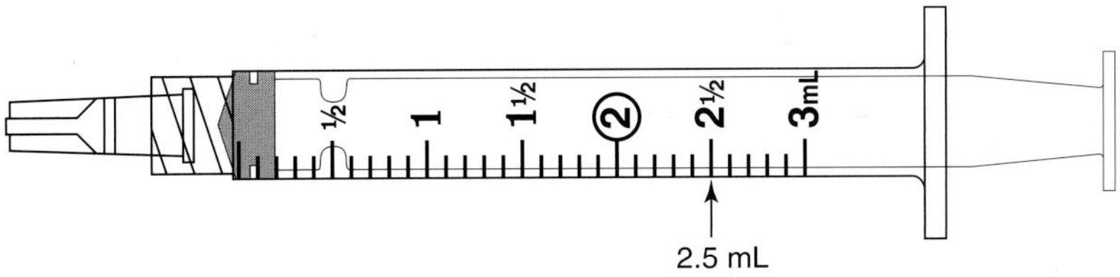

14) 0.5

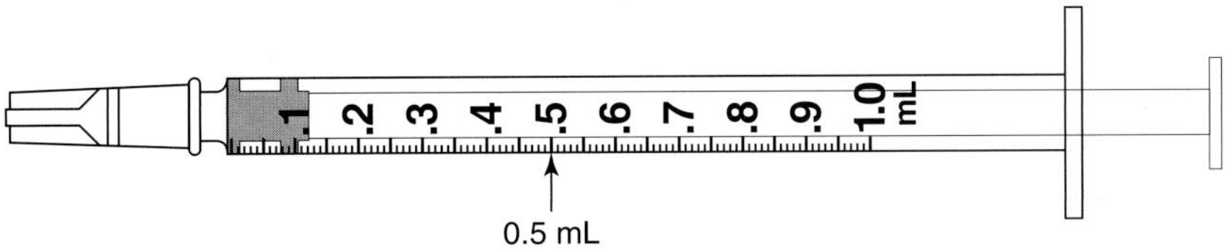

15) 100 mL. Metronidazole is available as a 100-mL premixed mini bag containing 5 mg/mL metronidazole in water for injection.

16) 1.5

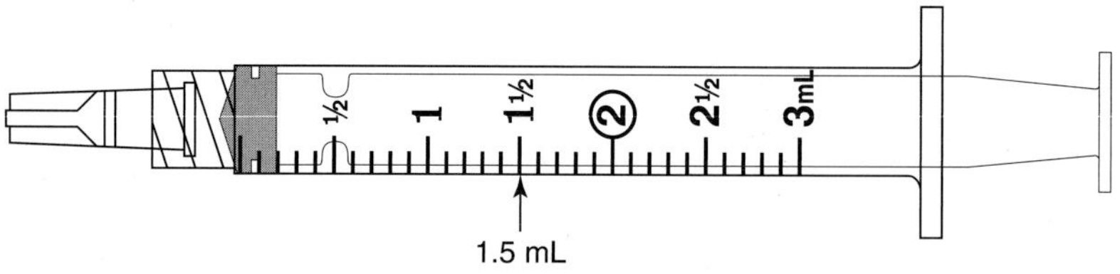

17) 0.5

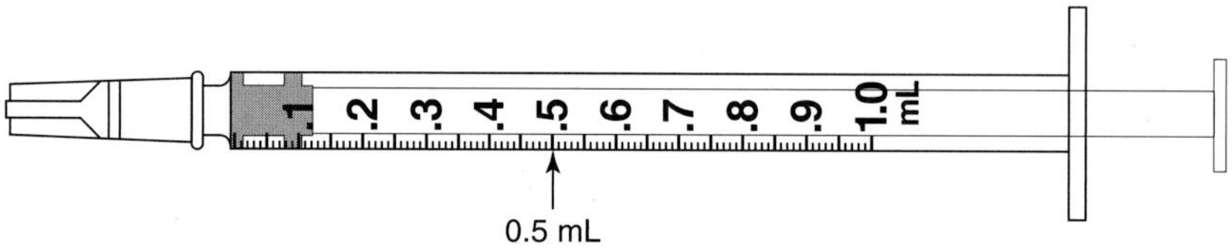

18) 1

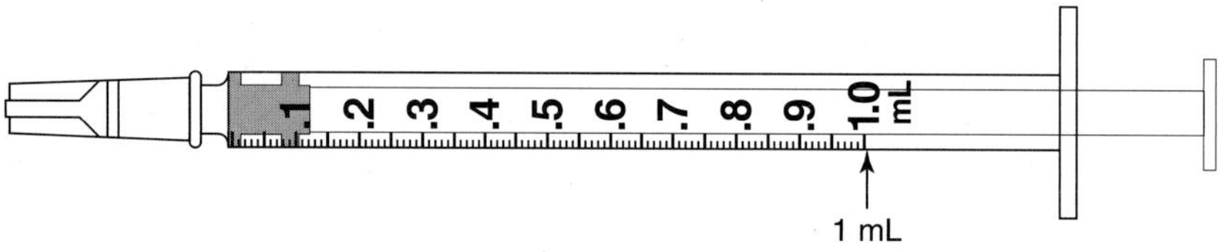

19) 0.5

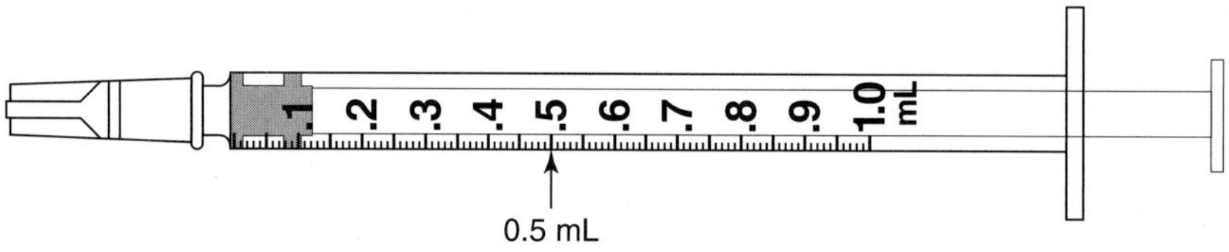

20) 1.5

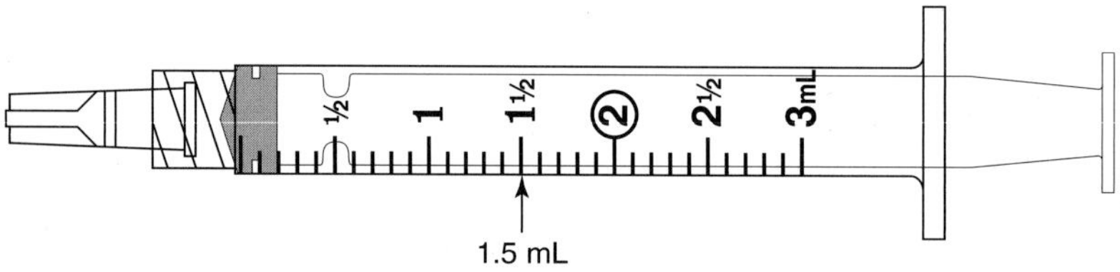

Selected Solutions—Review Set 22

1) Order: 100 mg

Supply: 150 mg/mL

$$\frac{D}{H} \times Q = \frac{10\not{0}\text{ mg}}{15\not{0}\text{ mg}} \times 1\text{ mL} = \frac{10}{15}\text{ mL} = 0.67\text{ mL}$$

2) Order: 2 400 000 units

Supply: 1 000 000 units/mL

$$\frac{D}{H} \times Q = \frac{\overset{2}{2\,\cancel{400\,000}}\text{ units}}{\underset{1}{1\,\cancel{200\,000}}\text{ units}} \times 1\text{ mL} = 2.4\text{ mL}$$

3) Order: 2 mg

Supply: 5 mg/mL

$$\frac{D}{H} \times Q = \frac{2\text{ mg}}{5\text{ mg}} \times 1 = \frac{2}{5}\text{ mL} = 0.4\text{ mL}$$

6) Order: 3500 units

Supply: 10 000 units/mL

$$\frac{D}{H} \times Q = \frac{35\cancel{00}\text{ units}}{10\,0\cancel{00}\text{ units}} \times 1\text{ mL} = \frac{35}{100}\text{ mL} = 0.35\text{ mL}$$

9) Order: 40 mg

Supply: 10 mg/mL

$$\frac{D}{H} \times Q = \frac{40}{10} \times 1\text{ mL} = 4\text{ mL}$$

10) Order: 15 mg

Supply: 15 mg/mL

$$\frac{D}{H} \times Q = \frac{\cancel{15\text{ mg}}}{\cancel{15\text{ mg}}} \times 1\text{ mL} = 1\text{ mL}$$

11) Order: 30 mg

Supply: 25 mg/mL

$$\frac{D}{H} \times Q = \frac{\overset{6}{\cancel{30 \text{ mg}}}}{\underset{5}{\cancel{25 \text{ mg}}}} \times 1 \text{ mL} = \frac{6}{5} \text{ mL} = 1.2 \text{ mL}$$

19) Order: 12.5 mg

Supply: 50 mg/2 mL

$$\frac{D}{H} \times Q = \frac{\overset{1}{\cancel{12.5 \text{ mg}}}}{\underset{4}{\cancel{50 \text{ mg}}}} \times 2 \text{ mL} = 0.5 \text{ mL}$$

Answers to Review Set 23 from pages 206–210

1) Humulin R, short-acting **2)** Novolin ge NPH, intermediate-acting **3)** Novo-Pen 4, long-acting **4)** Humalog, rapid-acting **5)** Premixed Humulin 30/70, short- and intermediate-acting **6)** Standard, dual-scale 100 unit/mL 100-unit syringe; lo-dose, 50 unit/0.5 mL 100-unit syringe; lo-dose, 30 unit/0.3 mL 100-unit syringe **7)** lo-dose, 30 unit 100-unit syringe **8)** lo-dose, 50 unit 100-unit syringe **9)** 0.6 **10)** 0.25 **11)** Standard dual-scale 100 unit 100-unit syringe **12)** False **13)** 73 **14)** 12 **15)** 32 **16)** 52

17)

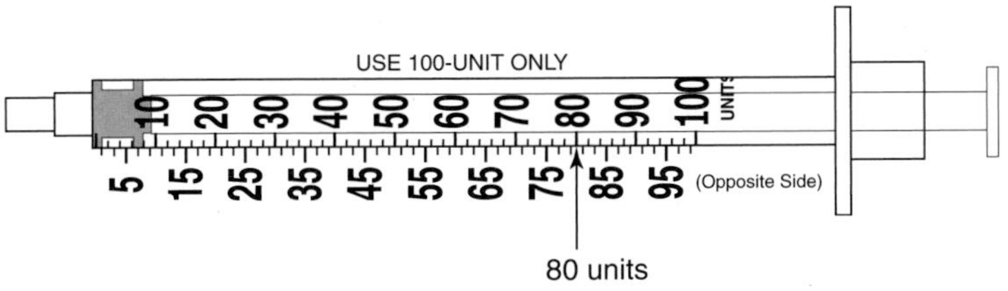

18)

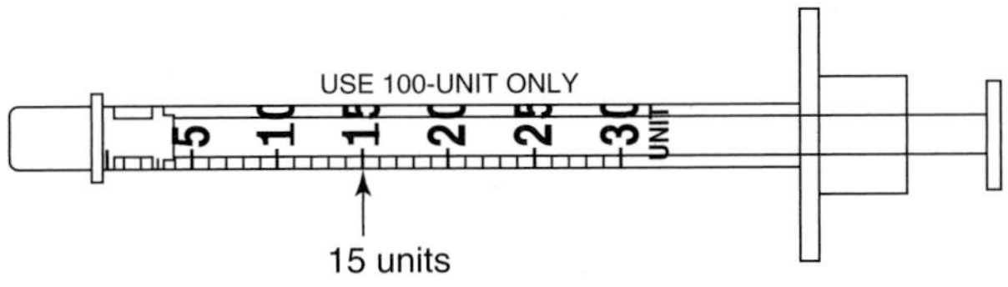

19)

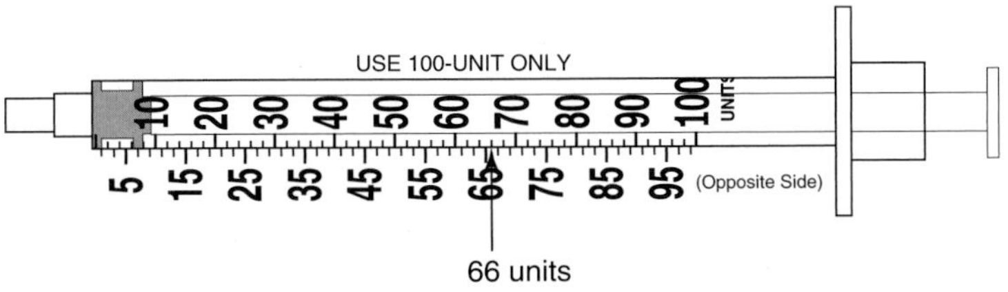

20)

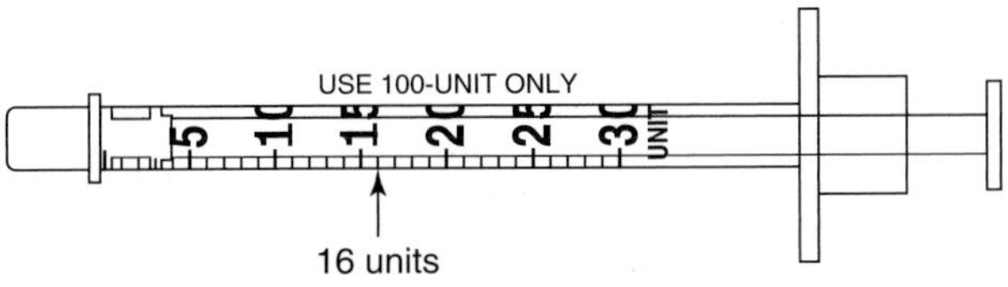

21)

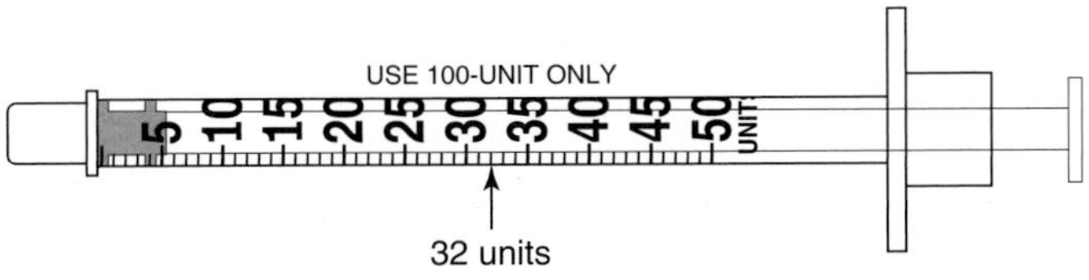

22)

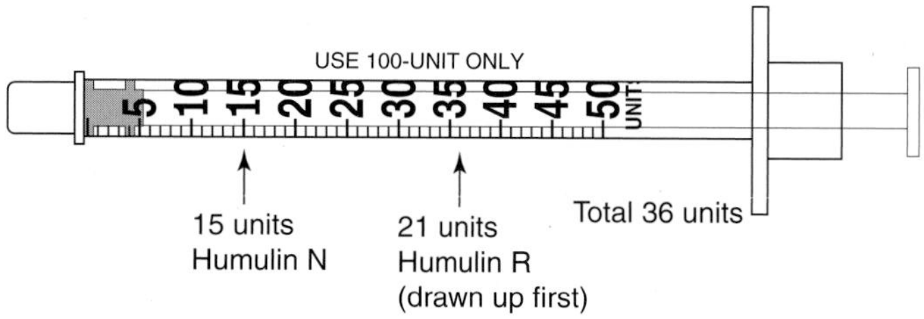
USE 100-UNIT ONLY
5 10 15 20 25 30 35 40 45 50 UNITS
15 units
Humulin N
21 units
Humulin R
(drawn up first)
Total 36 units

23)

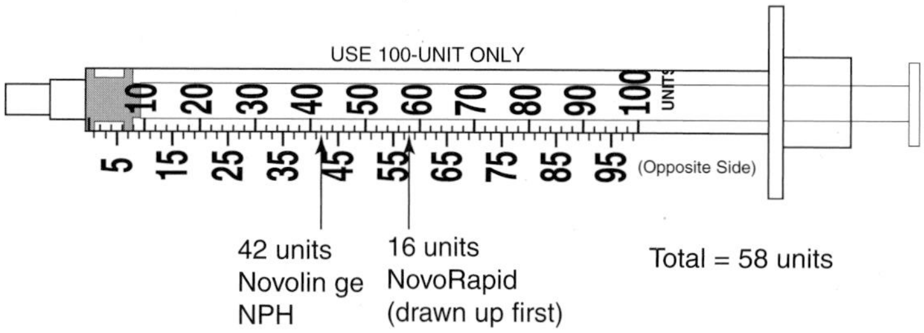
USE 100-UNIT ONLY
10 20 30 40 50 60 70 80 90 100 UNITS
5 15 25 35 45 55 65 75 85 95 (Opposite Side)
42 units
Novolin ge
NPH
16 units
NovoRapid
(drawn up first)
Total = 58 units

24)

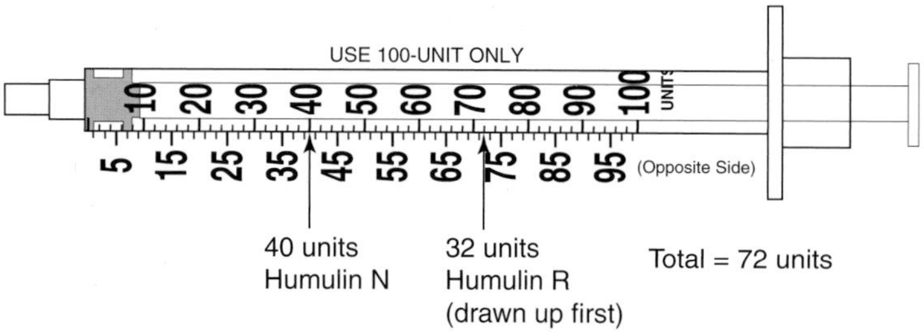
USE 100-UNIT ONLY
10 20 30 40 50 60 70 80 90 100 UNITS
5 15 25 35 45 55 65 75 85 95 (Opposite Side)
40 units
Humulin N
32 units
Humulin R
(drawn up first)
Total = 72 units

25)

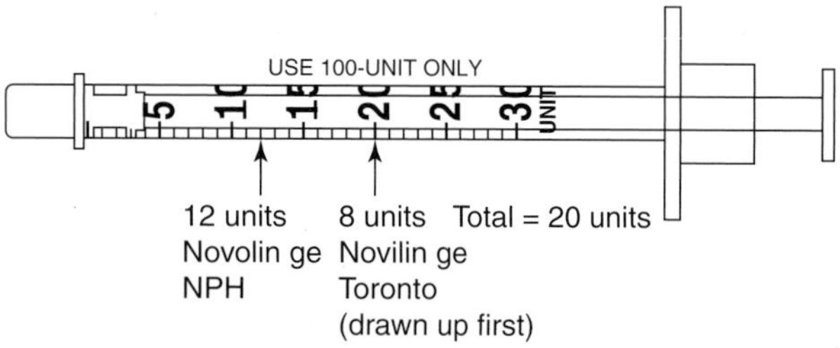
USE 100-UNIT ONLY
5 10 15 20 25 30 UNITS
12 units
Novolin ge
NPH
8 units
Novilin ge
Toronto
(drawn up first)
Total = 20 units

26) Before meals and before insulin administration.

27) Blood glucose levels of 8 to 20.

28) Administer 4 units of Humulin R 100-unit insulin.

29) None, do not administer insulin.

30) Administer 10 units of Humulin R 100-unit insulin.

Selected Solutions—Review Set 23

9) Recall 100 units = 100 units per mL

$$\frac{\overset{6}{\cancel{60}}\ \cancel{\text{units}}}{\underset{10}{\cancel{100}}\ \cancel{\text{units}}} \times 1\text{ mL} = 0.6\text{ mL}$$

Answers to Practice Problems—Chapter 9 from pages 211–219

1) 0.4; 1 mL tuberculin
The route is IM; the needle may need to be changed to an appropriate gauge and length.

2) 1.5; 3 mL

3) 0.5; 1 mL tuberculin

4) 0.4; 1 mL tuberculin

5) 2; 3 mL

6) 0.75; 1 mL tuberculin

7) 0.67; 1 mL tuberculin

8) 1; 1 mL or 3 mL

9) 4 mL; 10 mL

10) 1; 1 mL or 3 mL

11) 1; 1 mL or 3 mL

12) 0.6; 1 mL or 3 mL

13) 0.6; 1 mL or 3 mL

14) 1.9; 3 mL

15) 0.25; 1 mL tuberculin

16) 1; 1 mL or 3 mL

17) 0.13; 1 mL

18) 0.8; 1 mL tuberculin

19) 1.2; 3 mL

20) 0.2; 1 mL or 3 mL

21) 0.75; 1 mL tuberculin
The route is IM; the needle may need to be changed to an appropriate gauge and length.

22) 1.5; 3 mL

23) 0.7; 1 mL or 3 mL

24) 1; 1 mL or 3 mL

25) 0.75; 1 mL tuberculin

26) 0.5; 1 mL tuberculin

27) 6; 10 mL

28) 0.8; 1 mL or 3 mL

29) 1.5; 3 mL

30) 2.5; 3 mL

31) 1; 1 mL or 3 mL

32) 2; 3 mL

33) 0.5; 1 mL or 3 mL

34) 0.5 mg; 1 mL or 3 mL

35) 16; 30 units lo-Dose 100-unit insulin

36) 25; 50 units lo-Dose 100-unit insulin

37) 0.3

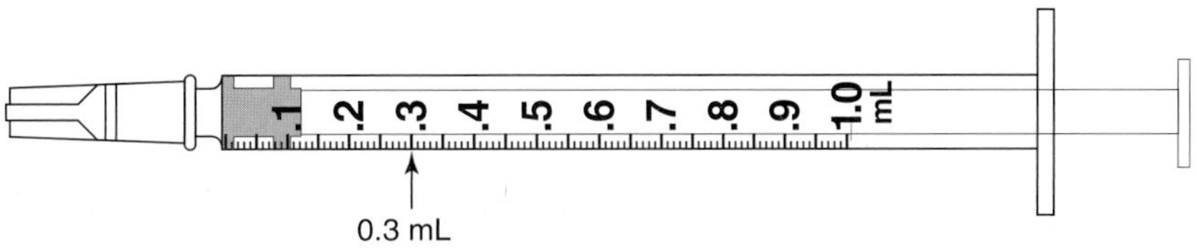

38) 1.6

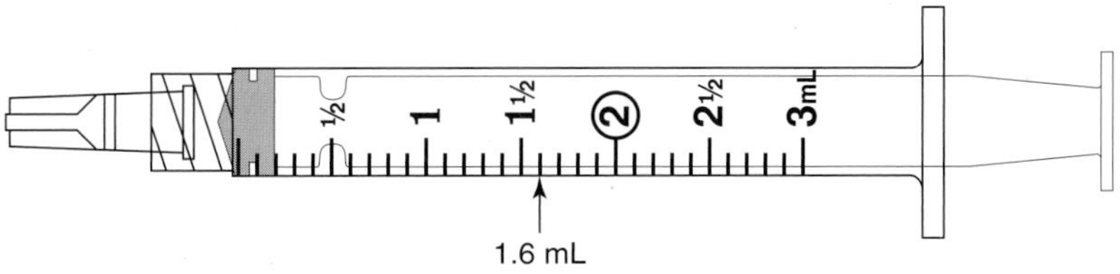

39) 1

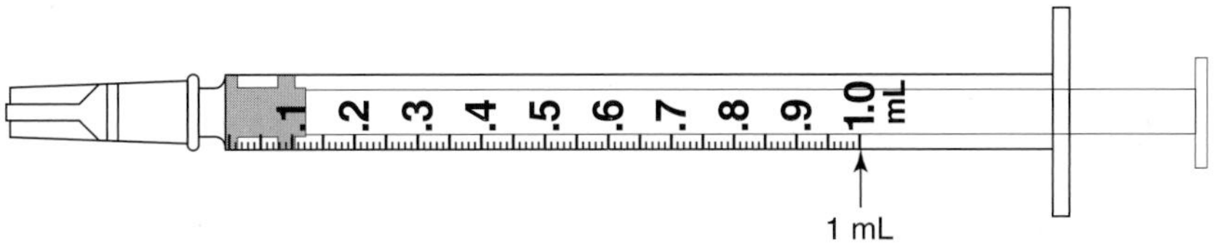

40) 2

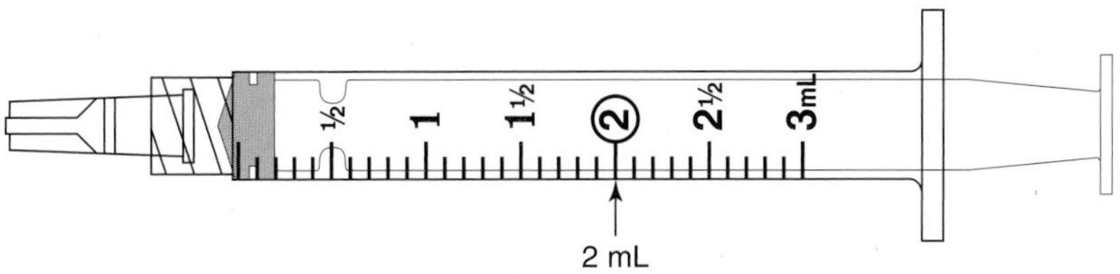

41) 1.2

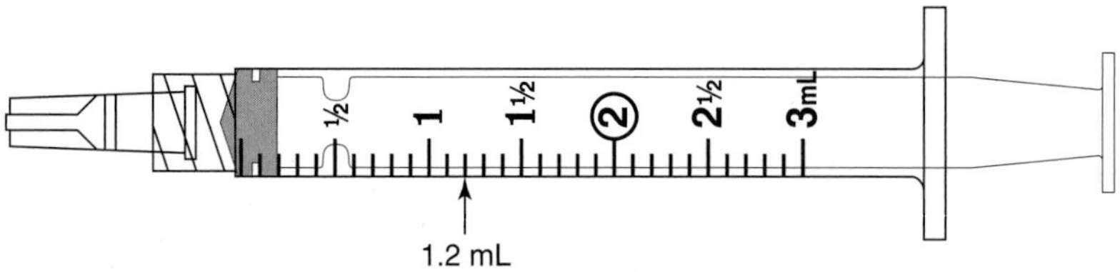

42) 22

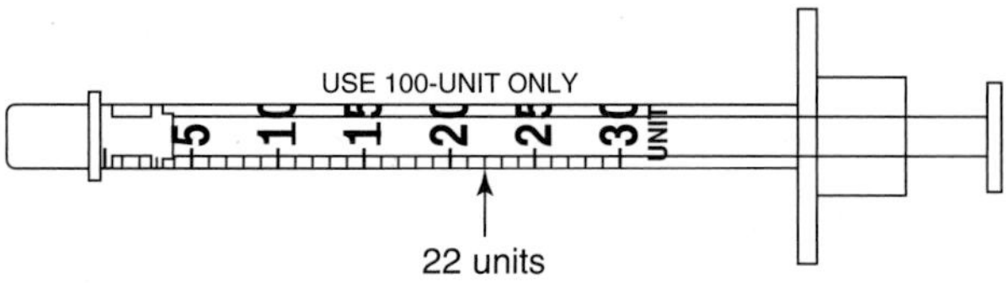

43) 0.8

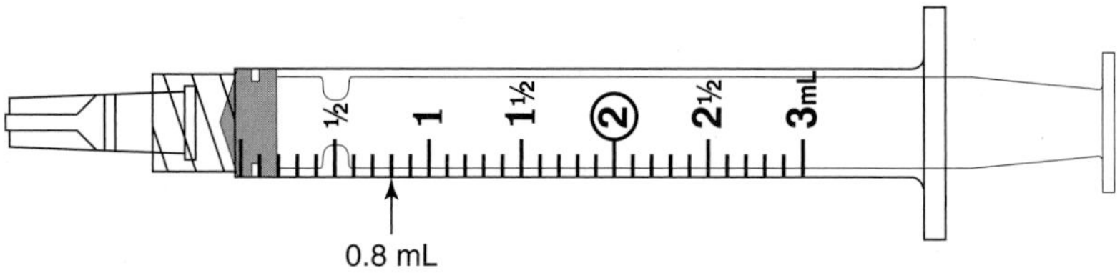

44) 0.6

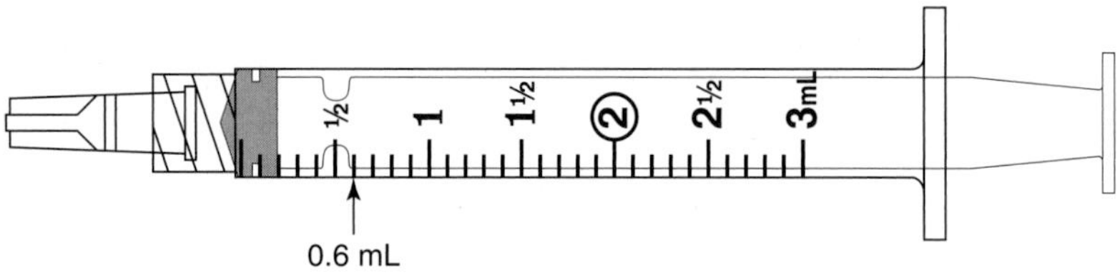

45) 1.4

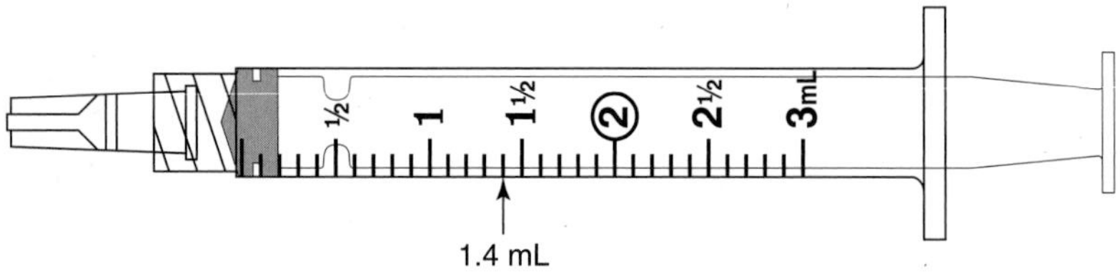

46) 0.75

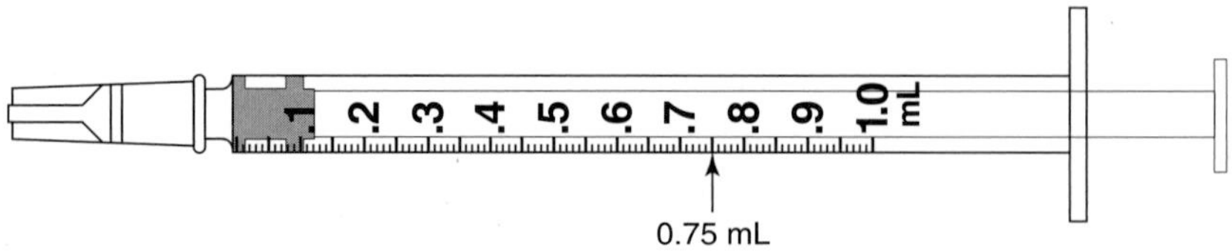

47) 86

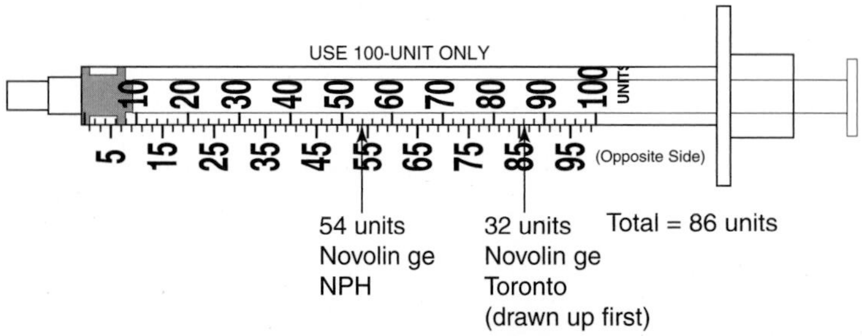

48) 46

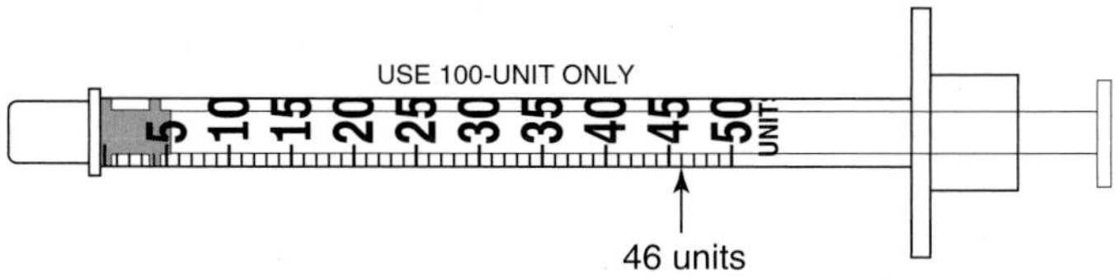

49) Critical Thinking: Prevention.

This error could have been avoided if? the nurse been more careful checking the label of the insulin vial and comparing the label to the order. The nurse should have checked the label three times as is taught in nursing school. In addition, the nurse should have asked another nurse to double-check her as she was drawing up the insulin, as required. Such hospital policies and procedures are written to protect the patient and the nurse.

50) Critical Thinking: Prevention.

This insulin error should never occur. It is obvious that the nurse did not use Step 2 of the three-step method. The nurse did not stop to think of the reasonable dosage. If so, the nurse would have realized that the supply dosage of 100-unit insulin is 100 units/mL, not 10 units/mL.

If you are unsure of what you are doing, you need to ask before you act. Insulin should only be given in an insulin syringe. The likelihood of the nurse needing to give insulin in a tuberculin syringe because an insulin syringe was unavailable is almost nonexistent today. The nurse chose the incorrect syringe. Whenever in doubt, the nurse should ask for help. Further, if the nurse had asked another nurse to double-check the dosage, as required, the error could have been found before the client received the wrong dosage of insulin. After giving the insulin, it is too late to rectify the error.

Selected Solutions—Practice Problems—Chapter 9

3) Order: 2.5 mg

Supply: 5 mg/mL

$$\frac{D}{H} \times Q = \frac{20 \text{ mg}}{50 \text{ mg}} \times 1 \text{ mL} = \frac{2.5 \cancel{\text{mg}}}{5 \cancel{\text{mg}}} \times 1 \text{ mL} = 0.5 \text{ mL}$$

4) Order: 20 mg

Supply: 50 mg/mL

$$\frac{D}{H} \times Q = \frac{\cancel{20} \cancel{\text{mg}}}{\cancel{50} \cancel{\text{mg}}} \times 1 \text{ mL} = \frac{2}{5} \times 1 \text{ mL} = 0.4 \text{ mL}$$

6) Order: 0.3 mg

Supply: 0.4 mg/mL

$$\frac{D}{H} \times Q = \frac{0.3 \text{ mg}}{0.4 \text{ mg}} \times 1 \text{ mL} = 0.75 \text{ mL}$$

14) Order: 75 mg

Supply: 80 mg/2 mL

$$\frac{D}{H} \times Q = \frac{75 \cancel{\text{mg}}}{\underset{40}{\cancel{80}} \cancel{\text{mg}}} \times \overset{1}{\cancel{2}} \text{ mL} = \frac{75}{40} \text{ mL} = 1.87 \text{ mL} = 1.9 \text{ mL}$$

15) Order: 12.5 mg

Supply: 50 mg/mL

$$\frac{D}{H} \times Q = \frac{12.5 \cancel{\text{mg}}}{50 \cancel{\text{mg}}} \times 1 \text{ mL} = 0.25 \text{ mL}$$

19) Order: 60 mg

Supply: 75 mg/1.5 mL

$$\frac{D}{H} \times Q = \frac{\overset{4}{\cancel{60}} \cancel{\text{mg}}}{\underset{5}{\cancel{75}} \cancel{\text{mg}}} \times 1.5 \text{ mL} = \frac{6}{5} \text{ mL} = 1.2 \text{ mL}$$

30) Order: 50 mg

Supply: 2% = 2 g/100 mL = 2000 mg/100 mL

= 20.000. = 20 mg/mL

$$\frac{D}{H} \times Q = \frac{\overset{5}{\cancel{50}} \cancel{\text{mg}}}{\underset{2}{\cancel{20}} \cancel{\text{mg}}} \times 1 \text{ mL} = \frac{5}{2} \text{ mL} = 2.5 \text{ mL}$$

33) Order: 0.5 mg

Supply: 1 mg/mL

1000 mg/2000 mL = 0.5 mg/mL

$$\frac{D}{H} \times Q = \frac{0.5 \text{ mg}}{1 \text{ mg}} \times 1 \text{ mL} = 0.5 \text{ mL}$$

41) Order: 12 000 units

Supply: 10 000 units/mL

$$\frac{D}{H} \times Q = \frac{\cancel{12\,000} \cancel{\text{unit}}}{\cancel{10\,000} \cancel{\text{unit}}} \times 1 \text{ mL} = \frac{12}{10} \text{ mL} = 1.2 \text{ mL}$$

Answers to Review Set 24 from pages 238–248

1) 3; 280; 0.7; 5.

Reconstitution Label

> 06/02/XX, 0800, reconstituted as 280 mg/mL. Expires 08/02/XX, 0800. Keep refrigerated. G.D.P

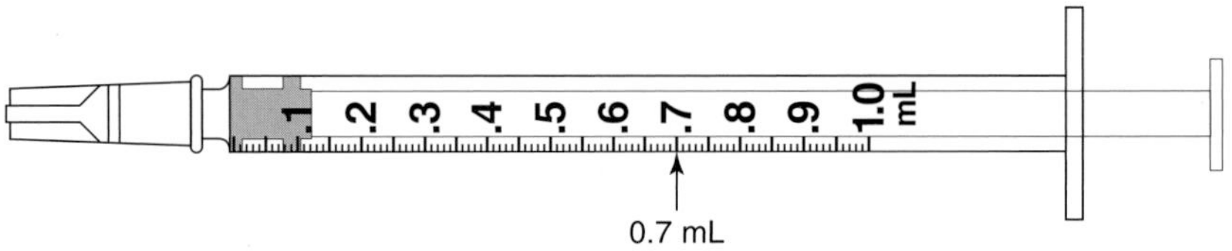

(Please note: Reconstituted solutions are to be used with 48 hours when refrigerated.)

2) 9.8; 5000; 0.5; 20

Reconstitution Label

> 06/02/XX, 0800, reconstituted as 5000 units/mL. Expires 13/02/XX, 0800. Keep refrigerated. G.D.P.

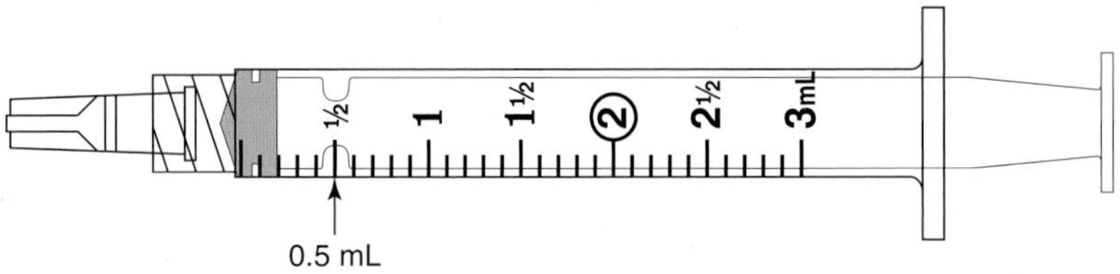

3) 1.1 mL

The vial contains 108 mg of enfuvirtide for delivery of 90 mg/mL when reconstituted. The vial is for single use. No reconstitution label is needed.

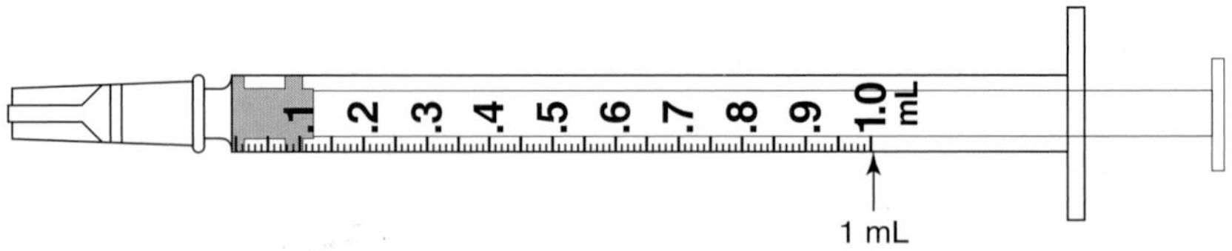

4) 4.8; 100; 5

No reconstitution label is required; all of the medication will be used for one dose.

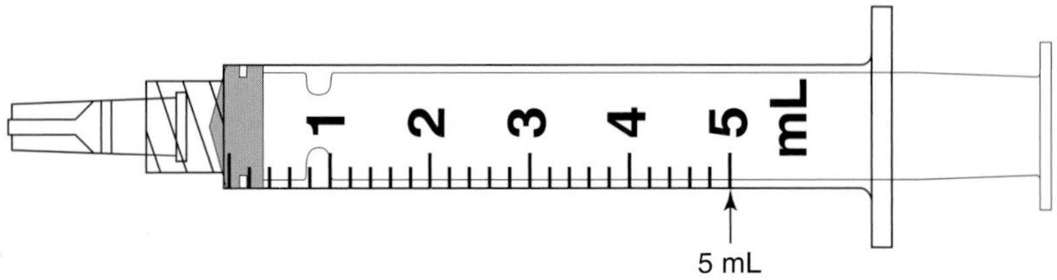

5) 2.2; 350; 2.1; 1

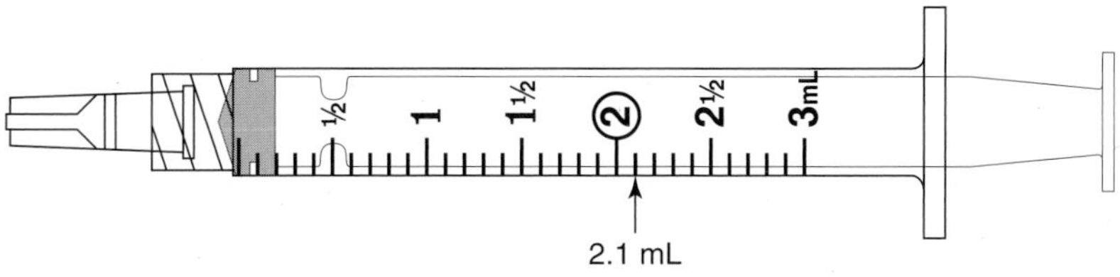

6) 8.2; 500 000; 2

3.1; 1 000 000; 1

Select 500 000 units/mL and give 2 mL. Either 1 mL or 2 mL is an appropriate amount to give IM depending on reconstitution, but 500 000 units/mL is less concentrated than 1 000 000 units/mL and is therefore less irritating to the muscle.

five doses available in vial

Reconstitution Label

06/02/XX, 0800, reconstituted as 500 000 units/mL. Expires 11/02/XX, 0800. Keep refrigerated. G.D.P.

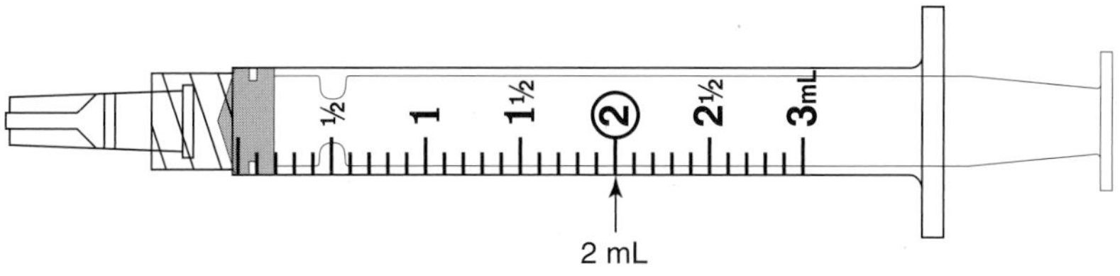

7) 7.8; 62.5; 2.8; 2

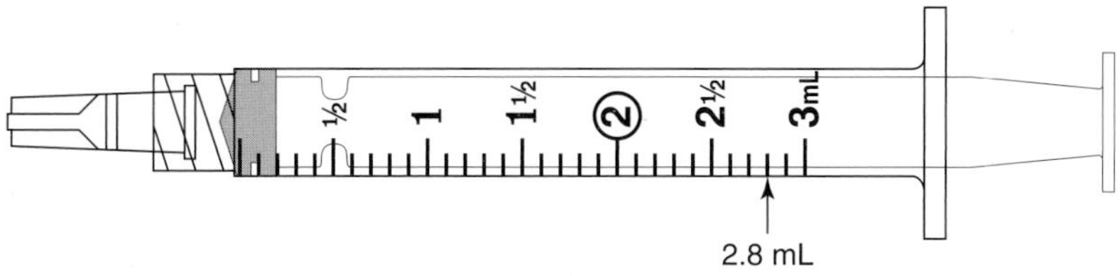

8) 4; 2 g/5 mL or 400 mg/mL; 0.5; single dose vial, discard unused portion

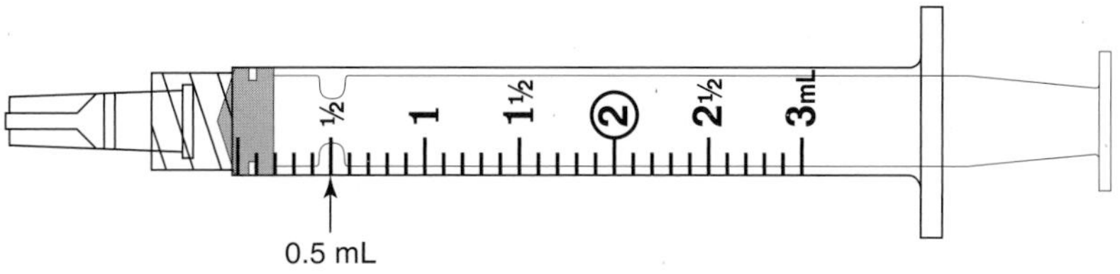

9) 1.8; 500 000; 2

3.8; 250 000; 4

Select 500 000 units/mL and give 1 mL. This is an appropriate IM dose and is less concentrated than the 1 000 000 units/mL dose. Therefore, it would be less irritating to the muscle.

two doses available.

Reconstitution Label

> *06/02/XX, 0800, reconstituted as 500 000 units/mL. Expires 11/02/XX, 0800. Keep refrigerated. G.D.P*

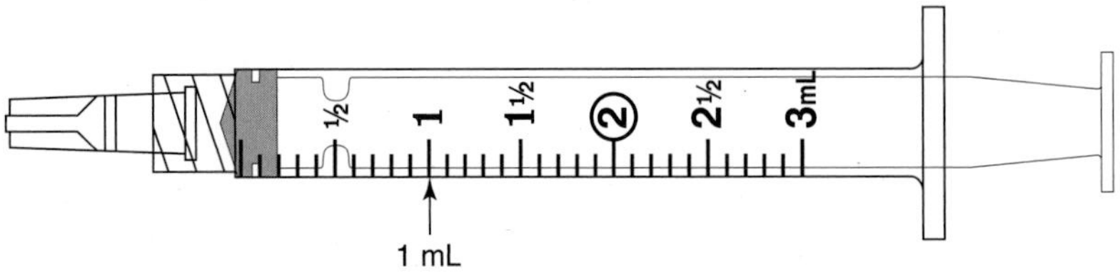

10) 10; 1.8; 180; 2.8; 4

(reconstituted, ampicillin is stable for 72 h)

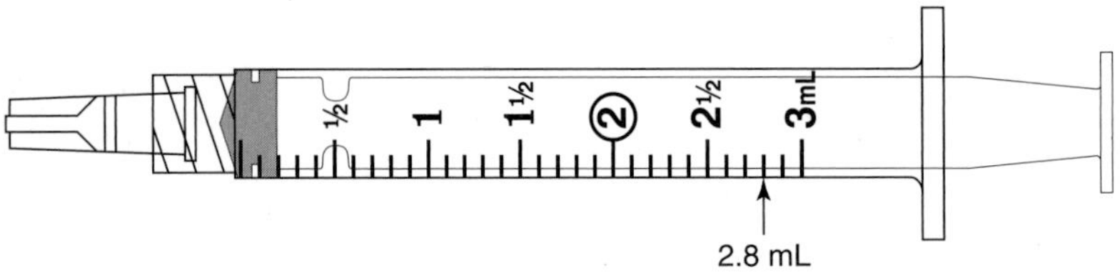

11) 1; 40; 0.6; 1

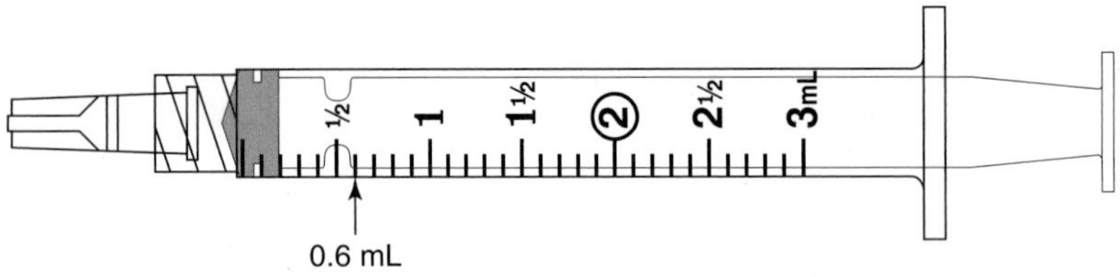

12) 10, 1800 mg/10 mL; 180; 1.4

Seven full doses of 1.4 mL are available.

No; the drug is ordered for administration twice a day; however, the solution is good for 48 hours under refrigeration. Therefore, only four doses can be used from this vial.

Reconstitution Label

> *06/02/XX, 0800, reconstituted as 180 mg/mL. Expires 08/02/XX, 0800. Keep refrigerated. G.D.P*

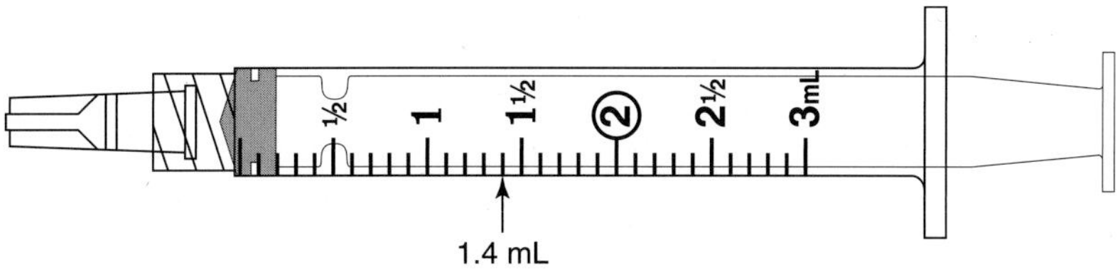

13) 9.6; 100; 7.5; 1; no label is necessary as one dose is available for use

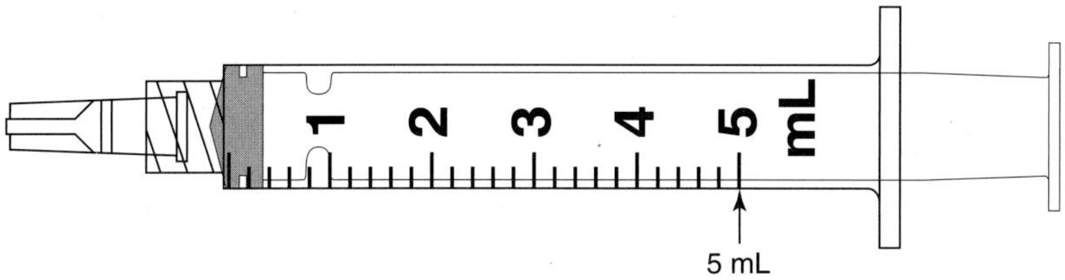

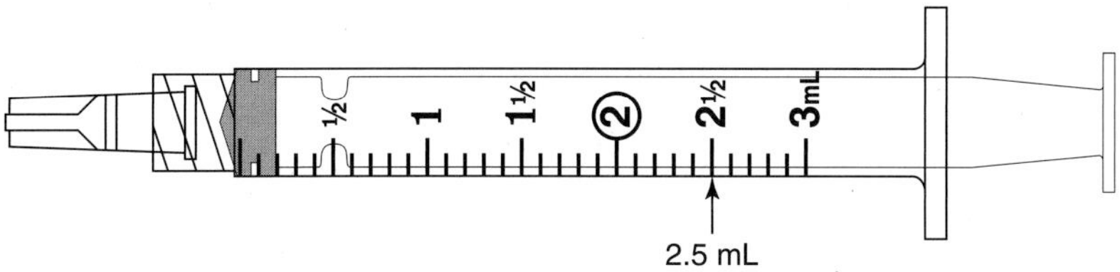

14) 30; 40; 2; 1; the solution should be used within 8 hours and the remaining unused portion discarded. No reconstitution label.

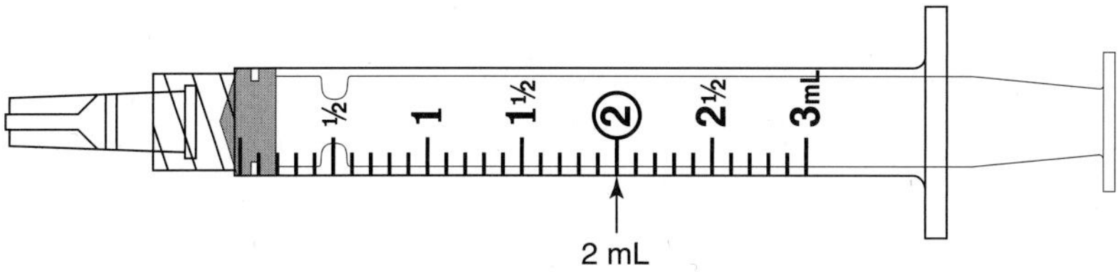

15) 2; 225; 1.1; 2.

Reconstitution Label

06/02/XX, 0800, reconstituted as 225 mg/mL. Expires 07/02/XX, 0800 when kept at room temperature. G.D.P

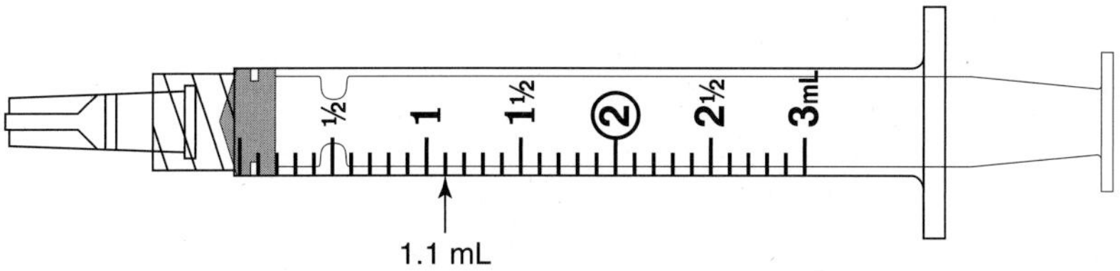

Selected Solutions—Review Set 24

1) Order: 200 mg

Supply: 280 mg/mL

$\frac{D}{H}\times Q = \frac{200\ \cancel{mg}}{280\ \cancel{mg}}\times 1\ mL = 0.714\ mL = 0.7\ mL$

1000 $\cancel{mg}$/vial ÷ 200 $\cancel{mg}$/dose = 5 doses/vial

2) Order: 2500 units

Supply: 5000 units/mL

$\frac{D}{H}\times Q = \frac{\overset{1}{\cancel{2500}}\ \cancel{units}}{\underset{2}{\cancel{5000}}\ \cancel{units}}\times 1\ mL = 0.5\ mL$

50 000 $\cancel{units}$/vial ÷ 2500 $\cancel{units}$/dose = 20 doses/vial

6) Order: 1 000 000 units

Supply: 250 000 units/mL

$\frac{D}{H}\times Q = \frac{\overset{4}{\cancel{1\,000\,000}}\ \cancel{units}}{\underset{1}{\cancel{250\,000}}\ \cancel{units}}\times 1\ mL = 4\ mL$

Order: 1 000 000 units

Supply: 500 000 units/mL

$\frac{D}{H}\times Q = \frac{\overset{2}{\cancel{1\,000\,000}}\ \cancel{units}}{\underset{1}{\cancel{500\,000}}\ \cancel{units}}\times 1\ mL = 2\ mL$

Order: 1 000 000 units

Supply: 1 000 000 units/mL

$\frac{D}{H}\times Q = \frac{\overset{1}{\cancel{1\,000\,000}}\ \cancel{units}}{\underset{1}{\cancel{1\,000\,000}}\ \cancel{units}}\times 1\ mL = 1\ mL$

5 000 000 $\cancel{units}$/vial ÷ 1 000 000 $\cancel{units}$/dose = 5 doses (available per vial)

8) Order: 200 mg

Supply: 400 mg/2.5 mL

$\frac{D}{H}\times Q = \frac{\overset{1}{\cancel{200}}\ \cancel{mg}}{\underset{2}{\cancel{400}}\ \cancel{mg}}\times 1\ mL = 0.5\ mL$

12) Order: 250 mg

Supply: 180 mg/mL

$\frac{D}{H}\times Q = \frac{25\cancel{0}\ \cancel{mg}}{18\cancel{0}\ \cancel{mg}}\times 1\ mL = \frac{25}{18}\ mL = 1.38\ mL = 1.4\ mL$

If looking at weight, there would be potentially 11 doses available—2000 $\cancel{mg}$/vial ÷ 180 $\cancel{mg}$/dose = 11 doses/vial. However, because the solution can be refrigerated for 48 hours only 4 doses would be obtained from this vial.

Answers to Review Set 25 from pages 254–255

1) 300 mL Ensure + 600 mL water = 900 mL $\frac{1}{3}$-strength Ensure; 2 cans; discard 170 mL.

2) 180 mL Isomil + 540 mL water = 720 mL $\frac{1}{4}$-strength Isomil; one 235-mL can; discard 55 mL.

3) 800 mL Boost Plus + 400 mL water = 1200 mL $\frac{2}{3}$-strength Boost Plus; 4 bottles; discard 148 mL.

4) 390 mL Ensure + 390 mL water = 780 mL $\frac{1}{2}$-strength Ensure; 2 cans; discard 80 mL.

5) 500 mL Boost Plus + 500 mL water = 1000 mL $\frac{1}{2}$-strength Boost Plus three 237-mL bottles. Discard 211 mL.

6) 1080 mL Isomil + 360 mL water = 1440 $\frac{3}{4}$-strength Isomil; use 5 cans. Discard 95 mL.

7) 120 mL Ensure + 60 water = 180 $\frac{2}{3}$-strength Ensure; use one 235-mL can. Discard 115 mL.

8) 120 mL Ensure + 360 mL water = 480 mL $\frac{1}{4}$-strength Ensure; use one can. Discard 115 mL.

9) 35 ml mouthwash + 15 mL water

10) 16 mL skin cleanser + 34 mL water

11) 1 mL sodium bicarbonate + 4 mL water

12) 120 mL hydrogen peroxide + 120 mL water

Selected Solutions—Review Set 25

1) $D\times Q = \frac{1}{\underset{1}{\cancel{3}}}\times \overset{300}{\cancel{900}}\ mL = 300\ mL$ Ensure

900 mL (total solution) − 300 mL (Ensure) = 600 mL (water)

one can = 235 mL

470 mL (two full cans) − 300 mL (Ensure needed) = 170 mL (discarded)

2) 120 mL q4h = 120 mL/feeding × 6 feedings = 720 mL total

$D \times Q = \frac{1}{\cancel{4}_{1}} \times \cancel{720}^{180} = 180$ mL (Isomil)

720 mL (solution) − 180 mL (Isomil) = 540 mL; use one 235-mL can; discard 55 mL.

8) $D \times Q = \frac{1}{4} \times 480$ mL = 120 mL Ensure

480 mL (solution) − 120 mL (Ensure) = 360 mL water; use one 235-mL can Ensure. Discard 115 mL.

Answers to Practice Problems—Chapter 10 from pages 256–262

1) 0.194.mL; 12.9; 20 mL or two syringes: 10 mL plus 3 mL; note that piperacillin sodium/tazobactam sodium is further diluted for intravenous administration **2)** 2; 3 mL **3)** 1.5; 3 mL **4)** 9.6; 100; 7.5; 1; 10 mL
5) 1.8; 3 mL; 2

> 06/02/XX, 0800, reconstituted as 280 mg/mL.
> Expires 09/02/XX, 0800. Keep refrigerated. G.D.P.

6) 3.8; 5 mL; 1 **7)** 2; 225; 1.3; 3 mL; 1; No **8)** 15.6; 62.5 mg/mL; 3.2; 10 mL; single-dose vial, no reconstitution label.
9) 2.5; 334; 1 mL; 3 mL; 2; Yes **10)** 9.8; 5000; 1.5; 3 mL; 6; Yes **11)** 10; 180/1; 6.9; 10 mL; 1; No
12) 30; 40; 1.5; 3 mL; potentially 8; however, this solution once reconstituted must be used within 8 h so no label.
13) 3.1; 1 000 000; 2; 3 mL; 2; Yes **14)** 1.8; 500 000; 2; 3 mL; 1; No **15)** 2; 225; 1.8; 3 mL; 1; No

16) 60 mL hydrogen peroxide + 420 mL normal saline = 480 mL $\frac{1}{8}$-strength solution.

17) 120 mL hydrogen peroxide + 200 mL normal saline = 320 mL $\frac{3}{8}$-strength solution.

18) 50 mL hydrogen peroxide + 30 mL normal saline = 80 $\frac{5}{8}$-strength solution.

19) 360 mL hydrogen peroxide + 180 mL normal saline = 540 mL $\frac{2}{3}$-strength solution.

20) 437.5 mL hydrogen peroxide + 62.5 mL normal saline = 500 mL $\frac{7}{8}$-strength solution.

21) 250 mL hydrogen peroxide + 750 mL normal saline = 1000 mL (1 L) $\frac{1}{4}$-strength solution.

22) 30 mL Enfamil + 90 mL water = 120 mL $\frac{1}{4}$-strength Enfamil; one 235-mL can. Discard 205 mL.

23) 270 mL Boost Plus + 90 mL water = 360 mL $\frac{3}{4}$-strength Boost Plus; two 237-mL bottles. Discard 204 mL.

24) 300 mL Ensure + 150 mL water = 450 mL $\frac{2}{3}$-strength Ensure; two 235-mL cans. Discard 170 mL.

25) 2880 mL Enfamil − 1800 mL water = 1080 mL $\frac{3}{8}$-strength Enfamil; five 235-mL cans. Discard 95 mL.

26) 20 mL Ensure + 140 mL water = 160 mL $\frac{1}{8}$-strength Ensure; one 235-mL can. Discard 215 mL.

27) 225 mL Ensure + 225 mL water = 550 mL $\frac{1}{2}$-strength Ensure; one 235-mL can. Discard 10 mL.

28) Use 2 cans; 120 mL discarded.

29) 1050

30) Critical Thinking: Prevention.

This type of error could have been prevented had the nurse read the label carefully for the correct amount of diluent for the dosage of medication to be prepared. Had the nurse read the label carefully before the medication was prepared, medication, valuable time, healthcare resources, and potential harm to the patient would have been avoided.

Selected Solutions—Practice Problems—Chapter 10

1) Concentration is 0.194/mL

Order: 2.5 g

Supply: 0.194/mL

$$\frac{D}{H}\times Q = \frac{2.5\ \cancel{g}}{0.195\ \cancel{g}}\times 1\ mL = 12.88\ mL = 12.9\ mL$$

4) Order: 750 mg

Supply: 100 mg/mL

$$\frac{D}{H}\times Q = \frac{750\ \cancel{mg}}{100\ \cancel{mg}}\times 1\ mL = 7.5\ mL$$

Vial has 2 g ceftriaxone sodium. Order is for 750 mg/dose.

2 g/vial = 2 × 1000 = 2000 mg/vial; 2000 ~~mg~~/vial ÷ 750 ~~mg~~/dose = 2.6 doses/vial = 2 full doses/vial

6) Order: 375 mg

Supply: 100 mg/mL

$$\frac{D}{H}\times Q = \frac{375\ \cancel{mg}}{100\ \cancel{mg}}\times 1\ mL = 3.75\ mL = 3.8\ mL$$

500 ~~mg~~/vial ÷ 375 ~~mg~~/dose = 1.3 doses/vial = 1 full dose/vial available.

9) Order: 350 mg

Supply: 334 mg/mL

$$\frac{D}{H}\times Q = \frac{350\ \cancel{mg}}{334\ \cancel{mg}}\times 1\ mL = 1.04\ mL = 1\ mL$$

1000 ~~mg~~/vial ÷ 334 ~~mg~~/dose = 2.9 doses/vial = 2 full doses/vial available.

14) Order: 1 000 000 units

Supply: 500 000 units/mL

$$\frac{D}{H}\times Q = \frac{\overset{20}{\cancel{1\,000\,000}}\ units}{\underset{1}{\cancel{500\,000}}\ units}\times 1\ mL = 20\ mL$$

(too much for IM dose)

Order: 1 000 000 units

Supply: 100 000 units/mL

$$\frac{D}{H}\times Q = \frac{\overset{10}{\cancel{1\,000\,000\ units}}}{\underset{1}{\cancel{100\,000\ units}}}\times 1\ mL = 10\ mL$$

(too much for IM dose)

Order: 1 000 000 units

Supply: 250 000 units/mL

$$\frac{D}{H}\times Q = \frac{\overset{4}{\cancel{1\,000\,000\ units}}}{\underset{1}{\cancel{250\,000\ units}}}\times 1\ mL = 4\ mL$$

(acceptable for IM dose)

Order: 1 000 000 units

Supply: 500 000 units/mL

$$\frac{D}{H}\times Q = \frac{\overset{2}{\cancel{1\,000\,000\ units}}}{\underset{1}{\cancel{500\,000\ units}}}\times 1\ mL = 2\ mL$$

(better for IM dose)

22) 12 mL every hour for 10 hours = 12 × 10 = 120 mL total;

$$D\times Q = \frac{1}{\underset{1}{\cancel{4}}}\times \overset{30}{\cancel{120}}\ mL = 30\ mL\ \text{Enfamil};$$

120 mL (solution) − 30 mL (Enfamil) = 90 mL (water); one 235-mL can available

30 mL Enfamil required

205 mL discarded

28) $D\times Q = \frac{1}{4}\times 1400\ mL = 350\ mL$ Enfamil.

Need 2 cans of 235 mL Enfamil; discard 470 ml − 350 mL = 120 mL

29) 1400 mL − 350 mL = 1050 mL water.

Answers to Review Set 26 from pages 276–283

1) 16.4; 820; 137; 1640; 273; No (underdose) **2)** Underdosed so contact prescriber **3)** 2.2; 55; 13.8; No (overdose) **4)** The ordered dosage is too high. The maximum daily dosage should be 55 mg. The child was ordered 55 mg every 12 hours. Contact the physician to clarify the order. **5)** 15; 120; Yes **6)** 6; 8 **7)** 32; 320; 480; Yes **8)** 15 **9)** 20; 500; 125; 1000; 250; Yes **10)** 5 **11)** 5; 20; 10; No (underdose)

12) The dosage ordered is slightly too low (underdose). Since this is an infant, contact the prescriber for clarification.

13) 3.4; 85; 170; No (underdose)

14) The dosage of ceftazidime 34 mg IV q12h is not within the recommended dosage of 85–170 mg (an underdose). Contact the prescriber for clarification.

15) 120; 60; 7.5; No (underdose)

16) The prescribed dose of 2.5 mL is below the recommended dose of 7.5 mL (based on the trimenthoprim component) and the patient would be underdosed. Contact the prescriber for clarification.

17) 1.8; 5.4; No (overdose)

18) The ordered dosage of 40 mg is excessively too high (eight times the recommended dose) and it is ordered to be given too frequently (q8h); total daily dose would be 120 mg (22 times the recommended dose!). The recommended dosage is 5.4 mg q12h. The prescribing practitioner should be notified and the order questioned.

19) 31.8; 0.22; 0.11; 0.32; 0.16; Yes

20) 3

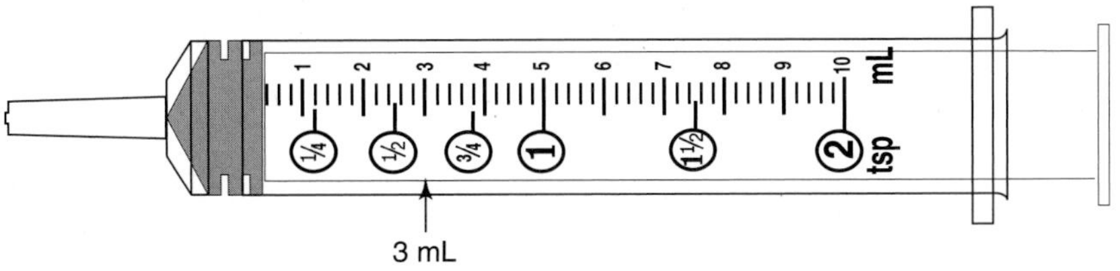

21) 17.7; 354; 118; 708; 236; No (underdose)

22) No, the dosage is slightly under the recommended dosage for this child. Contact the prescriber for instructions.

23) 25; 750; 250; 3000; 1000; Yes

24) 6.5 mL

25) No, the ordered dosage is not safe. The recommended range is 210–840 mg q8h. The amount prescribed is 275 mg but it is prescribed daily instead of every 8 hours. The physician should be contacted to clarify the order maximum of over 8 years of age. This child is only 7 and the order exceeds the maximum recommended dosage.

26) For patients weighing less than 60 kg, 200–300 mg/kg/day by IV infusion in divided doses every 4 or 6 hours, based on ticarcillin content.

27) 3.1 g every 4 to 6 hours.

28) 11.8; 17.7

29) 2; 3

30) 3; 4.4

Selected Solutions—Review Set 26

1) 1 kg = 2.2 lb; smaller → larger: (÷)

36 lb = 36 ÷ 2.2 = 16.4 kg

Minimum daily dosage:

$50 \text{ mg}/\cancel{\text{kg}}/\text{day} \times 16.4\ \cancel{\text{kg}} = 820 \text{ mg/day}$

820 mg ÷ 4 doses = 205 mg/dose

Maximum daily dosage:

$100 \text{ mg}/\cancel{\text{kg}}/\text{day} \times 16.4\ \cancel{\text{kg}} = 1640 \text{ mg/day}$

1640 mg ÷ 4 doses = 410 mg/dose

No, the dose is not safe, it is too low. Contact the prescriber to clarify the order.

Convert g to kg: 2200 g = 2200 ÷ 1000 = 2.2 kg

$50 \text{ mg}/\cancel{\text{kg}}/\text{day} \times 2.2\ \cancel{\text{kg}} = 110 \text{ mg/day}$

110 mg ÷ 6 doses = 18.3 mg/dose;

2) no, the dosage is not safe.

3) Convert g to kg: 2200 g = 2200   1000 = 2.2 kg

25 mg/kg/day × 2.2 kg = 55 mg/day

55 mg ÷ 4 doses = 13.8 mg/dose; no, the dosage is not safe.

4) The ordered dosage is too high. The maximum daily dosage should be 55 mg. The child was ordered 55 mg every 12 hours rather than the frequency of every 6 hours. Contact the physician to clarify the order.

13) 1 lb = 16 oz; 8 oz = 8 ÷ 16 = $\frac{1}{2}$ lb

7 lb 8 oz = $7\frac{1}{2}$ lb = 7.5 ÷ 2.2 = 3.4 kg

25 mg kg × 3.4 kg = 85 mg/dose

85 mg ÷ 2 doses = 42.5 mg/dose, if administered q12h

Ordered dosage of 34 mg q12h is not safe; it is a small amount below the recommended dose.

Confirm with the prerscriber; administer 0.8 mL if confirmed.

Maximum daily dosage: 50 mg/kg/day × 3.4 kg = 170 mg/day 170 mg ÷ 2 doses = 85 mg q12h

19) 70 lb = 70 ÷ 2.2 = 31.8 kg

Minimum daily dosage:

7 mcg/kg/day × 31.8 kg = 222.6 mcg/day

Convert mcg to mg; 222.6 mcg/day =

222.6 ÷ 1000 = 0.2226 mg/day = 0.22 mg/day

Minimum single dosage:

0.22 mg ÷ 2 doses = 0.11 mg/dose

Maximum daily dosage:

10 mcg/kg /day × 31.8 kg = 318 mcg/day

Convert mcg to mg; 318 mcg/day =

318 ÷ 1000 = 0.318 mg/day = 0.32 mg/day

Maximum single dosage:

0.32 mg ÷ 2 doses = 0.16 mg/dose

Yes, dosage ordered is safe.

21) 39 lb = 39 ÷ 2.2 = 17.72 kg = 17.7 kg

Minimum daily dosage:

20 mg/kg/day × 17.7 kg = 354 mg/day

Minimum single dosage:

354 mg ÷ 3 doses = 118 mg/dose

Maximum daily dosage:

40 mg/kg/day × 17.7 kg = 708 mg/day

Maximum single dosage:

708 mg ÷ 3 doses = 236 mg/dose

The dosage of 100 mg q8h is not safe. It is an underdosage and would not produce a therapeutic effect, as the recommended dosage range is 118–236 mg/dose.

28) 200 mg/kg/day × 59.1 kg = 11 800 mg/day

Convert mg to g: 11 800 mg/day =

11 800 ÷ 1000 = 11.8 g/day

300 mg/kg /day × 59.1 kg = 17 730 mg/day

Convert mg to g: 17 730 mg/day =

17 730 ÷ 1000 = 17.73 g/day

= 17.7 g/day

29) 11.8 g ÷ 6 doses = 2 g/dose

17.7 g ÷ 6 doses = 3 g/dose

30) 11.8 g ÷ 4 doses = 3 g/dose

17.7 g ÷ 4 doses = 4.4 g/dose

Answers to Practice Problems—Chapter 11 from pages 284–296

1) 5.5 **2)** 3.8 **3)** 1.6 **4)** 2.3 **5)** 15.5 **6)** 3 **7)** 23.6 **8)** 0.9 **9)** 240 **10)** 80 **11)** 19.5; 19.5; 39; No

12) It is not a safe dosage. The ordered amount is too low, therefore contact the physician to clarify.

13) 7.3; 1.8; 7.3; No

14) Do not administer. It is not a safe dosage. The ordered amount is too high. Contact the prescriber to clarify the order.

15) 22.7; 90.8; 45.4; 181.6; 90.8; No

16) The dosage order is too high; call the prescriber to clarify the order.

17) 29.1; 291; 145.5; 436.5; 218.3; Yes

18) 3

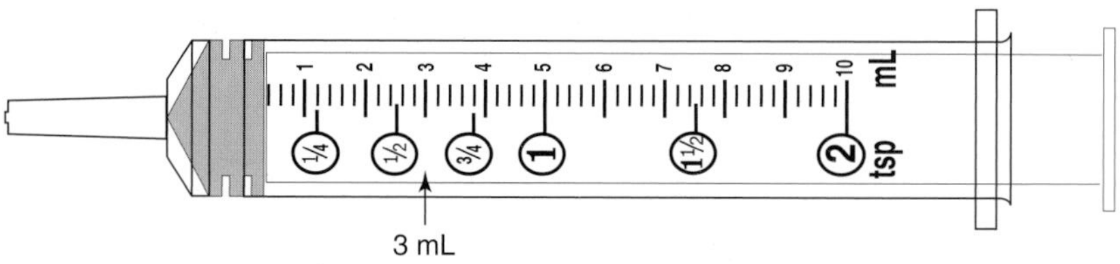

19) 2.5; 2250; 750; Yes

20) 9.8; 10; 5000; 0.15

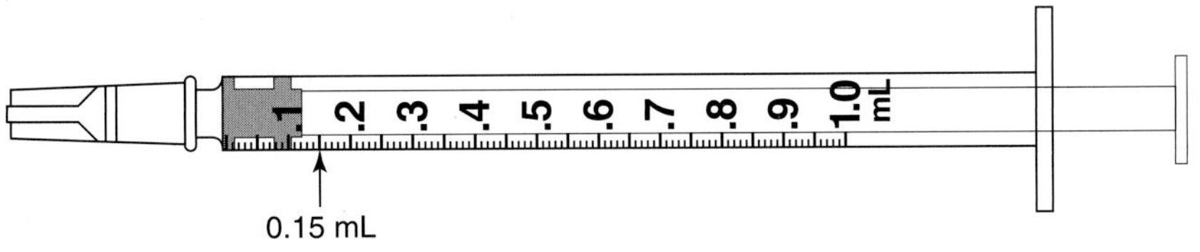

21) 18.6; 372; 124; 744; 248; Yes

22) 6

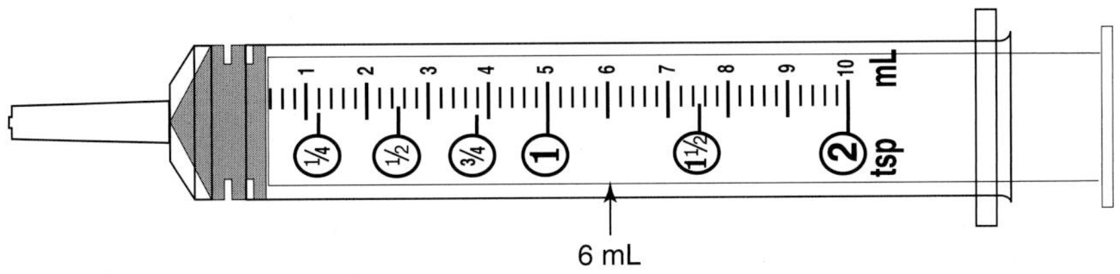

23) 9.3; 372; 186; Yes, the ordered dosage is reasonably safe; it is, however, 1 mg above the recommended dose.

24) 5

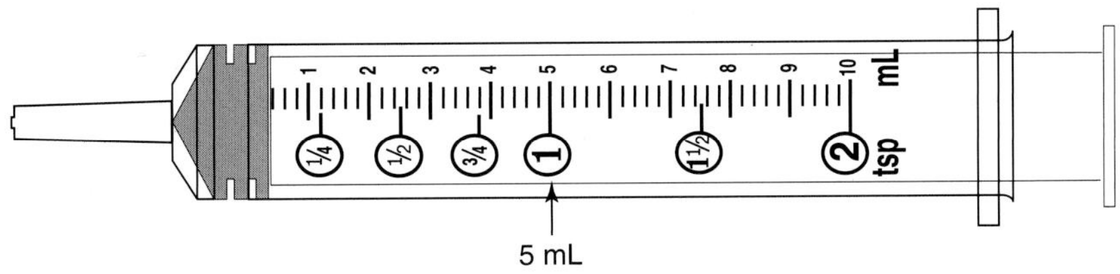

25) 10; 0.1; Yes

26) 0.25

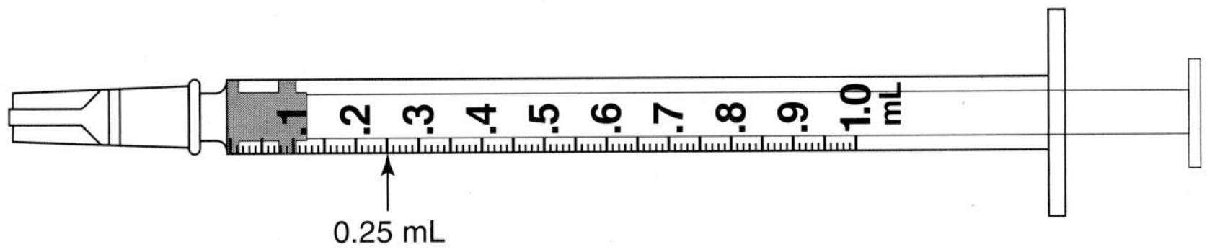

27) 28; 35; No

28) The safe range for the medication is 28–35 mg. The order is for 40 mg; therefore, the order is too high. Call the physician for clarification.

29) 9.1; 227.5; 341.3; No

30) The ordered dosage of 1 g is not safe. The recommended dosage range for a child of this weight is 227.5–341.3 mg/dose. The dose also exceeds the 50–75 mg/kg/day dose. Physician should be called for clarification.

31) 0.057; No, it is slightly underdosing the child.

32) The dose is slightly under the recommended dosage. Contact the prescriber.

33) 8.2; 82; 270.6; No

34) Dosage is not safe; recommended dose of 400 mg IV q8h exceeds the maximum recommended individual dose. The order should be clarified with the prescriber.

35) 20.5; 512.5; 256.3; No

36) The dosage ordered is not safe. It is too low compared to the recommended dosage. Call the prescriber and clarify the order.

37) 8.2; 164; 54.7; No

38) Dosage ordered is not safe. Call prescriber for clarification, as ordered dosage is higher than the recommended dosage.

39) 20.5; 512.5; 128.1; 1025; 256.3; No

40) No, the dosage is not safe. It is slightly below the recommended dosage; call the prescriber for clarification.

41) 23.2; 348; 174; Yes, dosage is reasonably safe. It is 1 mg below the recommended dose.

42) 3.5

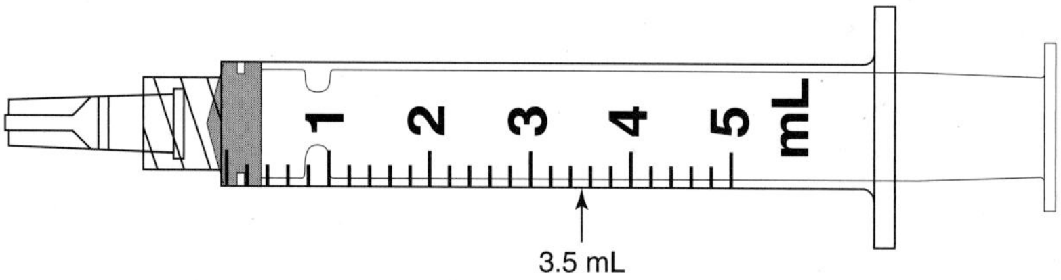

43) 0.25

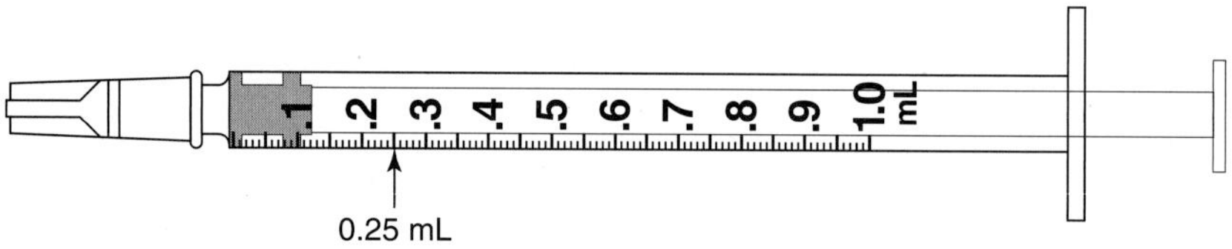

44) 3.5

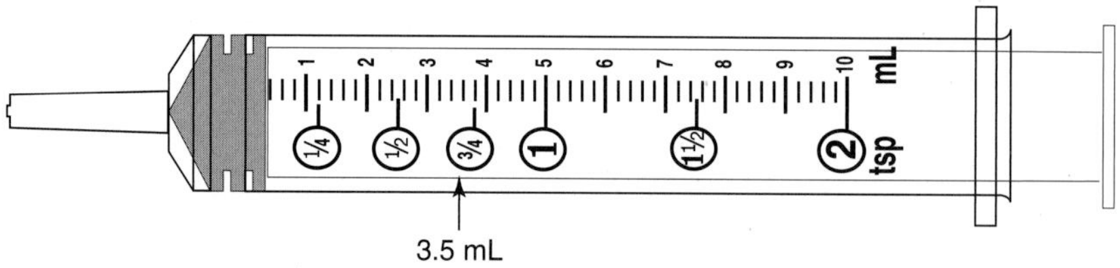

45) 500 000; 0.9

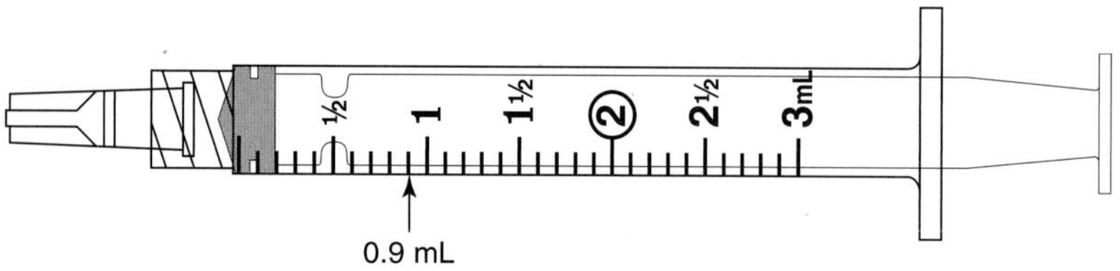

46) Dosage is not safe; this child is ordered a total of 2 mg/day, which is too high. Maximum daily dose is 1.275 mg. Prescriber should be called to clarify.

47) The ordered dosage of 20 mg q3–4h prn is too high when compared to the recommended dosage range for a child of this weight. The order should be clarified with the prescriber.

48) 0.75

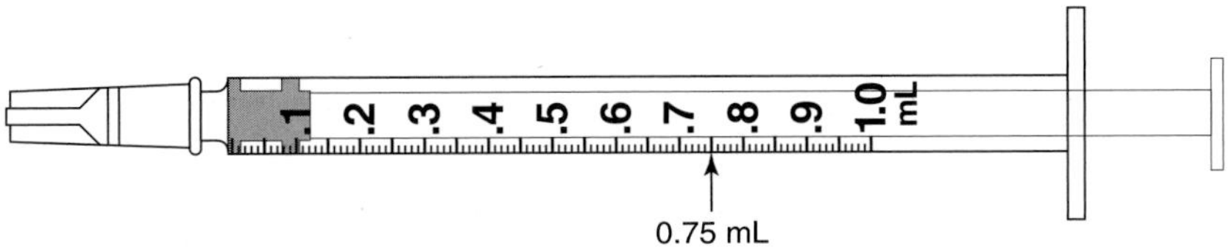

49) #45 (penicillin G sodium) and #48 (cefazolin sodium). (Note: #43 methylprednisolone is a single-dose vial. Check package insert to determine if storage after mixing is safe.)

50) Critical Thinking: Prevention.

The child should have received 75 mg a day and no more than 25 mg per dose. The child received more than four times the safe dosage of tobramycin sulfate. Had the nurse calculated the safe dosage, the error would have been caught sooner, the resident consulted, and the dosage could have been adjusted before the child ever received the first dose. The pharmacist also should have caught the error but did not. In this scenario the resident, pharmacist, and nurse all committed medication errors. If the resident had not noticed the error, one can only wonder how many doses the child would have received. The nurse is the last safety net for the child when it comes to a dosage error, because the nurse administers the drug.

In addition, the nurse has to reconcile the fact that she actually gave the overdose. The nurse is responsible for whatever dosage is administered and must verify the safety of the order and the client's rights. We are all accountable for our actions. Taking shortcuts in administering medications to children can be disastrous. The time the nurse saved by not calculating the safe dosage was more than lost in the extra monitoring, not to mention the cost of follow-up to the medication error, *and most importantly*, the risk to the child.

Selected Solutions—Practice Problems—Chapter 11

1) 1 kg = 2.2 lb; smaller → larger: (÷)

12 lb = 12 ÷ 2.2 = 5.45 kg = 5.5 kg

2) $8 \text{ lb } 4 \text{ oz} = 8\frac{4}{16} \text{ lb} = 8\frac{1}{4} \text{ lb} = 8.25 \text{ lb}$

8.25 lb = 8.25 ÷ 2.2 = 3.75 kg = 3.8 kg

3) 1570 g = 1570 ÷ 1000 = 1.57 kg = 1.6 kg

6) $1 \text{ lb} = 16 \text{ oz}; 10 \text{ oz} = 10 \div 16 = \frac{5}{8} \text{ lb}$

$6 \text{ lb } 10 \text{ oz} = 6\frac{5}{8} \text{ lb} = 6.625 \text{ lb}$

6.625 lb = 6.625 ÷ 2.2 = 3.01 kg = 3 kg

17) 64 lb = 64 ÷ 2.2 = 29.09 kg = 29.1 kg

Minimum daily dosage:

$10 \text{ mg/}\cancel{\text{kg}}\text{/day} \times 29.1\ \cancel{\text{kg}} = 291 \text{ mg/day}$

Minimum single dosage: (based on BID)

291 mg/2 doses = 145.5 mg/dose

Maximum daily dosage:

$15 \text{ mg/}\cancel{\text{kg}}\text{/day} \times 29.1\ \cancel{\text{kg}} = 436.5 \text{ mg/day}$

Maximum single dosage: (based on BID)

436.5 mg ÷ 2 doses = 218.25 = 218.3 mg/dose

Dosage ordered is safe. Child will receive 300 mg in a 24-hour period in divided doses of 150 mg BID. This falls within the recommended dosage range of 145.5 mg/dose to 218.3 mg/dose and does not exceed the maximum recommended single-dosage allowance of 250 mg/dose.

18) $\frac{D}{H} \times Q = \frac{\overset{3}{\cancel{150 \text{ mg}}}}{\underset{5}{\cancel{250 \text{ mg}}}} \times 5 \text{ mL} = \frac{3}{\cancel{5}} \times \cancel{5} \text{ mL} = 3 \text{ mL}$

19) 2500 g = 2500 ÷ 1000 = 2.5 kg

Recommended daily dosage:

900 units/~~kg~~/day × 2.5 ~~kg~~ = 2250 units/day

Recommended single dosage:

2250 units ÷ 3 doses = 750 units/dose

Ordered dosage is safe.

23) 20.5 lb = 20.5 ÷ 2.2 = 9.31 kg = 9.3 kg

Recommended daily dosage:

40 mg/~~kg~~/day × 9.3 ~~kg~~ = 372 mg/day

Recommended single dosage:

372 mg ÷ 2 doses = 186 mg/dose

The ordered dosage of 187 mg PO is reasonably safe for this child although it is 1 mg higher than the recommended dose.

24) $\frac{D}{H} \times Q = \frac{\overset{1}{\cancel{187\text{ mg}}}}{\underset{1}{\cancel{187\text{ mg}}}} \times 5 \text{ mL} = 5 \text{ mL}$

If we used the recommended single dosage of 186 mg/dose, the calculation would be:

$\frac{D}{H} \times Q = \frac{186 \cancel{\text{mg}}}{187 \cancel{\text{mg}}} \times 5 \text{ mL} = 4.9 \text{ mL};$

which is rounded to 5 mL to measure in the pediatric oral syringe; therefore, as indicated above, the ordered dosage is reasonably safe.

25) 22 lb = 22 ÷ 2.2 = 10 kg

0.01 mg/~~kg~~/dose 10 ~~kg~~ = 0.1 mg/dose

0.1 mg = 0.1 × 1000 = 100 mcg

Ordered dosage is safe.

29) 20 lb = 20 ÷ 2.2 = 9.1 kg

Recommended minimum daily dosage:

25 mg/~~kg~~/day × 9.1 ~~kg~~ = 227.5 mg/day

Recommended maximum daily dosage:

375 mg/~~kg~~/day × 9.1 ~~kg~~ = 341.3 mg/day

The dosage ordered (1 g q12h) is not safe. The recommended dosage range for a child of this weight is 227.5–341.3 mg/dose. Physician should be called for clarification.

41) 51 lb = 51 ÷ 2.2 = 23.2 kg

Recommended daily dosage:

15 mg/~~kg~~/day × 23.2 ~~kg~~ = 348 mg/day

Recommended single dosage:

348 mg ÷ 2 doses = 174 mg/dose

Ordered dosage of 175 mg is reasonably safe as an oral medication and should be given.

43) 95 lb = 95 ÷ 2.2 = 43.2 kg

0.5 mg/~~kg~~/day × 43.2 ~~kg~~ = 21.6 mg/day

Since the recommended dosage is not less than 21.6 mg/day and the order is for 10 mg q6h for a total of 40 mg/day, the order is safe.

$\frac{D}{H} \times Q = \frac{\overset{1}{\cancel{10\text{ mg}}}}{\underset{4}{\cancel{40\text{ mg}}}} \times 1 \text{ mL} = \frac{1}{4} \text{ mL} = 0.25 \text{ mL}$

Answers to Section 3—Self-Evaluation from pages 297–309

1) C; 2 **2)** A; 2 F; 1/2 **3)** J; 2 or G; 1/2 **4)** B; 7.5 **5)** H; 12 **6)** I; 2 **7)** E; 3 **8)** K; 1.5 **9)** M; 1.25 **10)** L; 3.5 **11)** E; 0.2 **12)** C; 0.5 **13)** G; 0.2 **14)** A; 0.8 **15)** D; 6 **16)** F; 0.8 **17)** B; 1.5 **18)** H; 0.75

19)

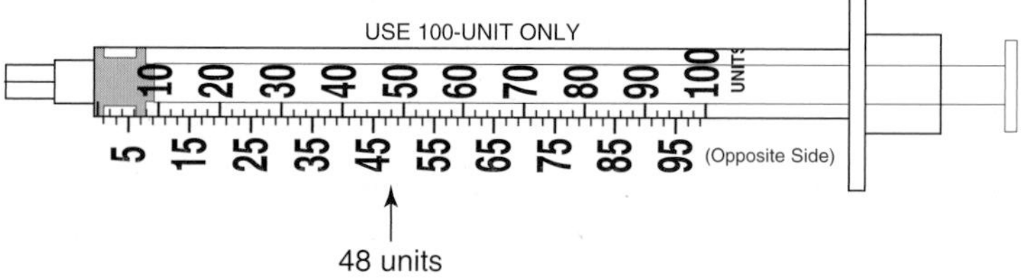

20)

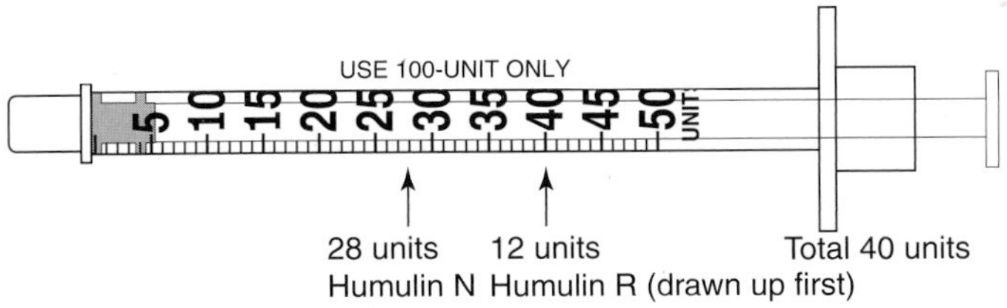
USE 100-UNIT ONLY
5 10 15 20 25 30 35 40 45 50 UNITS
28 units
Humulin N
12 units
Humulin R (drawn up first)
Total 40 units

21) 4.8; 5; 100; 4

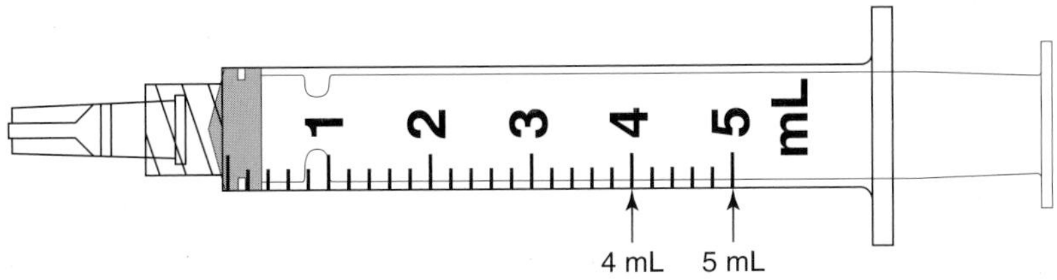
1 2 3 4 5 mL
4 mL
5 mL

22) 10; 50; 10

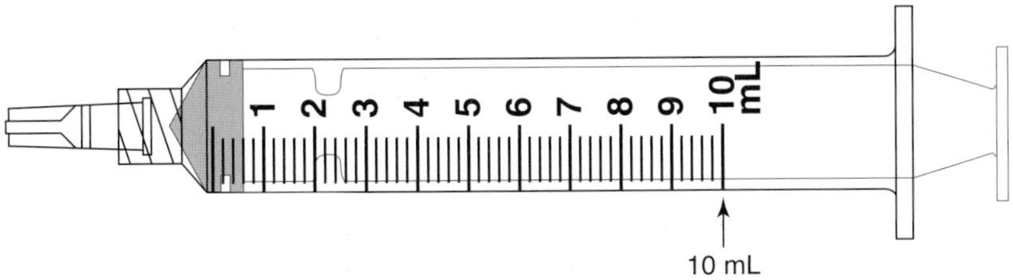
1 2 3 4 5 6 7 8 9 10 mL
10 mL

23) 3; 280; 0.71.

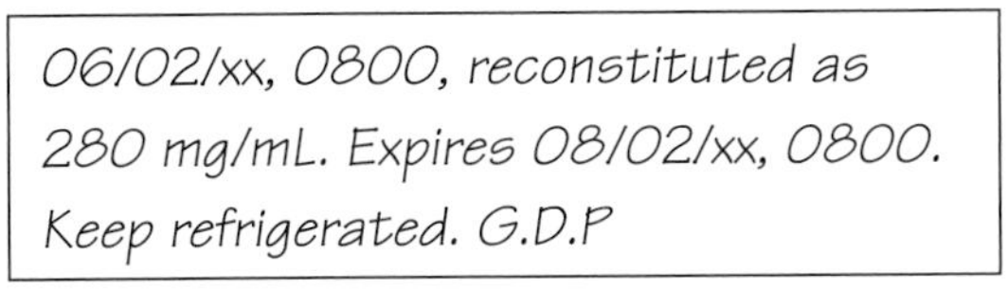
06/02/xx, 0800, reconstituted as
280 mg/mL. Expires 08/02/xx, 0800.
Keep refrigerated. G.D.P

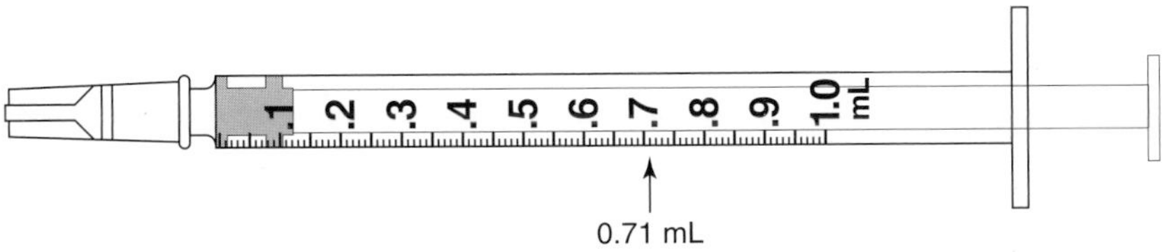
.1 .2 .3 .4 .5 .6 .7 .8 .9 1.0 mL
0.71 mL

24) 2.5; 334; 2.3

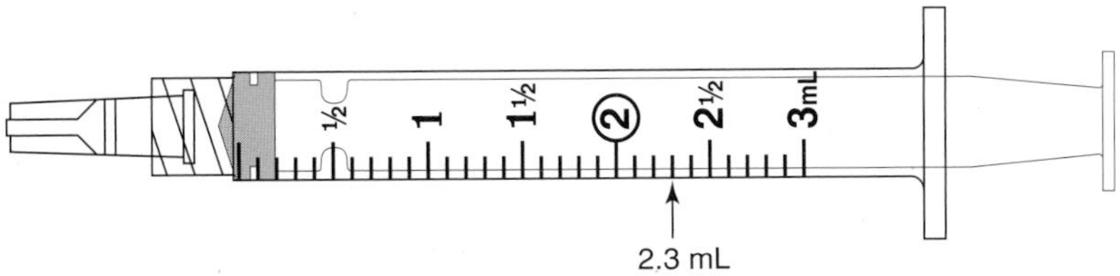
½ 1 1½ 2 2½ 3mL
2.3 mL

25) 7.8; 8; 62.5; 4; discard unused portion, no label required

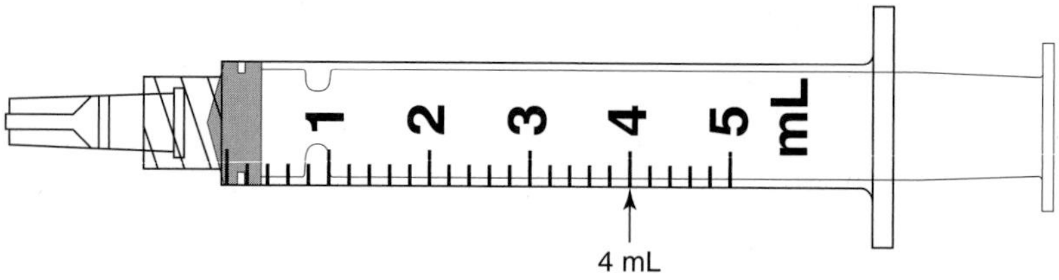

26) 30; 30; 40; 2.5

> *06/02/xx, 0800, reconstituted as 40 mg/mL. Expires 06/02/xx, 1600. Store at room temperature. G.D.P.*

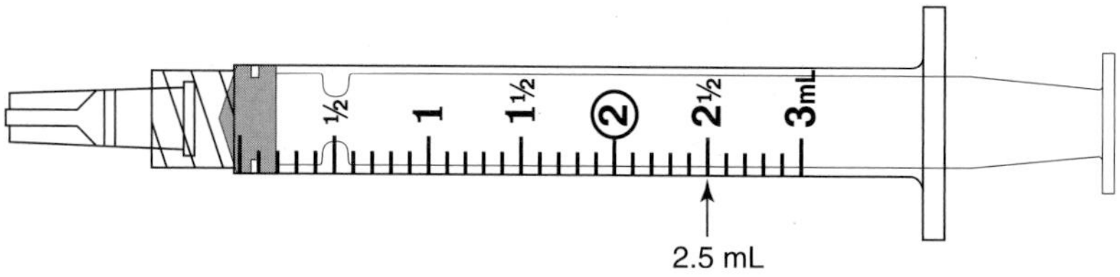

27) 12 doses are available, but the product is only good for 8 hours once reconstituted.

28) The medication will expire before all the doses are completed as the reconstituted vial of tobramycin is only stable for 8 hours at room temperature. The further diluted tobramycin within an IV infusion fluid is stable for 24 hours at room temperature or 36 hours refrigerated. Therefore, if the reconstituted tobramycin is added immediately to four different bags of the IV infusion liquid, the infusion fluid would be good for four doses if refrigerated.

29) 120; 240 **30)** 180; 60 **31)** 1280; 640 **32)** 6; 160 **33)** 3 **34)** 5407

35) 1.2

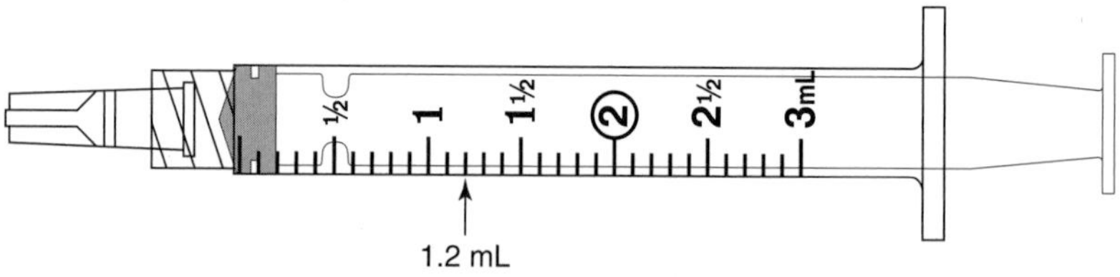

36) 129 mL; 5 mL; 1.5 mg/mL; 1.5 mL

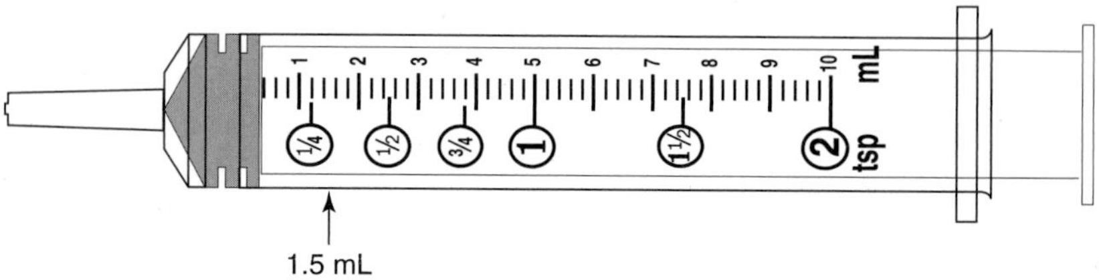

37) Order of 200 mg IV is insufficient for this child considering the circumstances. Physician should be called for clarification.

38) Order is too high and the maximum recommended dosage for this child is 292 mg/day. This order is for 748 mg/day. Recommended dosage is also twice daily and this order is for four times/day. This order is not safe. Physician should be called for clarification.

39) Order is too high and is not safe. The maximum recommended dosage for the child weighing 7.3 kg is 54.8 mg/day or 18.3 mg/dose. Physician should be called for clarification.

40) 250; 313

Selected Solutions—Section 3—Self-Evaluation

5) Order: 16 mEq

Supply: 20 mEq/15 mL

$$\frac{D}{H} \times Q = \frac{\overset{4}{\cancel{16}}\text{ mEq}}{\underset{5}{\cancel{20}}\text{ mEq}} \times 15\text{ mL} = \frac{4}{\underset{1}{\cancel{5}}} \times \overset{3}{\cancel{15}}\text{ mL} = 12\text{ mL}$$

7) Order: 75 mg

Supply: 25 mg/tab

$$\frac{D}{H} \times Q = \frac{\overset{3}{\cancel{75}}\ \cancel{\text{mcg}}}{\underset{1}{\cancel{25}}\ \cancel{\text{mcg}}} \times 1\text{ tab} = 3\text{ tab}$$

8) Order: 7.5 mg

Supply: 5 mg/tab

$$\frac{D}{H} \times Q = \frac{\overset{1.5}{\cancel{7.5}}\ \cancel{\text{mg}}}{\underset{1}{\cancel{5}}\ \cancel{\text{mg}}} \times 1\text{ tab} = 1.5\text{ tab}$$

9) Order: 12.5 mg

Supply: 10 mg/mL

$$\frac{D}{H} \times Q = \frac{12.5\ \cancel{\text{mg}}}{10\ \cancel{\text{mg}}} \times 1\text{ mL} = 1.25\text{ mL}$$

Answer should be left at 1.25 mL as the dropper supplied with the medication will measure 1.25 mL.

35) Recommended dosage:

$100\text{ mcg}/\cancel{\text{kg}}/\text{dose} \times 30.5\ \cancel{\text{kg}} =$ 3050 mcg (minimum) = 3 mg

$200\text{ mcg}/\cancel{\text{kg}}/\text{dose} \times 30.5\ \cancel{\text{kg}} =$ 6100 mcg (maximum) = 6.1 mg

Order: 6.0 mg

This dosage is safe.

$$\frac{D}{H} \times Q = \frac{6\ \cancel{\text{mg}}}{5\ \cancel{\text{mg}}} \times 1\text{ mL} = \frac{6}{5}\text{ mL} = 1.2\text{ mL}$$

36) Minimum daily dosage:

$25\text{ mg}/\cancel{\text{kg}}/\text{day} \times 6.8\ \cancel{\text{kg}} = 170\text{ mg/day}$

Minimum single dosage:

$170\text{ mg} \div 3\text{ doses} = 56.7\text{ mg/dose}$

Maximum daily dosage:

$40\text{ mg}/\cancel{\text{kg}}/\text{day} \times 6.8\ \cancel{\text{kg}} = 272\text{ mg/day}$

Maximum single dosage:

$272\text{ mg} \div 3\text{ doses} = 90.7\text{ mg/dose}$

Dosage ordered is safe.

$$\frac{D}{H} \times Q = \frac{75\ \cancel{\text{mg}}}{50\ \cancel{\text{mg}}} \times 1\text{ mL} = 1.5\text{ mL}$$

37) Recommended dosage:

$15\text{ mg}/\cancel{\text{kg}}/\text{day} \times 20\ \cancel{\text{kg}} = 300\text{ mg/day (minimum)}$

Order is insufficient to be effective. The prescriber should be contacted.

38) Recommended dosage:

$40\text{ mg}/\cancel{\text{kg}}/\text{day} \times 7.3\ \cancel{\text{kg}} = 292\text{ mg/day}$

Ordered dosage is not safe. The child would receive 187 mg × 4 doses or a total of 748 mg/day, which is over the recommended dosage of 292 mg/day.

39) Recommended dosage:

Minimum daily dosage:

$6\text{ mg}/\cancel{\text{kg}}/\text{day} \times 7.3\ \cancel{\text{kg}} = 43.8\text{ mg/day}$

Maximum daily dosage:

$7.5\text{ mg}/\cancel{\text{kg}}/\text{day} \times 7.3\ \cancel{\text{kg}} = 54.75 = 54.8\text{ mg/day}$

$54.8\text{ mg} \div 3\text{ doses} = 18.28 = 18.3\text{ mg/dose}$

Order is too high and is not safe. Recommended dosage is 14.5–18.3 mg/dose.

40) $7.5\text{ mg}/\cancel{\text{kg}}/\text{day} \times 125\ \cancel{\text{kg}} =$ 937.5 mg/day (maximum)

divided by 3 = 313 mg/dose

6 mg/kg/day × 125 mg = 750 mg/day (minimum)

divided by 3 = 250 mg/dose

Dosage range for this person would be between 250 mg to 313 mg per dose (maximum of 1.5 g/day or 1500 mg/day).

Answers to Review Set 27 from pages 317–319

1) C; sodium chloride 0.9%, 0.9 g/100 mL; 308 mOsm/L; isotonic
2) E; dextrose 5%, 5 g/100 mL; 252 mOsm/L; isotonic (Note: Although isotonic in the bag, D5W acts like a hypotonic solution once it enters the bloodstream because its low concentration of dextrose is quickly metabolized by the cells of the lining of the vein and the circulating cells in the bloodstream)
3) G; dextrose 5%, 5 g/100 mL; sodium chloride 0.9%, 0.9 g/100 mL; 560 mOsm/L; hypertonic
4) D; dextrose 5%, 5 g/100 mL, sodium chloride 0.45%, 0.45 g/100 mL; 406 mOsm/L; hypertonic
5) A; dextrose 5%, 5 g/100 mL, sodium chloride 0.225%, 0.225 g/100 mL; 329 mOsm/L; hypertonic
6) H; dextrose 5%, 5 g/100 mL; sodium lactate 0.31 g/100 mL, NaCl 0.6 g/100 mL; KCl 0.03 g/100 mL; CaCl 0.02 g/100 mL; 525 mOsm/L; hypertonic
7) B; dextrose 5%, 5 g/100 mL; sodium chloride 0.45%; 0.45 g/100 mL; potassium chloride 20 mEq per litre (0.149 g/100 mL); 447 mOsm/L; hypertonic
8) F; sodium chloride 0.45%, 0.45 g/100 mL; 154 mOsm/L; hypotonic

Answers to Review Set 28 from page 321

1) 50; 9 **2)** 25; 2.25 **3)** 25 **4)** 6.75 **5)** 25; 1.65 **6)** 150; 27 **7)** 50; 1.125 **8)** 36; 2.7 **9)** 100; 4.5 **10)** 3.375

Selected Solutions—Review Set 28

1) D_5 NS = 5 g dextrose per 100 mL and 0.9 g NaCl per 100 mL

Dextrose:

$$\frac{5\text{ g}}{100\text{ mL}} \times \frac{X\text{ g}}{1000\text{ mL}}$$

$$100X = 5000$$

$$\frac{100X}{100} = \frac{5000}{100}$$

$$X = 50\text{ g}$$

NaCl:

$$\frac{0.9\text{ g}}{100\text{ mL}} \times \frac{X\text{ g}}{1000\text{ mL}}$$

$$100X = 900$$

$$\frac{100X}{100} = \frac{900}{100}$$

$$X = 9\text{ g (NaCl)}$$

7) $D_{10}\frac{1}{4}$ NS = 10 g dextrose per 100 mL and 0.225 g NaCl per 100 mL

Dextrose:

$$\frac{10\text{ g}}{100\text{ mL}} \times \frac{X\text{ g}}{500\text{ mL}}$$

$$100X = 5000$$

$$\frac{100X}{100} = \frac{5000}{100}$$

$$X = 50\text{ g}$$

NaCl:

$$\frac{0.225\text{ g}}{100\text{ mL}} \times \frac{X\text{ g}}{500\text{ mL}}$$

$$100X = 112.5$$

$$\frac{100X}{100} = \frac{112.5}{100}$$

$$X = 1.125\text{ g (NaCl)}$$

Answers to Review Set 29 from page 330

1) 100 **2)** 120 **3)** 83 **4)** 200 **5)** 120 **6)** 125 **7)** 125 **8)** 200 **9)** 75 **10)** 125 **11)** 63 **12)** 24 **13)** 150 **14)** 125 **15)** 42

Selected Solutions—Review Set 29

1) 1 L = 1000 mL

$$\frac{\text{Total mL}}{\text{Total h}} = \frac{1000\text{ mL}}{10\text{ h}} = 100\text{ mL/h}$$

3) $$\frac{\text{Total mL}}{\text{Total h}} = \frac{2000\text{ mL}}{24\text{ h}} = 83.3\text{ mL/h} = 83\text{ mL/h}$$

4) $$\frac{100\text{ mL}}{\overset{}{\cancel{30\text{ min}}}_{1}} \times \frac{\overset{2}{\cancel{60\text{ min}}}}{\text{h}} = 200\text{ mL/h}$$

5) $$\frac{30\text{ mL}}{\cancel{15\text{ min}}_{1}} \times \frac{\overset{4}{\cancel{60\text{ min}}}}{\text{h}} = 120\text{ mL/h}$$

6) 2.5 L = 2.5 × 1000 = 2500 mL

$$\frac{\text{Total mL}}{\text{Total h}} = \frac{2500\text{ ml}}{20\text{ h}} = 125\text{ mL/h}$$

Answers to Review Set 30 from pages 332–333

1) 15 **2)** 10 **3)** 60 **4)** 60 **5)** 10

Answers to Review Set 31 from page 336

1) $\frac{V}{T} \times C = R$ **2)** 21 **3)** 50 **4)** 17 **5)** 25 **6)** 42 **7)** 26 **8)** 25 **9)** 50 **10)** 80 **11)** 20 **12)** 30 **13)** 8 **14)** 28 **15)** 40

Selected Solutions—Review Set 31

1) $\frac{V}{T} \times C = R$ or $\frac{\text{Volume}}{\text{Time in min}} \times \text{Drop Factor} = \text{Rate}$

Volume in mL divided by *time* in minutes, multiplied by the *drop factor calibration* in drops per millilitre, equals the flow *rate* in drops per minute.

2) $\frac{V}{T} \times C = \frac{125\ \cancel{\text{mL}}}{\cancel{60\ \text{min}}_{6}} \times \cancel{10}^{1}\ \text{gtt}/\cancel{\text{mL}}$

$= \frac{125\ \text{gtt}}{6\ \text{min}} = 20.8\ \text{gtt/min} = 21\ \text{gtt/min}$

3) $\frac{V}{T} \times C = \frac{50\ \cancel{\text{mL}}}{\cancel{60}_{1}\ \text{min}} \times \cancel{60}^{1}\ \text{gtt}/\cancel{\text{mL}} = 50\ \text{gtt/min}$

Recall that when drop factor is 60 mL/h, then mL/h = gtt/min.

4) $\frac{V}{T} \times C = \frac{100\ \cancel{\text{mL}}}{\cancel{60}_{6}\ \text{min}} \times \cancel{10}^{1}\ \text{gtt}/\cancel{\text{mL}}$

$= \frac{100\ \text{gtt}}{6\ \text{min}} = 16.6\ \text{gtt/min} = 17\ \text{gtt/min}$

6) Two 500 mL units of blood = 1000 mL total volume

$\text{mL/h} = \frac{1000\ \text{mL}}{4\ \text{h}} = 250\ \text{mL/h}$

$\frac{V}{T} \times C = \frac{250\ \cancel{\text{mL}}}{\cancel{60}_{6}\ \text{min}} \times \cancel{10}^{1}\ \text{gtt}/\cancel{\text{mL}}$

$= \frac{250\ \text{gtt}}{3\ \text{min}} = 41.6\ \text{gtt/min} = 42\ \text{gtt/min}$

7) $\frac{\text{Total mL}}{\text{Total h}} = \frac{1240\ \text{mL}}{12\ \text{h}} = 103.3\ \text{mL/h} = 103\ \text{mL/h}$

$\frac{V}{T} \times C = \frac{103\ \cancel{\text{mL}}}{\cancel{60}_{4}\ \text{min}} \times \cancel{15}^{1}\ \text{gtt}/\cancel{\text{mL}}$

$= \frac{103\ \text{gtt}}{4\ \text{min}} = 25.7\ \text{gtt/min} = 26\ \text{gtt/min}$

9) $\frac{150\ \cancel{\text{mL}}}{\cancel{45}_{3}\ \text{min}} \times \cancel{15}^{1}\ \text{gtt}/\cancel{\text{mL}} = \frac{\cancel{150}^{50}\ \text{gtt}}{\cancel{3}_{1}\ \text{min}} = 50\ \text{gtt/min}$

Answers to Review Set 32 from page 339

1) 60 **2)** 1 **3)** 4 **4)** 6 **5)** $\frac{\text{mL/h}}{\text{drop factor constant}} = \text{gtt/min}$ **6)** 50 **7)** 31 **8)** 28 **9)** 60 **10)** 8 **11)** 31 **12)** 14 **13)** 25 **14)** 11 **15)** 50

Selected Solutions—Review Set 32

3) $\frac{60}{15} = 4$

6) $\frac{\text{mL/h}}{\text{drop factor constant}} = \text{gtt/min}: \frac{200\ \text{mL/h}}{4}$

$= 50\ \text{gtt/min}$

7) $\frac{\text{mL/h}}{\text{drop factor constant}} = \text{gtt/min}: \frac{125\ \text{mL/h}}{4}$

$= 31.2\ \text{gtt/min} = 31\ \text{gtt/min}$

8) $\frac{\text{mL/h}}{\text{drop factor constant}} = \text{gtt/min}: \frac{165\ \text{mL/h}}{6}$

$= 27.5\ \text{gtt/min} = 28\ \text{gtt/min}$

9) $\frac{\text{mL/h}}{\text{drop factor constant}} = \text{gtt/min}: \frac{60\ \text{mL/h}}{1}$

$= 60\ \text{gtt/min}$

(Set the flow rate at the same number of gtt/min as the number of mL/h when the drop factor is 60 gtt/mL because the drop factor constant is 1.)

13) 0.5 L = 500 mL; $\frac{500\ \text{mL}}{20\ \text{h}} = 25\ \text{mL/h}$; since drop factor is 60 gtt/mL, then mL/h = gtt/min; so rate is 25 gtt/min.

14) 650 mL in 10 h $= \frac{650\ \text{mL}}{10\ \text{h}} = 65\ \text{mL/h}$

$\frac{\text{mL/h}}{\text{drop factor constant}} = \text{gtt/min}: \frac{65\ \text{mL/h}}{6}$

$= 10.8\ \text{gtt/min} = 11\ \text{gtt/min}$

Answers to Review Set 33 from pages 340–341

1) 125; 31 **2)** 100 **3)** 100; 17 **4)** 50 **5)** 125; 31 **6)** 125; 125 **7)** 18 **8)** 17 **9)** 25 **10)** 125 **11)** 83 **12)** 125 **13)** 200 **14)** 150 **15)** 200 **16)** 13.5 **17)** 20; 1.8 **18)** 22.5 **19)** 32.5; 2.145 **20)** 50; 2.25

Selected Solutions—Review Set 33

1) $\frac{\text{Total mL}}{\text{Total h}} = \frac{3000 \text{ mL}}{24 \text{ h}} = 125 \text{ mL/h}$

$\frac{V}{T} \times C = \frac{125 \cancel{\text{mL}}}{\underset{4}{\cancel{60}} \text{ min}} \times \overset{1}{\cancel{15}} \text{ gtt/}\cancel{\text{mL}} = \frac{125 \text{ gtt}}{4 \text{ min}}$

$= 31.3 \text{ gtt/min} = 31 \text{ gtt/min}$

7) $\frac{\text{mL/h}}{\text{drop factor constant}} = \text{gtt/min: } \frac{105 \text{ mL/h}}{6}$

$= 18 \text{ gtt/min}$

8) $\frac{\text{mL/h}}{\text{drop factor constant}} = \text{gtt/min: } \frac{100 \text{ mL/h}}{6}$

$= 16.6 \text{ gtt/min} = 17 \text{ gtt/min}$

10) $\frac{\text{Total mL}}{\text{Total h}} = \frac{1000 \text{ mL}}{8 \text{ h}} = 125 \text{ mL/h}$

13) $\frac{100 \text{ mL}}{\underset{1}{\cancel{30 \text{ min}}}} \times \frac{\overset{2}{\cancel{60 \text{ min}}}}{\text{h}} = 200 \text{ mL/h}$

15) $\frac{150 \text{ mL}}{\underset{3}{\cancel{45 \text{ min}}}} \times \frac{\overset{4}{\cancel{60 \text{ min}}}}{\text{h}} = 200 \text{ mL/h}$

16) $\frac{1}{2} \text{ NS} = 0.45\% \text{ NaCl} = 0.45 \text{ g NaCl per 100 mL}$

$\frac{0.45 \text{ g}}{100 \text{ mL}} \times \frac{X \text{ g}}{3000 \text{ mL}}$

$100X = 1350$

$\frac{100X}{100} = \frac{1350}{100}$

$X = 13.5 \text{ g (NaCl)}$

17) $D_{10}NS = 10\% \text{ dextrose} = 10 \text{ g dextrose per 100 mL and } 0.9\% \text{ NaCl} = 0.9 \text{ g NaCl per 100 mL}$

Dextrose:

$\frac{10 \text{ g}}{100 \text{ mL}} \times \frac{X \text{ g}}{200 \text{ mL}}$

$100X = 2000$

$\frac{100X}{100} = \frac{2000}{100}$

$X = 20 \text{ g (dextrose)}$

$\text{NS} = 0.9\% \text{ NaCl} = 0.9 \text{ g NaCl per 100 mL}$

NaCl:

$\frac{0.9 \text{ g}}{100 \text{ mL}} \times \frac{X \text{ g}}{200 \text{ mL}}$

$100X = 180$

$\frac{100X}{100} = \frac{180}{100}$

$X = 1.8 \text{ g (NaCl)}$

Answers to Review Set 34 from pages 344–346

1) 21; 6; 142; 24; 14%; reset to 24 gtt/min (14% increase is acceptable).

2) 42; 2; 180; 45; 7%; reset to 45 gtt/min (7% increase is acceptable).

3) 21; 4; 200; 33; 57%; recalculated rate 33 gtt/min (57% increase is unacceptable). Consult physician.

4) 28; 4; 188; 31; 11%; reset to 31 gtt/min (11% increase is acceptable).

5) 21; 4; 188; 31; 48% (48% increase is unacceptable). Consult physician.

6) 31; 1350; 10; 135; 34; 10%; reset to 34 gtt/min (10% increase is acceptable).

7) 25; 3; 233; 39; 56% (56% increase is unacceptable). Consult physician.

8) 17; 3; 83; 14; −18%; (−16% slower is acceptable). IV is ahead of schedule. Slow rate to 14 gtt/min, and observe patient's condition.

9) 13; 10; 60; 15; 15%; reset to 15 gtt/min (15% increase is acceptable).

10) 100; 5; 100; 100; 0%; IV is on time, so no adjustment is needed.

Selected Solutions—Review Set 34

1) $\frac{V}{T} \times C = \frac{125\ \cancel{mL}}{\underset{6}{\cancel{60}}\ min} \times \overset{1}{\cancel{10}}\ gtt/\cancel{mL} = \ = \frac{125\ gtt}{6\ min} = 20.8\ gtt/min = 21\ gtt/min$ (ordered rate)

$12\ h - 6\ h = 6\ h$

$\frac{\text{Remaining volume}}{\text{Remaining hours}} = \text{Recalculated mL/h}; \frac{850\ mL}{6\ h} = 141.6\ mL/h = 142\ mL/h$

$\frac{V}{T} \times C = \frac{142\ \cancel{mL}}{\underset{6}{\cancel{60}}\ min} \times \overset{1}{\cancel{10}}\ gtt/\cancel{mL} = \ = \frac{142\ gtt}{6\ min} = 23.5\ gtt/min = 24\ gtt/min$ (adjusted rate)

$\frac{\text{Adjusted gtt/min} - \text{Ordered gtt/min}}{\text{Ordered gtt/min}} = \text{\% of variation}; \frac{24 - 21}{21} = \frac{3}{21} = 0.14 = 14\%$ (within the acceptable % of variation); reset rate to 47 gtt/min

3) $\frac{V}{T} \times C = \frac{125\ \cancel{mL}}{\underset{6}{\cancel{60}}\ min} \times \overset{1}{\cancel{10}}\ gtt/\cancel{mL} = \ = \frac{125\ gtt}{6\ min} = 20.8\ gtt/min = 21\ gtt/min$ (ordered rate)

$8\ h - 4\ h = 4\ h$

$\frac{800\ mL}{4\ h} = 200\ mL/h; \frac{V}{T} \times C = \frac{200\ \cancel{mL}}{\underset{6}{\cancel{60}}\ min} \times \overset{1}{\cancel{10}}\ gtt/\cancel{mL} = \ = \frac{200\ gtt}{6\ min} = 33.3 = 33\ gtt/min$ (adjusted rate)

$\frac{\text{Adjusted gtt/min} - \text{Ordered gtt/min}}{\text{Ordered gtt/min}} = \text{\% of variation}; \frac{33 - 21}{21} = \frac{12}{21} = 0.3 = 57\%$ faster; unacceptable % of variation—call physician for a revised order

6) $\frac{V}{T} \times C = \frac{125\ \cancel{mL}}{\underset{4}{\cancel{60}}\ min} \times \overset{1}{\cancel{15}}\ gtt/\cancel{mL} = \ = \frac{125\ gtt}{4\ min} = 31.3\ gtt/min = 31\ gtt/min$ (ordered rate)

$2000\ mL - 650\ mL = 1350\ mL$ remaining; $16\ h - 6\ h = 10\ h$

$\frac{1350\ mL}{10\ h} = 135\ mL/h; \frac{V}{T} \times C = \frac{135\ \cancel{mL}}{\underset{4}{\cancel{60}}\ min} \times \overset{1}{\cancel{15}}\ gtt/\cancel{mL} = \frac{135\ gtt}{4\ min} = 33.7\ gtt/min = 34\ gtt/min$

$\frac{\text{Adjusted gtt/min} - \text{Ordered gtt/min}}{\text{Ordered gtt/min}} = \text{\% of variation}; \frac{34 - 31}{31} = \frac{3}{31} = 0.096 = 0.10 = 10\%$ (within acceptable % of variation); reset rate to 34 gtt/min

8) $\frac{V}{T} \times C = \frac{100\ \cancel{mL}}{\underset{6}{\cancel{60}}\ min} \times \overset{1}{\cancel{10}}\ gtt/\cancel{mL} = \frac{100\ gtt}{6\ min} = 16.7\ gtt/min = 17\ gtt/min$ (ordered rate)

$5\ h - 2\ h = 3\ h$

$\frac{250\ mL}{3\ h} = 83.3\ mL/h = 83\ mL/h; \frac{V}{T} \times C = \frac{83\ \cancel{mL}}{\underset{6}{\cancel{60}}\ min} \times \overset{1}{\cancel{10}}\ gtt/\cancel{mL} = \frac{83\ gtt}{6\ min} = 13.7\ gtt/min$

$= 14\ gtt/min$ (adjusted rate)

$\frac{\text{Adjusted gtt/min} - \text{Ordered gtt/min}}{\text{Ordered gtt/min}} = \text{\% of variation}; \frac{14 - 17}{17} = \frac{-3}{17} = -0.176 = -18\%$

(Remember the [−] sign indicates the IV is ahead of schedule and rate must be decreased.) Within the acceptable % of variation. Slow IV to 14 gtt/min, and closely monitor patient.

Answers to Review Set 35 from pages 352–354

1) 133 **2)** 133 **3)** 50 **4)** 200 **5)** 100 **6)** 25 **7)** 50 **8)** 200 **9)** 150 **10)** 167 **11)** 67 **12)** 25 **13)** 120 **14)** 63 **15)** 200 **16)** 12; 3; 1 **17)** 3; 3; 0.25 **18)** 0.6; 2; 24; 0.06 **19)** 2; 18; 10; 2.5 **20)** 1.5; 1.25; 0.3

Selected Solutions—Review Set 35

1) $\frac{V}{T} \times C = \frac{100 \cancel{mL}}{\overset{}{\cancel{45}}_{3} \text{ min}} \times \overset{4}{\cancel{60}} \text{ gtt}/\cancel{mL} = \frac{400 \text{ gtt}}{3 \text{ min}}$

$= 133.3 \text{ gtt/min} = 133 \text{ gtt/min}$

2) $\frac{100 \text{ mL}}{45 \text{ mn}} \times \frac{X \text{ mL}}{60 \text{ min}}$

$45X = 6000$

$\frac{45X}{45} = \frac{6000}{45}$

$X = 133.3 \text{ mL} = 133 \text{ mL}$

$133 \text{ mL}/60 \text{ min} = 133 \text{ mL/h}$

3) $\frac{V}{T} \times C = \frac{50 \cancel{mL}}{\cancel{15}_{1} \text{ min}} \times \overset{1}{\cancel{15}} \text{ gtt}/\cancel{mL} = 50 \text{ gtt/min}$

4) $\frac{50 \text{ mL}}{15 \text{ min}} \times \frac{X \text{ mL}}{60 \text{ min}}$

$15X = 3000$

$\frac{15X}{15} = \frac{3000}{15}$

$X = 200 \text{ mL}$

$200 \text{ mL}/60 \text{ min} = 200 \text{ mL/h}$

11) $\frac{V}{T} \times C = \frac{100 \cancel{mL}}{\cancel{15}_{3} \text{ min}} \times \overset{2}{\cancel{10}} \text{ gtt}/\cancel{mL} = \frac{200 \text{ gtt}}{3 \text{ min}}$

$= 66.6 \text{ gtt/min} = 67 \text{ gtt/min}$

16) $\frac{D}{H} \times Q = \frac{12\cancel{0} \cancel{mg}}{1\cancel{0} \cancel{mg}} \times 1 \text{ mL} = 12 \text{ mL}$

$\frac{D}{H} \times Q = \frac{\overset{3}{\cancel{120}} \text{ mg}}{\cancel{40}_{1} \text{ mg}} \times 1 \text{ min} = 3 \text{ min}$

Administer 12 mL over at least 3 min.

$1 \text{ min} = 60 \text{ sec}$

$3 \text{ min} = 3 \times 60 = 180 \text{ sec}$

$\frac{12 \text{ mL}}{180 \text{ sec}} \times \frac{X \text{ mL}}{15 \text{ sec}}$

$180X = 180$

$\frac{180X}{180} = \frac{180}{180}$

$X = 1 \text{ mL per 15 sec}$

17) $\frac{D}{H} \times Q = \frac{150 \cancel{mg}}{\cancel{250}_{50} \cancel{mg}} \times \overset{1}{\cancel{5}} \text{ mL} = = \frac{\overset{3}{\cancel{150}}}{\cancel{50}_{1}} \text{ mL} = 3 \text{ mL}$

$\frac{D}{H} \times Q = \frac{\overset{3}{\cancel{150}} \cancel{mg}}{\cancel{50}_{1} \cancel{mg}} \times 1 \text{ min} = 3 \text{ min}$

Administer 3 mL over 3 min.

$1 \text{ min} = 60 \text{ sec}$

$3 \text{ min} = 3 \times 60 = 180 \text{ sec}$

$\frac{3 \text{ mL}}{180 \text{ sec}} \times \frac{X \text{ mL}}{15 \text{ sec}}$

$180X = 45$

$\frac{180X}{180} = \frac{45}{180}$

$X = 0.25 \text{ mL (per 15 sec)}$

18) $\frac{D}{H} \times Q = \frac{6 \cancel{mg}}{10 \cancel{mg}} \times 1 \text{ mL} = \frac{6}{10} \text{ mL} = 0.6 \text{ mL}$

$\frac{D}{H} \times Q = \frac{6 \cancel{mg}}{2.5 \cancel{mg}} \times 1 \text{ min} = 2.4 \text{ min}$

$1 \text{ min} = 60 \text{ sec}$

$2 \text{ min} = 2 \times 60 = 120 \text{ sec}; 0.4 \text{ min} = 0.4 \times 60 =$ 24 sec

$120 \text{ sec} + 24 \text{ sec} = 144 \text{ sec}$

$\frac{0.6 \text{ mL}}{144 \text{ sec}} \times \frac{X \text{ mL}}{15 \text{ sec}}$

$144X = 9$

$\frac{144X}{144} = \frac{9}{144}$

$X = 0.06 \text{ mL (per 15 sec)}$

Answers to Review Set 36 from pages 357–359

1) 2 h and 47 min **2)** 6 h and 40 min **3)** 8 **4)** 6; 20 **5)** 4; 20 **6)** Approximately 11; 0300 the next morning **7)** 16; 0730 the next morning **8)** 3000 **9)** 1152 **10)** 3024 **11)** 260 **12)** 300 **13)** 600 **14)** 480, 320 **15)** 240, 1080

Selected Solutions—Review Set 36

1) $\frac{V}{T} \times C = R$; notice T is the missing quantity

$\frac{500 \text{ mL}}{T \text{ min}} \times 10 \text{ gtt/mL} = 30 \text{ gtt/min}$

$\frac{5000}{T} \times \frac{30}{1}$

$30T = 5000$

$\frac{30T}{30} = \frac{5000}{30}$

$T = 166.7 \text{ min}$

$166.7 \text{ min} = \frac{166.7}{60} = 2 \text{ h and } 47 \text{ min}$

2) $\frac{V}{T} \times C = R$; notice T is the missing quantity

$\frac{1000 \text{ mL}}{T \text{ min}} \times 10 \text{ gtt/mL} = 25 \text{ gtt/min}$

$\frac{10\,000}{T} = \frac{25}{1}$

$25T = 10\,000$

$\frac{25T}{25} = \frac{10\,000}{25}$

$T = 400 \text{ min}$

$400 \text{ min} = \frac{400}{60} = 6 \text{ h and } 40 \text{ min}$

4) Time: $\frac{\text{Total vol}}{\text{mL/h}} = \text{Total h}$

$\frac{120 \cancel{\text{mL}}}{20 \cancel{\text{mL}}/\text{h}} = 6 \text{ h}$

$\frac{V}{T} \times C = \frac{20 \cancel{\text{mL}}}{\cancel{60}_1 \text{ min}} \times \cancel{60}^1 \text{ gtt/}\cancel{\text{mL}} = 20 \text{ gtt/min}$

6) $\frac{V}{T} \times C = R$; notice T is the missing quantity

$\frac{1200 \text{ mL}}{T \text{ min}} \times 15 \text{ gtt/mL} = 27 \text{ gtt/min}$

$\frac{18\,000}{T} = \frac{27}{1}$

$27T = 18\,000$

$\frac{27T}{27} = \frac{18\,000}{27}$

$T = 667 \text{ min}; 667 \text{ min} = \frac{667}{60} = 11 \text{ h and } 7 \text{ min}$

or 11 h (rounded)

$1600 + 1100\ (11\text{h}) = 2700 - 2400 = 0300$

7) Time: $\frac{\text{Total vol}}{\text{mL/h}} = \text{Total h}$

$\frac{2000 \cancel{\text{mL}}}{125 \cancel{\text{mL}}/\text{h}} = 16 \text{ h}$

$1530 + 1600 = 3130 - 2400 = 0730$

8) Total hours × mL/h = Total volume

$24 \cancel{\text{h}} \times 125 \text{ mL/}\cancel{\text{h}} = 3000 \text{ mL}$

9) $\frac{V}{T} \times C = R$; notice V is the missing quantity

$\frac{V \text{ mL}}{1440 \text{ min}} \times 15 \text{ gtt/mL} = 12 \text{ gtt/min}$

$\frac{15V}{1440} = \frac{12}{}$

$15V = 17\,280$

$\frac{15V}{15} = \frac{17\,280}{15}$

$V = 1152 \text{ mL}$

11) $65 \text{ mL/}\cancel{\text{h}} \times 4 \cancel{\text{h}} = 260 \text{ mL}$

14) $8 \text{ h} = 8 \times 60 = 480 \text{ min}$

$\frac{V}{T} \times C = R$; notice V is the missing quantity

$\frac{V \text{ mL}}{480 \text{ min}} \times 60 \text{ gtt/mL} = 40 \text{ gtt/min}$

$\frac{60V}{480} = \frac{40}{1}$

$60V = 19\,200$

$\frac{60V}{60} = \frac{19\,200}{60}$

$V = 320 \text{ mL}$

15) $4 \text{ h} = 4 \times 60 = 240 \text{ min}$

$\frac{V}{T} \times C = R$; notice V is the missing quantity

$\frac{V \text{ ml}}{240 \text{ min}} \times 10 \text{ gtt/mL} = 45 \text{ gtt/min}$

$\frac{10V}{240} = \frac{45}{1}$

$10V = 10\,800$

$\frac{10V}{10} = \frac{10\,800}{10}$

$V = 1080 \text{ mL}$

Answers to Practice Problems—Chapter 12 from pages 360–363

1) 17 **2)** 42 **3)** 21 **4)** 8 **5)** 125 **6)** Assess patient. If stable, recalculate and reset to 114 mL/h, acceptable variation of 9%; observe patient closely. **7)** 31 **8)** 21 **9)** Assess patient. If stable, recalculate and reset to 50 gtt/min, acceptable variation of 19%; observe patient closely. **10)** 3000 **11)** Abbott Laboratories **12)** 15 gtt/mL **13)** 4

14) $\text{mL/h} = \frac{500 \text{ mL}}{4 \text{ h}} = 125 \text{ mL/h}$

$\frac{\text{mL/h}}{\text{drop factor constant}} = \text{gtt/min: } \frac{125 \text{ mL/h}}{4} = 31.2 \text{ gtt/min} = 31 \text{ gtt/min}$

15) $\frac{V}{T} \times C = \frac{125 \cancel{\text{mL}}}{\cancel{60}_4 \text{ min}} \times \cancel{15}^1 \text{ gtt/}\cancel{\text{mL}} = \frac{125 \text{ gtt}}{4 \text{ min}} = 31.3 \text{ gtt/min} = 31 \text{ gtt/min}$

16) 1930 **17)** 250 **18)** Recalculate 210 mL to infuse over remaining 2 hours, acceptable variation. Reset IV to 26 gtt/min and observe patient closely. **19)** 125 **20)** 100 **21)** Dextrose 2.5% (2.5 g/100 mL) and NaCl 0.45% (0.45 g/100 mL) **22)** 25; 4.5 **23)** A central line is a special catheter inserted to access a large vein in the chest. **24)** A primary line is the IV tubing used to set up a primary IV infusion. **25)** The purpose of a saline lock is to administer IV medications when the patient does not require continuous IV fluids. **26)** 10; 5; 0.5; 0.13 **27)** The purpose of the PCA pump is to allow the patient to safely self-administer IV pain medication without having to call the nurse for a prn medication. **28)** Advantages of the syringe pump are that a small amount of medication can be delivered directly from the syringe, and a specified time can be programmed in the pump. **29)** Phlebitis and infiltration **30)** q $\frac{1}{2}$ − 1 h, according to institution policy **31)** This IV tubing has two spikes—one for blood, the other for saline—that join at a common drip chamber or Y connection. **32)** 14 **33)** 21 **34)** 83 **35)** 17 **36)** 25 **37)** 100 **38)** 33 **39)** 50 **40)** 200 **41)** 8 **42)** 11 **43)** 45 **44)** 150. The IV will finish in 1 hour. **45)** 1250

46) Critical Thinking Skill: Prevention.

This error could have been prevented had the nurse carefully inspected the IV tubing package to determine the drop factor. Every IV tubing set has the drop factor printed on the package, so it is not necessary to memorize or guess the drop factor. The IV calculation should have looked like this:

$$\frac{125\ \cancel{mL}}{\cancelto{6}{60}\ min} \times \cancelto{1}{10}\ gtt/\cancel{mL} = \frac{125\ gtt}{6\ min} = 20.8\ gtt/min = 21\ gtt/min$$

With the infusion set of 10 gtt/mL, a flow rate of 21 gtt/min would infuse 125 mL/h. At the 125-gtt/min rate the nurse calculated, the patient received six times the IV fluid ordered hourly. Thus, the patient actually received 750 mL/h of IV fluids.

Selected Solutions—Practice Problems—Chapter 12

1) $\frac{\text{Total mL}}{\text{Total h}} = \frac{200\ mL}{2\ h} = 100\ mL/h$

$\frac{V}{T} \times C = \frac{100\ \cancel{mL}}{\cancelto{6}{60}\ min} \times \cancelto{1}{10}\ gtt/\cancel{mL} = \frac{100\ gtt}{6\ min}$

$= 16.6\ gtt/min = 17\ gtt/min$

2) $\frac{\text{Total mL}}{\text{Total h}} = \frac{1000\ mL}{24\ h} = 41.6\ mL/h = 42\ mL/h$

drop factor is 60 gtt/mL: 42 mL/h = 42 gtt/min

5) $\frac{\text{Total mL}}{\text{Total h}} = \frac{1000\ mL}{8\ h} = 125\ mL/h$

6) $\frac{\text{Total mL}}{\text{Total h}} = \frac{800\ mL}{7\ h} = 114.2\ mL/h = 114\ mL/h$

$\frac{\text{Adjusted gtt/min} - \text{Ordered gtt/min}}{\text{Ordered gtt/min}} = \%\ \text{variation:}$

$\frac{144 - 25}{125} = \frac{-11}{125} = -0.088 = -9\%\ \text{(decrease)};$

within safe limits of 25% variance.

Reset infusion rate to 114 mL/h.

7) 1000 mL + 2000 mL = 3000 mL;

$\frac{\text{Total mL}}{\text{Total h}} = \frac{3000\ mL}{24\ h} = 125\ mL/h$

$\frac{V}{T} \times C = \frac{125\ \cancel{mL}}{\cancelto{4}{60}\ min} \times \cancelto{1}{15}\ gtt/\cancel{mL} = \frac{125\ gtt}{4\ min}$

$= 31.3\ gtt/min = 31\ gtt/min$

8) $\frac{V}{T} \times C = \frac{125\ \cancel{mL}}{\cancelto{6}{60}\ min} \times \cancelto{1}{10}\ gtt/\cancel{mL} = \frac{125\ gtt}{6\ min}$

$= 20.6\ gtt/min = 21\ gtt/min$

9) $\frac{\text{Total mL}}{\text{Total h}} = \frac{1000\ mL}{6\ h} = 166.6\ mL/h = 167\ mL/h$

$\frac{V}{T} \times C = \frac{167\ \cancel{mL}}{\cancelto{4}{60}\ min} \times \cancelto{1}{15}\ gt/\cancel{mL} = \frac{167\ gtt}{4\ min}$

$= 41.7\ gtt/min = 42\ gtt/min$

6 h − 2 h = 4 h remaining;

$\frac{\text{Total mL}}{\text{Total h}} = \frac{\cancelto{200}{800}\ mL}{\cancelto{1}{4}\ h} = 200\ mL/h$

$\frac{V}{T} \times C = \frac{200\ \cancel{mL}}{\cancelto{4}{60}\ min} \times \cancelto{1}{15}\ gtt/\cancel{mL} = \frac{\cancelto{50}{200}\ gtt}{\cancelto{1}{4}\ min}$

$= 50\ gtt/min$

$\frac{\text{Adjusted gtt/min} - \text{Ordered gtt/min}}{\text{Ordered gtt/min}} = \%\ \text{variation:}$

$\frac{50 - 42}{42} = \frac{8}{42} = 0.19 = 19\%\ \text{increase};$

within safe limits of 25% variance

Reset infusion rate to 50 gtt/min.

10) q4h = 6 times/24 h; 6 × 500 mL = 3000 mL

13) $\frac{60}{15} = 4$

16) $1530 + 4\text{ h} = 1530 + 0400 = 1930$

17) $\frac{\text{Total mL}}{\text{Total h}} = \frac{500\text{ mL}}{4\text{ h}} = 125\text{ mL/h}$

$125\text{ mL/}\cancel{\text{h}} \times 2\,\cancel{\text{h}} = 250\text{ mL}$

18) $\frac{\text{Total mL}}{\text{Total h}} = \frac{210\text{ mL}}{2\text{ h}} = 105\text{ mL/h}$

$\frac{V}{T} \times C = \frac{105\,\cancel{\text{mL}}}{\cancel{60}^{4}\text{ min}} \times \cancel{15}^{1}\text{ gtt/}\cancel{\text{mL}} = \frac{105\text{ gtt}}{4\text{ min}}$

$= 26.2\text{ gtt/min} = 26\text{ gtt/min}$

$\frac{\text{Adjusted gtt/min} - \text{Ordered gtt/min}}{\text{Ordered gtt/min}} = \%\text{ variation:}$

$\frac{26 - 31}{31} = \frac{-5}{31} = 0.16 = -16\%$ decrease; within safe limits

Reset infusion rate to 26 gtt/min.

19) $\frac{\text{Total mL}}{\text{Total h}} = \frac{500\text{ mL}}{4\text{ h}} = 125\text{ mL/h}$

20) $\frac{50\text{ mL}}{30\text{ min}} \rightleftarrows \frac{X\text{ mL}}{60\text{ min}}$

$30X = 3000$

$\frac{30X}{30} = \frac{3000}{30}$

$X = 100\text{ mL/h}$

22) Dextrose 5% = 5 g/100 mL NaCl 0.9% = 0.9 g/100 mL

Dextrose:

$\frac{5\text{ g}}{100\text{ mL}} \rightleftarrows \frac{X\text{ g}}{500\text{ mL}}$

$100X = 2500$

$\frac{100X}{100} = \frac{2500}{100}$

$X = 25\text{ g}$

NaCl:

$\frac{0.9\text{ g}}{100\text{ mL}} \rightleftarrows \frac{X\text{ g}}{500\text{ mL}}$

$100X = 450$

$\frac{100X}{100} = \frac{450}{100}$

$X = 4.5\text{ g}$

26) $\frac{5\text{ mg}}{1\text{ min}} \rightleftarrows \frac{50\text{ mg}}{X\text{ min}}$

$5X = 50$

$\frac{5X}{5} = \frac{50}{5}$

$X = 10\text{ min}$

$\frac{D}{C} \times Q = \frac{\cancel{50}^{5}\,\cancel{\text{mg}}}{\cancel{10}_{1}\,\cancel{\text{mg}}} \times 1\text{ mL} = 5\text{ mL}$

Give 50 mg/10 min or 5 mL/10 min; 0.5 mL/min

$1\text{ min} = 60\text{ sec}$

$10\text{ min} = 10 \times 60 = 600\text{ sec}$

$\frac{5\text{ mL}}{600\text{ sec}} \rightleftarrows \frac{X\text{ mL}}{15\text{ sec}}$

$600X = 75$

$\frac{600X}{600} = \frac{75}{600}$

$X = 0.13\text{ mL/15 sec}$

32) $\frac{\text{Total mL}}{\text{Total h}} = \frac{1000\text{ mL}}{12\text{ h}} = 83.3\text{ mL/h}$

$= 83\text{ mL/h}; \frac{V}{T} \times C$

$= \frac{83\,\cancel{\text{mL}}}{\cancel{60}_{6}\text{ min}} \times \cancel{10}^{1}\text{ gtt/}\cancel{\text{mL}} = \frac{83\text{ gtt}}{6\text{ min}} = 13.8\text{ gtt/min}$

$= 14\text{ gtt/min}$

33) $\frac{V}{T} \times C = \frac{83\,\cancel{\text{mL}}}{\cancel{60}_{4}\text{ min}} \times \cancel{15}^{1}\text{ gtt/}\cancel{\text{mL}} = \frac{83\text{ gtt}}{4\text{ min}}$

$= 20.7\text{ gtt/min} = 21\text{ gtt/min}$

34) $\frac{V}{T} \times C = \frac{83\,\cancel{\text{mL}}}{\cancel{60}_{1}\text{ min}} \times \cancel{60}^{1}\text{ gtt/}\cancel{\text{mL}} = 83\text{ gtt/min}$

Remember, if drop factor is 60 gtt/mL, then mL/ h = gtt/min; so 83 mL/h = 83 gtt/min

44) $\frac{V}{T} \times C = R$; V is the unknown quantity

$\frac{V\text{ mL}}{60\text{ min}} \times 10\text{ gtt/mL} = 25\text{ gtt/min}$

$\frac{10V}{60} \rightleftarrows \frac{25}{1}$

$10V = 1500$

$\frac{10V}{10} = \frac{1500}{10}$

$V = 150\text{ mL}$

45) $\frac{400\,\cancel{\text{mL}}}{75\,\cancel{\text{mL}}\text{/h}} = 5\frac{1}{3}$ h or 5 h and 20 min

$0730 + 0520 = 1250$

Answers to Review Set 37 from page 368

1) 2.35 **2)** 0.69 **3)** 1.40 **4)** 2.03 **5)** 1.66 **6)** 1.69 **7)** 0.52 **8)** 0.78 **9)** 0.15 **10)** 0.78 **11)** 0.39 **12)** 0.64 **13)** 1.08 **14)** 0.5 **15)** 0.88

Selected Solutions—Review Set 37

1) Metric: $\text{BSA (m}^2) = \sqrt{\frac{\text{ht (cm)} \times \text{wt (kg)}}{3600}} = \sqrt{\frac{190 \times 105}{3600}} = \sqrt{\frac{19\,950}{3600}} = \sqrt{5.542} = 2.354 \text{ m}^2 = 2.35 \text{ m}^2$

Answers to Review Set 38 from pages 370–372

1) 1 640 000 **2)** 5.9; 11.8 **3)** 735 **4)** 1584; 6.34 **5)** 250 **6)** 0.48; 120; Yes; 2.4 **7)** 0.89; 2.9; Yes; 1.2 **8)** 66; 22; Yes; **9)**198; Yes; 990 **10)** 612; 612; 1224; 2448 **11)** 8.1; 24.7 **12)** 67–167.5; 33.5–83.8; Yes **13)** 8–14.4; Yes **14)** 0.82; 2050; Yes; 2.7; 102.7; 51 **15)** 1.62; 4050; Yes; 5.4; 105.4; 53

Selected Solutions—Review Set 38

1) $2\,000\,000 \text{ units}/\cancel{\text{m}^2} \times 0.82 \cancel{\text{m}^2} = 1\,640\,000 \text{ units}$

2) $10 \text{ mg}/\cancel{\text{m}^2}/\text{day} \times 0.59 \cancel{\text{m}^2} = 5.9 \text{ mg/day}$ (minimum safe dosage)

$20 \text{ mg}/\cancel{\text{m}^2}/\text{day} \times 0.59 \cancel{\text{m}^2} = 11.8 \text{ mg/day}$ (maximum safe dosage)

3) $500 \text{ mg}/\cancel{\text{m}^2} \times 1.47 \cancel{\text{m}^2} = 735 \text{ mg}$

4) $600 \text{ mg/m}^2/\text{dose} \times 2.64 \cancel{\text{m}^2} = 1584 \text{ mg/day}$

8) $900 \text{ mg}/\cancel{\text{m}^2}/\text{day} \times 0.22 \cancel{\text{m}^2} = 198 \text{ mg/day};$ dosage is safe

$198 \text{ mg/day} \times 5 \text{ days} = 990 \text{ mg}$

10) $600 \text{ mg}/\cancel{\text{m}^2} \times 1.02 \cancel{\text{m}^2} = 612 \text{ mg}$, initially

$300 \text{ mg}/\cancel{\text{m}^2} \times 1.02 \cancel{\text{m}^2} = 306 \text{ mg}$; for 2 doses:

$306 \text{ mg} \times 2 = 612 \text{ mg}$

q12h is 2 doses/day and

$2 \text{ doses}/\cancel{\text{day}} \times 2 \cancel{\text{days}} = 4 \text{ doses}$

$306 \text{ mg} \times 4 = 1224 \text{ mg}$

$612 \text{ mg} + 612 \text{ mg} + 1224 \text{ mg} = 2448 \text{ mg (total)}$

12) Metric: $\text{BSA (m}^2) = \sqrt{\frac{\text{ht (cm)} \times \text{wt (kg)}}{3600}} =$

$\sqrt{\frac{100 \times 24}{3600}} = \sqrt{\frac{2400}{3600}} = \sqrt{0.667} = 0.816 \text{ m}^2 = 0.82 \text{ m}^2$

$2500 \text{ units}/\cancel{\text{m}^2} \times 0.82 \cancel{\text{m}^2} = 2050 \text{ units}$; dosage is safe

$\frac{D}{H} \times Q = \frac{2050 \cancel{\text{U}}}{750 \cancel{\text{U}}} \times 1 \text{ mL} = 2.7 \text{ mL}$

$\frac{102.7 \text{ mL}}{2 \text{ h}} = 51.3 \text{ mL/h} = 51 \text{ mL/h}$

13) Metric: $\text{BSA (m}^2) = \sqrt{\frac{\text{ht (cm)} \times \text{wt (kg)}}{3600}} =$

$\sqrt{\frac{58.2 \times 162}{3600}} = \sqrt{\frac{9428.4}{3600}} = \sqrt{2.619} = 1.62 \text{ m}^2$

$2500 \text{ units}/\cancel{\text{m}^2} \times 1.62 \cancel{\text{m}^2} = 4050 \text{ units}$; dosage is safe

$\frac{D}{H} \times Q = \frac{4050 \cancel{\text{units}}}{750 \cancel{\text{units}}} \times 1 \text{ mL} = 5.4 \text{ mL}$

Total volume: 100 mL IV fluid + 5.4 mL med. = 105.4 mL

$\frac{105.4 \text{ mL}}{2 \text{ h}} = 52.7 \text{ mL/h} = 53 \text{ mL/h}$

Answers to Review Set 39 from pages 375–377

1) 87; 0.5; 50 **2)** 49.5; 5.6; 50 **3)** 120; 1.8; 25 **4)** 80; 6; 50 **5)** 60; 1; 32; 180 **6)** 2; 25 **7)** 0.5; 10 **8)** 12; 57 **9)** 7.2; 44 **10)** 10.5; 45

Selected Solutions—Review Set 39

1) Total volume: 50 mL + 15 mL = 65 mL

$\frac{V}{T} \times C = \frac{65 \cancel{\text{mL}}}{\cancelto{3}{45} \text{ min}} \times \cancelto{4}{60} \text{ gtt}/\cancel{\text{mL}} =$

$\frac{260 \text{ gtt}}{3 \text{ min}} = 86.6 \text{ gtt/min} = 87 \text{ gtt/min}$

$\frac{D}{H} \times Q = \frac{\cancel{125 \text{ mg}}}{\cancel{250 \text{ mg}}} \times 1 \text{ mL} = 0.5 \text{ mL (medication)}$

9.5

Add 0.5 mL amikacin to the chamber and fill with IV fluid to a volume of 50 mL. Follow with the 15-mL flush also set at 87 gtt/min

4) Total volume: 50 mL + 30 mL = 80 mL

80 mL/60 min = 80 mL/h

$$\frac{D}{H} \times Q = \frac{0.6\ \cancel{g}}{1\ \cancel{g}} \times 10\ mL = 6\ mL\ (medication)$$

Add 6 mL cefazolin sodium to the chamber and fill with IV fluid to a volume of 50 mL. Follow with the 30mL flush.

6)
$$\frac{50\ mL}{60\ min} \times \frac{X\ mL}{30\ min}$$

$$60X = 1500$$

$$\frac{60X}{60} = \frac{1500}{60}$$

$$X = 25\ mL\ (total\ volume)$$

$$\frac{D}{H} \times Q = \frac{\overset{2}{\cancel{250}}\ mg}{\underset{1}{\cancel{125}}\ mg} \times 1\ mL = 2\ mL\ (medication)$$

Add 2 mL cefazolin sodium to the chamber and fill with IV fluid to a volume of 25 mL.

8)
$$\frac{85\ mL}{60\ min} \times \frac{X\ mL}{40\ min}$$

$$60X = 3400$$

$$\frac{60X}{60} = \frac{3400}{60}$$

$$X = 56.6\ mL = 57\ mL\ (total\ volume)$$

$$\frac{D}{H} \times Q = \frac{\overset{12}{\cancel{600\ mg}}}{\underset{1}{\cancel{50\ mg}}} \times 1\ mL = 12\ mL\ (medication)$$

Add 12 mL erythromycin to the chamber and fill with IV fluid to a volume of 57 mL.

9)
$$\frac{66\ mL}{60\ min} = \frac{X\ mL}{40\ min}$$

$$60X = 2640$$

$$\frac{60X}{60} = \frac{2640}{60}$$

$$X = 44\ mL\ (total\ volume)$$

$$\frac{D}{H} \times Q = \frac{720\ \cancel{mg}}{\underset{100}{\cancel{1000}}\ \cancel{mg}} \times \overset{1}{\cancel{10}}\ mL$$

$$= \frac{720}{100}\ mL = 7.2\ mL\ (medication)$$

Add 7.2 mL ceftazidime to the chamber and fill with IV fluid to a volume of 44 mL.

Answers to Review Set 40 from pages 380–381

1) 4 **2)** 25 **3)** 1600; 67 **4)** 1150; 48 **5)** 1800; 75 **6)** 350; 15 **7)** 3.5 or 4; 11.6 or 12 **8)** 2.6 or 3; 65 **9)** 2.3 or 3; 35 **10)** This order should be questioned because normal saline is an isotonic solution and appears to be a continuous infusion for this child. This solution does not contribute enough electrolytes for the child and water intoxication may result. A 1000mL bag would last 20 h (too long to hang one bag; it is better to use a 250 mL or 500 mL bag for children)

Selected Solutions—Review Set 40

1)
$$\frac{100\ mg}{1\ mL} \times \frac{400\ mg}{X\ mL}$$

$$100X = 400$$

$$\frac{100X}{100} = \frac{400}{100}$$

$$X = 4\ mL$$

3)
100 mL/$\cancel{kg}$/day × 10 $\cancel{kg}$ = 1000 mL/day for first 10

50 mL/$\cancel{kg}$/day × 10 $\cancel{kg}$ = 500 mL/day for next 10

20 mL/$\cancel{kg}$/day × 5 $\cancel{kg}$ = 100 mL/day for remaining

1600 mL/day or per 24 h

$$\frac{1600\ mL}{24\ h} = 66.7\ mL/h = 67\ mL/h$$

4)
100 mL/$\cancel{kg}$/day × 10 $\cancel{kg}$ = 1000 mL/day for first 10 kg

150 mL/day × 3 $\cancel{kg}$ = 150 mL/day for next 10 kg

1150 mL/day or per 24 h

$$\frac{1150\ mL}{24\ h} = 47.9\ mL/h = 48\ mL/h$$

5)
$$77\ lb = \frac{77}{2.2} = 35\ kg$$

100 mL/$\cancel{kg}$/day × 10 $\cancel{kg}$ = 1000 mL/day for first 10

50 mL/kg/day × 10 kg = 500 mL/day for next 10

20 mL/kg/day × 15 kg = 300 mL/day for remaining

1800 mL/day or per 24 h

$$\frac{1800\ mL}{24\ h} = 75\ mL/h$$

7)
$$\frac{100\ mg}{1\ ml} \times \frac{350\ mg}{X\ mL}$$

$$100X = 350$$

$$\frac{100X}{100} = \frac{350}{100}$$

X = 3.5 or 4 mL (min. dilution volu me)

$$\frac{30\ mg}{1\ mL} \times \frac{350\ mg}{X\ mL}$$

$$30X = 350$$

$$\frac{30X}{30} = \frac{350}{30}$$

X = 11.6 or 12 mL (max. dilution volume)

Answers to Practice Problems—Chapter 13 from pages 381–386

1) 1.16; 1.7–2.3; Yes; 2; 0.5 **2)** 0.52; 42; 0.84 **3)** 0.43; 108 **4)** 2.2 **5)** 0.7 **6)** 0.78; 1950 **7)** 2.6 **8)** No **9)** 1.3; 26 **10)** 13 **11)** 0.32 **12)** 1.92 **13)** 1.63 **14)** 0.69 **15)** 1.67 **16)** 0.52 **17)** 560 000 **18)** 1085; 1.09 **19)** 1.9–3.8 **20)** 8 **21)** 40 **22)** 45; 90; 4.2; 30 **23)** 58.8 **24)** 60; 60; 1.9; 45 **25)** 22.8 **26)** 2; 22 **27)** 6.2; 44 **28)** 1520; 63 **29)** 1810; 75 **30)** 1250; 52 **31)** 240; 10 **32)** 1500–1875; 250–312.5; Yes; 2.8 **33)** 35; 2.8; 35 **34)** 123; Yes; 2 **35)** 100; 2; 100 **36)** 330–495; 110–165; Yes; 3.3 **37)** 25; 1.7; 23.3 **38)** 1800–2700; 300–450; No; exceeds maximum dose; do not give dosage ordered. **39)** 25 mL; 2.25 mL; 25 **40)** 500 000-6 250 000; 416 667–1 041 667 **41)** Yes; 2.6 **42)** 20; 2.6; 20.4

Selected Solutions—Practice Problems—Chapter 13

1) $\text{BSA (m}^2) = \sqrt{\frac{\text{ht (cm)} \times \text{wt (kg)}}{3600}} = \sqrt{\frac{127 \times 38}{3600}} =$

$\sqrt{\frac{4826}{3600}} = \sqrt{1} = 1.157\ \text{m}^2 = 1.16\ \text{m}^2$

Recommended dosage range:

$1.5\ \text{mg}/\cancel{\text{m}^2} \times 1.16\ \cancel{\text{m}^2} = 1.74\ \text{mg} = 1.7\ \text{mg}$

$2\ \text{mg}/\cancel{\text{m}^2} \times 1.16\ \cancel{\text{m}^2} = 2.32\ \text{mg} = 2.3\ \text{mg}$

Ordered dosage is safe.

$\frac{D}{H} \times Q = \frac{2\ \cancel{\text{mg}}}{1\ \cancel{\text{mg}}} \times 1\ \text{mL} = 2\ \text{mL}$

Give 2 mL/min

$\frac{2\ \text{mL}}{60\ \text{sec}} \times \frac{X\ \text{mL}}{15\ \text{sec}}$

$60X = 30$

$\frac{60X}{60} = \frac{30}{60}$

$X = 0.5\ \text{mL (per 15 sec)}$

2) $\text{BSA} = 0.52\ \text{m}^2$

$80\ \text{mg}/\cancel{\text{m}^2}/\text{day} \times 0.52\ \cancel{\text{m}^2} = 41.6\ \text{mg/day}$

$= 42\ \text{mg/day}$

$\frac{D}{H} \times Q = \frac{42\ \cancel{\text{mg}}}{50\ \cancel{\text{mg}}} \times 1\ \text{mL} = 0.84\ \text{mL}$

3) $\text{BSA} = 0.40\ \text{m}^2$

$250\ \text{mcg}/\cancel{\text{m}^2}/\text{day} \times 0.40\ \cancel{\text{m}^2} = 100\ \text{mcg/day}$

$= 100\ \text{mcg/day}$

4) $\frac{D}{H} \times Q = \frac{100\ \cancel{\text{mcg}}}{500\ \cancel{\text{mcg}}} \times 10\ \text{mL} = 2\ \text{mL}$

6) $\text{BSA} = 0.78\ \text{m}^2$

$2\,500\ \text{units}/\cancel{\text{m}^2} \times 0.78\ \cancel{\text{m}^2} = 1950\ \text{units}$

7) $\frac{D}{H} \times Q = \frac{1950\ \cancel{\text{units}}}{750\ \cancel{\text{units}}} \times 1\ \text{mL} = 2.6\ \text{mL}$

9) Metric: $\text{BSA (m}^2) = \sqrt{\frac{\text{ht (cm)} \times \text{wt (kg)}}{3600}}$

$= \sqrt{\frac{140 \times 43.5}{3600}} =$

$\sqrt{\frac{6090}{3600}} = \sqrt{1.69} = 1.3\ \text{m}^2$

$20\ \text{mg}/\cancel{\text{m}^2} \times 1.3\ \cancel{\text{m}^2} = 26\ \text{mg}$

10) $\frac{D}{H} \times Q = \frac{\overset{13}{\cancel{26}}\ \cancel{\text{mg}}}{\underset{1}{\cancel{2}}\ \cancel{\text{mg}}} \times 1\ \text{mL} = 13\ \text{mL}$

11) Metric:

$\text{BSA (m}^2) = \sqrt{\frac{\text{ht (cm)} \times \text{wt (kg)}}{3600}} = \sqrt{\frac{60 \times 6}{3600}} =$

$\sqrt{\frac{360}{3600}} = \sqrt{0.1} = 0.316\ \text{m}^2 = 0.32\ \text{m}^2$

15) $64\ \text{in} = 64 \times 2.5 = 160\ \text{cm}\ (1\ \text{in} = 2.5\ \text{cm})$

Metric: $\text{BSA (m}^2) = \sqrt{\frac{\text{ht (cm)} \times \text{wt (kg)}}{3600}}$

$= \sqrt{\frac{160 \times 63}{3600}}$

$= \sqrt{\frac{10\,080}{3600}} = \sqrt{2.8} = 1.673\ \text{m}^2 = 1.67\ \text{m}^2$

18) $500\ \text{mg}/\cancel{\text{m}^2} \times 2.17\ \cancel{\text{m}^2} = 1085\ \text{mg}$

$1085\ \text{mg} = 1085 \div 1000 = 1.085\ \text{g} = 1.09\ \text{g}$

20) $6\ \text{mg}/\cancel{\text{m}^2} \times 1.34\ \cancel{\text{m}^2} = 8.04 = 8\ \text{mg}$

21) $8.04\ \text{mg}/\cancel{\text{day}} \times 5\ \cancel{\text{days}} = 40.2\ \text{mg} = 40\ \text{mg}$

22) Total volume = 30 mL + 15 mL = 45 mL

Flow rate: $\frac{45\ \text{mL}}{\underset{1}{\cancel{30}}\ \text{min}} \times \frac{\overset{2}{\cancel{60}}\ \cancel{\text{min}}}{\text{h}} = 90\ \text{mL/h}$

$\frac{D}{H} \times Q = \frac{420\ \cancel{\text{mg}}}{\underset{100}{\cancel{500}}\ \cancel{\text{mg}}} \times \overset{1}{\cancel{5}}\ \text{mL} = \frac{420}{100}\ \text{mL}$

$= 4.2\ \text{mL medication}$

30 mL total solution − 4.2 mL med = 25.8 mL D_5NS

Note: Add 4.2 mL med. to chamber and fill with D_5NS to 30 mL.

23) $4.2\ \text{mL}/\cancel{\text{dose}} \times 2\ \cancel{\text{doses}}/\text{day} = 8.4\ \text{mL/day}$

$8.4\ \text{mL}/\cancel{\text{day}} \times 7\ \cancel{\text{days}} = 58.8\ \text{mL (total)}$

24) Total volume: 45 mL + 15 mL = 60 mL

Flow rate: $\frac{60\ \text{mL}}{60\ \text{min}} = 60\ \text{mL/h}$

$\frac{D}{H} \times Q = \frac{285\ \cancel{\text{mg}}}{75\ \cancel{\text{mg}}} \times 0.5\ \text{mL} = 1.9\ \text{mL (med)}$

Volume of IV fluid: 45 mL − 1.9 mL = 43.1 mL

25) 1.9 mL/~~dose~~ × 3 ~~doses~~/day = 5.7 mL/day

5.7 mL/~~day~~ × 4 ~~days~~ = 22.8 mL (total)

26) $\frac{D}{H} \times Q = \frac{\overset{2}{\cancel{500\text{ mg}}}}{\underset{1}{\cancel{250\text{ mg}}}} \times 1\text{ mL} = 2\text{ mL (med)}$

$\frac{65\text{ mL}}{60\text{ min}} = \frac{X\text{ mL}}{20\text{ min}}$

60X = 1300

$\frac{60X}{60} = \frac{1300}{60}$

X = 21.6 mL = 22 mL

22 mL total solution − 2 mL med

= 20 mL D_5 0.33% NaCl

28) 100 mL/~~kg~~/day × 10 ~~kg~~ = 1000 mL/day for first 10 kg

50 mL/~~kg~~/day × 10 ~~kg~~ = 500 mL/day for next 10 kg

20 mL/~~kg~~/day × 1 ~~kg~~

= 20 mL/day for remaining 1 kg

1520 mL/day or per 24 h

$\frac{1520\text{ mL}}{24\text{ h}} = 63.3\text{ mL/h} = 63\text{ mL/h}$

29) 78 lb = 78 ÷ 2.2 = 35.45 = 35.5 kg

100 mL/~~kg~~/day × 10 ~~kg~~ = 1000 mL/day for first 10 kg

50 mL/~~kg~~/day × 10 ~~kg~~ = 500 mL/day for next 10 kg

20 mL/~~kg~~/day × 15.5 ~~kg~~

= 310 mL/day for remaining 15.5 kg

1810 mL/day or per 24 h

$\frac{1810\text{ mL}}{24\text{ h}} = 75.4\text{ mL/h} = 75\text{ mL/h}$

31) 2400 g = 2400 ÷ 1000 = 2.4 kg

100 mL/~~kg~~/day × 2.4 ~~kg~~ = 240 mL/day

$\frac{240\text{ mL}}{24\text{ h}} = 10\text{ mL/h}$

32) Safe daily dosage range:

100 mg/~~kg~~ × 15 ~~kg~~ = 1500 mg

125 mg/~~kg~~ × 15 ~~kg~~ = 1875 mg

Safe single dosage range:

$\frac{1500\text{ mg}}{6\text{ doses}} = 250\text{ mg/dose}$

$\frac{1875\text{ mg}}{6\text{ doses}} = 312.5\text{ mg/dose}$

Yes, the dosage is safe.

1 g = 1000 mg

$\frac{D}{H} \times Q = \frac{275\,\cancel{\text{mg}}}{1000\,\cancel{\text{mg}}} \times 10\text{ mL} = 2.75\text{ mL} = 2.8\text{ mL}$

33) IV fluid volume:

$\frac{53\text{ mL}}{60\text{ min}} = \frac{X\text{ mL}}{40\text{ min}}$

60X = 2120

$\frac{60X}{60} = \frac{2120}{60}$

X = 35.3 mL = 35 mL

35 mL total − 2.8 mL med. = 32.2 mL D_5 0.45% NaCl

38) Safe daily dosage range:

200 mg/~~kg~~ × 9 ~~kg~~ = 1800 mg

300 mg/~~kg~~ × 9 ~~kg~~ = 2700 mg

Safe single dosage range:

$\frac{1800\text{ mg}}{6\text{ doses}} = 300\text{ mg/dose}$

$\frac{2700\text{ mg}}{6\text{ doses}} = 450\text{ mg/dose}$

Dosage is *not* safe; exceeds maximum safe dosage.

Do not give dosage ordered; consult with physician.

40) Safe daily dosage:

100 000 units/~~kg~~ × 25 ~~kg~~ = 2 500 000 units

250 000 units/~~kg~~ × 25 ~~kg~~ = 6 250 000 units

Safe single dosage:

$\frac{2\,500\,000\text{ units}}{6\text{ doses}} = 416\,666.6 = 416\,667\text{ units/dose}$

$\frac{6\,250\,000\text{ units}}{6\text{ doses}} = 1\,041\,666.6$

= 041 667 units/dose

41) Yes, dosage is safe.

$\frac{D}{H} \times Q = \frac{525\,\cancel{000\text{ units}}}{200\,\cancel{000\text{ units}}} \times 1\text{ mL}$

= 2.62 mL = 2.6 mL

42) $\frac{60\text{ mL}}{60\text{ min}} = \frac{X\text{ mL}}{20\text{ min}}$

60X = 1200

$\frac{60X}{60} = \frac{1200}{60}$

X = 20 mL

20 mL total − 2.6 mL med. = 17.4 mL D_5NS

Answers to Review Set 41 from pages 392–394

1) 40 **2)** 14 **3)** 10 **4)** 19 **5)** 48; consult physician **6)** 16 **7)** 000; 6; 1350; 14 **8)** 6000; 6; 1650; 17 **9)** 3000; 3; 1800; 18 **10)** Continue the rate at 1800 units/h or 18 mL/h **11)** 10 **12)** 50 **13)** 4 **14)** 20 **15)** 8

Selected Solutions—Review Set 41

1) $\frac{D}{H} \times Q = \frac{1000\ \cancel{\text{units}}/\text{h}}{\underset{25}{\cancel{25\,000}}\ \cancel{\text{units}}} \times \overset{1}{\cancel{1000}}\ \text{mL} = \frac{\overset{40}{\cancel{1000}}}{\underset{1}{\cancel{25}}}\ \text{mL/h}$

$= 40\ \text{ml/h}$

4) $\frac{D}{H} \times Q = \frac{1500\ \cancel{\text{units}}/\text{h}}{\underset{80}{\cancel{40\,000}}\ \cancel{\text{units}}} \times \overset{1}{\cancel{500}}\ \text{mL} = 18.7\ \text{mL/h}$

$= 19\ \text{mL/h}$

5) $\frac{D}{H} \times Q = \frac{1200\ \cancel{\text{units}}/\text{h}}{\underset{25}{\cancel{25\,000}}\ \cancel{\text{units}}} \times \overset{1}{\cancel{1000}}\ \text{mL} = 48\ \text{mL/h}$

The IV is infusing too rapidly. The physician should be called immediately for further action.

6) $\frac{D}{H} \times Q = \frac{800\ \cancel{\text{units}}/\text{h}}{\underset{50}{\cancel{25\,000}}\ \cancel{\text{units}}} \times \overset{1}{\cancel{500}}\ \text{mL} = \frac{\overset{16}{\cancel{800}}}{\underset{1}{\cancel{50}}}\ \text{mL/h}$

$= 16\ \text{mL/h}$

7) Initial heparin bolus: 80 units/$\cancel{\text{kg}}$ × 75 $\cancel{\text{kg}}$

$= 60\,000$ units

$\frac{D}{H} \times Q = \frac{6000\ \cancel{\text{units}}}{1000\ \cancel{\text{units}}} \times 1\ \text{mL} = 6\ \text{mL}$

Initial heparin infusion rate: 18 units/$\cancel{\text{kg}}$/h × 75 $\cancel{\text{kg}}$

$= 1350$ units/h

$\frac{D}{H} \times Q = \frac{1350\ \cancel{\text{units}}/\text{h}}{\underset{100}{\cancel{25\,000}}\ \cancel{\text{units}}} \times \overset{1}{\cancel{250}}\ \text{mL} = 13.5\ \text{mL/h}$

$= 14\ \text{mL/h}$

8) Rebolus: 80 units/$\cancel{\text{kg}}$ × 75 $\cancel{\text{kg}}$ = 6000 units

$\frac{D}{H} \times Q = \frac{6000\ \cancel{\text{units}}}{1000\ \cancel{\text{units}}} \times 1\ \text{mL} = 6\ \text{mL}$

Reset infusion rate: 4 units/$\cancel{\text{kg}}$/h × 75 $\cancel{\text{kg}}$

$= 300$ units/h (increase)

1350 units/h + 300 units/h = 1650 units/h

$\frac{D}{H} \times Q = \frac{1650\ \cancel{\text{units}}/\text{h}}{\underset{100}{\cancel{25\,000}}\ \cancel{\text{units}}} \times \overset{1}{\cancel{250}}\ \text{mL} = 16.5\ \text{mL/h}$

$= 17\text{mL/h}$

9) Rebolus: 40 units/$\cancel{\text{kg}}$ × 75 $\cancel{\text{kg}}$ = 3000 units

$\frac{D}{H} \times Q = \frac{3000\ \cancel{\text{units}}}{1000\ \cancel{\text{units}}} \times 1\ \text{mL} = 3\ \text{mL}$

Reset infusion rate: 2 units/$\cancel{\text{kg}}$/h × 75 $\cancel{\text{kg}}$

$= 150$ units/h (increase)

1650 units/h + 150 units/h = 1800 units/h

$\frac{D}{H} \times Q = \frac{1800\ \cancel{\text{units/h}}}{\underset{100}{\cancel{25\,000}}\ \cancel{\text{units}}} \times \overset{1}{\cancel{250}}\ \text{mL} = 18\ \text{mL/h}$

11) $\frac{D}{H} \times Q = \frac{10\ \cancel{\text{units}}/\text{h}}{\cancel{500\ \text{units}}} \times \cancel{500}\ \text{mL} = 10\ \text{mL/h}$

13) $\frac{D}{H} \times Q = \frac{5\ \cancel{\text{mg}}/\text{h}}{\underset{5}{\cancel{125}}\ \cancel{\text{mg}}} \times \overset{4}{\cancel{100}}\ \text{mL} = \frac{\overset{4}{\cancel{20}}}{\underset{1}{\cancel{5}}}\ \text{mL/h} = 4\ \text{mL/h}$

14) $\frac{D}{H} \times Q = \frac{10\ \cancel{\text{mg}}/\text{h}}{\underset{1}{\cancel{125}}\ \cancel{\text{mg}}} \times \overset{2}{\cancel{250}}\ \text{mL} = 20\ \text{mL/h}$

Answers to Review Set 42 from pages 403–404

1) 2; 120 **2)** 1; 60 **3)** 1.5; 90 **4)** 360; 0.4; 24 **5)** 1 050; 0.66; 40 **6)** 142–568 **7)** 0.14–0.57 **8)** Yes **9)** 4 **10)** Yes **11)** 100; 25 **12)** 1 **13)** 0.025

Selected Solutions—Review Set 42

1) $\frac{D}{H} \times Q = \frac{4\ \cancel{\text{mg}}/\text{min}}{\underset{2}{\cancel{2000}}\ \cancel{\text{mg}}} \times \overset{1}{\cancel{1000}}\ \text{mL}\ \frac{\overset{2}{\cancel{4}}}{\underset{1}{\cancel{2}}}\ \text{mL/min}$

$= 2\ \text{mL/min}$

2 mL/$\cancel{\text{min}}$ × 60 $\cancel{\text{min}}$/h = 120 mL/h

2) $\frac{D}{H} \times Q = \frac{2\ \cancel{\text{mg}}/\text{min}}{\underset{2}{\cancel{500}}\ \cancel{\text{mg}}} \times \overset{1}{\cancel{250}}\ \text{mL}\ \frac{\overset{1}{\cancel{2}}}{\underset{1}{\cancel{2}}}\ \text{mL/min}$

$= 1\ \text{mL/min}$

1 mL/$\cancel{\text{min}}$ × 60 $\cancel{\text{min}}$/h = 60 mL/h

3) $\frac{D}{H} \times Q = \frac{6\ \cancel{\text{mcg}}/\text{min}}{\underset{4}{\cancel{2000}}\ \cancel{\text{mcg}}} \times \overset{1}{\cancel{500}}\ \text{mL} = \frac{6}{4}\ \text{mL/min}$

$= 1.5\ \text{mL/min}$

1.5 mL/$\cancel{\text{min}}$ × 60 $\cancel{\text{min}}$/h = 90 mL/h

4) 4 mcg/$\cancel{\text{kg}}$/min × 90 $\cancel{\text{kg}}$ = 360 mcg/min

360 mcg/min = 360 ÷ 1000 = 0.36 mg/min

$\frac{D}{H} \times Q = \frac{0.36\ \cancel{\text{mg}}/\text{min}}{\underset{9}{\cancel{450}}\ \cancel{\text{mg}}} \times \overset{10}{\cancel{500}}\ \text{mL} = \frac{3.6}{9}\ \text{mL/min}$

$= 0.4\ \text{mL/min}$

0.4 mL/$\cancel{\text{min}}$ × 60 $\cancel{\text{min}}$/h = 24 mL/h

5) 15 mcg/$\cancel{\text{kg}}$/min × 70 $\cancel{\text{kg}}$ = 1050 mcg/min

1050 mcg/min = 1050 ÷ 1000 = 1.05 mg/min

$\frac{D}{H} \times Q = \frac{1.05\ \cancel{\text{mg}}/\text{min}}{\underset{8}{\cancel{800}}\ \cancel{\text{mg}}} \times \overset{5}{\cancel{500}}\ \text{mL} = \frac{5.25}{8}\ \text{mL/min}$

$= 0.656\ \text{mL/min} = 0.66\ \text{mL/min}$

0.66 mL/$\cancel{\text{min}}$ × 60 $\cancel{\text{min}}$/h = 39.6 mL/h = 40 mL/h

6) Minimum: 2.5 mcg/~~kg~~/min × 56.8 ~~kg~~

= 142 mcg/min

Maximum: 10 mcg/~~kg~~/min × 56.8 ~~kg~~

= 568 mcg/min

7) Minimum: 142 mcg/min = 142 ÷ 1000

= 0.14 mg/min

Maximum: 568 mcg/min = 568 ÷ 1000

= 0.57 mg/min

8) $\frac{500 \text{ mg}}{500 \text{ mL}} = \frac{\text{X mg/h}}{15 \text{ mL/h}}$

500X = 7500

$\frac{500X}{500} = \frac{7500}{500}$

X = 15 mg/h

$\frac{15 \text{ mg/}\cancel{\text{h}}}{60 \text{ min/}\cancel{\text{h}}} = 0.25 \text{ mg/min}$

Yes, the order is within the safe range of 0.14−0.57 mg/min.

9) $\frac{2000 \text{ mg}}{500 \text{ mL}} = \frac{\text{X mg/h}}{60 \text{ mL/h}}$

500X = 120 000

$\frac{500X}{500} = \frac{12\ 000}{500}$

X = 240 mg/h

$\frac{240 \text{ mg/}\cancel{\text{h}}}{60 \text{ min/}\cancel{\text{h}}} = 4 \text{ mg/min}$

11) Bolus:

$\frac{2\text{g}}{30 \text{ min}} = \frac{\text{Xg}}{60 \text{ min}}$

30X = 120

X = 4g (per 60 min or 4 g/h)

$\frac{20 \text{ mg}}{500 \text{ mL}} = \frac{4 \text{ g/h}}{\text{X mL/h}}$

20X = 2000

$\frac{20X}{20} = \frac{2000}{20}$

X = 100 mL/h

Continuous:

$\frac{20 \text{ mg}}{500 \text{ mL}} = \frac{1 \text{ g/h}}{\text{X mL/h}}$

20X = 500

$\frac{20X}{20} = \frac{500}{20}$

X = 25 mL/h

12) 1 milliunit = 1 ÷ 1000 = 0.001 units

$\frac{D}{H} \times Q = \frac{0.001 \cancel{\text{units}}/\text{min}}{15 \cancel{\text{units}}} \times 250 \text{ mL}$

= 0.017 mL/min

0.017 mL/~~min~~ × 60 ~~min~~/h = 1.02 mL/h = 1 mL/h

13) $\frac{10 \text{ mg}}{1000 \text{ mL}} = \frac{\text{X mg/h}}{150 \text{ mL/h}}$

1000X = 1500

$\frac{1000X}{1000} = \frac{1500}{1000}$

X = 1.5 mg/h

$X = \frac{1.5 \text{ mg/}\cancel{\text{h}}}{60 \text{ min/}\cancel{\text{h}}} = 0.025 \text{ mg/min}$

Answers to Review Set 43 from pages 406–408

1) 33; 19 **2)** 40; 42 **3)** 25; 32 **4)** 50; 90 **5)** 50; 40 **6)** 100; 100 **7)** 200; 76 **8)** 200; 122 **9)** 17; 21 **10)** 120; 112

Selected Solutions—Review Set 43

1) Step 1. IVPB rate: $\frac{V}{T} \times C = \frac{100 \cancel{\text{mL}}}{\cancel{30}_{3} \text{ min}} \times \cancel{10}^{1} \text{ gtt/}\cancel{\text{mL}} = \frac{100}{3}$ gtt/min = 33.3 gtt/min = 33 gtt/min

Step 2. Total IVPB time: q4h × 30 min = 6 × 30 min = 180 min = 180 ÷ 60 = 3 h

Step 3. Total IVPB volume: 6 × 100 mL = 600 mL

Step 4. Total Regular IV volume: 3000 mL − 600 mL = 2400 mL

Step 5. Total Regular IV time: 24 h − 3 h = 21 h

Step 6. Regular IV rate:

$\frac{2400 \text{ mL}}{21 \text{ h}} = 114 \text{ mL/h}$

$\frac{\text{mL/h}}{\text{drop factor constant}} = \text{gtt/min}; \frac{114 \text{ mL/h}}{6} = 19 \text{ gtt/min}$

2) Step 1. IVPB rate: When drop factor is 60 gtt/mL, then mL/h = gtt/min. Rate is 40 gtt/min.

Step 2. Total IVPB time: qid × 1 h = 4 × 1 h = 4 h

Step 3. Total IVPB volume: 4 × 40 mL = 160 mL

Step 4. Total regular IV volume: 1000 mL − 160 mL = 840 mL

Step 5. Total regular IV time: 24 h − 4 h = 20 h

Step 6. Total regular IV rate: $\text{mL/h} = \frac{840 \text{ mL}}{20 \text{ h}} = 42 \text{ mL/h}$. When drop factor is 60 gtt/mL, then mL/h = gtt/min. Rate is 42 gtt/min.

3) Step 1. IVPB rate: $\frac{V}{T} \times C = \frac{50 \cancel{\text{mL}}}{\cancel{30}_{2} \text{ min}} \times \cancel{15}^{1} \text{ gtt}/\cancel{\text{mL}} = \frac{50}{2} \text{ gtt/min} = 25 \text{ gtt/min}$

Step 2. Total IVPB time: q6h × 30 min = 4 × 30 min = 120 min = 120 ÷ 60 = 2 h

Step 3. Total IVPB volume: 4 × 50 mL = 200 mL

Step 4. Total regular IV volume: 3000 mL − 200 mL = 2800 mL

Step 5. Total regular IV time: 24 h − 2 h = 22 h

Step 6. Total regular IV rate:

$$\frac{2800 \text{ mL}}{22 \text{ h}} = 127 \text{ mL/h}$$

$$\frac{\text{mL/h}}{\text{drop factor constant}} = \text{gtt/min}; \frac{127 \text{ mL/h}}{4} = 31.7 \text{ gtt/min} = 32 \text{ gtt/min}$$

4) Step 1. IVPB rate: 50 mL/h or 50 gtt/min (because drop factor is 60 gtt/mL)

Step 2. Total IVPB time: q6h × 1 h = 4 × 1 h = 4 h

Step 3. Total IVPB volume: 4 × 50 mL = 200 mL

Step 4. Total regular IV volume: 2000 mL − 200 mL = 1800 mL

Step 5. Total regular IV time: 24 h − 4 h = 20 h

Step 6. Regular IV rate: $\frac{1800 \text{ mL}}{20 \text{ h}} = 90 \text{ mL/h}$ or 90 gtt/min (because drop factor is 60 gtt/mL)

5) Step 1. IVPB rate: 50 mL/h or 50 gtt/min (because drop factor is 60 gtt/mL)

Step 2. IVPB time: q8h × 1 h = 3 × 1 h = 3 h

Step 3. IVPB volume: 3 × 50 mL = 150 mL

Step 4. Total regular IV volume: 1000 mL − 150 mL = 850 mL

Step 5. Total regular IV time: 24 h − 3 h = 21 h

Step 6. Regular IV rate: $\frac{850 \text{ mL}}{21 \text{ h}} = 40.4 \text{ mL/h} = 40 \text{ gtt/min}$ (because drop factor is 60 gtt/mL)

6) Step 1. IVPB rate

$$\frac{50 \text{ mL}}{30 \text{ min}} \times \frac{X \text{ mL}}{60 \text{ min}}$$

$$30X = 3000$$

$$\frac{30X}{30} = \frac{3000}{30}$$

X = 100 mL;100 mL/60 min = 100 mL/h

Step 2. IVPB time: q6h × 30 min = 4 × 30 min = 120 min = 120 ÷ 60 = 2 h

Step 3. IVPB volume: 4 × 50 mL = 200 mL

Step 4. Total regular IV volume: 2400 mL − 200 mL = 2200 mL

Step 5. Total regular IV time: 24 h − 2 h = 22 h

Step 6. Regular IV rate: $\frac{2200 \text{ mL}}{22 \text{ h}} = 100 \text{ mL/h}$

7) Step 1. IVPB rate:

$$\frac{100 \text{ mL}}{30 \text{ min}} \times \frac{X \text{ mL}}{60 \text{ min}}$$

$$30 X = 6000$$

$$\frac{30 X}{30} = \frac{6000}{30}$$

$$X = 200 \text{ mL}; 200 \text{ mL}/60 \text{ min} = 200 \text{ mL/h}$$

Step 2. IVPB time: q8h $\times$ 30 min = 3 $\times$ 30 min = 90 min = 90 $\div$ 60 = $1\frac{1}{2}$ h

Step 3. IVPB volume: 3 $\times$ 100 mL = 300 mL

Step 4. Total regular IV volume: 2000 mL − 300 mL = 1700 mL

Step 5. Total regular IV time: 24 h − $1\frac{1}{2}$ h=22 $\frac{1}{2}$ h

Step 6. Regular IV rate: $\frac{1700 \text{ mL}}{22.5 \text{ h}} = 75.5 \text{ mL/h} = 76 \text{ mL/h}$

8) Step 1. IVPB rate

$$\frac{50 \text{ mL}}{15 \text{ min}} \times \frac{X \text{ mL}}{60 \text{ min}}$$

$$15 X = 3000$$

$$\frac{15 X}{5} = \frac{3000}{15}$$

$$X = 200 \text{ mL}; 200 \text{ mL}/60 \text{ min} = 200 \text{ mL/h}$$

Step 2. IVPB time: q6h $\times$ 15 min = 4 $\times$ 15 min = 60 min = 1 h

Step 3. IVPB volume: 4 $\times$ 50 mL = 200 mL

Step 4. Total regular IV volume: 3000 mL − 200 mL = 2800 mL

Step 5. Total regular IV time: 24 h − 1 h = 23 h

Step 6. Regular IV rate: $\frac{2800 \text{ mL}}{23 \text{ h}} = 121.7 \text{ mL/h} = 122 \text{ mL/h}$

Answers to Practice Problems—Chapter 14 from pages 409–415

1) 60 **2)** 5.5 **3)** 19.5 **4)** 50 **5)** 1 **6)** 12 **7)** 50 **8)** 63 **9)** 35 **10)** 6; 15 **11)** 60 **12)** 45 **13)** 60 **14)** 24 **15)** Yes **16)** 17; 22 **17)** 100; 127 **18)** 102 **19)** 8 mEq **20)** 2 **21)** 15 **22)** 50; 50 **23)** 75; 75 **24)** 7.4 **25)** 12; 18 **26)** 150; 50 **27)** 2 **28)** 35 **29)** 8 **30)** 63 **31)** 80 **32)** 0.4 **33)** 4 **34)** 4 **35)** 0.1; 100 **36)** 60 **37)** 200; 50 **38)** 5 **39)** 550 **40)** 2450 **41)** 19 **42)** 129 **43)** 13; 39 **44)** (Worksheet is on the next page.) 80 **45)** 8000; 1000; 8 **46)** 18; 1800; 100; 18 **47)** 6; 4000; 4; increase; 200; 2; 20 **48)** Decrease rate by 2 units/kg/h; 18

49) Critical Thinking Skill: Prevention.

The nurse who prepares any IV solution with an additive should *carefully* compare the order and medication three times: before beginning to prepare the dose, after the dosage is prepared, and just before it is administered to the client. Further, the nurse should verify the safety of the dosage using the three-step method (convert, think, and calculate). It was clear that the nurse realized the error when a colleague questioned what was being prepared and the nurse verified the actual order. Also taking the time to do the calculation on paper helps the nurse to "see" the answer and avoid a potentially life-threatening error.

Standard Weight-Based Heparin Protocol Worksheet

Round Client's Total Body Weight to Nearest 10 kg: *100* kg
DO NOT Change the Weight Based on Daily Measurements

FOUND ON THE ORDER FORM				
Initial Bolus (80 units/kg)	*8000*	units	*8*	mL
Initial Infusion Rate (18 units/kg/h)	*1800*	units/h	*18*	mL/h

Make adjustments to the heparin drip rate as directed by the order form.
ALL DOSES ARE ROUNDED TO THE NEAREST 100 UNITS

Date	Time	APTT	Bolus	Rate Change units/h	Rate Change mL/h	New Rate	RN 1	RN 2
10/05/XX	*1730*	*37 sec (4 mL)*	*4000 units*	*+200 units/h*	*+2 mL/h*	*20 mL/h*	*G.P.*	M.S.
10/05/XX	*2330*	*77 sec*		*–200 units/h*	*–2 mL/h*	*18 mL/h*	*G.P.*	*M.S.*

Signatures	Initials
G. Pickar, RN	*G.P.*
M. Smith, RN	*M.S.*

Selected Solutions—Practice Problems—Chapter 14

3) $\frac{50 \text{ mL}}{60 \text{ min}} = \frac{X \text{ mL}}{30 \text{ min}}$

$60X = 1500$

$\frac{60X}{60} = \frac{1500}{60}$

$X = 25 \text{ mL total volume}$

$25 \text{ mL(total)} - 5.5 \text{ mL(med)} = 19.5 \text{ mL}(D_5W)$

4) $\frac{\text{mL/h}}{\text{drop factor constant}} = \frac{50 \text{ mL/h}}{1} = 50 \text{ gtt/min};$

when drop factor is 60 gtt/mL, then mL/h = gtt/min

6) $\frac{D}{H} \times Q = \frac{1200 \text{ units/h}}{25\,000 \text{ units}} \times 250 \text{ mL} = \frac{1200}{100} \text{ mL/h}$

$= 12 \text{ mL/h}$

7) $\frac{D}{H} \times Q = \frac{5 \text{ mg/h}}{100 \text{ mg}} \times 1000 \text{ mL} = 50 \text{ mL/h}$

8) $\frac{D}{H} \times Q = \frac{500 \text{ mg/h}}{4000 \text{ mg}} \times 500 \text{ mL} = \frac{500}{8} \text{ mL/h}$

$= 62.5 \text{ mL/h} = 63 \text{ mL/h}$

9) $\frac{D}{H} \times Q = \frac{1400 \text{ units/h}}{20\,000 \text{ units}} \times 500 \text{ mL} = \frac{1400}{40} \text{ mL/h}$

$= 35 \text{ mL/h}$

10) $1.5\text{L} = 1.5 \times 1000 = 1500 \text{ mL}$

$\frac{1500 \text{ mL}}{4 \text{ mL/min}} = 375 \text{ min}$

$375 \text{ min} \div 60 \text{ min/h} = 6.25 = 6\frac{1}{4} \text{ h} = 6 \text{ h } 15 \text{ min}$

11) $\frac{D}{H} \times Q = \frac{4 \text{ mg/min}}{2000 \text{ mg}} \times 500 \text{ mL} = \frac{4}{4} \text{ mL/min}$

$= 1 \text{ mL/min},$

which is the same as 60 mL/60 min or 60 mL/h

12) $\frac{D}{H} \times Q = \frac{3 \text{ mg/min}}{1000 \text{ mg}} \times 250 \text{ mL} = \frac{3}{4} \text{ mL/min}$

$= 0.75 \text{ mL/min}$

$0.75 \text{ mL/min} \times 60 \text{ min/h} = 45 \text{ mL/h}$

13) $\frac{D}{H} \times Q = \frac{2 \text{ mg/min}}{1000 \text{ mg}} \times 500 \text{ mL} = \frac{2}{2} \text{ mL/min}$

$= 1 \text{ mL/min},$

which is the same as 60 mL/60 min or 60 mL/h

14) $5 \text{ mcg/kg/min} \times 80 \text{ kg} = 400 \text{ mcg/min}$

$400 \text{ mcg/min} = 400 \div 1000 = 0.4 \text{ mg/min}$

$\frac{D}{H} \times Q = \frac{0.4 \text{ mg/min}}{250 \text{ mg}} \times 250 \text{ mL} = 0.4 \text{ mL/min}$

$0.4 \text{ mL/min} \times 60 \text{ min/h} = 24 \text{ mL/h}$

15) $$\frac{2000\text{ mg}}{1000\text{ mL}} = \frac{X\text{ mg/h}}{75\text{ mL/h}}$$

$$1000X = 150\,000$$

$$\frac{1000X}{1000} = \frac{15\,000}{1000}$$

$$X = 150\text{ mg/h}$$

$150\text{ mg/}\cancel{h} \div 60\text{ min/}\cancel{h} = 2.5\text{ mg/min}$,

within normal range of 1–5 mg/min

16) IVPB flow rate: $\frac{\text{mL/h}}{\text{drop factor constant}} = \frac{100\text{ mL/h}}{6}$

$= 16.6\text{ gtt/min} = 17\text{ gtt/min}$

Total IVPB time:q6h $\times$ 1 h $= 4 \times 1\text{ h} = 4\text{ h}$

Total IVPB volume:$4 \times 100\text{ mL} = 400\text{ mL}$

Total regular IV volume: $3000\text{ mL} - 400\text{ mL}$

$= 2600\text{ mL}$

Total regular IV time: $24\text{ h} - 4\text{ h} = 20\text{ h}$

Regular IV rate: $\text{mL/h} = \frac{2600\text{ mL}}{20\text{ h}} = 130\text{ mL/h}$;

$$\frac{\text{mL/h}}{\text{drop factor constant}} = \frac{130\text{ mL/h}}{6} = 21.6\text{ gtt/min}$$

$= 22\text{ gtt/min}$

17) IVPB rate:

$$\frac{50\text{ mL}}{30\text{ min}} = \frac{X\text{ mL}}{60\text{ min}}$$

$$30X = 3000$$

$$\frac{30X}{30} = \frac{3000}{30}$$

$X = 100\text{ mL}$; $100\text{ mL/60 min} = 100\text{ mL/h}$

Total IVPB time: qid $\times$ 30 min $= 4 \times 30\text{ min}$

$= 120\text{ min} = 120 \div 60 = 2\text{ h}$

Total IVPB volume:$4 \times 50\text{ mL} = 200\text{ mL}$

Total regular IV volume: $3000\text{ mL} - 200\text{ mL}$

$= 2800\text{ mL}$

Total regular IV time: $24\text{ h} - 2\text{ h} = 22\text{ h}$

Regular IV rate: $\frac{2800\text{ mL}}{22\text{ h}} = 127.2\text{ mL/h}$

$= 127\text{ mL/h}$

18) $125\text{ lb} = \frac{125}{2.2} = 56.81\text{ kg} = 56.8\text{ kg}$

$3\text{ mcg/}\cancel{\text{kg}}\text{/min} \times 56.8\ \cancel{\text{kg}} = 170.4\text{ mcg/min}$

$170.4\text{ mcg/min} = 170.4 \div 1000 = 0.17\text{ mg/min}$

$$\frac{D}{H} \times Q = \frac{0.17\ \cancel{\text{mg}}\text{/min}}{\cancelto{1}{50}\ \cancel{\text{mg}}} \times \cancelto{10}{500}\text{ mL} = 1.7\text{ mL/min}$$

$1.7\text{ mL/min} \times 60\ \text{min/h} = 102\text{ mL/h}$

19) $1000\text{ mL} - 800\text{ mL} = 200\text{ mL infused}$

$$\frac{40\text{ mEq}}{1000\text{ mL}} = \frac{X\text{ mEq}}{200\text{ mL}}$$

$$1000X = 8000$$

$$\frac{1000X}{1000} = \frac{8000}{1000}$$

$$X = 8\text{ mEq}$$

20) $\frac{125\text{ mL}}{60\text{ min}} = 2.1\text{ mL/min} = 2\text{ mL/min}$

21) $\frac{1500\ \cancel{\text{mL}}}{100\ \cancel{\text{mL}}\text{/h}} = 15\text{ h}$

22) $\frac{D}{H} \times Q = \frac{2\ \cancel{\text{mEq}}\text{/h}}{\cancelto{1}{40}\ \cancel{\text{mEq}}} \times \cancelto{25}{1000}\text{ mL} = 50\text{ mL/h}$ or,

50 gtt/min (because drop factor is 60 gtt/mL)

23) $\frac{D}{H} \times Q = \frac{3750\ \cancel{\text{units}}\text{/h}}{\cancelto{50}{50\,000}\ \cancel{\text{units}}} \times \cancelto{1}{1000}\text{ mL} = \frac{3750}{50}\text{ mL/h}$

$= 75\text{ mL/h}$;

75 gtt/min (because drop factor is 60 gtt/mL)

24) $$\frac{5\text{ mg}}{1\text{ mL}} = \frac{37\text{ mg}}{X\text{ mL}}$$

$$5X = 37$$

$$\frac{5X}{5} = \frac{37}{5}$$

$$X = 7.4\text{ mL}$$

25) $10\text{ units} = 10 \times 1000 = 10\,000\text{ milliunits}$

$$\frac{D}{H} \times Q = \frac{4\ \cancel{\text{milliunits}}\text{/min}}{\cancelto{20}{10\,000}\ \cancel{\text{milliunits}}} \times \cancelto{1}{500}\text{ mL}$$

$= \frac{4}{20}\text{ mL/min} = 0.2\text{ mL/min}$ (for first 20 min)

$0.2\text{ mL/min} \times 60\ \text{min/h} = 12\text{ mL/h}$

$$\frac{D}{H} \times Q = \frac{6\ \cancel{\text{milliunits}}\text{/min}}{\cancelto{20}{10\,000}\ \cancel{\text{milliunits}}} \times \cancelto{1}{500}\text{ mL}$$

$= \frac{6}{20}\text{ mL/min} = 0.3\text{ mL/min}$ (for next 20 min)

$0.3\text{ mL/}\cancel{\text{min}} \times 60\ \cancel{\text{min}}\text{/h} = 18\text{ mL/h}$

26) Bolus:

$$\frac{3\text{ g}}{30\text{ min}} = \frac{X\text{ g}}{60\text{ min}}$$

$$\frac{30X}{30} = \frac{180}{30}$$

$$X = 6\text{ g}$$

$6\text{ g/60 min} = 60\text{ g/h}$

$$\frac{D}{H} \times Q = \frac{6\ \cancel{\text{g}}\text{/h}}{\cancelto{1}{20}\ \cancel{\text{g}}} \times \cancelto{25}{500}\text{ mL} = 150\text{ mL/h}$$

Continuous infusion:

$$\frac{D}{H} \times Q = \frac{2\ \cancel{g}/h}{\underset{1}{\cancel{20}}\ \cancel{g}} \times \overset{25}{\cancel{500}}\ mL = 50\ mL/h$$

29) $\dfrac{\overset{8}{\cancel{4000}}\ mg}{\underset{1}{\cancel{500}}\ mL} = 8\ mg/mL$

30) $\dfrac{D}{H} \times Q = \dfrac{500\ \cancel{mg}/h}{\underset{8}{\cancel{4000}}\ \cancel{mg}} \times \overset{1}{\cancel{500}}\ mL = \dfrac{500}{8}\ mL/h$

$= 62.5\ mL/h = 63\ mL/h$

31) 80 units $= 80 \times 1000 = 80\,000$ milliunits

$\dfrac{\overset{80}{\cancel{80\,000}}\ milliunits}{\underset{1}{\cancel{1000}}\ mL} = 80\ milliunits/mL$

32) $\dfrac{2450\ mL}{19\ h} = 128.9\ mL/h = 129\ mL/h$

33) $4\ mg = 4 \times 1000 = 4000\ mcg$

$\dfrac{\overset{4}{\cancel{4000}}\ mcg}{\underset{1}{\cancel{1000}}\ mL} = 4\ mcg/mL$

35) $\dfrac{\overset{1}{\cancel{10}}\ mg}{\underset{10}{\cancel{100}}\ mL} = \dfrac{1}{10}\ mg/mL = 0.1\ mg/mL$

$0.1\ mg/mL = 0.1 \times 1000 = 100\ mcg/mL$

36) $1\ mcg/\cancel{kg}/min \times 100\ \cancel{kg} = 100\ mcg/min$

$\dfrac{D}{H} \times Q = \dfrac{100\ \cancel{mcg}/min}{\underset{200}{\cancel{20\,000}}\ \cancel{mcg}} \times \overset{1}{\cancel{100}}\ mL = \dfrac{100}{200}\ mL/min$

$= 0.5\ mL/min$

$0.5\ mL/\cancel{min} \times 60\ \cancel{min}/h = 30\ mL/h$

37) IVPB rates:

$\dfrac{100\ mL}{30\ min} \times \dfrac{X\ mL}{60\ min}$ (cross-multiply)

$30X = 6000$

$\dfrac{30X}{30} = \dfrac{6000}{30}$

$X = 200$ mL (per 60 min)

200 mL/60 min = 200 mL/h (ampicillin sodium)

gentamicin sulfate: 50 mL/h

38) ampicillin sodium: q6h × 30 min = 4 × 30 min

= 120 min = 120 ÷ 60 = 2 h

gentamicin sulfate: q8h × 1h = 3 × 1 h = 3 h

Total IVPB time: 2 h + 3 h = 5 h

39) ampicillin sodium:

$4\ \cancel{doses} \times 100\ mL/\cancel{dose} = 400\ mL$

gentamicin sulfate:

$3\ \cancel{doses} \times 50\ mL/\cancel{dose} = 150\ mL$

Total IVPB volume: 400 mL + 150 mL = 550 mL

40) 3000 mL − 500 mL = 2450 mL

41) 24 h − 5 h = 19 h

43) $4\ mcg/\cancel{kg}/min \times 86.4\ \cancel{kg} = 345.6\ mcg/min$

$345.6\ mcg/\cancel{min} \times 60\ \cancel{min}/h = 20\,736\ mcg/h =$

$20\,736\ mcg/h = 20\,736 \div 1000 = 20.736\ mg/h$

$= 21\ mg/h$

$\dfrac{D}{H} \times Q = \dfrac{21\ \cancel{mg}/h}{\underset{8}{\cancel{800}}\ \cancel{mg}} \times \overset{5}{\cancel{500}}\ mL = \dfrac{105}{8}\ mL/h =$

13.1 mL/h = 13 mL/h (initial rate)

$12\ mcg/\cancel{kg}/min \times 86.4\ \cancel{kg} = 1036.8\ mcg/min$

$1036.8\ mcg/\cancel{min} \times 60\ \cancel{min}/h = 62\,208$

$62\,208\ mcg/h = 62\,208 \div 1000 = 62\ mg/h$

$\dfrac{D}{H} \times Q = \dfrac{62\ \cancel{mg}/h}{\underset{8}{\cancel{800}}\ \cancel{mg}} \times \overset{5}{\cancel{500}}\ mL = \dfrac{310}{8}\ mL/h =$

38.7 mL/h = 39 mL/h (after titration)

45) $80\ units/\cancel{kg} \times 100\ \cancel{kg} = 8000\ units$

1000 units/mL

$\dfrac{D}{H} \times Q = \dfrac{\cancel{8000\ units}}{\cancel{1000\ units}} \times 1\ mL = 8\ mL$

46) 18 units/kg/h

$18\ units/\cancel{kg}/h \times 100\ \cancel{kg} = 1800\ units/h$

25 000 units/250 mL or 100 units/mL

$\dfrac{D}{H} \times Q = \dfrac{\cancel{1800\ units}/h}{\cancel{100\ units}} \times 1\ mL = 18\ mL/h$

47) q6h

$40\ units/\cancel{kg} \times 100\ \cancel{kg} = 4000\ units$

$\dfrac{\cancel{4000\ units}}{\cancel{1000\ units}} \times 1\ mL = 4\ mL$

Increaserate: $2\ units/\cancel{kg}/h \times 100\ \cancel{kg} = 200\ units/h$

Increaserate: $\dfrac{\overset{2}{\cancel{200}}\ \cancel{units}/h}{\underset{1}{\cancel{100}}\ \cancel{units}} \times 1\ mL = 2\ mL/h$

18 mL/h + 2 mL/h = 20 mL/h (newinfusionrate)

48) Decrease rate by 2 units/kg/h.

$2\ units/\cancel{kg}/h \times 100\ \cancel{kg} = 200\ units/h$

$\dfrac{200\ \cancel{units}/h}{100\ \cancel{units}} \times 1\ mL = 2\ mL/h$

20 mL/h − 2 mL/h = 18 mL/h (new infusion rate)

Answers to Section 4—Self-Evaluation from pages 416–420

1) 0.9% NaCl **2)** 0.9 g NaCl/100mL **3)** 0.45 g NaCl/100 mL **4)** 50 **5)** 3.3 **6)** 2.25 **7)** 75 **8)** 6.75 **9)** mL/h **10)** 21 **11)** 83 **12)** 1940 h **13)** 1 536 **14)** Give a total of 3000 mL IV solution per day to include 5% normal saline (0.9% NaCl) with 20 milliequivalents of potassium chloride added per litre (1000 mL) *and* a piggyback IV solution of 250 mg cefazolin added to 100 mL of normal saline (0.9% NaCl) every 8 hours. To administer the order each day, give 900 mL NS with KCl over $7\frac{1}{2}$ hours × 3 administrations and 100 mL NS with cefazolin over $\frac{1}{2}$ hour × 3 administrations, q8h **15)** 120 **16)** 200 **17)** Reset rate to 118 mL/min, if policy and patient's condition permit. **18)** 1 410 **19)** 59 **20)** 120 **21)** 5 **22)** 0.48 **23)** 1.30 **24)** 0.47 **25)** 17.4–35.3 **26)** Yes **27)** 18.5 **28)** 37 mL **29)** 120 **30)** 18.5 **31)** 0.8 **32)** 1.6 **33)** Yes **34)** 1.6 **35)** 18; 2 **36.** 12.5–37.5 mg/dose not to exceed 50 mg/dose. **37.** No the dose ordered is above the recommended dose. Do not administer and contact the prescriber. **38)** 43 **39)** 200 **40)** 43 **41)** 200 **42)** 50 **43)** 12 **44)** 15 **45)** 0.13 **46)** 8 **47)** 80 **48)** 20 **49)** 61 **50)** 38

Selected Solutions—Section 4—Self-Evaluation

4) D_5 0.33% NaCl = 5% dextrose = 5g dextrose/100mL

$$\frac{5\text{g}}{100\text{mL}} \times \frac{X\text{ g}}{1000\text{mL}}$$

$$100X = 5000$$

$$\frac{100X}{100} = \frac{5000}{100}$$

$$X = 50\text{g}$$

5) D_5 0.33% NaCl = 0.33% Nacl = 0.33g NaCl/100mL

$$\frac{0.33\text{g}}{100\text{mL}} \times \frac{X\text{ g}}{1000\text{mL}}$$

$$100X = 3300$$

$$\frac{100X}{100} = \frac{3300}{100}$$

$$X = 3.3\text{g}$$

10) $\frac{2000\text{ mL}}{24\text{ h}} = 83.3\text{ mL/h} = 83\text{ mL/h}$

$$\frac{\text{mL/h}}{\text{drop factor constant}} = \text{gtt/min}$$

$$\frac{83\text{mL/h}}{4} = 20.7\text{ gtt/min} = 21\text{ gtt/min}$$

12) $\frac{V}{T} \times C = R: \frac{400\text{ mL}}{T\text{ min}} \times 15\text{ gtt/mL} = 24\text{ gtt/min}$

$$\frac{400}{T} \times 15 = 24$$

$$\frac{6000}{T} \times \frac{24}{1}$$

$$24T = 6000$$

$$\frac{24T}{24} = \frac{6000}{24}$$

$$T = 250\text{min}$$

$250\text{ min} = 250 \div 60 = 4\frac{1}{6}\text{ h} = 4\text{ h }10\text{ min}$

1530 hours
+410 hours
1940 hours

13) $\frac{V}{T} \times C = R: \frac{V\text{ mL}}{60\text{ min}} \times 10\text{ gtt/mL} = 32\text{ gtt/min}$

$$\frac{10V}{60} \times \frac{32}{1}$$

$$10V = 1920$$

$$\frac{10V}{10} = \frac{1920}{10}$$

$V = 192$ mL/h; 192mL/~~h~~ × 8 ~~h~~ = 1536mL (administered during your 8 h shift)

15) $\frac{2700\text{ mL}}{22.5\text{ h}} = 120\text{ mL/h}$

16) $\frac{100\text{ mL}}{30\text{ min}} \times \frac{X\text{ mL}}{60\text{ min}}$

$$30X = 6000$$

$$\frac{30X}{30} = \frac{6000}{30}$$

$$X = 200\text{mL}$$

200 mL/60min = 200 mL/h

17) $\frac{1200\text{ mL}}{100\text{ mL/h}} = 12$ h (total time ordered to infuse 1200 mL) (mL struck out)

2200 hours (current time)
−1530 hours (start time)
0630 = 6 h 30 min (elapsed time)

$6\frac{1}{2}$ ~~h~~ × 100 mL/ ~~h~~ = 650mL

After $6\frac{1}{2}$ h, 650 mL should have been infused, with 550 mL remaining. IV is behind schedule.

1200 mL − 650 mL = 550 mL (should be remaining)

$$\frac{\text{remaining volume}}{\text{remaining time}} = \frac{650\text{ mL}}{5.5\text{ h}} = 118\text{ mL/h}$$

(adjusted rate)

$$\frac{\text{Adjusted gtt/min} - \text{Ordered gtt/min}}{\text{Ordered gtt/min}} = \text{\% of variation;}$$

$$\frac{118 - 100}{100} = \frac{18}{100} = 0.18 = 18\%\text{(variance is safe)}$$

If policy and client's condition permit, reset rate to 118 mL/h.

18) 1st 10 kg: $100\text{ mL/}\cancel{\text{kg}}\text{/day} \times 10\ \cancel{\text{kg}} = 1000\text{ mL/day}$

Remaining 8.2 kg: $50\text{mL/}\cancel{\text{kg}}\text{/day} \times 8.2\ \cancel{\text{kg}} = \underline{410\text{ mL/day}}$

1410mL/day

19) $\frac{1410\text{ mL}}{24\text{ h}} = 58.7\text{ mL/h} = 59\text{ mL/h}$

20) $1185\text{ g} = 1185 \div 1000 = 1.185\text{ kg} = 1.2\text{ kg}$

1st 10 kg: $100\text{mL/}\cancel{\text{kg}}\text{/day} \times 1.2\ \cancel{\text{kg}} = 120\text{mL/day}$

21) $\frac{120\text{ mL}}{24\text{ h}} = 5\text{ mL/h}$

$$\text{BSA (m}^2\text{)} = \sqrt{\frac{\text{ht (cm)} \times \text{wt (kg)}}{3600}} = \sqrt{\frac{76 \times 11}{3600}} =$$

$$\sqrt{\frac{836}{3600}} = \sqrt{0.232} = 0.48\text{ m}^2$$

23) $\text{BSA (m}^2\text{)} = \sqrt{\frac{\text{ht (cm)} \times \text{wt (kg)}}{3600}} = \sqrt{\frac{155 \times 39}{3600}} =$

$\sqrt{1.679} = 1.295\text{ m}^2 = 1.30\text{ m}^2$

25) Minimum safe dosage: $37\text{ mg/}\ \cancel{\text{m}^2} \times 0.47\ \cancel{\text{m}^2} =$ 17.4 mg

Maximum safe dosage: $75\text{mg/}\cancel{\text{m}^2} \times 0.47\ \cancel{\text{m}^2} =$ 35.3 mg

27) $\frac{D}{H} \times Q = \frac{18.5\ \cancel{\text{mg}}}{1\ \cancel{\text{mg}}} \times 1\text{ mL} = 18.5\text{ mL}$

28) $2\text{ mL/}\cancel{\text{mg}} \times 18.5\ \cancel{\text{mg}} = 37\text{ mL}$

29) $\frac{D}{H} \times Q = \frac{1\ \cancel{\text{mg}}\text{/min}}{18.5\ \cancel{\text{mg}}} \times 37\text{ mL} = 2\text{ mL/min}$

$2\text{ mL/}\cancel{\text{min}} \times 60\ \cancel{\text{min}}\text{/h} = 120\text{ mL/h}$

30) At 1 mg/min, 18.5 mg will infuse in 18.5 min.

$$\frac{1\text{ mg}}{1\text{ min}} \times \frac{18.5\text{ mg}}{X\text{ min}}$$

$X = 18.5\text{ min}$

32) $2\text{ mg/}\cancel{\text{m}^2} \times 0.8\ \cancel{\text{m}^2} = 1.6\text{ mg}$

35) $\frac{D}{H} \times Q = \frac{\cancel{250}\ \cancel{\text{mg}}}{\cancel{125}\ \cancel{\text{mg}}} \times 1\text{ mL} = 2\text{ mL (cefazolin)}$

$$\frac{40\text{ mL}}{60\text{ min}} \times \frac{X\text{ mL}}{30\text{ min}}$$

$60X = 1200$

$$\frac{60X}{60} = \frac{1200}{60}$$

$X = 20\text{ mL}$

20 mL (total IV solution) −2 mL (cefazolin)= 18 mL (NS)

36) $25\text{ kg} \times 0.5\text{ mg/kg/dose} = 12.5\text{ mg/dose}$

$25\text{ kg} \times 1.5\text{ mg/kg/dose} = 37.5\text{ mg/dose}$

Maximum dose $= 25\text{ mg} \times 2\text{ mg/kg/dose} =$ 50 mg/dose

Recommended dose is 12.5–37.5 mg to maximum of 50 mg/dose.

38) Total IVPB volume: $100\text{ mL} \times 6 = 600\text{ mL}$

Regular IV volume: $1500\text{ mL} - 600\text{ mL} = 900\text{ mL}$

Total IVPB time of q4h: 30 min: $6 \times 30\text{ min} =$ $180\text{ min} = 180 \div 60 = 3\text{ h}$

Total regular IV time: $24\text{ h} - 3\text{ h} = 21\text{ h}$

Regular IV rate: $\text{mL/h} = \frac{900\text{ mL}}{21\text{ h}} = 42.8\text{ mL/h} =$ 43 mL/h

or 43 gtt/min because mL/h = gtt/min when drop factor is 60 gtt/mL.

$$\frac{\text{mL/h}}{\text{drop factor constant}} = \text{gtt/min;}\ \frac{43\text{ mL/h}}{1} = 43\text{ gtt/min}$$

39) $\frac{100\text{ mL}}{30\text{ min}} \times \frac{X\text{ mL}}{60\text{ min}}$

$30X = 6000$

$$\frac{30X}{30} = \frac{6000}{30}$$

X = 200 mL; 200 mL/60 min = 200 mL/h or 200 gtt/min (because drop factor is 60 gtt/mL)

40) See #38, regular IV rate calculated at 42.8 mL/h or 43 mL/h.

41) See #39, IVPB rate calculated at 200 mL/h.

42) $\frac{D}{H} \times Q = \frac{\overset{1}{\cancel{2}}\ \cancel{\text{mEq}}\text{/ h}}{\underset{20}{\cancel{40}}\ \cancel{\text{mEq}}} \times 1000\text{ mL} = 50\text{ mL/h}$

43) $\frac{25\text{ mg}}{1\text{ L}} = \frac{25.000.}{1.000.} = \frac{25\,000\text{ mcg}}{1000\text{ mL}} = \frac{25\,000\text{ mcg}}{1000\text{ mL}} =$ 25 mcg/mL

$\frac{D}{H} \times Q = \frac{\overset{1}{\cancel{5}\ \cancel{mcg}}/min}{\underset{5}{\cancel{25}}\ \cancel{mcg}} \times 1\ mL = \frac{1}{5}\ mL/min =$

0.2 mL/min

$0.2\ mL/\cancel{min} \times 60\ \cancel{min}/h = 12\ mL/h$

44) $\frac{15\ units}{1\ L} = \frac{15.000.}{1.000.} = \frac{15\ \cancel{000}\ \cancel{milliunits}}{1\cancel{000}\ mL} =$

$15\ \cancel{milliunits}/mL$

45) $\frac{D}{H} \times Q = \frac{2\ \cancel{milliunits}/min}{15\ \cancel{milliunits}} \times 1\ mL =$

$\frac{2}{15}\ mL/min = 0.13\ mL/min$

46) $0.13\ mL/\cancel{min} \times 60\ \cancel{min}/h = 7.8 = 8\ mL/h$

47) $\frac{\overset{4}{\cancel{20}}\ \cancel{milliunits}/min}{\underset{3}{\cancel{15}}\ \cancel{milliunits}} \times 1\ mL = \frac{4}{3}\ mL/min =$

1.33 mL/min

$1.33\ mL/\cancel{min} \times 60\ \cancel{min}/h = 80\ mL/h$

48) $4\ mcg/\cancel{kg}/min \times 68\ \cancel{kg} = 272 = 272\ mcg/min$

$272\ mcg/\cancel{min} \times 60\ \cancel{min}/h = 16380\ mcg/h$

$0.5\ L = 0.5\ 1000 = 500\ mL$

$\frac{400\ mg}{0.5\ L} = \frac{40\cancel{0}\ mg}{50\cancel{0}\ mL}$

$= 0.8\ mg/mL$

$0.8\ mg/mL = 0.8 \times 1000 = 800\ mcg/mL$

$\frac{D}{H} \times Q = \frac{16\ 380\ \cancel{mcg}/h}{800\ \cancel{mcg}} \times 1\ mL = 20.47\ mL/h =$

20 mL/h

49) $12\ mcg/kg/min \times 68.2\ kg = 818.4\ mcg/min =$

818 mcg/min

$818\ mcg/min \times 60\ min/h = 49\ 080\ mcg/h$

$\frac{D}{H} \times Q = \frac{49\ 080\ \cancel{mcg}/h}{800\ \cancel{mcg}} \times 1\ mL = 61.4\ mL/h =$

61 mL/h

50) $\frac{D}{H} \times Q = \frac{750\ \cancel{units}/h}{\underset{20}{\cancel{10\ 000}}\ \cancel{units}} \times \cancel{500}\ mL = \frac{750}{20}\ mL/h =$

$\frac{D}{H} \times Q = \frac{750\ \cancel{units}/h}{\underset{20}{\cancel{10\ 000}}\ \cancel{units}} \times \overset{1}{\cancel{500}}\ mL = \frac{750}{20}\ mL/h =$

$37.5\ mL/h = 38\ mL/h$

Answers to Essential Skills Evaluation from pages 421–436

1) 0.5

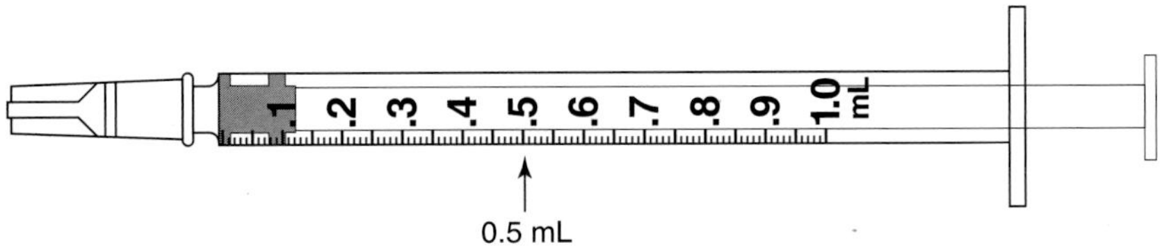

2) 1.4

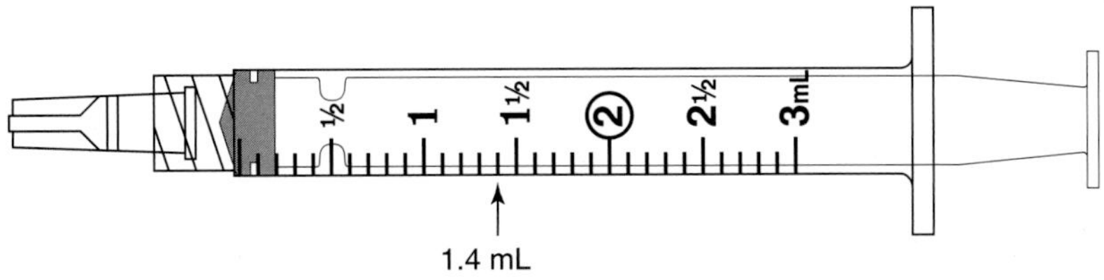

3) 1.5, 1, 0.25

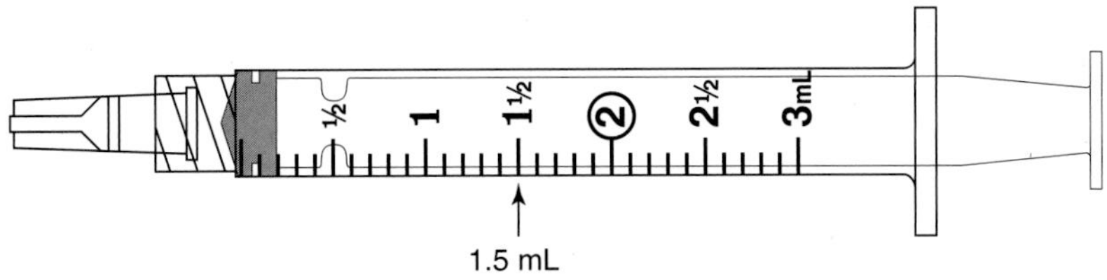

4) 1

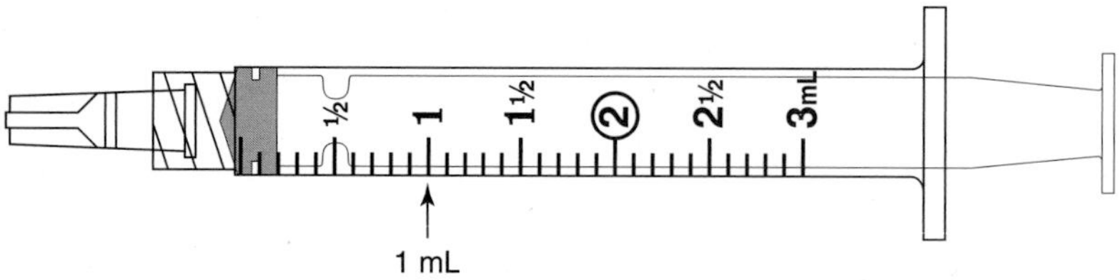
1 mL

5) $1\frac{1}{2}$

6) 0.5

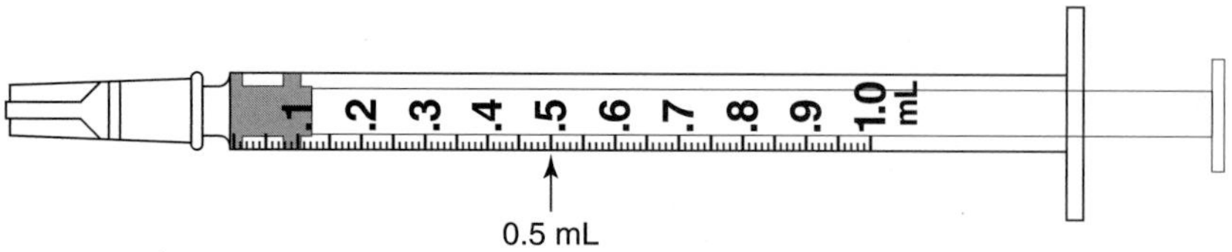
0.5 mL

7) $\frac{1}{2}$

8) 1.4

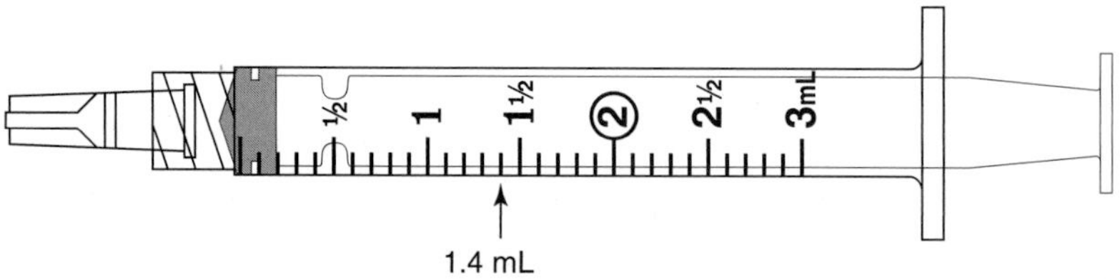
1.4 mL

9) 68

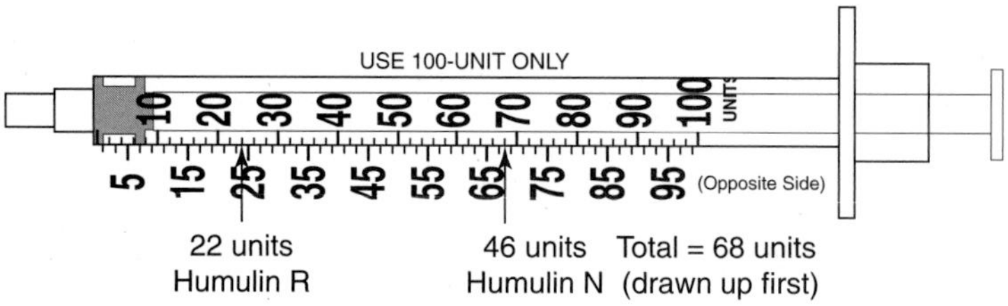
USE 100-UNIT ONLY
(Opposite Side)
22 units
Humulin R
46 units
Humulin N
Total = 68 units
(drawn up first)

10) 4 tabs **11)** 1; $\frac{1}{2}$ **12)** 2 tabs

13) 0.8

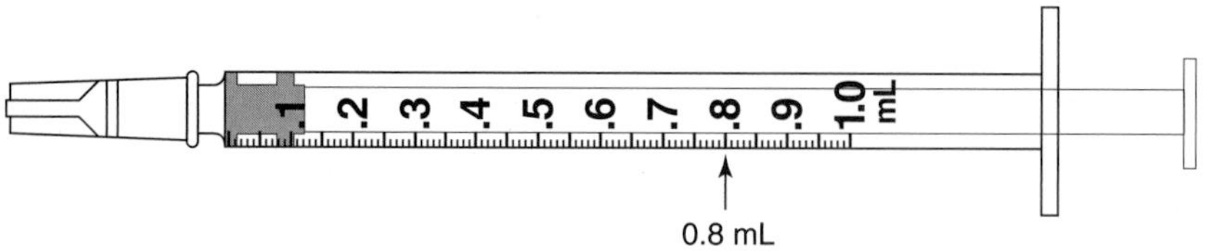
0.8 mL

14) 0.75

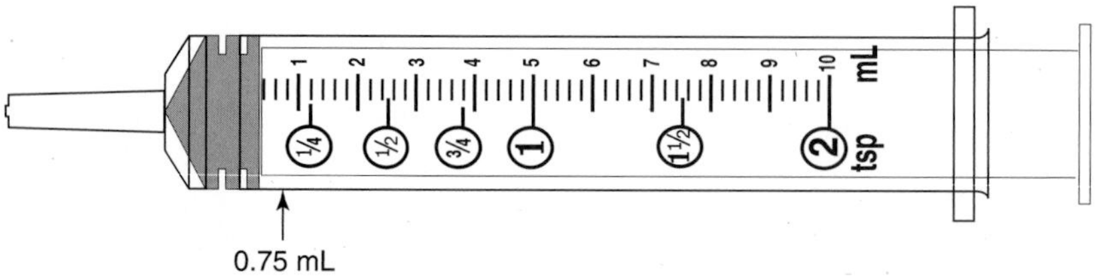
mL
tsp
0.75 mL

15) 2

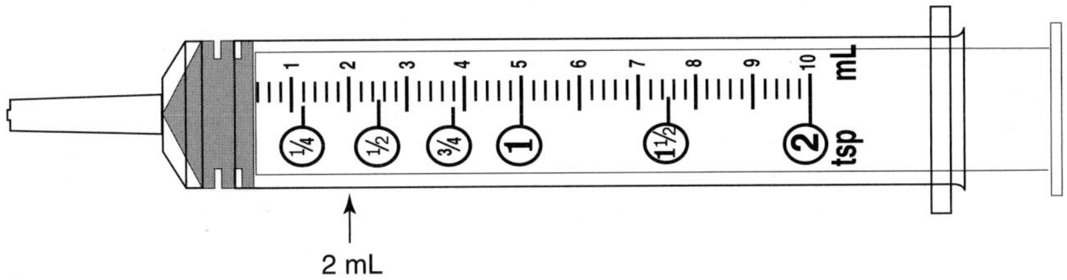

16) 1.5

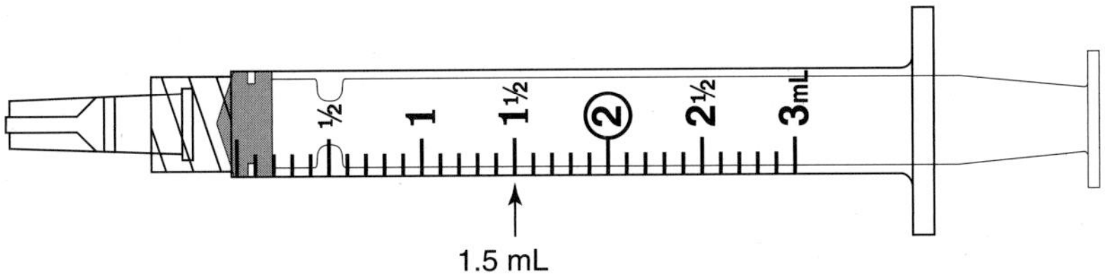

17) 1.4; 75

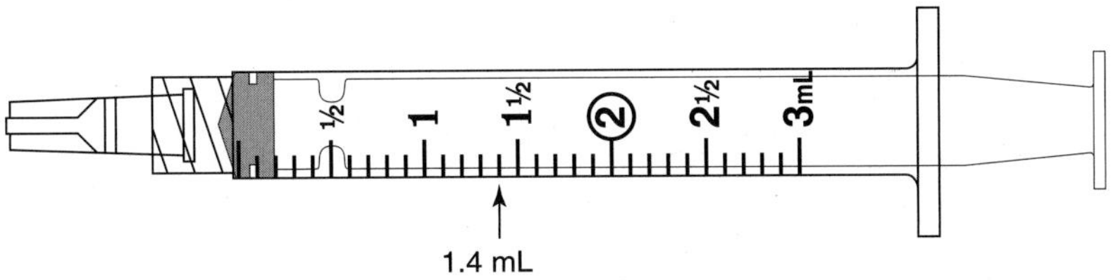

18) Yes. Her temperature is 39°C. Acetaminophen is indicated for fever over 38.3°C every 4 hours. It has been 5 hours and 5 minutes since her last dose.

19) 2 **20)** 0.5 mL

21) diphenhydramine; capsule

22) naloxone hydrochloride; 1

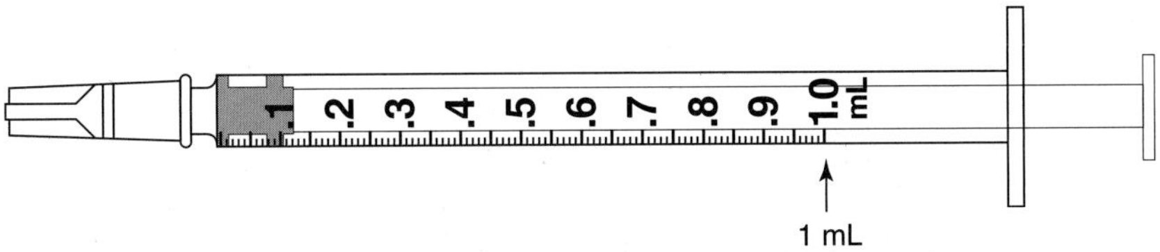

23)80; 30; 160 **24)** 125 **25)** 1.8; 2.5 **26)** 1; 0700, 1100, 1700, 2200

27) 10; subcutaneous

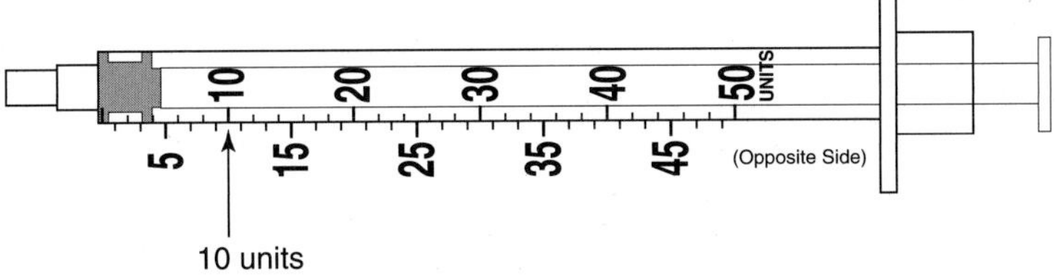

28) Yes; 6.8 × 40 mg/kg/day divided by three doses/day is 91 mg/dose. **29)** 116 mL water **30)** 3.6 **31)** 3.6; every 8 hours **32)** 25–75; Yes; 2; 26 **33)** 1000 **34)** Yes **35)** 1; dosage is safe **36)** 38 **37)** 280–420 **38)** 13 **39)** 29.5; No **40)** Do not administer; consult with physician before giving drug. **41)** 1 **42)** 50; 5 **43)** 30 **44)** 2030; 8:30 PM **45)** 500 **46)** 11 **47)** 180 **48)** 2.8

49)

30/01/XX, 1400, reconstituted as 180 mg/mL. Expires 02/02/XX, 1400. Keep refrigerated. G.D.P.

50) The importance of checking a medication label at least three times to verify supply dosage cannot be overemphasized. It is also important NEVER to assume that the supply dosage is the same as a supply dosage used to calculate previously. Always read the label carefully. Writing the calculation down will also help improve accuracy.

Selected Solutions—Essential Skills Evaluation

1) $\frac{D}{H} \times Q = \frac{12.5\ \cancel{mg}}{25\ \cancel{mg}} \times 1\text{ mL} = 0.5\text{ mL}$

2) $\frac{D}{H} \times Q = \frac{\overset{7}{\cancel{35}}\ \cancel{mg}}{\underset{5}{\cancel{25}}\ \cancel{mg}} \times 1\text{ mL} = \frac{7}{5}\text{ mL} = 1.5\text{ mL}$

3) $\frac{D}{H} \times Q = \frac{7.5\ \cancel{mg}}{5\ \cancel{mg}} \times 1\text{ mL} = 1.5\text{ mL}$

5 mg/min × 1.5 mL/7.5 mg = 1 mL/min

$$\frac{1\text{ mL}}{60\text{ sec}} \times \frac{X\text{ mL}}{15\text{ sec}}$$

$60X = 15$

$$\frac{60X}{60} = \frac{15}{60}$$

X = 1.5 mL at 1 mL (per 60 sec)

or 0.25 mL (per 15 sec)

Note: 1-mL syringe is the better choice because measurement of 0.25-mL increments is clearly visible. However, 1.5 mL is to be administered so a 2-mL syringe would be used.

4) 0.4 mg = 0.4 × 1000 = 400 mcg

$\frac{D}{H} \times Q = \frac{200\ \cancel{mcg}}{\underset{200}{\cancel{400}}\ \cancel{mcg}} \times \overset{1}{\cancel{2}}\text{ mL} = \frac{\overset{1}{\cancel{200}}}{\underset{1}{\cancel{200}}} \times 1\text{ mL} = 1\text{ mL}$

5) $\frac{D}{H} \times Q = \frac{7.5\ \cancel{mg}}{5\ \cancel{mg}} \times 1\text{ tab} = 1.5\text{ tab} = 1\frac{1}{2}\text{ tab}$

6) 0.125 mg = 0.125 × 1000 = 125 mcg

$\frac{D}{H} \times Q = \frac{125\ \cancel{mcg}}{\underset{250}{\cancel{500}}\ \cancel{mcg}} \times \overset{1}{\cancel{2}}\text{ mL} = \frac{\overset{1}{\cancel{125}}}{\underset{2}{\cancel{250}}} \times 1\text{ mL} = 0.5\text{ mL}$

7) $\frac{D}{H} \times Q = \frac{7.5\ \cancel{mg}}{15\ \cancel{mg}} \times 1\text{ tab} = 0.5\text{ tab} = \frac{1}{2}\text{ tab}$

8) $\frac{D}{H} \times Q = \frac{\overset{7}{\cancel{350}}\text{ mg}}{\underset{10}{\cancel{500}}\text{ mg}} \times 2\text{ mL} = \frac{14}{10}\text{ mL} = 1.4\text{ mL}$

9) 46 units + 22 units = 68 units (total)

10) 0.3 mg = 0.3 × 1000 = 300 mcg

$\frac{D}{H} \times Q = \frac{\overset{2}{\cancel{300}}\ \cancel{mcg}}{\underset{1}{\cancel{150}}\ \cancel{mcg}} \times 1\text{ tab} = 2\text{ tab}$

11) $\frac{D}{H} \times Q = \frac{\overset{1}{\cancel{125}}\ \cancel{mg}}{\underset{2}{\cancel{250}}\ \cancel{mg}} \times 1\text{ tab} = \frac{1}{2}\text{ tab}$

12) $\frac{D}{H} \times Q = \frac{\overset{3}{\cancel{375}}\ \cancel{mg}}{\underset{2}{\cancel{250}}\ \cancel{mg}} \times 1\text{ tab} = \frac{3}{2}\text{ tab} = 1\frac{1}{2}\text{ tab}$

13) $\frac{D}{H} \times Q = \frac{\overset{4}{\cancel{40}}\ \cancel{mg}}{\underset{5}{\cancel{50}}\ \cancel{mg}} \times 1\text{ mL} = \frac{4}{5}\text{ mL} = 0.8\text{ mL}$

14) $\frac{D}{H} \times Q = \frac{15\ \cancel{mg}}{20\ \cancel{mg}} \times 1\text{ mL} = \frac{3}{4}\text{ mL} = 0.75\text{ mL}$

You will need 2 vials of the drug, because each vial contains 1 mL.

15) $\frac{D}{H} \times Q = \frac{\overset{4}{\cancel{100}}\text{ mg}}{\underset{10}{\cancel{250}}\text{ mg}} \times 5\text{ mL} = \frac{4}{10} \times 5\text{ mL} = 2\text{ mL}$

16) $\frac{D}{H} \times Q = \frac{\overset{3}{\cancel{0.6}}\ \cancel{mg}}{\underset{2}{\cancel{0.4}}\ \cancel{mg}} \times 1\text{ mL} = \frac{3}{2}\text{ mL} = 1.5\text{ mL}$

17) $\frac{D}{H} \times Q = \frac{35\ \cancel{mg}}{\underset{25}{\cancel{50}}\ \cancel{mg}} \times \overset{1}{\cancel{2}}\text{ mL} = \frac{\overset{7}{\cancel{35}}}{\underset{5}{\cancel{25}}} \times 1\text{ mL} = \frac{7}{5}\text{ mL} = 1.4\text{ mL}$

$\frac{D}{H} \times Q = \frac{35\ \cancel{mg}}{\underset{25}{\cancel{50}}\ \cancel{mg}} \times \overset{1}{\cancel{2}}\text{ mL} = \frac{\overset{7}{\cancel{35}}}{\underset{5}{\cancel{25}}} \times 1\text{ mL} = \frac{7}{5}\text{ mL} = 1.4\text{ mL}$

$\frac{V}{T} \times C = \frac{\overset{5}{\cancel{100}}\ \cancel{mL}}{\underset{1}{\cancel{20}}\text{ min}} \times 15\text{ gtt}/\cancel{mL} = 75\text{ gtt/min}$

18) 2400 − 2150 = 0250 or 2 h 50 min; 0215 = 2 h 15 min after 2400; 2 h 50 min +2 h 15 min = 5 h 5 min; yes; temperature is greater than 38.3°C and more than 4 hours has passed since last dosage of acetaminophen

19) $\frac{D}{H} \times Q = \frac{\overset{2}{\cancel{650}}\ \cancel{mg}}{\underset{1}{\cancel{325}}\ \cancel{mg}} \times 1 \text{ tab} = 2 \text{ tab}$

20) $\frac{\overset{1}{\cancel{30}}\ \cancel{mg}}{\underset{2}{\cancel{60}}\ \cancel{mg}} \times 1 \text{ mL} = 0.5 \text{ mL}$

21) $\frac{D}{H} \times Q = \frac{50\ \cancel{mg}}{50\ \cancel{mg}} \times 1 \text{ capsule} = 1 \text{ capsule}$

22) $\frac{D}{H} \times Q = \frac{\cancel{0.4\ mg}}{\cancel{0.4\ mg}} \times 1 \text{ mL} = 1 \text{ mL}$

23) 0.8 mg/mL = 100 mg/x mL; x = 80 mL of theophylline in D5W solution.

$\frac{80\ \cancel{mL}}{\cancel{30}\text{ min}} \times \overset{2}{\cancel{60}} \text{ gtt}/\cancel{mL} = 160 \text{ gtt/min}$

24) 160 gtt/min = 160 mL/h, because gtt/min = mL/h when drop factor is 60 gtt/mL

25) $\frac{D}{H} \times Q = \frac{125 \text{ mg}}{250 \text{ mg}} \times 2 \text{ mL} = 1 \text{ mL}$ and use 1 vial

One vial will be used.

26) $\frac{D}{H} \times Q = \frac{\cancel{1 g}}{\cancel{1 g}} \times 1 \text{ tab} = 1 \text{ tab}$

29) Recommended dosage for ear infection

$40 \text{ mg}/\cancel{kg}/\text{day} \times 6.8\ \cancel{kg} = 272 \text{ mg/day}$

$\frac{272 \text{ mg}}{3 \text{ doses}} = 90.6 \text{ mg/dose} = 91 \text{ mg/dose}$

30) Yes, safe 91 mg/125 kg × 5 mL = 3.64 = 3.6 mL

$\frac{D}{H} \times Q = \frac{91\cancel{mg}}{125\ \cancel{mg}} \times 5 \text{ mL} = 3.64 - 3.64\text{mL}$

32) 50 kg × 2mg/kg/day = 100 mg/day divided by 4 doses = 25 mg/dose

50 kg × 6 mg/kg/day = 300 mg/day divided by 4 = 75 mg/dose

Yes, safe.

50 mg/25 mg × 1 mL = 2 mL in 50 mL of D5W

52 mL/20 min × 10 gtt/mL = 26 gtt/min

33)

IV fluid = 200 ml

gelatin = 120 mL = 4 × 30 = 120 mL

water = 90 mL × 2 = (3 × 30) × 2 = 90 × 2 = 180 mL

apple juice = 500 mL = 500 mL

Total = 1000 mL

34) $40 \text{ mg}/\cancel{kg}/\text{day} \times 18.2\ \cancel{kg} = 728 \text{ mg}$

$\frac{728 \text{ mg}}{3 \text{ doses}} = 242.6 \text{ mg} = 243 \text{ mg}$; close approximation to ordered dosage of 240 mg; dosage is safe.

35) $\frac{D}{0.96 \text{ tablet} = 1 \text{ tablet H}} \times Q = \frac{240\ \cancel{mg}}{\underset{50}{\cancel{250}}\ \cancel{mg}} \times 1 \text{ table}$

36) $\text{mL/h} = \frac{\overset{150}{\cancel{600}} \text{ mL}}{\underset{1}{\cancel{4}} \text{ h}} = 150 \text{ mL/h}$

$\frac{V}{T} \times C = \frac{150\ \cancel{mL}}{\underset{4}{\cancel{60}} \text{ min}} \times \overset{1}{\cancel{15}} \text{ gtt}/\cancel{mL} = \frac{150 \text{ gtt}}{4 \text{ min}} =$

37.5 gtt/min

= 38 gtt/min

37) Minimum dosage: $10 \text{ mg}/\cancel{kg} \times 28\ \cancel{kg} = 280 \text{ mg}$

Minimum dosage: $15 \text{ mg}/\cancel{kg} \times 28\ \cancel{kg} = 420 \text{ mg}$

38) $\frac{D}{H} \times Q = \frac{420\ \cancel{mg}}{160\ \cancel{mg}} \times 5 \text{ mL} = 13.1 \text{ mL} = 13 \text{ mL}$

= 13.1 mL = 13 mL

39) $5 \text{ mg}/\cancel{kg}/\text{day} \times 23.6\ \cancel{kg} = 118 \text{ mg/day}$

$\frac{118 \text{ mg}}{4 \text{ doses}} = 29.5 \text{ mg/dose}$; dosage is too low to be therapeutic and is not safe.

41) $\frac{D}{H} \times Q = \frac{10\ \cancel{mg}}{\underset{10}{\cancel{300}}\ \cancel{mg}} \times \overset{1}{\cancel{30}} \text{ mL} = \frac{\overset{1}{\cancel{10}}}{\underset{1}{\cancel{10}}} \text{ mL} = 1 \text{ mL}$

42) $10 \text{ mg}/\cancel{dose} \times 5\ \cancel{doses} = 50 \text{ mg}$

$1 \text{ mL}/\cancel{dose} \times 5\ \cancel{doses} = 5 \text{ mL}$

43) $\frac{\overset{3}{\cancel{300}}\ \cancel{mg}}{\underset{1}{\cancel{10}}\ \cancel{mg}/\text{does}} = 30 \text{ doses}$

44) $\frac{30\ \cancel{doses}}{5\ \cancel{doses}/\text{h}} = 6 \text{ h}$

$$\begin{array}{r} 1430 \text{ h} \\ +\ 600 \text{ h} \\ \hline 2030 \text{ h} \end{array} \qquad \begin{array}{r} 2030 \\ -1200 \\ \hline 8{:}30 \text{ PM} \end{array}$$

45) $\frac{250 \text{ mL}}{30 \text{ min}} \times \frac{X \text{ mL}}{60 \text{ min}}$ (cross-multiply)

$30X = 15\,000$

$\frac{30X}{30} = \frac{15\,000}{30}$

$X = 500 \text{ mL}$

500 mL/60 min = 500 mL/h

Answers to Comprehensive Skills Evaluation from pages 437–449

1) 1 **2)** Sublingual. The medication is to be administered under the tongue. Buccal means against the inside of the cheek. **3)** 2; 2; 0.5 **4)** 1

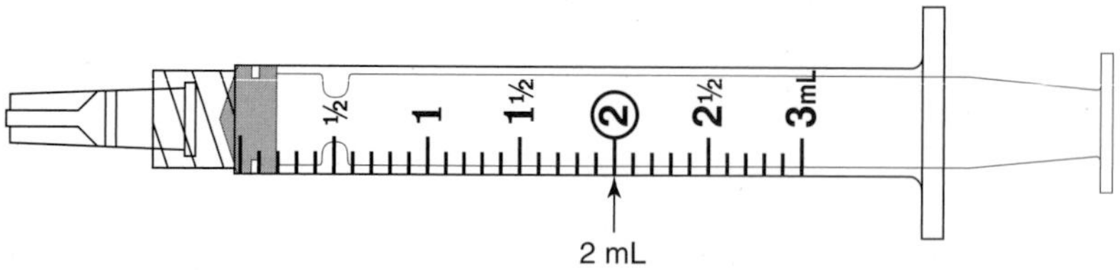

5) 1; 1; 0.25

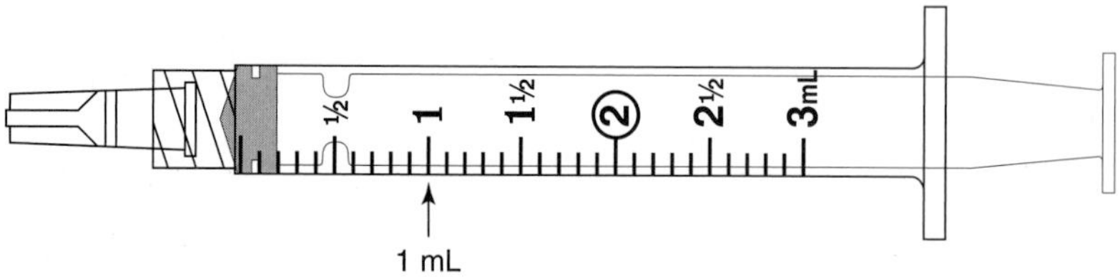

6) 6 **7)** 80

8) 0.8 **9)** 1920 **10)** 0500; 04/09/XX **11)** 2 **12)** 80 **13)** all: nitroglycerin, furosemide, digoxin, potassium chloride, and acetaminophen

14) 5

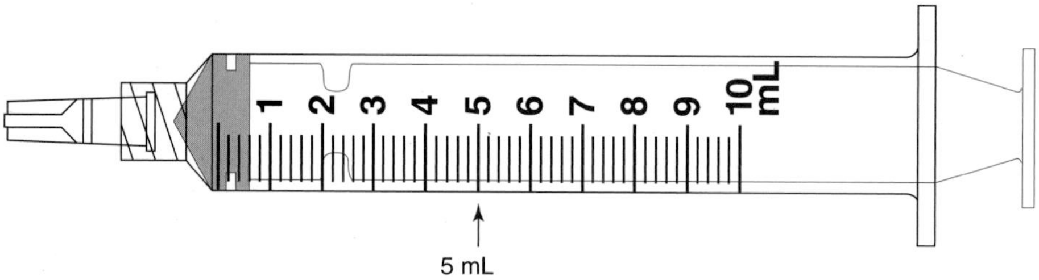

15) 30

16) Dosage ordered is safe.

17) 19 **18)** 30 000 mcg/h or 30 mg/h; 30 **19)** 60 **20)** No, the maximum recommended dosage for this child is 112.5 mg/day in three divided doses or 37.5 mg/dose. The ordered dosage is 114 mg/day. This is slightly more than the maximum recommended dosage; 3.8; 96.2 (add sufficient 0.9% NS to make 100 mL); 115 mL/h **21)** 12 **22)** Yes, safe dosage for this child is 300 mg/dose, which is the same as the order; 6; 44 (or add IV solution to 50 mL); 1200 **23)** 0.8 **24)** 0.4 **25)** 1.2 **26)** 2.5

27)

> 06/02/xx, 0800, 3304 mg/mL. Expires 07/02/xx, 0800. Keep at room temperature. G.D.P.

28) 1.5; 48.5 (or add D5W to 50 mL)

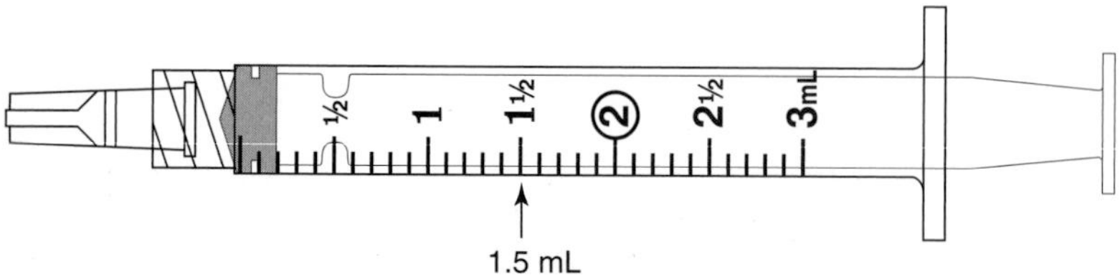

29) 130

30) 1; 60

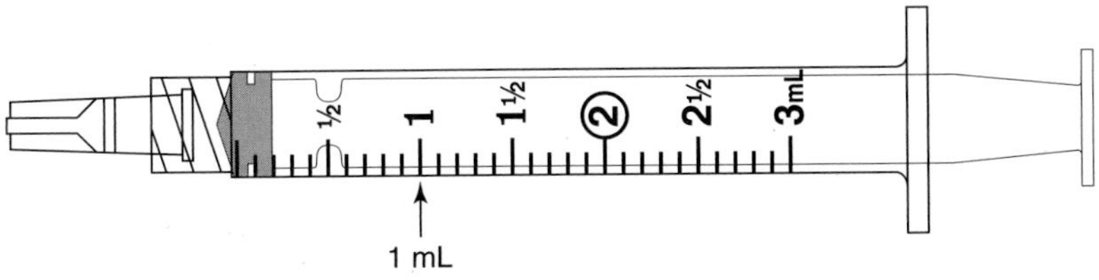

31) 4544; 4.5; 1022; 10 **32)** Decrease rate by 2 units/kg/h; 908; 9

33) 8; 0.08

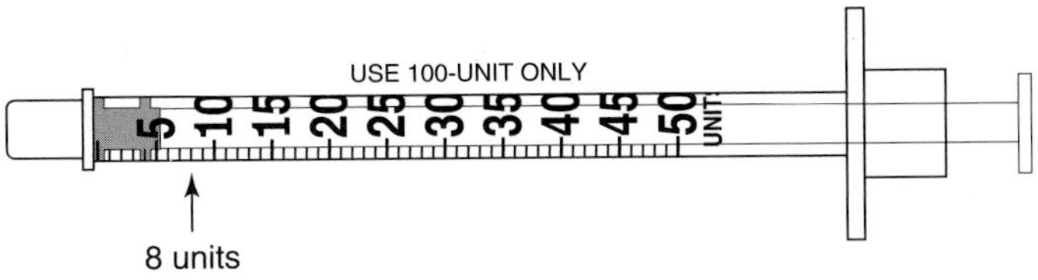

34) 60

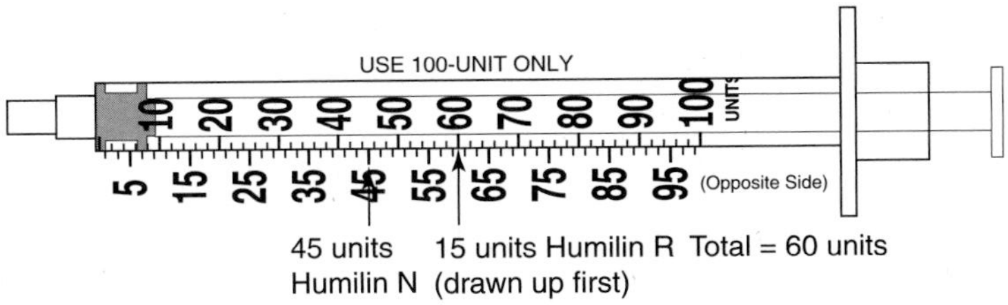

35) 20 **36)** 80 mL Isomil; 240 mL water **37)** 730; 30 **38)** 1.43 **39)** 14.3–28.6; Yes; 0.5; 56; 5.6; 1.4 **40)** 50; 3.3 **41)** 10; 90 (or add IV solution to 100 mL) **42)** Yes; the minimal amount of IV fluid to safely dilute this med is 50 mL. The order calls for 100 mL total, or 90. **43)** 1 600 000; Yes, the minimum daily dosage is 1 000 000 units/day and the maximum is 4 000 000 units/day. The ordered dosage falls within this range; 8.2; 500 000; 0.8

Reconstitution Label

14/01/xx; 0800, reconstituted as 500 000 units/mL. Expires 19/01/xx; 0800. Keep refrigerated. G.D.P.

44) 102 **45)** 2145 h **46)** 1; 1; 0.25 **47)** 8.3 **48)** 216

49) Either the route or the frequency of this order is missing or is unclear. If the student actually gave this medication in the eye, it would cause a severe reaction. The medication particles could scratch the eyes, or cause a worse reaction, such as blindness.

To prevent this from occurring, the student nurse should always ensure that each medication order is complete. Every order should include the name of the drug, the dose, the route, and the time. When any of these are missing, the order should be clarified. The student nurse should also look up medications and know the safe use for each medication ordered. Had this student looked up digoxin in a drug guide, it would have been discovered that the medication is never given in the eye. In addition, OD is an abbreviation that ISMP-Canada recommends not be used because of this type of potential for error. OD should be written out in full as "daily."

50) The student nurse took the correct action with this order. The nurses who had given the medication previously should have looked up the medication if they were unfamiliar with it to safely identify whether it was ordered by an appropriate route, correct dose, and correct time. There was also an error made by the pharmacist who supplied the medication to the nursing unit. It is extremely important to be familiar with the medications being given. If there is a question or any doubt, the medication should be looked up in a drug guide or the prescriber questioned. Also, close reading of the label and matching it to the order is also extremely important. Remember the rights of medication administration.

Selected Solutions—Comprehensive Skills Evaluation

1) $\frac{D}{H} \times Q = \frac{\cancel{0.5\text{ mg}}}{\cancel{0.5\text{ mg}}} \times 1\text{ tablet} = 1\text{ tablet}$

3) $\frac{D}{H} \times Q = \frac{\overset{2}{\cancel{20\text{ mg}}}}{\underset{1}{\cancel{10\text{ mg}}}} \times 1\text{ mL} = 2\text{ mL}$

$\frac{40\text{ mg}}{2\text{ min}} \times \frac{20\text{ mg}}{X\text{ min}}$

$40X = 40$

$\frac{40X}{40} = \frac{40}{40}$

$X = 1$ min Give 2 mL over 1 min

$\frac{2\text{ mL}}{60\text{ sec}} \times \frac{X\text{ mL}}{15\text{ sec}}$

$60X = 30$

$\frac{60X}{60} = \frac{30}{60}$

$X = 0.5$ Give 0.5 mL over 15 sec

4) $\frac{D}{H} \times Q = \frac{\overset{1}{\cancel{20\text{ mcg}}}}{\underset{1}{\cancel{20\text{ mcg}}}} \times 1\text{ tab} = 1\text{ tab}$

5) 0.25 mg = 1 mL added to 4 mL NS = 5 mL total

$\frac{\overset{1}{\cancel{5}}\text{ mL}}{\underset{1}{\cancel{5}}\text{ min}} = 1\text{ mL/min}$

$\frac{1\text{ mL}}{60\text{ sec}} \times \frac{X\text{ mL}}{15\text{ sec}}$

$60X = 15$

$\frac{60X}{60} = \frac{15}{60}$

$X = 0.25$ mL (per 15 sec)

6) 0.25 mg = 0.25 × 1000 = 250 mcg

$\frac{D}{H} \times Q = \frac{\overset{2}{\cancel{250\text{ mcg}}}}{\underset{1}{\cancel{125\text{ mcg}}}} \times 1\text{ tab} = 2\text{ tab}$

"daily" means once per day; need 3 days' supply; therefore need 6 tablets

7) $\frac{\text{mL/h}}{\text{drop factor constant}} = \text{gtt/min}$

$\frac{80\text{ mL/h}}{1} = 80\text{ gtt/min}$ or

80 mL/h = 80 gtt/min (because drop factor is 60 gtt/mL)

8) The total fluid volume is:

1000 mL $D_5\frac{1}{2}$ NS + 5 mL KCl = 1005 mL

$\frac{10\text{ mEq}}{1005\text{ mL}} \times \frac{X\text{ mEq/h}}{80\text{ mL/h}}$

$1005X = 800$

$\frac{1005X}{1005} = \frac{800}{1005}$

$X = 0.8$ mEq/h

9) $80\text{ mL/}\cancel{h} \times 24\ \cancel{h} = 1920\text{ mL}$

10) $\frac{1000\ \cancel{\text{mL}}}{80\ \cancel{\text{mL}}\text{/h}} = 12.5\text{ h} = 12\text{ h }30\text{ min}$

1630 h + 12 h 30 min later = 0500 h the next day; 04/09/XX

11) 1 g = 1000 mg

$\frac{D}{H} \times Q = \frac{\overset{2}{\cancel{1000\text{ mg}}}}{\underset{1}{\cancel{500\text{ mg}}}} \times 1\text{ tab} = 2\text{ tab}$

12) Order is for 80 mL/h.

14) $\frac{D}{H} \times Q = \frac{\overset{5}{\cancel{50\text{ mg}}}}{\underset{1}{\cancel{10\text{ mg}}}} \times 1\text{ mL} = 5\text{ mL}$

15) $\frac{D}{H} \times Q = \frac{2\ \cancel{\text{mg}}\text{/min}}{\underset{4}{\cancel{2000\text{ mg}}}} \times \overset{1}{\cancel{500}}\text{ mL} = \frac{\overset{1}{\cancel{2}}}{\underset{2}{\cancel{4}}} = 0.5\text{ mL/min}$

$0.5\text{ mL/}\cancel{\text{min}} \times 60\ \cancel{\text{min}}\text{/h} = 30\text{ mL/h}$

16) Minimum: $5\text{ mcg/}\cancel{\text{kg}}\text{/min} \times 50\ \cancel{\text{kg}} = 250\text{ mcg/min}$

Maximum: $10\text{ mcg/}\cancel{\text{kg}}\text{/min} \times 50\ \cancel{\text{kg}} = 500\text{ mcg/min}$

Ordered dosage is safe.

17) 500 mcg/min = 500 ÷ 1000 = 0.5 mg/min

$\frac{D}{H} \times Q = \frac{0.5\ \cancel{\text{mg}}\text{/min}}{\underset{8}{\cancel{400\text{ mg}}}} \times \overset{5}{\cancel{250}}\text{ mL} = \frac{2.5\text{ mL}}{8\text{ min}}$

= 0.312 mL/min = 0.31 mL/min

$0.31\text{ mL/}\cancel{\text{min}} \times 60\ \cancel{\text{min}}\text{/h} = 18.6\text{ mL/h} = 19\text{ mL/h}$

18) $500\text{ mcg/}\cancel{\text{min}} \times 60\ \cancel{\text{min}}\text{/h} = 30\,000\text{ mcg/h}$

30 000 mcg/h = 30 000 ÷ 1000 = 30 mg/h

19) $\frac{D}{H}\times Q = \frac{4\ \cancel{mg}/min}{\underset{4}{\cancel{2000}}\ mg}\times \overset{1}{\cancel{500}}\ mL = \frac{\overset{1}{\cancel{4}}}{\underset{1}{\cancel{4}}} = 1\ mL/min$

$1\ mL/\cancel{min}\times 60\ \cancel{min}/h = 60\ mL/h$

20) $7.5\ mg/\cancel{kg}/day\times 15\ \cancel{kg} = 112.5\ mg/day$

Maximum: $\frac{112.5\ mg}{3\ doses} = 37.5\ mg/dose$

The order is safe.

$\frac{D}{H}\times Q = \frac{\overset{1}{\cancel{38\ mg}}}{\underset{1}{\cancel{30\ mg}}}\times 3\ mL = 3.8\ mL$

100 N/S − 3.8 mL gentamicin sulfate = 96.2 mL

$D_5\frac{1}{2}$ NS for

100 mL total solution + 15 mL flush = 115 mL

total in 1 h

115 mL over 1 h is 115 mL/h.

21) $\frac{D}{H}\times Q = \frac{\overset{3}{\cancel{15}}\ \cancel{mg}/h}{\underset{25}{\cancel{125}}\ \cancel{mg}}\times 100\ mL =$

$\frac{3\ h}{\underset{1}{\cancel{25}}}\times \overset{4}{\cancel{100}}\ mL = 12\ mL/h$

22) $66\ lb = \frac{66}{2.2} = 30\ kg$

$40\ mg/\cancel{kg}/day\times 30\ \cancel{kg} = 1200\ mg/day$

$\frac{1200\ mg}{4\ doses} = 300\ mg/dose$

$\frac{D}{H}\times Q = \frac{300\ \cancel{mg}}{\underset{50}{\cancel{500}}\ mg}\times \overset{1}{\cancel{10}}\ mL = \frac{300}{50}\ mL = 6\ mL$

50 mL (total IV volume) − 6 mL (Vancocin) =

44 mL$\left(D_5\frac{1}{2}NS\right)$; 50 mL/$\cancel{h}$ × 24 $\cancel{h}$ = 1,200 mL

24) $\frac{D}{H}\times Q = \frac{60\ mg}{75\ mg}\times 1\ mL = \frac{12}{15} = 0.8\ mL$

$\frac{D}{H}\times Q = \frac{0.12\ mg}{0.3\ mg}\times 1\ mL = 0.4\ mL$

25) 0.8 mL + 0.4 mL = 1.2 mL

26) Select smallest quantity diluent (2.5 mL) to obtain most concentrated solution because 50 mL IV fluid is ordered for each Prostaphlin dose.

28) $\frac{D}{H}\times Q = \frac{500\ mg}{330\ mg}\times 1\ mL = \frac{500}{330} = 1.5\ mL$

50 mL (total IV volume) − 1.5 mL (cefazolin) =

48.5 mL (D_5W)

29) 50 mL (total IV solution) + 15 mL (flush)

= 65 mL (total)

65 mL over 30 min = 130 mL/h

30) $\frac{D}{H}\times Q = \frac{\overset{1}{\cancel{10\,000}}\ \cancel{unit}}{\underset{1}{\cancel{10\,000}}\ \cancel{unit}}\times 1\ mL = 1\ mL$

$\frac{D}{H}\times Q = \frac{1200\ \cancel{unit}/h}{\underset{20}{\cancel{10\,000}}\ \cancel{unit}}\times \overset{1}{\cancel{500}}\ mL$

$= \frac{\overset{60}{\cancel{1200}}}{\underset{1}{\cancel{20}}}\ mL/h = 60\ mL/h$

31) $80\ \cancel{units}/kg\times 56.8\ \cancel{kg} = 4{,}544\ units$

$\frac{D}{H}\times Q = \frac{4544\ \cancel{units}}{1000\ \cancel{units}}\times 1\ mL = 4.554\ mL = 4.5\ mL$

18 units/kg/h × 56.8 kg = 1022.4 units/h

= 1022 units/h

$\frac{D}{H}\times Q = \frac{1022\ units/h}{\underset{100}{\cancel{25\,000}}\ units}\times \overset{1}{\cancel{250}}\ mL = 10.22\ mL/h$

= 10 mL/h

32) Decrease rate by 2 units/kg/h

$2\ units/\cancel{kg}/h\times 56.8\ \cancel{kg} = 113.6\ units/h$

= 114 units/h

1022 units/h − 114 units/h = 908 units/h

$\frac{D}{H}\times Q = \frac{908\ \cancel{units}/h}{\underset{100}{\cancel{25\,000}}\ \cancel{units}}\times \overset{1}{\cancel{250}}\ mL$

= 9.08 mL/h = 9 mL/h

33) $\frac{100\ units}{1\ mL} \rightleftarrows \frac{8\ units}{X\ mL}$

$100X = 8$

$\frac{100X}{100} = \frac{8}{100}$

$X = 0.08\ mL$

34) 15 units + 45 units = 60 units

35) 100-unit insulin: 100 units/mL

$\frac{100\ units}{1\ mL} \rightleftarrows \frac{300\ units}{X\ mL}$

$100X = 300$

$\frac{100X}{100} = \frac{300}{100}$

$X = 3\ mL$

Total IV volume: 150 mL NS + 3 mL insulin = 153 mL

$\frac{300\ units}{153\ mL} \rightleftarrows \frac{X\ units/h}{10\ mL/h}$

$153X = 3000$

$\frac{153X}{153} = \frac{3000}{153}$

$X = 19.6\ units/h = 20\ units/h$

36) 240 mL

80 mL × 4 feedings = 320 mL

$\frac{1}{4}\times 320\ mL = 80\ mL$ Isomil

320 mL total − 80 mL Isomil = 240 mL water

37) 100 mL/kg/day × 7.3 kg = 730 mL/day

730 mL/day ÷ 24 h/day = 30 mL/h

38) $\text{BSA}(\text{m}^2) = \sqrt{\dfrac{\text{ht (cm)} \times \text{wt (kg)}}{3600}} = \sqrt{\dfrac{157.5 \times 46.8}{3600}}$

$= \sqrt{2.05} = 1.43 \text{ m}^2$

39) 10 mg/m² × 1.43 m² = 14.3 mg

20 mg/m² × 1.43 m² = 28.6 mg

Yes, the order is safe.

Concentration: 20 mg/40 mL = 0.5 mg/mL

$\frac{D}{H} \times Q = \frac{28 \text{ mg}}{0.5 \text{ mg}} \times 1 \text{ mL} = 56 \text{ mL}$

$\frac{56 \text{ mL}}{10 \text{ min}} \quad \frac{X \text{ mL}}{1 \text{ min}}$

$10X = 56$

$\frac{10X}{10} = \frac{56}{10}$

$X = 5.6 \text{ mL/min}$

$\frac{5.6 \text{ mL}}{60 \text{ sec}} \quad \frac{X \text{ mL}}{15 \text{ sec}}$

$60X = 84$

$\frac{60X}{60} = \frac{84}{60}$

X = 1.4 mL (per 15 sec)

40) Dextrose:

$\frac{5 \text{ g}}{100 \text{ mL}} = \frac{X \text{ g}}{1000 \text{ mL}}$

$100X = 5000$

$\frac{100X}{100} = \frac{5000}{100}$

$X = 50 \text{ g}$

NaCl:

$\frac{0.33 \text{ g}}{100 \text{ mL}} = \frac{X \text{ g}}{1000 \text{ mL}}$

$100X = 330$

$\frac{100X}{100} = \frac{330}{100}$

$X = 3.3 \text{ g}$

41) $\frac{D}{H} \times Q = \frac{500 \text{ mg}}{500 \text{ mg}} \times 10 \text{ mL} = 10 \text{ mL}$

100 mL − 10 mL = 90 mL (IV fluid). Note: Add the med to the chamber, and then add IV fluid up to 100 mL.

42) $\frac{10 \text{ mg}}{1 \text{ mL}} = \frac{500 \text{ mg}}{X \text{ mL}}$

$10X = 500$

$\frac{10X}{10} = \frac{500}{10}$

$X = 50 \text{ mL}$

43) 400 000 units/dose × 4 dose/day = 1 600 000 units/day

Minimum: 100 000 units/kg/day × 10 kg

= 1 000 000 units/day

Maximum: 400 000 units/kg/day × 10 kg

4 000 000 units/day

Reconstitute with 8.2 mL for a concentration of 500 000 units/mL. This concentration is selected because the amount desired is convenient for accurate measurement. This dose is safe.

$\frac{D}{H} \times Q = \frac{400\,000 \text{ units}}{500\,000 \text{ units}} \times 1 \text{ mL} = 0.8 \text{ mL penicillin}$

14/01/XX, 0800, reconstituted as 500 000 units/mL. Expires 19/01/XX, 0800 if at room temperature. G.D.P.

44) 50 mL (NS) + 0.8 mL (penicillin) = 50.8 or 101.6 mL to be infused in 60 min or 1 h. Set IV pump at 102 mL/h.

45) The primary IV will infuse for 8 hours. The IVPB will infuse for 30 minutes. Therefore, the primary IV will be interrupted by the IVPB and then will resume. The IV will be completely infused in 8 hours and 30 min. (1315 + 8 h 30 min = 1315 + 0830 = 2145)

46) $\frac{D}{H} \times Q = \frac{\overset{1}{25 \text{ mg}}}{\underset{2}{50 \text{ mg}}} \times 2 \text{ mL} = 1 \text{ mL}$

Give 1 mL/min or

$\frac{1 \text{ mL}}{60 \text{ sec}} = \frac{X \text{ mL}}{15 \text{ sec}}$

$60X = 15$

$\frac{60X}{60} = \frac{15}{60}$

X = 0.25 mL (per 15 sec)

47) $\frac{D}{H} \times Q = \frac{1500 \text{ mg}}{180 \text{ mg}} \times 1 \text{ mL} = \frac{150}{18} \times 1 \text{ mL} = 8.3 \text{ mL}$

48) $\frac{108 \text{ mL}}{\underset{1}{30} \text{ min}} \times \frac{\overset{2}{60 \text{ min}}}{1 \text{ h}} = 216 \text{ mL/h}$

APPENDIX A

Systems of Measurement

The apothecary system was the first system of medication measurement used by pharmacists and physicians. It originated in Greece and made its way to Europe via Rome and France. The English used it during the late 1600s, and the colonists brought it to North America. A modified system of measurement for everyday use evolved and is now recognized as the household system.

Apothecary System

New learners consider apothecary notations complicated. First, instead of using the Arabic number system with symbols called digits (e.g., 1, 2, 3, 4, 5), the apothecary system uses the Roman numeral system and quantities are represented by symbols (e.g., i, v, x). The Roman numeral system uses seven basic symbols and various combinations of these symbols to represent all the numbers in the Arabic number system. The most common numeral symbols used in dosage calculations are i, v, and x.

For further information regarding the apothecary system of measurement and its use in medication dosages, refer to Appendix B.

Household System

Household units are likely to be used by the patient at home where hospital measuring devices are not available. The healthcare professional who is familiar with the household system will be able to do patient education in an understandable language. Even though there is no standardized system of notation, usually the quantity, in Arabic numbers and fractions, is expressed first. An abbreviation of the unit usually follows the quantity. For the purpose of medication dosages, common household units and International System of Units (SI) equivalent units are given below.

Household Unit	Equivalent SI Unit (abbreviated)
1 teaspoon	5 mL
1 tablespoon	15 mL
1 fluid ounce	30 mL
1 cup	250 mL*
1 quart	1 L*

* not exact equivalents but are commonly used as such

For further information regarding the household system of measurement and its use in medication dosages, refer to Appendix C.

International System of Units (SI)[1]

BASE QUANTITIES AND BASE UNITS USED IN SI

Base Quantity	Base Unit	Symbol
length	metre	m
mass	kilogram	kg
time, duration	second	s
electric current	ampere	A
thermodynamic temperature	Kelvin	K
amount of substance	mole	mol
luminous intensity	candela	cd

[1] Bureau International des Poids et Mesures. (2011) The international system of units (SI). Retrieved from http://www.bipm.org/en/si/

SI PREFIXES

Factor	Name	Symbol	Factor	Name	Symbol
10^{1}	deca	da	10^{-1}	deci	d
10^{2}	hecto	h	10^{-2}	centi	c
10^{3}	kilo	k	10^{-3}	milli	m
10^{6}	mega	M	10^{-6}	micro	μ, mc*
10^{9}	giga	G	10^{-9}	nano	n
10^{12}	tera	T	10^{-12}	pico	p
10^{15}	peta	P	10^{-15}	femto	f
10^{18}	exa	E	10^{-18}	atto	a
10^{21}	zeta	Z	10^{-21}	zepto	z
10^{24}	yotta	Y	10^{-24}	yocto	y

* The official SI symbol of micro is μ but in the health sector, in order to lessen the possibility for transcribing error, the preferred form is mc.

APPENDIX B

Apothecary System of Measurement

COMMON ROMAN NUMERALS USED IN MEDICATION DOSAGES

Arabic Numeral	Roman Notation	Apothecary Number	Arabic Numeral	Roman Notation	Apothecary Number
1	I	i, $\overline{\text{i}}$	8	VIII	viii, $\overline{\text{viii}}$
2	II	ii, $\overline{\text{ii}}$	9	IX	ix, $\overline{\text{ix}}$
3	III	iii, $\overline{\text{iii}}$	10	X	x, $\overline{\text{x}}$
4	IV	iv, $\overline{\text{iv}}$	15	XV	xv, $\overline{\text{xv}}$
5	V	v, $\overline{\text{v}}$	20	XX	xx, $\overline{\text{xx}}$
6	VI	vi, $\overline{\text{vi}}$	25	XXV	xxv, $\overline{\text{xxv}}$
7	VII	vii, $\overline{\text{vii}}$	30	XXX	xxx, $\overline{\text{xxx}}$

RULE

To accurately write apothecary notation:

1. **The unit or abbreviation precedes the amount. Example: gr v, NOT v gr**
2. **Lowercase Roman numerals are used to express whole numbers, 1–10, 15, 20, and 30. Arabic numbers are used for other quantities. Examples: ℥ iii (three ounces), gr 12 (twelve grains), and gr xx (twenty grains)**
3. **Fractions are used to designate amounts less than 1. Example: gr $\frac{1}{4}$, NOT 0.25 gr**
4. **The fraction $\frac{1}{2}$ is designated by the symbol *ss*. Example: ℥ iiss (two and one-half ounces)**

MATH TIP

To decrease errors in interpretation of medical notation, a line can be drawn over the lowercase Roman numerals to distinguish them from other letters in a word or phrase. The lowercase *i* is dotted above, not below, the line.

Example:

℥ iii or $\overline{\text{iii}}$

Because Canada sometimes uses the same manufacturers as our southern neighbour, the United States, healthcare professionals may occasionally encounter syringes and medicine cups that identify the minim and dram scales. Special care is needed to avoid confusing the markings for minims and drams with the medication doses required.

In the apothecary system, weight, length, and a couple of volume units have no readily used equivalents in medication calculations. The following table lists the apothecary units of measurement and essential equivalents of volume that may be encountered in reading drug dosages.

APOTHECARY UNITS OF MEASUREMENT AND EQUIVALENTS

	APOTHECARY	
Unit	**Abbreviation**	**Equivalents**
grain	gr	
quart	qt	qt i = pt ii
pint	pt	pt i = ℥ 16
ounce or fluid ounce	℥	qt i = ℥ 32
dram	ʒ	
minim	♏	

NOTE: The minim (♏) and fluid dram (ʒ) are given only so that you will be able to recognize them.

MATH TIP

The ounce (℥) is a larger unit, and its symbol has one more loop than the dram (ʒ), or there is "more bounce to the ounce."

CAUTION

Notice that the abbreviations for the apothecary grain (**gr**) and the metric gram (**g**) can be confusing. The rule of indicating the abbreviation or symbol before the quantity in apothecary measurement further distinguishes it from a metric measurement. If you are ever doubtful about the meaning that is intended, be sure to ask the writer for clarification.

QUICK REVIEW

In the apothecary system:

- The common units for dosage calculation are grain (gr) and ounce (℥).
- The quantity is best expressed in lowercase Roman numerals. Amounts greater than ten may be expressed in Arabic numbers, *except* 15 (xv), 20 (xx), and 30 (xxx).
- Quantities of less than one are expressed as fractions, *except* $\frac{1}{2}$. One-half ($\frac{1}{2}$) is expressed by the symbol *ss*.
- The abbreviation or unit symbol is clearly written *before* the quantity.
- If you are unsure about the exact meaning of any medical notation, do not guess or assume. Ask the writer for clarification.

APPENDIX C

COMMON HOUSEHOLD UNITS, ABBREVIATIONS, AND THEIR EQUIVALENTS

HOUSEHOLD		
Unit	**Abbreviation**	**Equivalents**
drop	gtt	
teaspoon	t (or tsp)	
tablespoon	T (or Tbs)	1 T = 3 t
ounce (fluid)	oz (ʒ)	2 T = 1 oz
ounce (weight)	oz	1 pound (lb) = 16 oz
cup	cup	1 cup = 8 oz
pint	pt	1 pt = 2 cups
quart	qt	1 qt = 4 cups = 2 pt

NOTE: Like the minim (D) and dram (ʒ), the drop (gtt) unit is given only for the purpose of recognition. There are no standard equivalents for *drop* to learn. The amount of each drop varies according to the diameter of the utensil used for measurement. (See Figure 5-2 Calibrated Dropper and Figure 12-16 Intravenous Drip Chambers.)

MATH TIP

Tablespoon is the larger unit, and the abbreviation is expressed with a capital *T*. Teaspoon is the smaller unit, and the abbreviation is expressed with a lowercase or small *t*. To avoid confusion and minimize error, using *Tbs* for *tablespoon* and tsp for *teaspoon* is preferred.

CAUTION

There is wide variation in household measures and common household measuring devices, such as tableware teaspoons. Therefore, using the household system or household measures for dosage measurement can constitute a safety risk. Advise patients and their families to use the measuring devices packaged with the medication or provided by the pharmacy, rather than using common household measuring devices.

QUICK REVIEW

In the household system:

- The common units used in healthcare are teaspoon, tablespoon, ounce, cup, pint, quart, and pound.
- The quantity is typically expressed in Arabic numbers with the unit abbreviation following the amount. Example: 5 t
- Quantities of less than 1 are preferably expressed as common fractions. Example: $\frac{1}{2}$ cup
- When in doubt about the exact amount or the abbreviation used, do not guess or assume. Ask the writer to clarify.

APPENDIX D

Units of Measurement for Temperature

Knowing and recognizing significant temperatures is important in the healthcare system for a number of reasons, for example, to:

1. Recognize healthy body temperatures.
2. Diagnose some disease states.
3. Accurately ensure certain aseptic and sterilizing procedures.
4. Recognize the safe maintenance of a "cold chain" in transporting and storing some medications, such as vaccines.

Three temperature scales are available today: Fahrenheit, Celsius, and Kelvin. The oldest scale is Fahrenheit. In 1724, it was proposed by and named for a German physicist who described water freezing at 32°F and boiling at 212°F at normal atmospheric pressure.

Less than 20 years later, Celsius, a Swedish astronomer, proposed a scale in which the difference between the freezing and boiling temperatures of pure water was divided into 100°. The Celsius scale is used most commonly throughout the world today.

The Kelvin scale is the newest scale, developed in the mid 1800s. It is the base unit in the SI. It is based on an *absolute zero* that is the equivalent of 2273.16°C. Its intervals are equivalent to the Celsius scale.

On April 1, 1975, weather reports and forecasts started using the SI, with Celsius temperatures replacing Fahrenheit. By September of that year, Canadians had rain dropping in millimetres and snow falling in centimetres.

The United States is a notable world exception in its continued use of the Fahrenheit scale. Since the United States is one of Canada's largest trading partners, many of Canada's household tools and equipment still indicate temperature in Fahrenheit. In addition, a number of healthcare tools and instruments still use the Fahrenheit scale. Although it is hoped that all health tools and instruments used by today's Canadian healthcare professionals provide the option of using the Celsius scale, the topic of temperature measurements is included here as a resource.

One final note is regarding the term, *centigrade,* which is sometimes used interchangeably with the Celsius scale. *Centigrade* means *divided into 100* and is based on the Latin words *centrum* meaning hundred, and *gradus,* meaning degree.

Since scientists mainly use the Kelvin scale, conversion between temperature scales will focus on the Fahrenheit and Celsius scales. Simple formulas are used for conversions.

Refer to Figure D-1 and note the 180° difference between the freezing and boiling points on the Fahrenheit thermometer while the difference between freezing and boiling on the Centigrade thermometer is 100°. The ratio of the difference between the Fahrenheit and Celsius scales can be expressed as 180:100 or 180/100. When reduced, this ratio is equivalent to 9/5 or 1.8. One or the other of these constants is used in temperature conversions. When converting between Fahrenheit and Celsius, if necessary, carry the math process to hundredths and round to tenths.

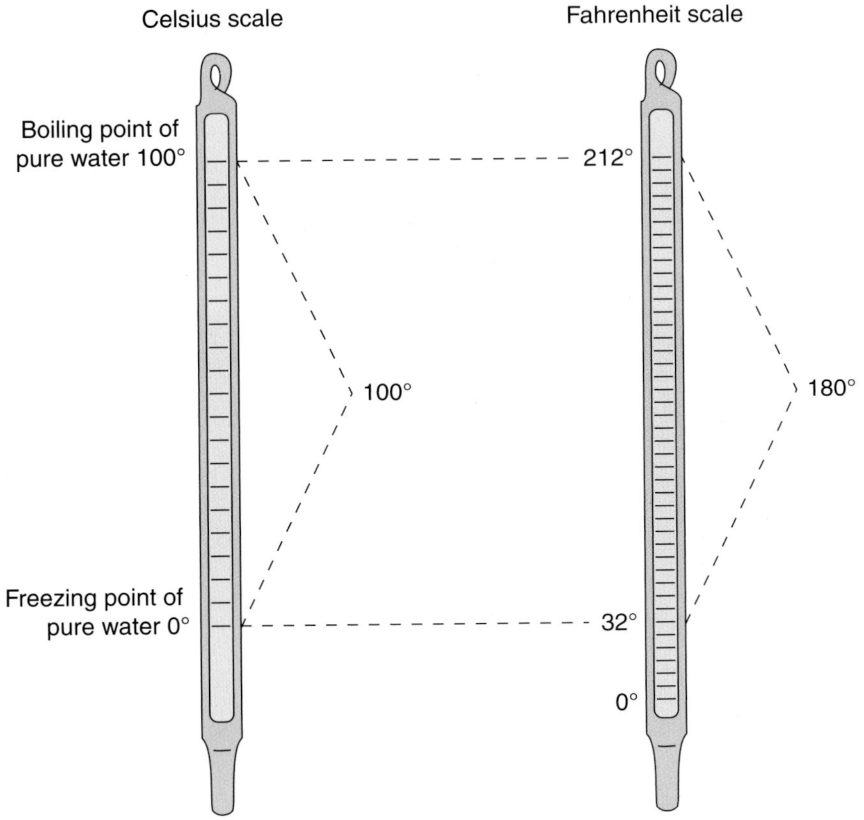
Celsius scale
Fahrenheit scale
Boiling point of pure water 100°
212°
100°
180°
Freezing point of pure water 0°
32°
0°

NOTE: Glass thermometers pictured in Figure D-1 are for demonstration purposes. Electronic digital temperature devices are more commonly used in healthcare settings. Most electronic devices can instantly convert between the two scales, freeing the healthcare provider from doing the actual calculations. However, the healthcare provider's ability to understand the difference between Celsius and Fahrenheit remains important.

FIGURE D-1 Comparison of Celsius and Fahrenheit Temperature Scales

RULE

To convert Fahrenheit temperature to Celsius, subtract 32 and then divide the result by 1.8, or multiply by $\frac{5}{9}$.

$$°C = \frac{°F - 32}{1.8} \text{ or } °C = °F - 32 \times \frac{5}{9}$$

Example:

Convert 98.6°F to °C

$$°C = \frac{98.6 - 32}{1.8}$$

$$°C = \frac{66.6}{1.8}$$

$$°C = 37$$

RULE

To convert Celsius temperature to Fahrenheit, multiply by 1.8 or $\frac{9}{5}$ and add 32.

$$°F = 1.8°C + 32 \text{ or } °F = \left(\frac{9}{5} \times °C\right) + 32$$

Note: One conversion is the reverse operation in the reverse order from the other.

Example:

Convert 35°C to °F

$°F = 1.8 \times 35 + 32$

$°F = 63 + 32$

$°F = 95$

QUICK REVIEW

Use these formulas to convert between Fahrenheit and Celsius temperatures:

- $°C = \dfrac{°F - 32}{1.8}$
- $°F = 1.8°C + 32$

or

- $°C = (°F - 32) \times \dfrac{5}{9}$
- $°F = \left(°C \times \dfrac{9}{5}\right) + 32$

Index